Surgical Spinal Oncology

Kern Singh • Matthew Colman
Editors

Surgical Spinal Oncology

Contemporary Multidisciplinary Strategies

Springer

Editors
Kern Singh
Department of Orthopaedic Surgery
Rush University Medical Center
Chicago, IL
USA

Matthew Colman
Department of Orthopaedic Surgery
Rush University Medical Center
Chicago, IL
USA

ISBN 978-3-030-50721-3 ISBN 978-3-030-50722-0 (eBook)
https://doi.org/10.1007/978-3-030-50722-0

This Springer imprint is published by the registered company Springer Nature Switzerland AG
The registered company address is: Gewerbestrasse 11, 6330 Cham, Switzerland

I would like to dedicate this book to three groups. First, to my wife Kathryn and our family, for the constant support making this project and others possible. Next, to my current partners and past mentors for the wisdom, guidance, and mentorship which has helped make me the surgeon and physician I am today. Lastly, to my patients and their families: I have had the privilege to live your struggles with you, and both the successes and failures along the way are carried forward to the next patient in need.

Matthew Colman, MD
Spine Surgery & Musculoskeletal Oncology
Director, Midwest Orthopaedics Spine Tumor Institute
Assistant Professor
Rush University Medical Center

This book represents a herculean effort on the part of my partner and colleague Matt Colman. I am proud to watch him transform a concept into reality. Without him, this book would never have been completed. I write this dedication in a very challenging time in the world. We are struck with a global pandemic that has altered our very existence. I am fortunate that my wife, two children, family, and parents are all healthy and safe. Simple things in life make a huge difference and only in times of despair do you truly realize what is important.

Kern Singh, MD
Co-Director, Minimally Invasive Spine Institute
Professor, Department of Orthopaedic Surgery
Rush University Medical Center

Preface

Springer's Spine Oncology contains the expert knowledge base of our field's most experienced practitioners in the field of extradural bone and soft tissue malignancy. We are passionate about spine tumors because of the complexity of disease, multidisciplinary nature, collaborative approach, and potential for life-quality-extending interventions in very difficult situations.

Since spine tumors are rarer than other musculoskeletal conditions, one might hypothesize that research and advancements in the field move slowly. Quite to the contrary, the care of spine tumors involves a complex interplay between medical, radiotherapy, and surgical fields. Within each one of these disciplines, small advancements occur on a regular basis, thereby opening the door for parallel or symbiotic progress in other areas. This text is an effort by our team to present the reader with a technology-forward state of the art in each of the important sub-disciplines of extradural spine oncology.

We wanted the reader to gain insight into the treatment of a spine tumor patient. As such, we created the chapters on modern classification, advanced anatomy, imaging, and the concepts around multidisciplinary approach. Further, we recognize that treating primary tumors requires very different strategies than those used in metastatic tumors, and have devoted separate sections to each sub-discipline. For primary tumors, the text covers both benign and malignant entities and addresses unique anatomic zones such as the sacrum and skull base, which require special technical expertise. For metastatic disease, we address the ever-important concept of prognosis and discuss how to answer the eternal question: "How much should we do, and for whom?" We also explore the state of the art of treatment for the "big 5" histologies (renal cell, lung, breast, prostate, thyroid), with a special chapter emphasis on separation surgery and the now-standard combinatorial care between radiation and surgery.

Although these topics are essential and shouldn't be omitted from any spine tumor text, our volume has unique features. We present an entire section on evolving surgical technology which covers the use of minimally invasive techniques, navigation, robotics, 3D-printing, and other evolving technologies for spine tumor care. We also present infrequently considered topics such as how to evaluate a lesion, which may be a tumor-mimic, and how to think about economic value in spine tumor surgery.

Our sincere hope is that this text will leave the reader more prepared to approach difficult clinical scenarios with a thoughtful, collaborative approach that leverages the best technology and thinking the field of spine oncology has to offer.

Chicago, IL, USA Matthew Colman, MD
Chicago, IL, USA Kern Singh, MD

Contents

Contributors

Ilyas S. Aleem, MD, MSc, FRCSC Department of Orthopaedic Surgery, University of Michigan, Ann Arbor, MI, USA

Department of Neurosurgery, University of Michigan, Ann Arbor, MI, USA

Bulent Arslan, MD, FSIR Rush University Medical Center, Rush Oak Park Hospital, Chicago, IL, USA

Gideon Blumstein, MD Department of Orthopaedic Surgery, David Geffen School of Medicine at the University of California Los Angeles, Los Angeles, CA, USA

Michiel E. R. Bongers, MD Department of Orthopaedic Surgery, Orthopaedic Oncology Service, Massachusetts General Hospital – Harvard Medical School, Boston, MA, USA

Raphaële Charest-Morin, MD, FRCSC Division Spine, Department of Orthopaedic Surgery, University of British Columbia, Vancouver General Hospital, Vancouver, BC, Canada

Mehee Choi, MD Department of Radiation Oncology, Rush Copley, Chicago, IL, USA

Matthew Colman, MD Department of Orthopaedic Surgery, Rush University Medical Center, Chicago, IL, USA

Andrew T. Dailey, MD Department of Neurological Surgery, Clinical Neurosciences Center, University of Utah, Salt Lake City, UT, USA

Aidnag Z. Diaz, MD, MPH Department of Radiation Medicine, University of Arizona Cancer Center at Dignity Health, Phoenix, AZ, USA

Srikanth N. Divi, MD Department of Orthopaedic Surgery, Rothman Institute, Thomas Jefferson University Hospital, Philadelphia, PA, USA

Ilyas M. Eli, MD Department of Neurological Surgery, Clinical Neurosciences Center, University of Utah, Salt Lake City, UT, USA

Michael G. Fehlings, MD, PhD Division of Neurosurgery, Toronto Western Hospital, University Health Network, Toronto, ON, Canada

Luis G. Fernandez III, MD Department of Neurological Surgery, Northwestern Memorial Hospital, Chicago, IL, USA

Marco L. Ferrone, MD Department of Orthopaedic Surgery, Brigham and Women's Hospital, Harvard Medical School, Boston, MA, USA

Alessandro Gasbarrini, MD Department of Oncologic and Degenerative Spine Surgery, IRCCS Istituto Ortopedico Rizzoli, Bologna, Italy

Riccardo Ghermandi, MD Department of Oncologic and Degenerative Spine Surgery, IRCCS Istituto Ortopedico Rizzoli, Bologna, Italy

Marco Girolami, MD Department of Oncologic and Degenerative Spine Surgery, IRCCS Istituto Ortopedico Rizzoli, Bologna, Italy

Matthew L. Goodwin, MD, PhD Department of Orthopaedics, Washington University, Barnes-Jewish Hospital, Saint Louis, MO, USA

Varan Haghshenas, MD Department of Orthopedic Surgery, Houston Methodist Hospital, Houston, TX, USA

Waqaas A. Hassan, MBBS Department of Orthopaedic Surgery, Rothman Institute, Thomas Jefferson University Hospital, Philadelphia, PA, USA

Francis Hornicek, MD Department of Orthopaedic Surgery, David Geffen School of Medicine at the University of California Los Angeles, Los Angeles, CA, USA

Benjamin Kelley, MD Department of Orthopaedic Surgery, David Geffen School of Medicine at the University of California Los Angeles, Los Angeles, CA, USA

Mena G. Kerolus, MD Department of Neurosurgery, Rush University Medical Center, Chicago, IL, USA

Philip Louie, MD Department of Orthopaedics and Neurosurgery, Virginia Mason Neuroscience Institute, Seattle, WA, USA

Sreekumar Madassery, MD Rush University Medical Center, Rush Oak Park Hospital, Chicago, IL, USA

Brett M. Mahon, MD Tempus Laboratories, Chicago, IL, USA

Rex A. W. Marco, MD Department of Orthopedic Surgery, Houston Methodist Hospital, Houston, TX, USA

Elie Massaad, MD Department of Neurosurgery, Massachusetts General Hospital, Harvard Medical School, Boston, MA, USA

Aditya Mazmudar, BA Department of Orthopaedic Surgery, Feinberg School of Medicine, Northwestern University, Chicago, IL, USA

Addisu Mesfin, MD Department of Orthopaedics & Rehabilitation, University of Rochester School of Medicine & Dentistry, Rochester, NY, USA

Ira J. Miller, MD Rush University Medical Center, Chicago, IL, USA

Ahmad Nassr, MD Department of Orthopaedic Surgery, Mayo Clinic, Rochester, MN, USA

Anick Nater, MD, PhD Division of Neurosurgery, Toronto Western Hospital, University Health Network, Toronto, ON, Canada

Scott Nelson, MD Department of Orthopaedic Surgery, David Geffen School of Medicine at the University of California Los Angeles, Los Angeles, CA, USA

Department of Pathology, David Geffen School of Medicine at the University of California Los Angeles, Los Angeles, CA, USA

Michael T. Nolte, MD Department of Orthopaedic Surgery, Rush University Medical Center, Chicago, IL, USA

John E. O'Toole, MD, MS Department of Neurosurgery, Rush University Medical Center, Chicago, IL, USA

Don Young Park, MD Department of Orthopaedic Surgery, David Geffen School of Medicine at the University of California Los Angeles, Los Angeles, CA, USA

Alpesh A. Patel, MD, FACS Department of Orthopaedic Surgery, Feinberg School of Medicine, Northwestern University, Chicago, IL, USA

Bowen Qui, MD Department of Orthopaedics & Rehabilitation, University of Rochester School of Medicine & Dentistry, Rochester, NY, USA

Arash J. Sayari, MD Department of Orthopaedic Surgery, Rush University Medical Center, Chicago, IL, USA

Nathaniel E. Schaffer, MD, PhD Department of Orthopaedic Surgery, University of Michigan, Ann Arbor, MI, USA

Andrew J. Schoenfeld, MD, MSc Department of Orthopaedic Surgery, Brigham and Women's Hospital, Harvard Medical School, Boston, MA, USA

Joseph H. Schwab, MD, MS Department of Orthopaedic Surgery, Orthopaedic Oncology Service, Massachusetts General Hospital – Harvard Medical School, Boston, MA, USA

Daniel M. Sciubba, MD Department of Neurosurgery, Johns Hopkins Hospital, Baltimore, MD, USA

Lubdha M. Shah, MD Department of Radiology, University of Utah, Salt Lake City, UT, USA

Ahmed N. Shehabeldin, MD Department of Anatomic and Clinical Pathology, Houston Methodist Hospital, Houston, TX, USA

John H. Shin, MD Department of Neurosurgery, Massachusetts General Hospital, Harvard Medical School, Boston, MA, USA

Kern Singh, MD Department of Orthopaedic Surgery, Rush University Medical Center, Chicago, IL, USA

Brittany L. Siontis, MD Department of Medical Oncology, Mayo Clinic, Rochester, MN, USA

David M. Tabriz, MD Rush University Medical Center, Rush Oak Park Hospital, Chicago, IL, USA

Alexander R. Vaccaro, MD, PhD, MBA Department of Orthopaedic Surgery, Rothman Institute, Thomas Jefferson University Hospital, Philadelphia, PA, USA

Eric Vess, MD Department of Orthopaedics & Rehabilitation, University of Rochester School of Medicine & Dentistry, Rochester, NY, USA

Dian Wang, MD, PhD Department of Radiation Oncology, Rush University Medical Center, Chicago, IL, USA

Jean-Paul Wolinsky, MD Department of Neurological Surgery, Northwestern Memorial Hospital, Chicago, IL, USA

Oren Zarnett, MD Department of Orthopaedic Surgery, University of British Columbia, Vancouver General Hospital, Vancouver, BC, Canada

Part I

Diagnostic Approach, Applied Anatomy, and Multidisciplinary Care

Joshua Patt

Advanced Spinal Anatomy and Applications for the Spine Tumor Surgeon

1

Elie Massaad and John H. Shin

Introduction

There is a wide spectrum of tumors that affect the spinal column, spinal cord, and central nervous system. These include intradural tumors, primary spinal column tumors, and metastatic tumors. Intradural tumors may consist of intramedullary or extramedullary tumors. Intramedullary tumors are tumors that arise from the substance of the spinal cord and include tumors such as astrocytoma and ependymoma. Extramedullary tumors are tumors that are found within the dura, but do not arise from the spinal cord itself. These tumors may originate from the dura itself, nerve, or nerve sheath. Examples of such tumors include meningioma, schwannoma, and neurofibroma. The anatomy specific to intradural tumors and their associated surgical approaches are outside the scope of this text.

The most common forms of tumor that affect the spinal column are metastatic tumors. Tumors that metastasize to the spine most commonly come from the breast, lung, prostate, and kidney, though any cancer affecting a solid organ can metastasize to the spine. Because of the nature of metastatic spread, these tumors may involve one, several, or multiple vertebrae of the spine based on the physiology of the disease and can affect all regions of the spinal column. This makes surgery, when indicated, a challenge, as surgeons must consider the morbidity of intervention and the potential complications associated with the surgery. The most direct access to the pathology in the spine may also be the most complicated, so careful consideration must be given to the approach-related morbidity in the decision-making process.

This is also true for cases of primary spinal column tumors which are not as common as metastases. With primary spinal column tumors such as sarcomas, the type of surgery and the extent of resection required differ significantly from the metastatic patient. In these cases, wide en bloc resections are often utilized to maximize local tumor control and survival. A full discussion of the surgical techniques for these types of tumors is beyond the scope of this chapter, but the conceptual framework is introduced, as it helps establish the importance of understanding why and when to consider the various approaches.

Spine tumor surgeries as a whole are complex and require not only mastery with decompression, stabilization, and reconstruction techniques, but also an appreciation for the anatomy in each region. In general, the spine can be approached through either anterior, lateral, or posterior approaches. The anterior approach can be more challenging given the complex anatomy of the

E. Massaad · J. H. Shin (✉)
Department of Neurosurgery, Massachusetts General Hospital, Harvard Medical School, Boston, MA, USA
e-mail: emassaad@mgh.harvard.edu; shin.john@mgh.harvard.edu

K. Singh, M. Colman (eds.), *Surgical Spinal Oncology*,
https://doi.org/10.1007/978-3-030-50722-0_1

vessels, nerves, and internal organs in the field of dissection. For these approaches, the spine surgeon is usually assisted by an access surgeon (head and neck, vascular, thoracic, or general surgeon) who can help secure access to the desired spine level. However, it is critical that the spine surgeon be knowledgeable of the anatomical considerations of the anticipated approach in order to minimize vascular injury, nerve injury, intraoperative and postoperative complications. Communication with the access surgeon is critical.

With advances in surgical technologies and minimal access surgery, the lateral approach to the thoracic and lumbar spine has made anterior column access and reconstruction less morbid while obviating the need for extensive soft tissue dissection and resection. On the other hand, the posterior approach to the entire spine is familiar to most surgeons, is the cornerstone of spine tumor surgery, and eliminates the need for an access surgeon. In the proper clinical setting, a number of different approaches can be utilized to achieve the goals of the operation which are usually neural decompression and stabilization. Given the myriad list of pathologies that affect the central nervous system and spinal column, a thorough understanding of the surgical techniques, approaches, and their relevant anatomic relationships is essential.

This chapter discusses the anatomy of the most common approaches relevant to spine tumor surgery and provides practical tips for the spine surgeon.

Cervical Approaches

Each region of the cervical spine has important anatomic considerations to consider. Whether addressing pathology at the craniovertebral junction, the subaxial cervical spine, or cervicothoracic junction, each area has potential structural "landmines" that can subvert any well-intentioned and well-planned operation.

Anterior Cervical

The anterior approach to the cervical spine is common in spine surgery and is familiar to most surgeons, given the routine use of this approach for degenerative and traumatic conditions of the spine. Because of the direct access to the spine, this is a versatile approach to the subaxial spine, typically between C3 and C7. To perform safe dissection and exposure of the anterior subaxial cervical region, surgeons should be familiar with the anatomic properties and surgical considerations of the important structures in this region, mainly the carotid sheath, trachea, and esophagus.

The anterior cervical approach gives access primarily to the subaxial cervical levels [1]. Transoral, transmandibular, and submandibular approaches to the craniovertebral junction and C2 are discussed elsewhere in this textbook. The laterality of the surgical approach is decided by the surgeon and may be influenced by the course of the recurrent laryngeal nerve (RLN). The left RLN has a more direct ascent in the tracheoesophageal groove compared to the right RLN which has a more oblique course outside the tracheoesophageal groove [2].

The anatomy of the cervical fascial layers is crucial in the anterior cervical approach. The cervical fascia helps compartmentalize the structures of the neck. Most anteriorly, the superficial layer of the cervical fascia surrounds the platysma muscle [3]. The platysma muscle may be either split longitudinally or divided in the direction of the skin incision. Then, the medial border of the sternocleidomastoid (SCM) is identified. The SCM is retracted laterally to allow further dissection. The omohyoid muscle can be also divided if it crosses the plane of the dissection. This is most commonly performed between C5 and C7. Dividing the omohyoid in this region helps visualize the lower cervical levels without excessively retracting or pulling on the surrounding soft tissue. When divided, it is not necessary to reapproximate the portion of the omohyoid that is divided, as it results in little cosmetic or swallowing issues. The most superficial layer of the deep cervical fascia is the investing fascia [2, 3]. It covers the SCM anteriorly and the trapezius muscle posteriorly. The dissection is carried along the anteromedial border of the sternocleidomastoid muscle until the carotid sheath is reached. The carotid sheath should be carefully mobilized in order to minimize the risk of carotid artery injury and cerebrovascular events [4]. It is usually not necessary to enter the carotid sheath and avoiding such will limit the possibility of injury to the vagus nerve. Particularly in elderly patients who are more likely to have atherosclerotic plaque in the carotid vessels, careful attention should be paid to avoid excessive retraction or manipulation of the carotid sheath. It is helpful to palpate the sheath to confirm orientation in the field.

On the medial side of the dissection plane, the trachea, the esophagus, and the strap muscles are identified. These structures are covered by the medial visceral layer of the deep cervical fascia, also known as the pre-tracheal fascia [5]. The RLN is usually posterior to the pre-tracheal fascia. These structures, along with RLN should be mobilized and retracted gently with caution in order to avoid nerve injury [6]. After retraction, the plane of dissection is bordered by the carotid sheath laterally, the esophagus and trachea medially. The spine can be palpated, and the anatomic level identified with intraoperative radiography. Access to the vertebral body is obtained after dissection and mobilization of the prevertebral muscles which are located between the prevertebral fascia and the vertebral body. The sympathetic trunk courses over the anterior surface of the longus colli lateral to the uncinate processes and is often difficult to visualize [7]. Prolonged or forceful retraction of the longus colli may cause damage to the sympathetic trunk and produce transient or irreversible Horner's syndrome [8, 9]. The incidence of Horner syndrome is around 0.1–0.3% in ACDF series, but is far more common in anterolateral approaches [10].

For most anterior approaches for spinal metastases, for instance, extensive resection or retraction of the longus colli on either side is usually not necessary, as the goal of surgery is palliative. In these situations, the anterior approach is excellent for direct access to the disc, vertebral body, and epidural space to achieve maximal decompression, reconstruction, and stabilization. In the metastatic tumor setting, the anterior approach is typically used to address spinal cord compression or pain from pathologic fracture or collapse of the vertebrae.

In the case of primary tumors such as chordoma, however, extensive resection or mobilization of the longus either at single or at multiple levels may be required. In cases of large tumors, this may be required bilaterally. In such cases, because of distortion of the anatomy by tumor, the sympathetic chain may not be readily identifiable. In these cases, the most concerning anatomic structure is the vertebral artery. When planning and preparing for such cases, it is essential to identify and anticipate where the vertebral artery will be both proximal and distal to the levels of interest. It is critical in any cervical spine operation to know the location and course of the vertebral arteries.

Posterior Cervical

The posterior cervical approach is considered safer than the anterior approach because of the absence of major blood vessels and organs during the dissection and the relative ease of exposure. It allows excellent exposure of the spinous processes, lamina, and facets. The spine is exposed after dividing and retracting the fascia of the trapezius, latissimus dorsi, rhomboids, and the ligamentum nuchae. The paraspinal muscles are elevated subperiosteally from the underlying laminae, using a Cobb elevator and/or electrocautery. With this approach, decompression including laminectomy, facetectomy, and instrumentation can be performed all through the same approach (Fig. 1.1). Because a number of levels can be easily and rapidly exposed with the posterior approach, multilevel decompression and instrumentation can be performed expeditiously. In the subaxial cervical spine, lateral mass screws are an excellent way to fixate the cervical spine. Similarly, if the facets are not suitable for fixation due to destruction by tumor, the cervical pedicles can be instrumented.

Cervical Spine Vascular Considerations

Blood supply to the spinal cord is delivered by two arterial systems: the anterior spinal artery and paired posterior spinal arteries. In the cervical

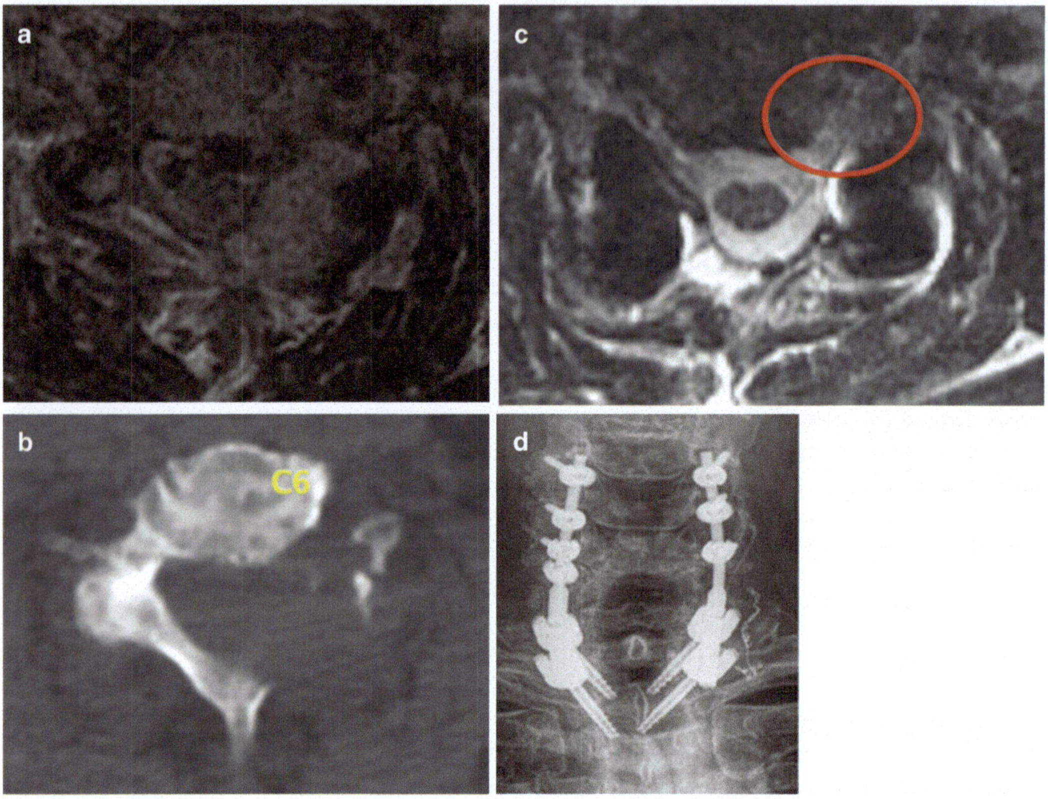

Fig. 1.1 (**a**) A 67-year-old patient with metastatic renal cell carcinoma presents with severe neck pain, left arm pain, and weakness affecting elbow extension. Axial T2 MRI shows metastatic destruction of the left lamina, facet, and pedicle with epidural and foraminal extension. The MRI shows complete obliteration of the neural foramen on the left side at the level of C6-7, compressing the C7 nerve root. (**b**) The preoperative axial CT shows the extent of lytic destruction. The lytic destruction extends to the vertebral foramen on the left side. (**c**) Postoperative MRI, axial T2 image shows restoration of the foramen on the left at C6-7 after separation surgery, tumor resection, and decompression of the central canal and left C7 nerve root. Cerebrospinal fluid is now seen in the central canal as well as bilateral foramen. (**d**) Postoperative AP standing radiograph demonstrating the construct from C3-T2, all performed through a posterior midline approach

region, the anterior spinal artery receives blood supply mainly from the vertebral artery and the costocervical trunk [7]. It also forms arterial anastomoses with the occipital artery, deep cervical artery, and the ascending cervical artery [11].

The vertebral artery (VA) arises from the right and left subclavian arteries. It usually enters the foramina at the C6 level but may enter at C5 or C7, and it exits the foramina in the area of the transverse process of the atlas [7]. The anatomy of the VA is very important in cervical spine tumors, especially when considering embolization before surgical resection. The complex arterial connections and anastomosis between the VA, the carotid arteries, and the tumor arterial feeders can result in iatrogenic intracranial vessel occlusion [12, 13]. Pre-evaluation of the vertebral arteries, subclavian arteries, the thyrocervical and the costocervical trunk by diagnostic angiography is paramount before and during an embolization procedure. Still, there are no clear anatomic definitions or indications regarding the need for permanent embolization of the VA and reports of such are highly variable. Vetter et al. (1997) occluded one vertebral artery by coiling in 23 out of 38 cervical spine tumors [14]. In contrast, Patsalides et al. performed very few permanent vertebral artery occlusions in a series of 49 cervical spine tumors [13].

The key is to understand that embolization of a spinal tumor is not without risk and one must consider the true potential benefit of such intervention. When obtaining a spinal angiogram, it is helpful to elucidate the vascular anatomy before embolization to minimize the risk of occluding essential vessels such as the anterior and posterior spinal arteries [15]. It is important to discuss what the intended surgical plan is with the angiographer so that if embolization is planned, it is done in such a way that facilitates the execution of surgery. For example, if an anterior or lateral approach is planned for the thoracic or lumbar spine, embolization of the segmental and feeding vessels contralateral to the side of the approach can be very helpful, as this is the side that will be deep and blind to the surgeon.

Upper Thoracic Approaches

Supraclavicular Approach

The supraclavicular approach allows exposure to the lower cervical levels and the T1 and T2 vertebral levels [16]. A transverse incision is made above the clavicle from the midline to the posterior border of the sternocleidomastoid (SCM). The platysma is incised perpendicularly to its fibers [16]. The external jugular vein courses superficial to and obliquely across the SCM [2, 17]. The spinal accessory nerve runs on the posterior aspect of the SCM toward its insertion in the trapezius. Identification of the spinal accessory nerve is necessary to preserve the function of the trapezius muscle [18]. The SCM and infrahyoid muscles cover the internal jugular vein, as it passes under the clavicle within the carotid sheath. The SCM should be divided medially and laterally while taking care of the internal jugular vein underneath the muscle. The floor of the incision, at this point, consists of the middle cervical fascia, which contains the omohyoid and the sternohyoid muscles. One can identify the anterior scalene muscle next. The superficial surfaces of the anterior scalene are composed of the outer layer of the prevertebral fascia [2, 11]. The phrenic nerve should be identified along its length on the ventral aspect of the anterior scalene muscle. It is important to carefully mobilize the phrenic nerve to preserve the function of the diaphragm [19]. Sometimes, the phrenic nerve cannot be easily identified because the prevertebral fascia is very thick. In this case, it is advised to perform a nerve stimulation of the phrenic nerve over the surface of the anterior scalene muscle [20]. The carotid sheath should be identified and mobilized medially with care.

The anterior scalene muscle originates from the anterior tubercles of the transverse process C3-C6 and inserts on the upper face of the first rib [2, 21]. This anatomical property can be used to locate the C3 vertebra. The fascia on the deep surface of the anterior scalene is called Sibson's fascia. It forms the suprapleural membrane which is an extension of the endothoracic fascia that covers the cervical surface of the pleura [22]. The spine will be reached after dissection of the anterior scalene muscle at its proximal origin, and also incising the Sibson's fascia at the transverse processes. The brachial plexus and the subclavian artery can be identified between the anterior and middle scalene muscles [2]. At the level of the spine, the proximal segment of the vertebral artery (VA) V1 can be identified at the C6 level. The VA enters into the transverse foramina of C6, between the medial longus colli and the lateral anterior scalene [23]. If the procedure is done on the left side, it is critical to not injure the thoracic duct. Over the dome of the pleura, the thoracic duct is anterior to the VA and vertebral. It enters the angle between the left internal jugular vein and the left subclavian vein.

Sternotomy and the Anteromedial Approach

The anteromedial approach extends the surgical field to give anterior access to the cervicothoracic junction. A median sternotomy or sternal osteotomy allows better exposure to the T3 and T4 levels when anterior access is needed. These approaches are rarely used in cases of metastatic spine tumor surgery given the morbidity associated with the approaches. These approaches are typically utilized for the resection of primary tumors such as chordoma and chondrosarcoma.

The sternohyoid and sternothyroid muscles have their origin at the dorsal surface of the sternoclavicular joint and manubrium, respectively. These muscles are liberated from their origin to allow better access to the spine, and a part of the manubrium sterni and medial clavicle is resected. Sternoclavicular osteotomies should be performed with care in order to avoid injury to the left or right subclavian artery. In fact, the right subclavian artery originates from the brachiocephalic artery at the base of the neck, posterior to the sternoclavicular junction. The left subclavian artery originates from the aortic arch and ascends to the base of the neck. The recurrent laryngeal nerve (RLN) also has different anatomical courses. The RLN turns around the right subclavian artery on the right side, and around the aortic arch on the left side. Therefore, a left-sided approach is usually recommended in order to avoid injury to the recurrent laryngeal nerve. The cervicothoracic approach has limited access to the T3 and T4 vertebra due to the location of the aortic arch and the left brachiocephalic vein in the superior mediastinum. The T3 and T4 levels are usually reached between the esophagus and trachea medially and the left common carotid or the brachiocephalic artery (BCA) laterally.

Standard Thoracotomy

The rib cage is formed by 12 ribs on each side which are connected posteriorly by the 12 thoracic vertebrae. On the anterior side, the first 7 ribs are attached to the sternum and are called the true ribs. The last 5 ribs are called the false ribs. Ribs 8–10 articulate with the seventh costal cartilage. Ribs 11 and 12 are free-floating and do not have any anterior connection. The neurovascular bundle runs along the inferior aspect of each rib and includes from top to bottom, the intercostal artery, vein, and nerve. The intercostal muscles are arranged in three layers (external intercostalis, internal intercostalis, and the innermost intercostalis), with their fibers perpendicular to the ribs.

The T4–T12 levels can be reached anteriorly by a standard thoracotomy. During this procedure, the patient is usually in the left decubitus position, and the thoracotomy is done from the right site, in order to avoid any injury to the aorta on the left side. The thoracotomy is usually cephalad to the lesion, and usually, the resected rib is 1 or 2 levels above the level of the lesion which allows better exposure. A more direct approach is to choose the rib that is directly horizontal to the vertebral body on the AP X-ray view. After removing the rib, the parietal pleura is incised along the line of the rib. The lung could be retracted medially and ventrally or could be collapsed by shifting ventilation from the right lung to the left lung by anesthesia assistance.

On the right side, the azygous vein runs superiorly and rightward to the vertebral column. The hemiazygous vein crosses from left to right at the level of the T9 vertebra and terminates into the azygous vein. The sympathetic chain has 11 ganglia located at each level of the rib neck. The splanchnic nerves course along with the lateral aspects of the middle and lower thoracic vertebral bodies.

Mini-open Lateral Approach to the Thoracic Spine

Thoracic corpectomy can also be achieved through a minimally invasive technique. The patient is positioned in the adequate lateral position, and the vertebral orientation is confirmed by fluoroscopy. A small incision 2–3 cm is made over the rib that corresponds to the vertebral body of interest. The rib is exposed and is resected while taking care of the neurovascular bundle on the inferior side of the rib. Resection of the rib should be as posterior as possible to allow maximal exposure to the posterior spine. The thoracic pleura is dissected along the wall of the rib and a space is created between the endothoracic fascia and the pleura. A blunt dissection is carried in this space, along the rib, to the corresponding vertebral body. The correct vertebral body can be confirmed by intraoperative fluoroscopy. The rib head articulating with the corresponding vertebral body should be identified. The rib head is drilled using a high-speed drill. This exposes the lateral aspect of the pedicle which is located underneath the resected rib head. The segmental vessels are exposed and coagulated. Partial discectomies are performed to better delineate the vertebral bodies. It is critical to identify the neural foramen posteriorly to avoid any nerve injury. A high-speed drill is also used to decompress the neural foramen and expose the epidural space. The posterior and inferior endplates of the adjacent vertebra should be preserved after the corpectomy.

Anterolateral Approach to the Thoracolumbar Junction

The anterior approach to the thoracolumbar junction is done by performing a T10 or T11 thoracotomy. The 11th rib is a floating rib and therefore can be more difficult to reconstruct the thoracic cage after an 11th rib osteotomy than after a tenth rib osteotomy. The surgeon can access the T12 vertebral level with a supra-diaphragmatic approach. However, mobilization of the diaphragm is needed to have access more caudally, to the L1–L2 levels [24]. The diaphragm is attached to the undersurface of the 11th and 12th ribs. It separates the thoracic and the retroperitoneal cavities. The dissection of the diaphragm is done along with its insertion at the 11th and 12th ribs. The phrenic nerve is easily damaged with this approach [25]. After reflection of the diaphragm ventrally, the lateral and medial arcuate ligaments are identified. The medial arcuate ligament passes over the psoas major muscle and has its insertion at the L1 vertebral body. In parallel, the lateral arcuate ligament passes over the quadratus lumborum muscle and has its insertion on the transverse process of the L1 vertebra. Given their anatomic insertion on L1, both the lateral and medial arcuate ligaments need to be undermined in order to have access to the thoracolumbar junction.

Preoperative assessment and description of the origin and path of the artery of Adamkiewicz are an essential step that helps avoid any vascular injury and morbid consequences during surgery. Most often, the artery of Adamkiewicz arises from the left segmental intercostal and lumbar arteries (80% of cases), between the T9 and T12 (75% of cases), but still can arise between L1 and L2 (10%).

Posterior Thoracic Approaches

The posterior thoracic approaches to the spine are the "workhorse" approaches for the spine tumor surgeon. This approach affords access to the spinal cord as well as the dorsal spinal anatomy for multilevel fixation and reconstruction (Figs. 1.2, 1.3, and 1.4).

Transpedicular Approach

The transpedicular approach is an extension of the laminectomy and allows ventral access to pathologies such as disc herniations and epidural tumor. After adequate localization, pedicle screws are usually placed two levels above and below the pathologic level. Depending on the quality of the bone, additional screws may need to be inserted above and below. Wide decompression and laminectomies expose the spinal cord and the exiting nerve roots. The pedicle is often identified at the junction of the transverse process and the superior articulating process. Sometimes, sacrificing a nerve root might be necessary to increase the working plane. When performing a vertebrectomy through a unilateral or bilateral transpedicular approach, the disks above and below the pathologic vertebrae are removed to prepare the adjacent endplates. The pedicle may be entered by a rongeur or a high-speed drill.

During this procedure, navigation can also be used to navigate the drill inside the pedicle and avoid injury to the anterior structures, such as the aorta, anterior vessels, diaphragm, and visceral organs. It is an application of navigation technology that can help guide the extent of resection and drilling. Also, the anterior longitudinal ligament and the anterior cortex provide important anatomical landmarks for the protection of the anterior visceral structures. After removal of the vertebral body, placing a cage for reconstruction requires having enough access. This often entails drilling or resecting part of the proximal rib head on that side to allow for enough space to safely introduce the cage into the vertebrectomy defect. Chou et al. described a technique called "trap door osteotomy for expandable cage placement" that mobilizes the rib at the thoracovertebral junction by perform-

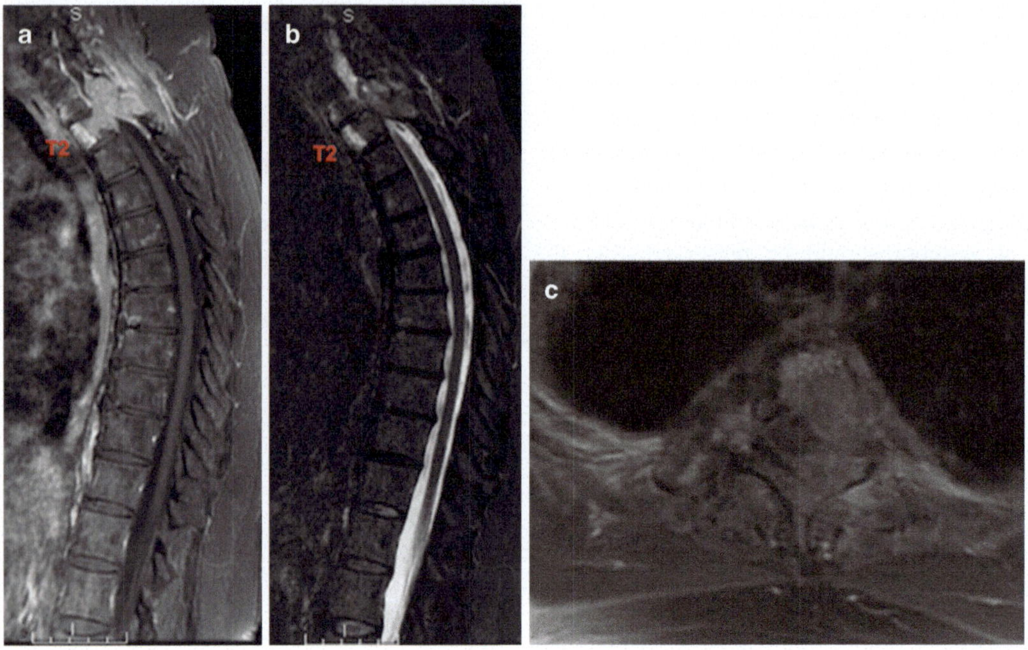

Fig. 1.2 (**a**) A 64-year-old EGFR+, non-small-cell lung cancer patient presents with severe back pain, leg weakness 3/5, inability to ambulate, and severe spinal cord compression. The patient previously underwent radiation to the thoracic spine as well as the chest for lung cancer. (**a**) Preoperative MRI and sagittal T1 post-contrast demonstrate T2 pathologic fracture and high-grade spinal cord compression. There is both anterior and posterior involvement of the spinal column with circumferential compression of the spinal cord. (**b**) Preoperative MRI, sagittal T2. The degree of spinal cord compression is evident. (**c**) Preoperative MRI, axial T1-post-contrast. High-grade epidural spinal cord compression with complete obliteration of the cerebrospinal fluid and distortion of the spinal cord

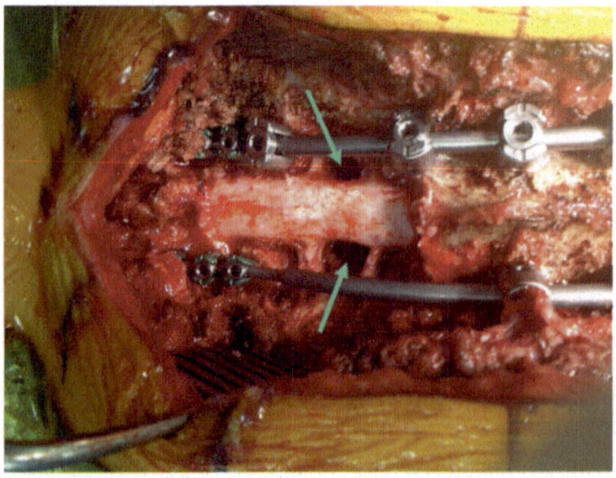

Fig. 1.3 Intraoperative photograph illustrating the bilateral transpedicular drilling at T2 and circumferential decompression of the spinal cord at that level. Spinal instrumentation has been performed above and below the level of compression, T2. The arrows point to the cavity created by the transpedicular drilling into the T2 vertebral body. This photograph is with the patient in the prone position. The top part of the photograph is the right side of the patient and the bottom is the left side. Cranial is left and caudal is right. The spinal cord is maximally decompressed above and below the level of compression

ing a small osteotomy lateral to the costovertebral junction [26]. This allows the rib head to move more anteriorly. The cage can be pushed in the corridor between the spinal cord and the rib head. The rib is then allowed to swing back posteriorly into proper position [26]. This approach can also be performed in a minimally invasive fashion [27]. The screws are placed percutaneously through multiple skin incisions, or through the fascia via a single incision. The single skin incision approach may prevent wound dehiscence at multiple incision sites [28].

Costotransversectomy and Lateral Extracavitary Approach

Costotransversectomy (CTE) allows simultaneous anterior and posterior exposure of the spine, in addition to circumferential decompression which is an advantage in spine tumor surgery. It is commonly used for T2-L1 levels. The lateral extracavitary approach (LECA) is a very similar

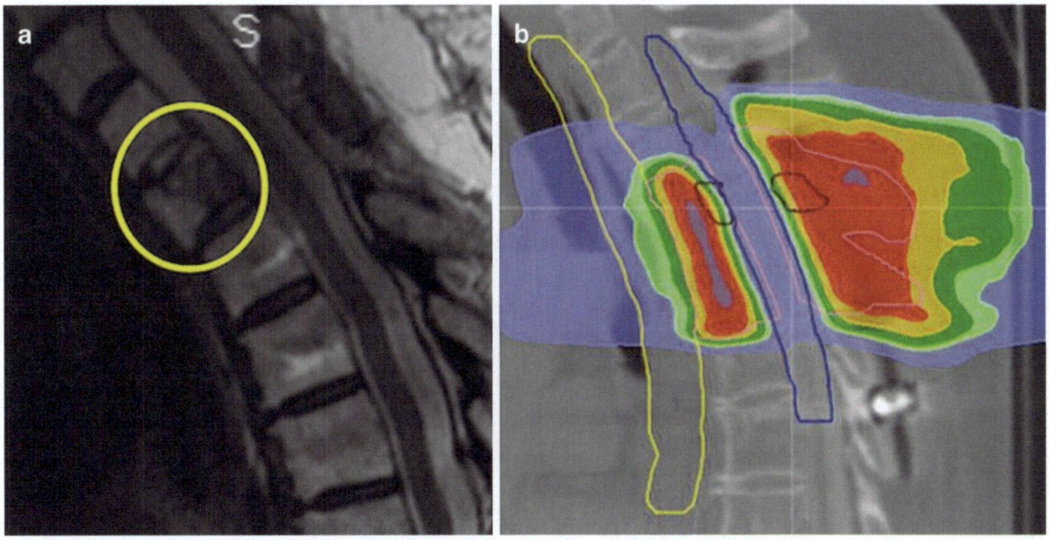

Fig. 1.4 (**a**) Postoperative MRI Sagittal T2 image showing residual T2 vertebral body after surgery and clear resection of epidural tumor. The cerebrospinal fluid has been reconstituted after surgery, further achieving the goal of separating the tumor away from the dura and the spinal cord. (**b**) Screenshot from the radiation treatment plan from postoperative stereotactic radiosurgery. With maximal decompression and separation of tumor away from the spinal cord, a dose of 24 Gy was administered in 2 fractions postoperatively. The spinal cord is contoured in dark blue

procedure to CTE, except for the extent of rib resection and access strategy to the spine. In CTE, the access is medial to the erector spinae muscles, more lateral or through the muscles in LECA. The access to the spine in both approaches requires resection of the rib head. In CTE, the length of rib resection is less than 6 cm; in LECA, it is between 6 and 12 cm. Given that, LECA involves a more lateral exposure than CTE with retraction or transection of the paraspinous thoracic muscles. LECA is very convenient for a total corpectomy. It allows placement of a graft or cage anteriorly and posterior instrumentation in the same sitting. At the T3 level, access to the spine in LECA can be restricted by the scapula, which can be rotated laterally by positioning of the arm preoperatively for adequate access.

The CTE approach is an excellent method to decompress and reconstruct the thoracic spinal column through a posterior approach. By resecting the transverse processes, the proximal rib heads, and the pedicles, complete vertebrectomy can be achieved. This can be done with a unilateral or bilateral approach. Sacrifice of the thoracic nerve root can help facilitate vertebrectomy and resection of the posterior longitudinal ligament (Figs. 1.5 and 1.6). It is important to know where the disc spaces are with this approach so that the endplates above and below are not violated. This has significant consequences with regard to anterior column reconstruction and interbody cage placement. If the inferior endplate is violated, this can lead to graft subsidence and potential hardware failure. Because the thoracic disc spaces may be calcified or narrow, meticulous dissection is required. A surgical pearl is to drill within the vertebral body toward the disc space. Once the drill goes from vertebral body to disc, the consistency of the disc material is an obvious change and indication that the disc space has been entered and that the next endplate is near. At this point, a down angled curette can be very helpful to start preparing the endplate for arthrodesis and graft placement.

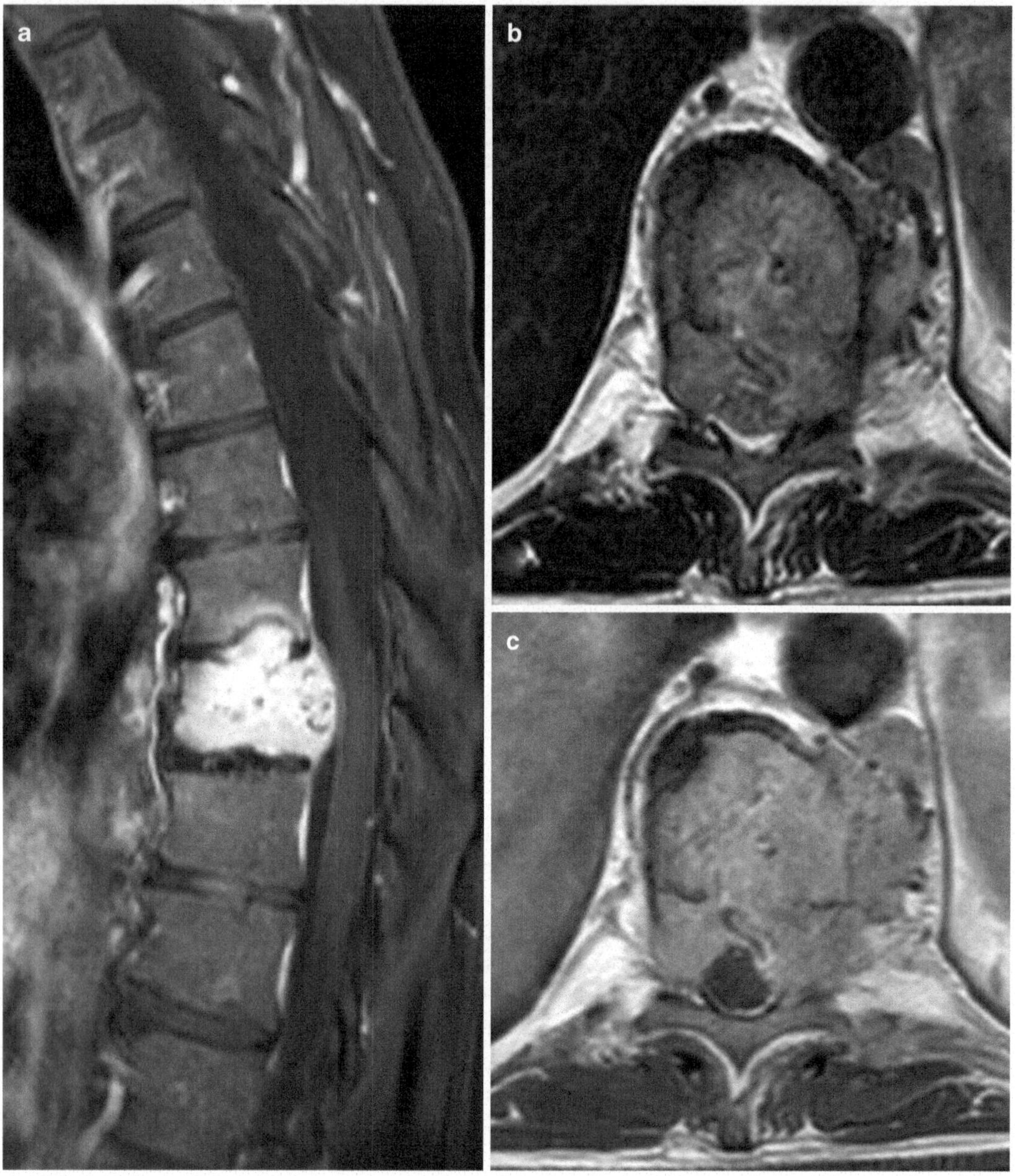

Fig. 1.5 A 49-year-old patient with metastatic renal cell carcinoma s/p nephrectomy 10 years ago presents with severe back pain and leg weakness 3/5. The patient is unable to ambulate due to pain and weakness. (**a**) Preoperative MRI, T1-sagittal post-contrast demonstrates T10 pathologic fracture and spinal cord compression. (**b**) Axial T2 image and (**c**) Axial T1-post-contrast image demonstrate the extent of spinal cord compression. Note the T2 dark flow voids on the axial image through the vertebral body and left paravertebral extension of tumor. The vascularity of such a lesion and its proximity to the aorta should not be underestimated

Lateral Retroperitoneal Approach

The lateral retroperitoneal approach gives the surgeon access to the lumbar vertebral levels. Planning the incision is very important in order to get direct access to the desired level. To expose L1–L2 levels, the incision should begin above the level of exposure and terminate at the lateral border of the rectus sheath above the midpoint of the costal margin and the umbili-

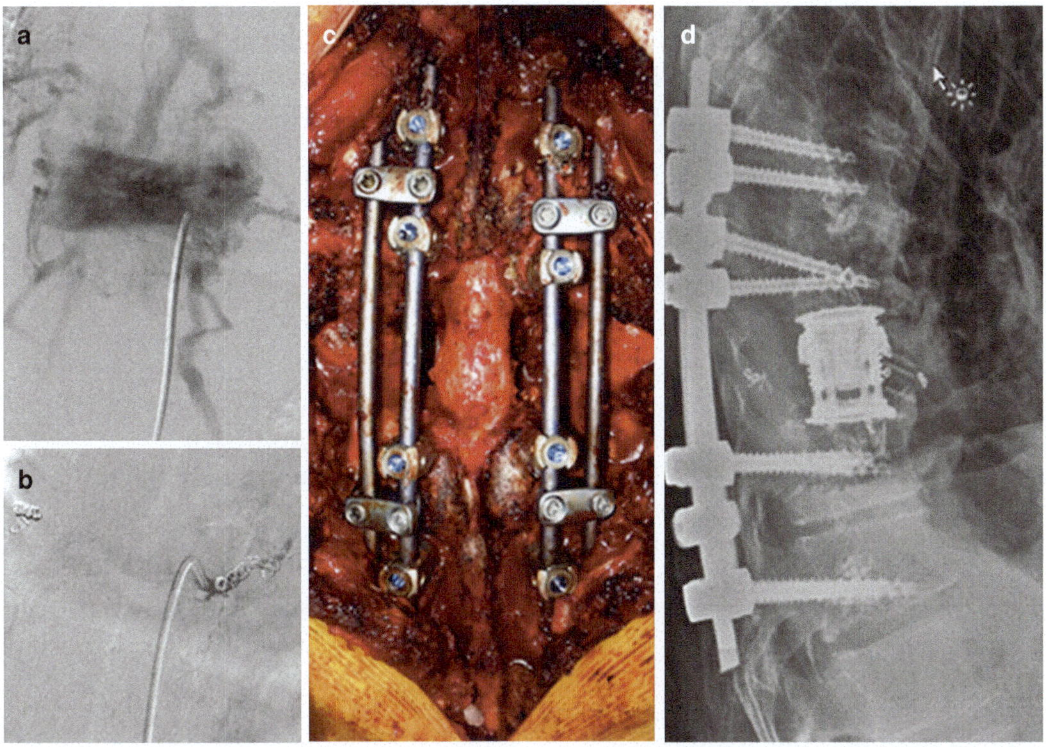

Fig. 1.6 (**a**) Preoperative angiogram demonstrating selective catheterization of a segmental vessel into the T10 vertebral body. Note the hyper-vascularity and the extent of tumor blush with contrast injection. (**b**) Post-embolization injection demonstrating the lack of contrast blush after embolization with coils. (**c**) Intraoperative photograph demonstrating the reconstruction and decompression achieved through a bilateral costotransversectomy approach. The T10 vertebral body has been resected and the anterior column has been reconstructed with an expandable titanium cage. (**d**) Standing postoperative lateral radiograph demonstrating the instrumentation and reconstruction

cus. The incision for an L2–L5 exposure starts at the posterior axillary line between the costal margin and the superior iliac crest and extends toward the umbilicus for L2–L4 and between the umbilicus and the pubic symphysis for L4–L5 [29]. The incision is usually directed by fluoroscopy. Next, dissection of the abdominal wall muscles (internal oblique, external oblique, and transversalis) should be done along their anatomical planes. After the opening of the transversalis fascia, the structures of the retroperitoneal cavity should be identified and retracted carefully. Blunt dissection of the retroperitoneal plane between the renal fascia ventrally and the quadratus lumborum/psoas muscle group posteriorly leads to the vertebral column.

The psoas major muscle arises from the anterolateral portions of the T12-L5 vertebral bodies, the intervertebral discs, and the transverse processes of the lumbar vertebrae [2]. The psoas minor is absent in 40% of patients, but, when present, lies anterior to the psoas major [30]. The lumbar plexus runs through the substance of the psoas major. The lateral femoral cutaneous nerve exits the psoas at the L3–L4 level and travels on the lateral margin of the psoas. The genitofemoral nerve is commonly identified on the medial side of the psoas [31]. For this reason, the psoas muscle should be reflected dorsally and not ventrally, to avoid stretching and injury to the lumbar plexus. Also, the abdominal portion of the ureter is located at the level of the L2 transverse process [32]. It is usually found in relation to the genitofemoral nerve and can be easily identified by the ureter peristalsis, known as the Kelly sign [33]. After identifying the psoas muscle, major retroperitoneal structures need to be identified by blunt dissection of the retroperitoneal sac. The common iliac arteries run inferolateral on the medial surface of the psoas to their bifurcation into the internal and external iliac arteries at the lumbosacral level. The iliac vessels usually bifurcate at the caudal L4 level, but it is better to check on preoperative images if they bifurcate at a more cephalad or caudal level [34]. On the right side, the inferior vena cava is lateral to the right common iliac artery. The lumbar sympathetic chain lies anterior to the vertebra bodies and medial to the psoas major muscle [30, 35]. The lumbar veins lie in the angle of the vertebral bodies and transverse processes, deep to the psoas muscle [36].

Anterior Retroperitoneal Approach

The anterior retroperitoneal approach is usually adopted for lower anterior access to the lower lumbar vertebral levels when the iliac crest limits access through a lateral approach [37, 38]. A midline vertical abdominal incision is made. Dissection to the anterior rectus sheath and linea alba exposes the peritoneum cavity. The transverse colon can be seen and should be packed and retracted superiorly with the small intestine in order to expose the posterior peritoneum [39]. The aortic bifurcation and the sacral promontory are identified through the dorsal peritoneum [40]. At this point, it is very important to identify the ureter and the hypogastric plexus in order to avoid the injury of these structures. In fact, both the right and left common iliac arteries are crossed by the ureter at their termination [32]. The superior hypogastric plexus is situated in front of the sacral promontory, anterior, and slightly inferior to the bifurcation of the abdominal aorta. The inferior part of the plexus can be found posterior to the sigmoid mesocolon and upper mesorectum. It continues into the right and left inferior hypogastric nerves [41]. In order to access the L5-S1 levels, one must mobilize the great vessels. The aorta and the inferior vena cava can be mobilized medially. The approach to L4–L5 is more challenging because the aortic bifurcation and the iliac vessels are anterior to the vertebral body. There is a high risk of tearing a vessel or causing an iliac artery or vein thrombosis. Therefore, the safest approach to the L4–L5 vertebrae is typically to identify and ligate the iliolumbar vein [42].

Minimally Invasive Lateral (MIS), Retroperitoneal Approach to Thoracolumbar and Lumbar Spine

In cancer patients with short life expectancy, anterior lumbar interbody fusion for spine stabilization can still be achieved with minimal postoperative complications by a mini-open retroperitoneal approach, laparoscopic transperitoneal approach, or an endoscopic lateral retroperitoneal approach [43, 44] (Figs. 1.7, 1.8, 1.9, and 1.10). Many factors need to be taken into consideration before and during an MIS approach, to avoid injuries and complications. First, patient positioning to obtain direct lateral access to the adequate spine level should be confirmed by AP fluoroscopy imagine. On AP, the spinous processes should be perfectly centered between their respective pedicles, and the endplates should be parallel. This is very important specifically in patients who have spinal deformity such as scoliosis. Next, the iliohypogastric and ilioinguinal nerves need to be identified during blunt dissection of abdominal muscles and the retroperitoneum. Note that the iliohypogastric nerve emerges from the upper lateral border of the psoas muscle and then courses inferolateral over the quadratus lumborum to the crest of the ilium; there, it pierces the transverses abdominis muscle near the anterior superior iliac spine (ASIS). Below the ASIS, the iliohypogastric nerve is just lateral to the rectus abdominus [45]. The ilioinguinal nerve usually runs adjacent to the iliohypogastric. Injury to these nerves will cause postoperative abdominal asymmetry, pseudohernia, or genital numbness [46].

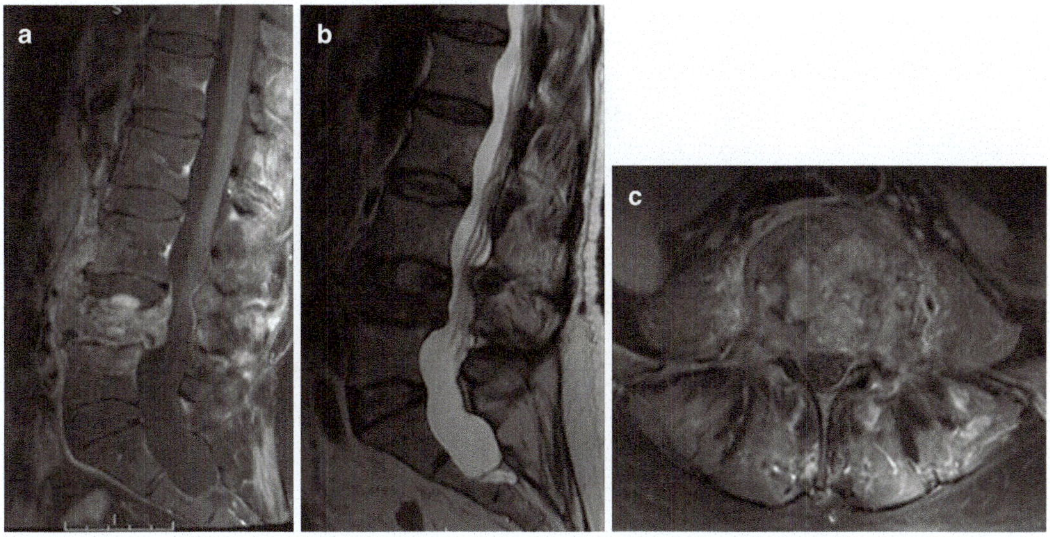

Fig. 1.7 A 56-year-old patient with metastatic breast cancer presents with severe back and left leg pain. (**a**) Preoperative T1-post-contrast and (**b**) T2 sagittal shows L4 pathologic fracture and (**c**) severe left L4 nerve root compression

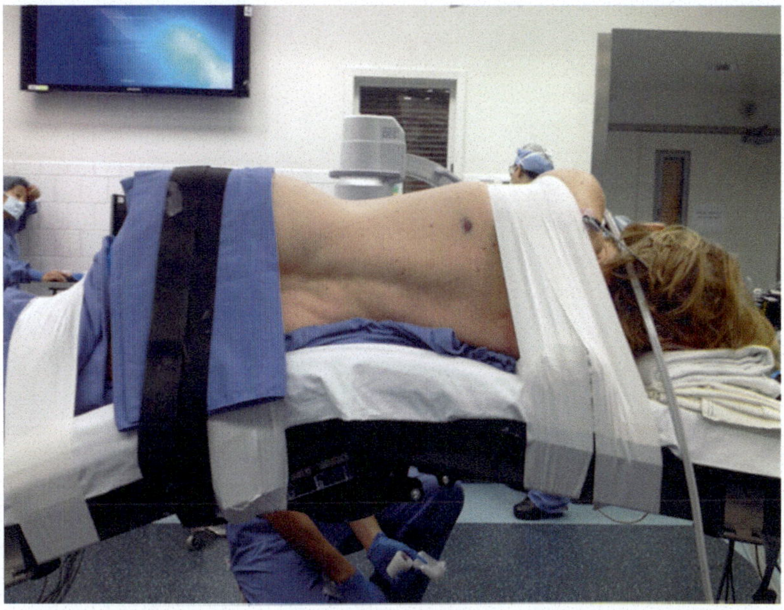

Fig. 1.8 Patient is positioned lateral for a minimally invasive left side, retroperitoneal approach to L4

Neuromonitoring (EMG nerve root mapping) is essential in the procedure to help avoid nerve injury. Also, pre-assessment of the anatomy of the psoas muscle by looking at preoperative imaging is required for a safe procedure. Uribe et al. defined safe surgical corridors and safe working zones away from the lumbar plexus in lumbar fusion [47]. They relied on radiographic and cadaveric studies to study the safety of the vertebral bodies zones I, II, III, and IV. According to this study, Zone 3 is safe for dissection between L1 and L4. The AP midpoint of the body is safest for dissection at the L4–L5 level [47]. The shallow docking technique is a useful technique that allows for the identification of nerves and vessels while carrying on the dissection through the psoas muscle [48].

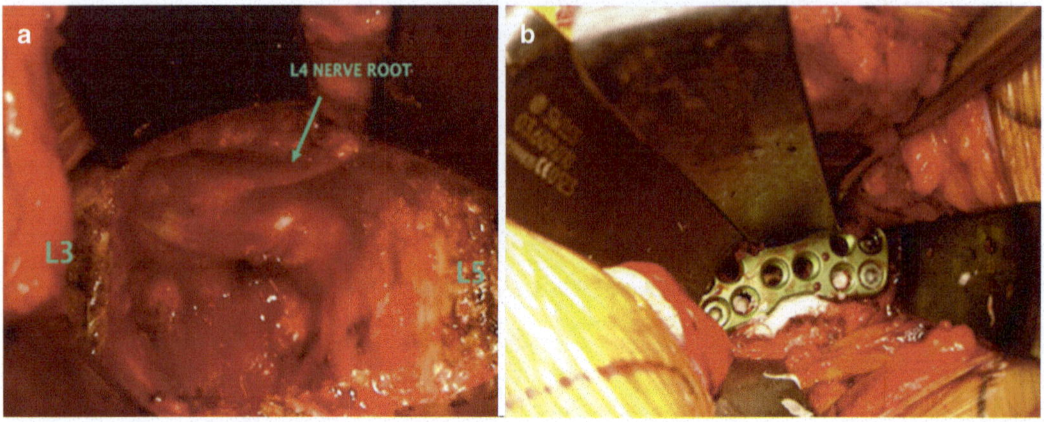

Fig. 1.9 (**a**) Intraoperative view showing the decompressed thecal sac and nerve roots. (**b**) Intraoperative view of the reconstruction using an expandable cage and cement with anterior plate and screws

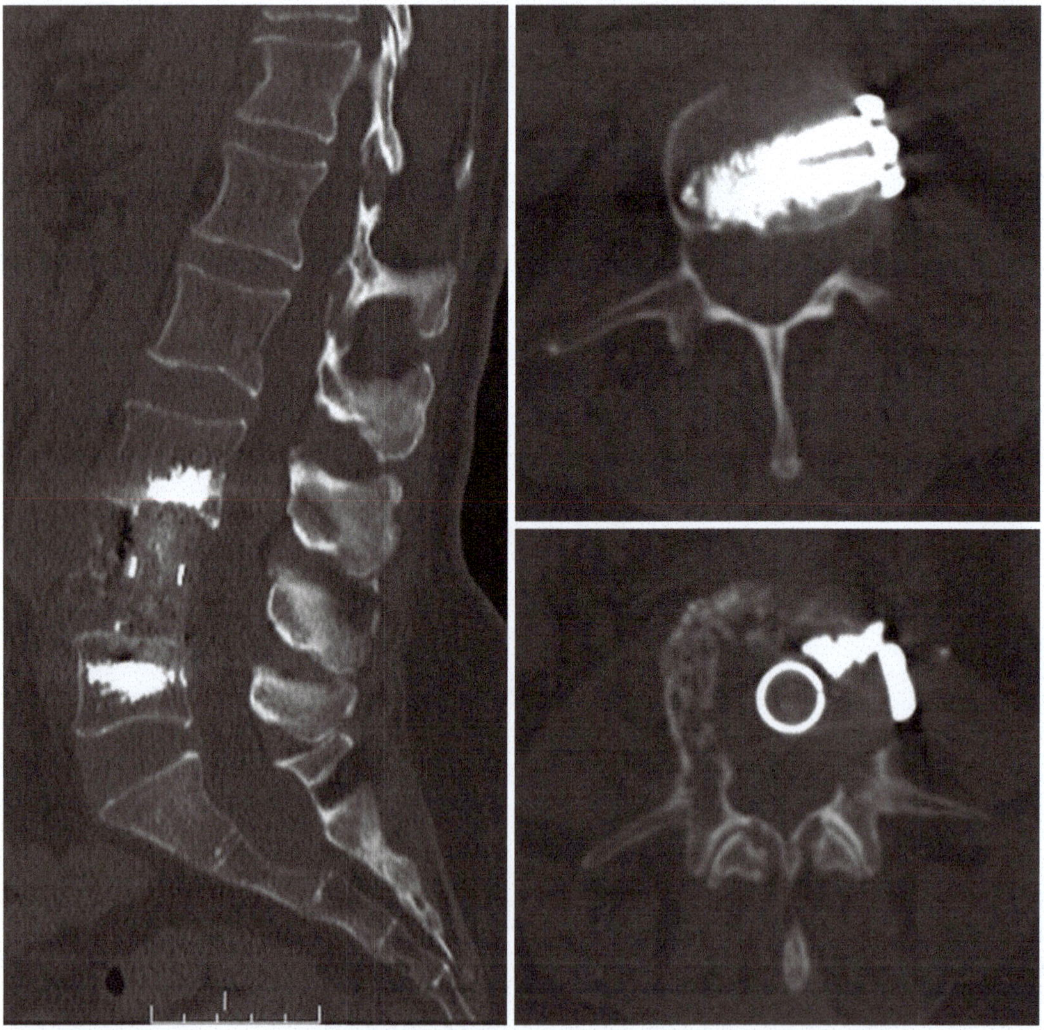

Fig. 1.10 Postoperative CT showing the extent of decompression and reconstruction. Cement was used to reinforce the anterior screw fixation

Retraction of the psoas muscle should be done in a very delicate and timely fashion, as the time of retraction is associated with increased risk of postoperative nerve injury or palsy [49]. For example, a prolonged retraction time at the L4–L5 level can be associated with a higher risk of femoral nerve injury at L4–L5 and subsequent neuropathic quadriceps muscle dysfunction [49]. In contrast to the transpsoas approach, an anterior psoas approach carries less risk of nerve injury. For the anterior psoas approach, a more anterior skin incision is required. In relation to the psoas, the genitofemoral nerve is at risk of injury here, because it runs on the anterior surface of the muscle [31]. Also, anterior docking carries a risk to anterior vascular structures as well as the sympathetic chain.

Posterior Approach to the Lumbar Spine

The posterior approach in the lumbar spine affords the spine surgeon considerable access to the cauda equina, nerve roots, as well as numerous bony landmarks for fixation options.

The main advantage of the posterior approach is the access to multiple lumbar levels for decompression, stabilization, and instrumentation through a single approach. It allows complete intralesional decompression of metastatic tumors whether posterior or anterior structures are involved by tumor. Ventral decompression and access to the space is easily achieved by removal of the facets and pedicles. Transpedicular drilling allows access to the vertebral body and other anatomy ventral to the neural elements. In this way, the posterior approach provides anterior access to the spine and helps avoid the potential complications that follow an anterior approach. The surgeon is compelled to choose a posterior approach when anatomic considerations are present which can complicate an anterior approach including visceral metastatic disease extent, previous surgical scar tissue, and use of chemo or radiotherapy adjuvants. For example, the lumbar spine might be accessed more easily from a posterior approach in cases of abdominal ascites, distention, venous hypertension, and lymphadenopathy, excessive scar tissue, difficult identification of major vessels, and other possible reasons. Posterior approaches are familiar to most spine surgeons and avoid the need for an access surgeon. For most situations involving metastatic tumors to the spine, an intralesional tumor debulking strategy is used to decompress the nerve roots, separate tumor from the dura, and simultaneously stabilize the spine. The advantage of the posterior approach is that this can all be done in the same setting without nerve sacrifice.

Unlike the curative en bloc resections commonly used for malignant primary spinal column tumors, in the metastatic setting, the intent is not usually curative. Thus, the scope and extent of surgery required in this region are usually limited. The posterior approach is effective in this regard, as it minimizes the surgical morbidity associated with either anterior or lateral approaches to the lumbar spine and sacrum. Given the goals of addressing cancer-related biologic and mechanical pain in the least destructive manner in the palliative setting, the posterior approach helps minimize the potential complications associated with the other approaches.

Conclusion

Patients with spine tumors may require neural decompression, stabilization, and reconstruction for pain and quality of life. Though many surgical treatment options exist, the majority are performed through a posterior approach. The posterior approach is most familiar to spine surgeons and affords the surgeon the ability to decompress and instrument the spine as needed through a single approach. In spine tumor surgery, the goals are primarily to decompress the nerve roots, separate tumor from the dura, and stabilize the spine. In the metastatic patient, this is often done through an intralesional technique with de-cancellation of the vertebral body and piecemeal resection of the vertebral body and tumor. Because the goal of surgery is not curative resection for these patients, an intralesional strategy is safe and effective. Thus, it is possible to avoid the anterior and lateral approaches which introduce a wider spectrum of potential complications involving other soft tissue organs and vascular structures.

In cases of primary tumor resections where an en bloc resection is planned, staging the resection and incorporating either anterior or lateral access may be advantageous. Staging these types of operations allows for careful planning of osteotomies and intended cuts through bone and soft tissue to maximize margins of resections and the surgical visibility. In these situations, the morbidity of such approaches may be justified considering the challenges of local tumor control with transgression through the tumor. In these cases, an intralesional approach must be avoided and therefore meticulous planning is required.

For patients with cancer and metastatic disease, anterior approaches may not be ideal, as patients may already be suffering from other side effects of chemotherapy or treatment, thereby affecting their other organ systems. For example, patients with liver metastases may have recurring ascites, abdominal distension, and venous hypertension requiring frequent peritoneal drainage among other issues, so avoiding the abdomen is paramount. Patients with diffuse adenopathy may also have venous congestion affecting venous return and circulation. For patients with previous bowel surgery or retroperitoneal surgery, the scar tissue associated with those approaches also make the anterior approach less inviting and potentially more dangerous, as dissection of the large vascular structures may present a contraindication to anterior approach.

Similarly, the lateral approach is an excellent way to access the lumbar spine, but in the metastatic patient, careful consideration of the regional anatomy is required. The lateral approach is an excellent way to reconstruct and instrument the lumbar spine for many spinal conditions. With the development of minimal access techniques, there is certainly a role for lateral approaches to the lumbar spine in tumor cases, but this is usually more difficult at the lumbosacral junction due to the anatomical relationship of this region to the iliac crest and the iliac vessels. Tumor that involves the lumbar vertebrae also involves the surrounding psoas muscles as well and that is a major consideration, especially for vascular tumors such as renal cell carcinoma. It is typically difficult to control bleeding in tumor that diffusely involves the psoas muscles. Practically, it is also technically difficult to work at L5 and S1 from this lateral position due to the position of the spine and the distance from the surgeon. It is also difficult to instrument the sacrum from this approach given the orientation and anatomy of the sacrum. The iliac crest is often in the way, limiting access to the sacrum from a lateral approach.

In conclusion, despite advances in radiation technology and cancer therapies, surgeons still need to be able to circumferentially work around the thecal sac and nerve roots. Careful selection of the least-morbid and least-invasive surgical approach to accomplish the surgical goals is the standard of care when managing tumors of the spinal axis.

References

1. Soliman H, Fridley J, Oyelese A, Gokaslan ZL. 32 – Management of spinal metastatic tumors. In: Ellenbogen RG, Sekhar LN, Kitchen ND, da Silva HB, editors. Principles of neurological surgery. 4th ed. Philadelphia: Elsevier; 2018. p. 510–7.e2.
2. Williams DJ. Grant's atlas of anatomy, Eleventh Edition by Anne M.R. Agur and Arthur F. Dalley. Clin Anat. 2006;19(6):575.
3. Petruzzelli GJ. Surgical anatomy of the head and neck. Otol Neurotol. 2002;23(2):237–8.
4. Hartl R, Alimi M, Abdelatif Boukebir M, Berlin CD, Navarro-Ramirez R, Arnold PM, et al. Carotid artery injury in anterior cervical spine surgery: Multicenter Cohort Study and Literature Review. Global Spine J. 2017;7(1 Suppl):71S–5S.
5. Thompson JC, Netter FH. Netter's concise orthopaedic anatomy E-book, updated edition. 2nd ed. Philadelphia: Elsevier; 2015.
6. Gokaslan ZL, Bydon M, De la Garza-Ramos R, Smith ZA, Hsu WK, Qureshi SA, et al. Recurrent laryngeal nerve palsy after cervical spine surgery: a Multicenter AOSpine Clinical Research Network Study. Global Spine J. 2017;7(1 Suppl):53S–7S.
7. Spetzler RF, George B, Bruneau M. Pathology and surgery around the vertebral artery. Paris: Springer; 2011.
8. Balak N, Baran O, Denli Yalvac ES, Esen Aydin A, Tanriover N. Surgical technique for the protection of

the cervical sympathetic trunk in anterolateral oblique corpectomy: a new cadaveric demonstration. J Clin Neurosci. 2019;63:267–71.
9. Than KD, Mummaneni PV, Smith ZA, Hsu WK, Arnold PM, Fehlings MG, et al. Brachial plexopathy after cervical spine surgery. Global Spine J. 2017;7(1 Suppl):17S–20S.
10. Traynelis VC, Malone HR, Smith ZA, Hsu WK, Kanter AS, Qureshi SA, et al. Rare complications of cervical spine surgery: Horner's syndrome. Global Spine J. 2017;7(1 Suppl):103S–8S.
11. Goodwin CR, Boone C, Sciubba DM. 31 – Anterior cervical spine surgery complications. In: Kumar M, Kofke WA, Levine JM, Schuster J, editors. Neurocritical care management of the neurosurgical patient. London: Elsevier; 2018. p. 315–22.
12. George B, Laurian C. Surgical approach to the whole length of the vertebral artery with special reference to the third portion. Acta Neurochir. 1980;51(3–4):259–72.
13. Patsalides A, Leng LZ, Kimball D, Marcus J, Knopman J, Laufer I, et al. Preoperative catheter spinal angiography and embolization of cervical spinal tumors: outcomes from a single center. Interv Neuroradiol. 2016;22(4):457–65.
14. Vetter SC, Strecker EP, Ackermann LW, Harms J. Preoperative embolization of cervical spine tumors. Cardiovasc Intervent Radiol. 1997;20(5):343–7.
15. Kee ST, Madoff DC, Murthy R. Clinical interventional oncology E-book: expert consult. London: Elsevier; 2013.
16. Neal A, David LF, Merwyn B. Anterior cervical fusion by the Smith-Robinson approach. J Neurosurg. 1968;29(4):397–404.
17. Dalip D, Iwanaga J, Loukas M, Oskouian RJ, Tubbs RS. Review of the variations of the superficial veins of the neck. Cureus. 2018;10(6):e2826.
18. Kierner AC, Zelenka I, Heller S, Burian M. Surgical anatomy of the spinal accessory nerve and the trapezius branches of the cervical plexus. JAMA Surg. 2000;135(12):1428–31.
19. Felten DL, O'Banion MK, Maida MS. 9 – Peripheral nervous system. In: Felten DL, O'Banion MK, Maida MS, editors. Netter's atlas of neuroscience. 3rd ed. Philadelphia: Elsevier; 2016. p. 153–231.
20. Malessy MJA, Pondaag W. Chapter 9 – Nerve repair/reconstruction strategies for neonatal brachial plexus palsies. In: Chung KC, Yang LJS, McGillicuddy JE, editors. Practical management of pediatric and adult brachial plexus palsies. Philadelphia: W.B. Saunders; 2012. p. 86–102.
21. Bordoni B, Varacallo M. Anatomy, head and neck, scalenus muscle. Treasure Island: StatPearls Publishing; 2018.
22. Bennett EE, Benzel EC. Procedure 34 – The lateral extracavitary approach for vertebrectomy. In: Baron EM, Vaccaro AR, editors. Operative techniques: spine surgery. 3rd ed. Philadelphia: Elsevier; 2018. p. 311–6.
23. Jabbour PM. Neurovascular surgical techniques. New Delhi: Jaypee Brothers Medical Publishers; 2013.
24. Schuchert MJ, McCormick KN, Abbas G, Pennathur A, Landreneau JP, Landreneau JR, et al. Anterior thoracic surgical approaches in the treatment of spinal infections and neoplasms. Ann Thorac Surg. 2014;97(5):1750–6; discussion 6-7.
25. Fell SC. Surgical anatomy of the diaphragm and the phrenic nerve. Chest Surg Clin N Am. 1998;8(2):281–94.
26. Chou D, Wang VY. Trap-door rib-head osteotomies for posterior placement of expandable cages after transpedicular corpectomy: an alternative to lateral extracavitary and costotransversectomy approaches. J Neurosurg Spine. 2009;10(1):40–5.
27. Chou D, Lu DC. Mini-open transpedicular corpectomies with expandable cage reconstruction. Technical note. J Neurosurg Spine. 2011;14(1):71–7.
28. Phillips FM, Lieberman I, Polly D. Minimally invasive spine surgery: surgical techniques and disease management. Springer New York: New York; 2014.
29. Fessler RG, Sekhar LN. Atlas of neurosurgical techniques: spine and peripheral nerves. New York: Thieme; 2016.
30. Cramer GD, Darby SA. Clinical anatomy of the spine, spinal cord, and ANS. 3rd ed. St. Louis: Mosby; 2013.
31. Tubbs RS, Loukas M, Hanna AS. Surgical anatomy of the lumbar plexus. New York: Thieme Medical Publishers, Incorporated; 2018.
32. Smith AD, Badlani GH, Preminger GM, Kavoussi LR. Ureteral anatomy. In: Smith's textbook of endourology. Hoboken: Wiley; 2019. p. 355–64.
33. Joffre F, Otal P, Soulie M. In: Springerlink, editor. Radiological imaging of the ureter: Berlin, Heidelberg, Springer Berlin Heidelberg; 2003.
34. Tezuka F, Sakai T, Nishisho T, Takata Y, Higashino K, Takao S, et al. Variations in arterial supply to the lower lumbar spine. Eur Spine J. 2016;25(12):4181–7.
35. Hansen JT, Netter FH, Machado CAG, Craig JA, Perkins JA. Netter's clinical anatomy. 3rd ed. Philadelphia: Saunders; 2014.
36. Valentine RJ, Wind GG. Anatomic exposures in vascular surgery. 3rd ed. Philadelphia: Wolters Kluwer Health/Lippincott Williams & Wilkins; 2013.
37. Lane JD Jr, Moore ES Jr. Transperitoneal approach to the intervertebral disc in the lumbar area. Ann Surg. 1948;127(3):537–51.
38. Kawahara N, Tomita K, Murakami H, Demura S, Yoshioka K, Kato S. Total en bloc spondylectomy of the lower lumbar spine: a surgical techniques of combined posterior-anterior approach. Spine (Phila Pa 1976). 2011;36(1):74–82.
39. RFM W, Snooks SJ. Fundamental anatomy for operative general surgery. London/New York: Springer-Verlag; 1989.
40. Benzel EC, Steinmetz MP. Benzel's spine surgery: techniques, complication avoidance, and management. 4th ed. Philadelphia: Elsevier; 2017.
41. Eid S, Iwanaga J, Chapman JR, Oskouian RJ, Loukas M, Tubbs RS. Superior hypogastric plexus and its

surgical implications during spine surgery: a review. World Neurosurg. 2018;120:163–7.

42. Dardis RM, Saxena A, Shad A, Chitnavis B, Gullan R. Chapter 154 – Disc replacement Technologies in the cervical and lumbar spine. In: Quiñones-Hinojosa A, editor. Schmidek and sweet operative neurosurgical techniques. 6th ed. Philadelphia: W.B. Saunders; 2012. p. 1777–88.
43. Wong AP, Lall RR, Dahdaleh NS, Lawton CD, Smith ZA, Wong RH, et al. Comparison of open and minimally invasive surgery for intradural-extramedullary spine tumors. Neurosurg Focus. 2015;39(2):E11.
44. Pennington Z, Ahmed AK, Molina CA, Ehresman J, Laufer I, Sciubba DM. Minimally invasive versus conventional spine surgery for vertebral metastases: a systematic review of the evidence. Ann Transl Med. 2018;6(6):103.
45. Craig A. Chapter 48 – Nerve compression/entrapment sites of the lower limb. In: Tubbs RS, Rizk E, Shoja MM, Loukas M, Barbaro N, Spinner RJ, editors. Nerves and nerve injuries. San Diego: Academic Press; 2015. p. 755–70.
46. Elias D, Tien VL, Ali AB, Anh XL, William DS, Behrooz AA, et al. Abdominal wall paresis as a complication of minimally invasive lateral transpsoas interbody fusion. Neurosurg Focus. 2011;31(4):E18.
47. Uribe JS, Arredondo N, Dakwar E, Vale FL. Defining the safe working zones using the minimally invasive lateral retroperitoneal transpsoas approach: an anatomical study. J Neurosurg Spine. 2010;13(2):260–6.
48. Wang MY, Sama AA, Uribe JS. Lateral access minimally invasive spine surgery. Cham: Springer International Publishing; 2017.
49. Matthew DC, Steven V, Allan DL, Yong Y, Michael YW. An analysis of postoperative thigh symptoms after minimally invasive transpsoas lumbar interbody fusion. J Neurosurg. 2011;15(1):11–8.

Modern Pathology in Spinal Tumors

2

Brett M. Mahon and Ira J. Miller

Introduction

Accurate pathological diagnosis is a team effort that is facilitated by advanced communication with the pathologist to ensure appropriate biopsy modality and tissue preservation for a particular lesion given the clinical and radiographic features and the relative need for pathological certainty [1]. For example, with classic cases of osteoid osteoma, sampling the lesion during a radio frequency ablation procedure may be of secondary importance to pragmatic treatment, while lesions with broad radiographic diagnostic considerations require representative, undistorted material. In difficult cases, repeat biopsy may be required. In general, nonmineralized solid lesions can be effectively sampled by image-guided core needle biopsy. Densely sclerotic bone lesions, however, usually require open biopsy or gentle, large bore drills to preserve the non-osseous component. In some cases, complete imaging workup may reveal an extra osseous component that is more amenable to biopsy than the osseous component.

B. M. Mahon (✉)
Tempus Laboratories, Chicago, IL, USA
e-mail: Brett.Mahon@tempus.com

I. J. Miller
Rush University Medical Center, Chicago, IL, USA
e-mail: Ira_J_Miller@rush.edu

K. Singh, M. Colman (eds.), *Surgical Spinal Oncology*,
https://doi.org/10.1007/978-3-030-50722-0_2

Technical and Procedural Considerations

A variety of tools are available for the proper diagnosis of pathology specimens in a modern laboratory. For example, most hospital laboratories offer intraoperative pathologic consultation by evaluation of immediately prepared cytologic fluid or "frozen section" analysis. The former allows for staining and immediate interpretation of aspirated fluids and touch imprints of tissues under the microscope. Diff-Quik or Wright-Giemsa staining of dried cytology specimens can easily be done under 20 minutes and allows for the determination of specimen adequacy and, frequently, diagnostic assessment. These can be particularly helpful for diagnosis of lymphoma. Some procedural rooms are equipped to allow for the slide staining and microscopic assessment of specimen adequacy. Intraoperative frozen section analysis allows a pathologist to freeze a portion of tissue in a medium that may be cut into thin sections of tissue. This tissue may then be fixed to a slide and stained for interpretation under the microscope. Immediate analysis can include assessment of diagnosis, involvement of margins, and adequacy of material for further specialized testing. Additional sections of frozen tumor made at that time and stored in methanol/acetic acid are ideal for subsequent FISH testing.

Prior to submission of material to the pathology department, the pathologist should be made aware of all prior tumor diagnoses from the patient, and given an opportunity to review the prior diagnostic material if deemed relevant. Communication of the pre-biopsy differential can aid the pathologist and at times expedite the diagnosis by ordering particular IHC stains during initial processing. Suspicion of residual tumor and the ability to distinguish between a tumor with a bland cytological appearance and a reparative process may require the use of immunohistochemistry (IHC), the choice of which is often informed by the prior tumor pathology. Metastasis from tumors of low grade or uncertain malignancy may resemble normal tissue and not provoke specific pathological interrogation without review of prior pathology. Appropriate microbiological culture also requires consideration prior to biopsy. In cases with relative certainty of diagnosis of metastatic tumor, fine-needle aspiration (FNA) alone may be sufficient to simply confirm the diagnosis. If treatment options are to be guided by tumor-genetic features or immunophenotype, then communication with the pathologist and oncologist upfront may be required to obtain useful material as testing requirements evolve. For example, decalcification of a bony sample may preclude accurate assessment of hormone receptor status in breast cancer.

Tissue biopsies, excisions, and resections are routinely submitted from operating rooms to pathology laboratories for diagnostic workup. These tissues are handled by pathologists, pathology assistants, and often residents to determine the areas of tissue to be sampled. Triage of the pathological specimen after receipt in the laboratory requires consideration to balance laboratory resources and the need to avoid waste against the need to maximize the use of the tissue. Many oncologic surgeons will actually carry the specimen to pathology personally to orient the specimen and review it with the pathologist. The mainstay of pathological diagnosis remains formalin-fixed paraffin-embedded (FFPE) routine hematoxylin and eosin (H&E) sections and should be the first priority. Because of the abundance of FFPE tissue blocks, immunohistochemistry and genetic testing has been developed to use this material routinely despite its limitations. Touch preps of fresh material may be helpful in some situations where cytological appearance can limit the need for a broad immunohistochemistry panel. Flow cytometry and karyotyping are occasionally of use, but rarely an absolute requirement in diagnosis of bone lymphomas; therefore, if multiple samples are to be taken, the best pieces should be placed promptly in formalin. Additional pieces may be sent fresh for pathological examination. These pieces should be placed on a lined pad moistened with saline in a tightly closed container to prevent them from drying. However, submerging the fragments in excess saline will cause tissue swelling and distortion of the morphology that can lead to misdiagnosis. If intraoperative analysis is performed to ensure adequacy of sampling, a definitive final pathological diagnosis may not be possible without additional formalin-fixed tumor even if a diagnosis of malignancy is certain on frozen section analysis. For flow cytometry and karyotyping, placing the material directly in sterile tissue culture medium is appropriate.

Once the biopsy or sections of a tissue resection are chosen, they are placed into tissue processors that, depending on the technology used, can provide H&E-stained slides in 6.5–21 hours [2, 3]. After processing and embedding tissue in paraffin wax, the tissue block is faced off on the microtome and sections are taken when the central third is reached [4]. In a good histology lab, a 0.75 mm diameter core of tissue will allow for an H&E section and 10–15 serial unstained sections for additional testing, if they are sliced off the block at the time of the initial sectioning. If only an H&E is requested initially, then, since refacing the block is required prior to taking additional sections, the diameter of remaining tumor will be much narrower, and fewer sections can be cut before depleting the tissue entirely. This may cause a need for repeat biopsy, especially when additional specialized testing is necessary. For larger bore samples, there is a little more leeway. Foresight and good intra-laboratory communication is essential to maximize the use of the tissue obtained by minimizing the number or rounds of sectioning the block.

Immunohistochemistry is performed on sections of FFPE tissue. Different antibodies are used to assess the expression of antigens on tumor cells. IHC may be used to determine the tissue of origin of metastases, lineage of differentiation and specific subtypes of sarcomas, prognosis, and as predictive therapeutic biomarkers [5]. The adequacy of IHC depends on the presence of sufficient tissue for testing, proper formalin fixation and tissue processing, and selection of the appropriate immunostains. For example, a poorly differentiated tumor in the bone may not resemble any normal tissue type and a clinical history of a primary tumor is unknown. Even the distinction between carcinoma and sarcoma may not be possible with microscopy alone. Positivity for thyroid transcription factor 1 (TTF-1), cytokeratin 7 (CK7), and mucicarmine would be consistent with a metastatic lung cancer in this situation, whereas positivity for CDX-2 and cytokeratin 20 (CK20) would be suggestive of a lower gastrointestinal, likely colonic, tumor. Similarly, positivity for programmed death ligand 1 (PD-L1) may be predictive of response to immunotherapy [5]. Further, a high proliferative index (ki-67) is typically associated with more aggressive behavior in lymphoma [6]. The usefulness of IHC depends on the selection of appropriate stains, the preservation of sufficient tissue for testing, and the correlation of clinical, radiologic, and surgical history.

One example of the power of IHC is in chordoma. Chordoma is a locally aggressive tumor that occurs in the clivus and vertebral bodies, primarily in the sacrum. This tumor usually has myxoid stroma containing cords, nests, and lobules of characteristic large cells with abundant, frothy, eosinophilic cytoplasm and mildly pleomorphic nuclei, the so-called physaliferous cells. In some cases, the matrix may be chondroid and tumor may mimic a cartilaginous neoplasm, or the tumor cells may be spindled without matrix and raise a broad histological differential. Chordomas and benign notochordal tumors show nuclear staining for brachyury (see Fig. 2.1) [7] and can therefore easily be distinguished from other entities.

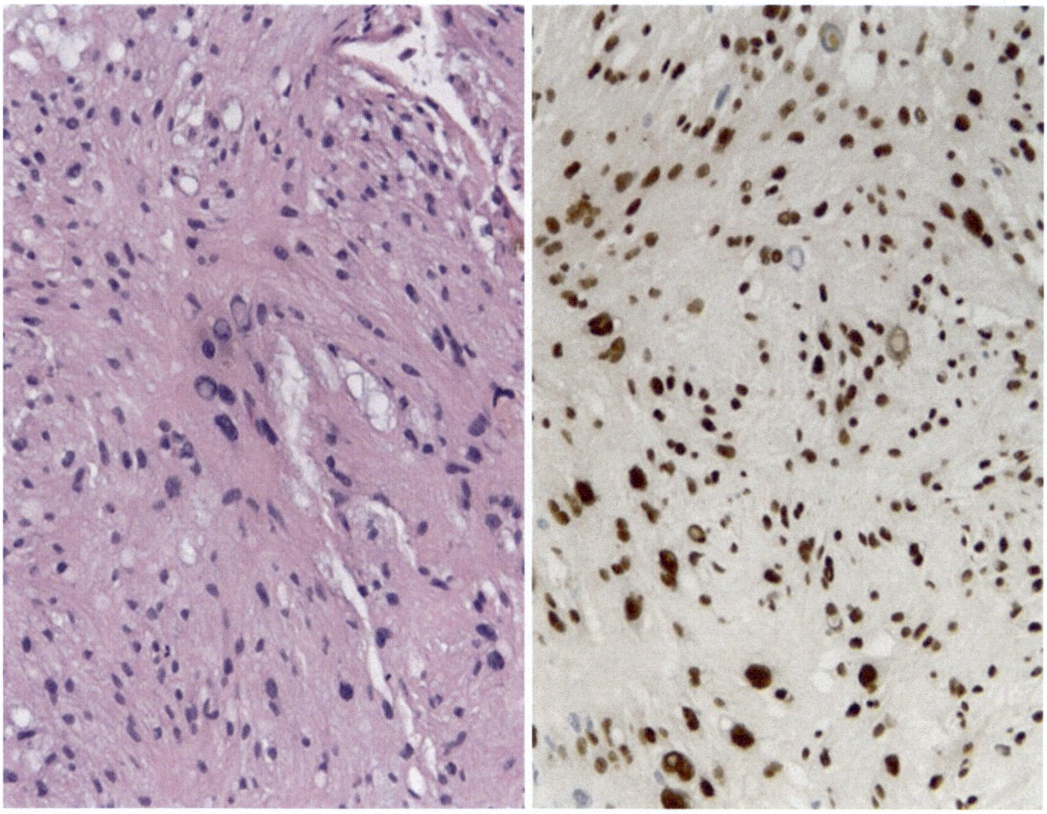

Fig. 2.1 (Left) H&E stain of a chordoma with spindle cell morphology and nuclear atypia. Physaliferous cells were not seen in the biopsy (425×). (Right) Immunohistochemical staining for the specific marker brachyury is positive, establishing the diagnosis of chordoma (425×)

Cytogenetics and Molecular Testing

Cytogenetics and molecular testing may generically refer to multiple different methods of testing, but important distinctions should be made. Karyotyping and fluorescence in situ hybridization (FISH) are typically referred to as "cytogenetic" testing, while sequencing of tumor tissue is referred to as "molecular" testing. The karyotype of a tumor is visual interpretation of a cell's chromosomes and any large alterations that may be present. Fresh tissue is required and the cells must be stimulated to grow before staining and interpretation can occur. FISH may be performed on fresh or fixed tissue and, using specific probes, can identify gene amplifications, deletions, and specific translocations (i.e., HER2 gene amplification in metastatic breast carcinoma or EWSR1-FLI1 gene rearrangement in Ewing sarcoma). FISH-prepared slides are read under a microscope with specialized light sources and filters. It is important to consider a differential diagnosis for FISH testing, as one must specify the probes to be tested.

Modern molecular testing broadly falls into two categories: single gene assays and next-generation sequencing (NGS) panels. A single gene assay requires less tissue and is simple to interpret, but only assesses for the presence or absence of a single alteration. Next-generation sequencing generally requires more tissue, but can be used to assess a large panel of genes and may be used to interrogate the entire genome, providing an overall tumor mutational burden (TMB) [8]. Interpretation of NGS results, however, may be complex, requiring the input of specialized computational scientists. Moreover, sequencing may uncover germline alterations associated with disease predisposition, requiring assistance from a genetic counselor. The use of NGS has allowed for the comprehensive assessment of tumor genetics and has assisted in the discovery of targetable biomarkers and markers of therapeutic resistance [8, 9]. Many spinal tumors are now known to harbor specific genetic alterations (see Table 2.1) [7, 10–13]. The same sequencing platforms used for DNA sequencing may also be used for RNA sequencing, allowing one to interrogate the "functional" aspect of spinal tumors including fusion analysis and gene expression profiling [14].

The utility of ancillary testing is helpful in small biopsies or cytologic specimens, especially in cases arising from unusual anatomic sites. For example, small biopsies of giant cell tumors with atypical features arising from the spine may be difficult to distinguish from other tumors including osteosarcomas [15, 16]. The distinction, however, is of critical therapeutic/prognostic importance. H3F3A and H3F3B driver mutations have been found in the vast majority of giant cell tumors and chondroblastomas but not aneurysmal bone cysts or giant cell-rich osteosarcomas [15]. Moreover, the vast majority are detected using an immunohistochemical stain (see Fig. 2.2) [15, 17].

Table 2.1 Common spinal tumors with immunohistochemistry markers and genetic findings

Diagnosis	Immunohistochemistry	Genetics
Giant cell tumor of bone	H3.3 G34W	H3F3A mutations
Chondroblastoma	H3.3 K36M	H3F3 mutations
Chordoma	Brachyury	PIK3, LYST, brachyury (T) mutations
Primary aneurysmal bone cyst		CDH11-USP6 translocation
Low-grade osteosarcoma	MDM2 and CDK4	MDM2/CDK4 amplification
Fibrous dysplasia		GNAS mutations

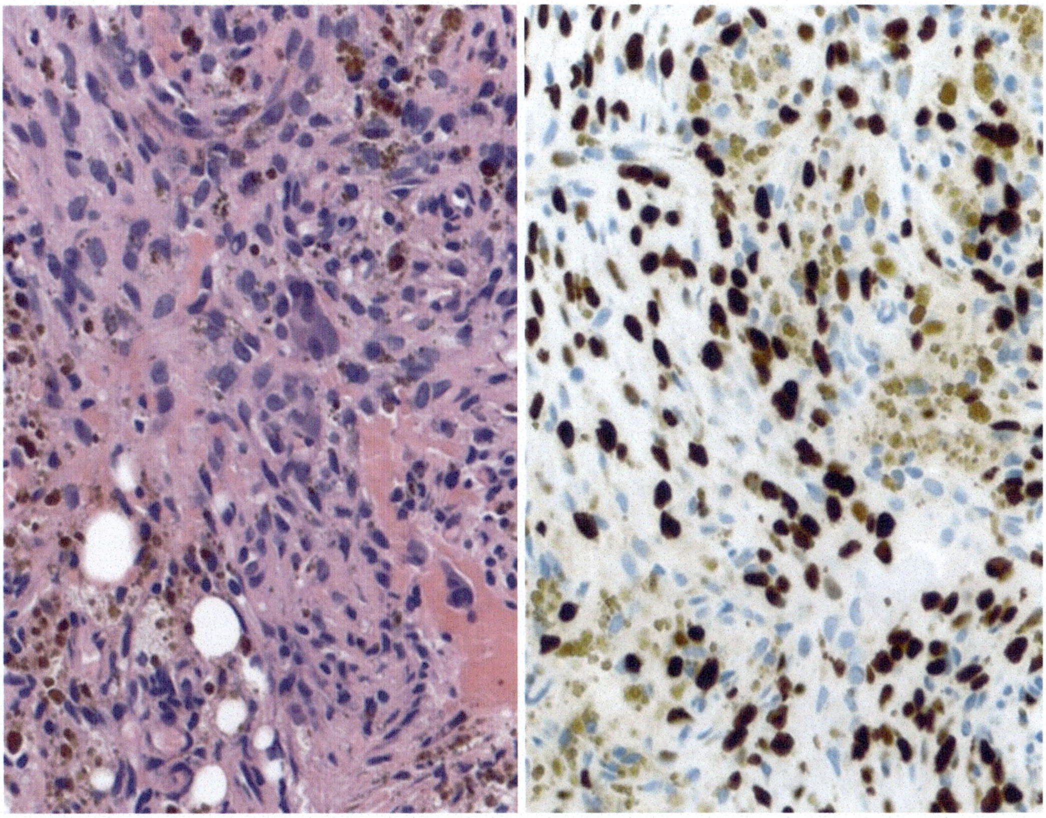

Fig. 2.2 (Left) H&E stain of the core needle biopsy of this tumor showed a nonspecific spindle cell proliferation with extensive hemosiderin deposition (850×). (Right) The neoplastic cell nuclei show expression of the H3AG34W immunostain, confirming the diagnosis of giant cell tumor of bone (850×)

Conclusion

As techniques and discoveries continue to grow in the fields of laboratory diagnosis and tumor profiling, the need for a collaborative approach to the workup of every spinal tumor patient will become increasingly important.

References

1. Burke MD. Laboratory medicine in the 21st century. Am J Clin Pathol. 2000;114(6):841–6.
2. Devi RB, Subhashree AR, Parameaswari PJ, Parijatham BO. Domestic microwave versus conventional tissue processing: a quantitative and qualitative analysis. J Clin Diagn Res. 2013;7(5):835–9.
3. Leong AS, Price D. Incorporation of microwave tissue processing into a routine pathology laboratory: impact on turnaround times and laboratory work patterns. Pathology. 2004;36(4):321–4.
4. Spencer LT, Bancroft J. Microtome: paraffin and frozen. In: Bancroft's theory and practice of histological technique. 7th ed. London: Churchill Livingstone; 2013.
5. Patel SP, Kurzrock R. PD-L1 expression as a predictive biomarker in cancer immunotherapy. Mol Cancer Ther. 2015;14(4):847–56.
6. Naz E, Mirza T, Aziz S, Ali A, Danish F. Correlation of Ki 67 proliferative index with clinical and pathological features on tissue sections of non Hodgkins lymphoma by immunostaining. J Pak Med Assoc. 2011;61(8):748–52.
7. Tirabosco R, Mangham DC, Rosenberg AE, Vujovic S, Bousdras K, Pizzolitto S, De Maglio G, den Bakker MA, Di Francesco L, Kalil RK, Athanasou NA, O'Donnell P, McCarthy EF, Flanagan AM. Brachyury expression in extra-axial skeletal and soft tissue chordomas: a marker that distinguishes chordoma from mixed tumor/myoepithelioma/parachordoma in soft tissue. Am J Surg Pathol. 2008;32(4):572–80.

8. Goodman AM, Kato S, Bazhenova L, Patel SP, Frampton GM, Miller V, Stephens PJ, Daniels GA, Kurzrock R. Tumor mutational burden as an independent predictor of response to immunotherapy in diverse cancers. Mol Cancer Ther. 2017;16(11):2598–608.
9. Norberg SM, Movva S. Role of genetic and molecular profiling in sarcomas. Curr Treat Options in Oncol. 2015;16(5):24.
10. Oliveira AM, Perez-Atayde AR, Inwards CY, Medeiros F, Derr V, Hsi BL, Gebhardt MC, Rosenberg AE, Fletcher JA. USP6 and CDH11 oncogenes identify the neoplastic cell in primary aneurysmal bone cysts and are absent in so-called secondary aneurysmal bone cysts. Am J Pathol. 2004;165(5):1773–80.
11. Amary MF, Berisha F, Mozela R, Gibbons R, Guttridge A, O'Donnell P, Baumhoer D, Tirabosco R, Flanagan AM. The H3F3 K36M mutant antibody is a sensitive and specific marker for the diagnosis of chondroblastoma. Histopathology. 2016;69(1):121–7.
12. Cleven AH, Höcker S, Briaire-de Bruijn I, Szuhai K, Cleton-Jansen AM, Bovée JV. Mutation analysis of H3F3A and H3F3B as a diagnostic tool for giant cell tumor of bone and chondroblastoma. Am J Surg Pathol. 2015;39(11):1576–83.
13. Tarpey PS, Behjati S, Young MD, Martincorena I, Alexandrov LB, Farndon SJ, Guzzo C, Hardy C, Latimer C, Butler AP, Teague JW, Shlien A, Futreal PA, Shah S, Bashashati A, Jamshidi F, Nielsen TO, Huntsman D, Baumhoer D, Brandner S, Wunder J, Dickson B, Cogswell P, Sommer J, Phillips JJ, Amary MF, Tirabosco R, Pillay N, Yip S, Stratton MR, Flanagan AM, Campbell PJ. The driver landscape of sporadic chordoma. Nat Commun. 2017;8(1):890.
14. Zhang H, He L, Cai L. Transcriptome sequencing: RNA-Seq. Methods Mol Biol. 1754;2018:15–27.
15. Schaefer IM, Fletcher JA, Nielsen GP, Shih AR, Ferrone ML, Hornick JL, Qian X. Immunohistochemistry for histone H3G34W and H3K36M is highly specific for giant cell tumor of bone and chondroblastoma, respectively, in FNA and core needle biopsy. Cancer Cytopathol. 2018;126(8):552–66.
16. Behjati S, Tarpey PS, Presneau N, Scheipl S, Pillay N, Van Loo P, Wedge DC, Cooke SL, Gundem G, Davies H, Nik-Zainal S, Martin S, McLaren S, Goodie V, Robinson B, Butler A, Teague JW, Halai D, Khatri B, Myklebost O, Baumhoer D, Jundt G, Hamoudi R, Tirabosco R, Amary MF, Futreal PA, Stratton MR, Campbell PJ, Flanagan AM. Distinct H3F3A and H3F3B driver mutations define chondroblastoma and giant cell tumor of bone. Nat Genet. 2013;45(12):1479–82.
17. Amary F, Berisha F, Ye H, Gupta M, Gutteridge A, Baumhoer D, Gibbons R, Tirabosco R, O'Donnell P, Flanagan AM. H3F3A (Histone 3.3) G34W immunohistochemistry: a reliable marker defining benign and malignant giant cell tumor of bone. Am J Surg Pathol. 2017;41(8):1059–68.

Tumor Classification and Staging Systems in Orthopaedic Spine Surgery

3

Michael T. Nolte and Matthew Colman

Introduction

The objectives of cancer staging and classification, as defined by the International Union Against Cancer, are to (1) aid in planning the course of treatment, (2) provide insight to the prognosis, (3) assist in evaluating the results of treatment, (4) facilitate effective interinstitutional communication, and (5) contribute to the continuing study of malignancies [1]. The goals of these systems in orthopaedic oncology, especially as they pertain to spine surgery, are similar. Given the complex anatomy of the spine, the critical role of spine physiology in everyday life, the variety of treatment options available, and involvement of multiple highly specialized teams, these staging and classification systems are especially important. Ideally, staging and classification in spine oncology should be practical, reproducible, and offer prognostic significance. They should ultimately enable physicians from unique disciplines to effectively communicate and formulate a treatment plan that can include chemotherapy, radiation, and/or surgery.

Several primary musculoskeletal tumor classification systems have been developed which apply to both the axial and appendicular skeleton. Historically, the most utilized and widely recognized of these are the Enneking Staging Systems for both malignant and benign neoplasms. In the modern era, the American Joint Commission on Cancer staging systems have emerged for classifying bone and soft tissue sarcoma. One classification unique to primary *spinal* lesions is the Weinstein-Boriani-Biagini (WBB) classification, which seeks to delineate the detailed anatomic distribution of spine tumors. Classification systems, which describe the anatomy and biologic behavior of metastatic disease, as distinct from primary tumors, have also emerged. These include the Spinal Instability Neoplastic Score (SINS), Neurologic Oncologic Mechanical and Systemic (NOMS) decision framework, and Metastatic Epidural Spinal Cord Compression (MESCC) or Blisky Scale.

Despite the benefits of these staging and classification systems, there are a number of inherent challenges. Rarity of the underlying condition, heterogeneity of biologic behavior of tumors, variability of the multiple treatment modalities, and lack of long-term follow-up given the competing risk of mortality from disease all limit the reliability of the data which help form these systems. Most systems were initially developed based upon expert opinion, clinical experience over an extended time period, and a limited number of patients. Fortunately, many subsequent studies have analyzed the reliability, reproducibility, and validity of these systems. An understanding of the available classification and staging systems, the

M. T. Nolte (✉) · M. Colman
Department of Orthopaedic Surgery, Rush University Medical Center, Chicago, IL, USA

K. Singh, M. Colman (eds.), *Surgical Spinal Oncology*,
https://doi.org/10.1007/978-3-030-50722-0_3

level of evidence to support their utilization, and their overall strengths and weaknesses is critical. The goal of this chapter is to provide a brief overview of the most widely recognized systems and their potential value to the reader.

Primary Spine Pathology

Enneking Stage of Primary Benign Tumors

Dr. William Enneking published his initial system for the staging of musculoskeletal tumors in 1977, based on data collected from 1968 to 1976 at the University of Florida. There are separate staging systems for benign and malignant tumors. The staging system for benign tumors is made up of three categories that are based on the radiographic characteristics of the tumor-host margin [2]. These are (1) latent, (2) active, and (3) aggressive (Table 3.1). Lesions with well-demarcated borders and quiescent biologic behavior comprise latent stage 1 lesions, whereas loss of a defined border, biologic activity, and some permeation into host bone are more consistent with a stage 2 tumor. The highest-grade tumors (grade 3) are aggressive-behaving lesions, which typically involve an extraosseous soft tissue component and relative rapidity of growth. As the stage increases, so too do the local aggressiveness and incidence of recurrence for these lesions [3]. In general, metastasis is uncommon for these benign lesions, but can occur for giant cell tumor and chondroblastoma in particular [4].

Enneking Stage of Primary Malignant Tumors

The Enneking staging system for malignant tumors takes into consideration three key factors:

Table 3.1 Enneking stage of primary benign tumors

Stage	Definition
1	Latent lesion
2	Active lesion
3	Aggressive lesion

Table 3.2 Enneking stage of primary malignant tumors

Stage	Grade	Site	Metastasis
IA	G1	T1	M0
IB	G1	T2	M0
IIA	G2	T1	M0
IIB	G2	T2	M0
III	G1 or G2	T1 or T2	M1

G1 low grade, *G2* high grade, *T1* intracompartmental, *T2* extracompartmental, *M0* no regional or distant metastasis, *M1* regional or distal metastasis

(1) surgical grade, (2) local extent of the lesion (intra- vs. extraosseous), and (3) presence of metastases [2]. These factors combine to help characterize the lesion into one of three stages (Table 3.2). Stages I and II refer to lesions without metastatic disease, and are determined based on the histologic grade of the tumor, which may either be "low" (I) or "high" (II). Both stages are subdivided into categories A and B based on the local extent of the tumor: intracompartmental (A) versus extracompartmental (B). Stage III lesions represent any tumor with distant metastatic lesions. The overall stage is the chief determinant of the extent of surgical resection, the surgical margin, and overall prognosis.

The first step in tumor staging according to the Enneking system is identifying a lesion as either low (G1) or high (G2) grade. A low-grade lesion is characterized by low rates of mitosis, low nuclear to cytoplasmic ratio, and limited degree of pleomorphism (Broder's Grade 1 or 2) [2]. These lesions carry a low risk for distant spread, typically less than 25%. High-grade lesions, on the other hand, are characterized by high rates of mitosis, prominent nucleoli, and high degree of pleomorphism (Broder's Grade 3 or 4). These lesions carry a significantly higher rate of metastasis. Although histology is the primary determinant of tumor grade, some tumors, such as dedifferentiated chondrosarcoma, are high grade by definition [5].

Tumor staging according to the Enneking system also considers the local extent of the tumor based on axial radiographic features. Local extent is interpreted in regard to containment within the anatomic boundaries of a musculoskeletal compartment. These compartments feature natural barriers to tumor spread, including fascial layers and bone structures. The degree of local extent, and whether a tumor is intracompartmental versus extracompartmental, is critical in determining surgical approach and the surgical margin goal. According to the Enneking classification, the overarching goal is that the tumor should not be entered during resection. A wide resection refers to when the tumor is removed with a margin of normal tissue around the tumor. A marginal resection refers to when the tumor is removed along with pseudocapsule of the tumor. When the tumor itself is entered during surgical resection, it is referred to as an intralesional resection.

Following the initial publication of their landmark staging system, Enneking et al. validated their approach through an analysis of 258 patients treated at the University of Florida, and 139 patients treated at 13 institutions overseen by the Musculoskeletal Tumor Society [2]. They found that the probability of survival for the combined group of 397 patients was lower for each subsequent Enneking stage, for every year that the patient was followed ($P < 0.01$). Of note, difficulty was reported in 5.5% of the cases studied at outside institutions, with nearly all problems relating to assessing the intra- versus extra-compartmental local extent of the tumor. Based on these findings, they suggested that use of the system was successful in helping determine patient prognosis based on stage, appropriately guiding treatment, and enabling efficient and effective communication between providers at different institutions.

Although the Enneking system was developed primarily for extremity tumors, it has been applied to the axial skeleton. Fisher et al. completed a multicenter cohort analysis of 147 patients with a primary bone tumor involving the spine who underwent surgical resection of the lesion between 1982 and 2008 [6]. Based on a retrospective review of operative documentation and the final pathology report, patients were labeled as either "Enneking Appropriate" (surgical margin as recommended by the Enneking classification) or "Enneking Inappropriate" (surgical margin not recommended by the Enneking classification). They found that 57 of the 77 patients in the inappropriate group and 14 of the 70 patients in the appropriate group experienced local recurrence of their tumor. They also found that an Enneking Inappropriate surgical approach resulted in a significantly higher risk of mortality compared to the Appropriate approach (Hazard Ratio = 3.10, $P = 0.0485$), lending additional support to the use of this pivotal system.

In regard to the reliability and reproducibility of the system, Chan et al. surveyed 15 members of the Spine Oncology Study Group with radiographic records of 18 patients in order to determine the intra- and interobserver reliability coefficients, and further guide use of the system [7]. They found that Enneking grade ($K = 0.82$), tumor extent ($K = 0.22$), stage ($K = 0.57$), and Enneking-recommended surgical margin ($K = 0.47$) had near-perfect, fair, moderate, and moderate interobserver reliability, respectively. These findings suggest that while tumor grade is reliable between observers, difficulty in determining Enneking stage is driven by disagreement on local extent of tumor, which in turn drives disagreement on the plan for surgical resection as recommended by the Enneking system.

American Joint Committee on Cancer (AJCC) Bone and Soft Tissue Sarcoma Staging System

The AJCC is a group comprised of leading scientists and clinicians across a number of medical fields. One of the central goals of the committee is to publish cancer staging systems unique to specific areas of medicine to help guide diagnosis, prognosis, and treatment options. The system for bone and soft tissue sarcoma staging is based on three key factors: the extent of the tumor (T), the spread to nearby lymph nodes (N), and the spread to distant sites (M). Unlike the Enneking system, the AJCC staging system now includes criteria unique to osseous lesions of the spine (Table 3.3) [8]. These are reflected in the T category. A tumor is graded as T1 if it is confined to one vertebral segment or two adjacent segments, T2 for three adjacent segments, T3 for four or

Table 3.3 American Joint Committee on Cancer (AJCC) Bone and Soft Tissue Sarcoma Staging System for the spine

T category	Criteria
TX	Primary tumor cannot be assessed
T0	No evidence of primary tumor
T1	Tumor confined to one vertebral segment or two adjacent segments
T2	Tumor confined to three adjacent vertebral segments
T3	Tumor confined to four or more adjacent vertebral segments, or any nonadjacent segments
T4	Extension into the spinal canal or great vessels
T4a	Extension into the spinal canal
T4b	Evidence of gross vascular invasion or tumor thrombus in the great vessels
N category	
NX	Regional lymph nodes cannot be assessed
N0	No regional lymph node metastasis
N1	Regional lymph node metastasis
M category	
M0	No distant metastasis
M1	Distant metastasis
M1a	Lung
M1b	Bone or other distant sites

more adjacent segments, or for any tumors with nonadjacent vertebral segment involvement. Finally, a tumor is graded as T4 if it features extension into the spinal canal (T4a) or great vessels (T4b). Given the recency of the AJCC spine-specific staging guidelines, there have not yet been any studies analyzing the efficacy or reproducibility of the system.

Although the AJCC and Enneking staging systems share a common goal, they feature unique differences. One fundamental difference is that the general AJCC system grades the tumor based on size, whereas the Enneking system grades based on compartment status. The latter strategy to subclassify tumors using compartment status was based on the surgical concept that a patient with a small tumor with extraosseous extension may still require a larger procedure than a patient with a large tumor that is entirely intraosseous. In order to compare the two systems, Heck et al. performed a retrospective analysis of 250 patients with sarcomas of the bone treated over a 12 year-period at the University of Chicago [9]. The group found that both systems were highly effective at predicting prognosis, with increasing stage accompanied by decreased survival. In comparing the two systems directly, however, they found that there were no significant advantages of one system over the other in regard to predicting prognosis. Future work is needed to determine the effectiveness of the AJCC spine-specific staging guidelines.

Weinstein-Boriani-Biagini (WBB) Classification

Initially published in 1997, the Weinstein-Boriani-Biagini (WBB) system was devised to effectively stage primary spinal tumors while recognizing the anatomic complexity of the spine. The main usefulness of this system is to describe the feasibility and type of necessary surgical resection for primary spine tumors. It implies and cues issues such as technique of approach, necessity of bony ring opening, and management of dural margins, all of which are critical to the planning of surgical management of primary spine tumors. The staging of a lesion is based primarily on axial location within the vertebral segment using a clock-face convention with radial depth modifiers [10]. Doctors Hart, Boriani, Biagini, and Weinstein based their classification system on their experience pertaining to 24 patients with primary giant cell tumors of the spine. Despite the common histology, they found different rates of local recurrence of the tumors based on their location within the spinal column. Specifically, recurrence rates were higher for tumors that involved both the vertebral body and posterior elements in comparison to those located only in the anterior elements (24% versus 0%). They also found that extraosseous extension into the canal or paraspinal musculature was associated with a higher rate or recurrence. Based on these findings, the study group concluded that the axial location of the lesion should serve as a chief determinant for the specific surgical procedure and approach and extent. For lesions in the vertebral body, they recommended vertebrectomy via dual anterior and posterior approach as the optimal treatment. Similarly, lesions involving the lateral aspect of the vertebral unit, specifically from the posterolateral aspect of the vertebral body to the ipsilateral facet joint are indicated for a sagittal resection via dual anterior and posterior approach. Lastly, lesions in the posterior elements alone are indicated for a posterior arch resection via isolated posterior approach. The fundamental goal guiding these principles is to spare the spinal cord without compromising the surgical tumor margins.

The use of this system has been shown to be both safe and feasible [11, 12]. Boriani et al. published the preliminary results on 29 patients who underwent surgical resection of a spinal lesion in accordance with the WBB classification [12]. Of these patients, there were 13 with lesions in the vertebral body, 9 with lesions in the posterior arch, and 7 with lesions in both part of the body and part of the arch. Twenty patients had a successful wide margin, whereas eight had a marginal margin, and one had an intralesional margin. Importantly, no patient had neurologic compromise as a result of the resection (unless nerve root was resected for oncologic purposes), and no local recurrence was found at an average follow-up of 30 months. Similarly, Yamazaki and the Spine Oncology Study Group performed a systematic review of patients undergoing *en bloc* resection of primary spine tumors in accordance with both the WBB and Enneking classifications [13]. Their primary goal was to determine the rate of achievement of disease-free margins, morbidity, mortality, and health resource utilization. Among 300 patients from 6 studies meeting inclusion criteria, they found that WBB staging accurately predicted the attainment of a wide or marginal resection in 88% of cases. Moreover, successful attainment of a wide margin was associated with decreased likelihood of recurrence and reduced mortality. More recently, Amendola et al. published their experience with 103 consecutive, prospectively enrolled patients with primary spinal tumors treated with resection in accordance with the WBB and Enneking classification [14]. At a mean follow-up of 39 months after surgery, 22 patients had experienced local recurrence of their tumor. They found that marginal and intralesional resection were significant independent predictors of local recurrence (HR 9.45 and 38.62, respectively). Furthermore, WBB surgical staging predicted surgical margins in 75.7% of cases.

As previously highlighted, Chan et al. surveyed 15 members of the Spine Oncology Study Group in regard to the radiographic records of 18 patients in order to determine the reliability of the Boriani-Biagini classifications [7]. They found that interobserver reliability for WBB zones ($K = 0.31$), WBB layers ($K = 0.58$), and WBB recommended surgical procedure ($K = 0.54$) was fair, moderate, and moderate, respectively. The group suggested that difficulty with the use of the system most commonly stems from limitations of the axial imaging, rotation or asymmetry of the vertebral unit, and inherent difficulty in determining the precise zones of involvement. Despite these shortcomings, the system offers moderate-to-substantial value in guiding surgical approach and procedure.

Spinal Metastatic Disease

The prevalence of metastatic disease to osseous structures is staggering, affecting an estimated 300,000 patients in the United States alone [15, 16]. Approximately 60% of osseous metastases are spinal metastases, and spinal metastases occur in 20–40% of all patients diagnosed with cancer. Furthermore, nearly 20% of patients with spinal metastases experience symptomatic spinal cord compression [17]. This metastatic disease most commonly affects the thoracic spine (70%), followed by the lumbar spine (20%), and lastly the cervical spine (10%) [16, 18]. Given the relative growth of the aging population at risk for cancer, targeted therapies extending survival for many patients with cancer, and the improved capabilities of diagnostic modalities, the prevalence of patients with metastatic spinal disease is only expected to grow [19].

Treatment goals for patients with spine metastases involve optimization of neurologic function, maintenance or restoration of spinal stability, effective local tumor control, and improvement in overall quality of life. Due to advances in technology, myriad treatment options now exist, including surgery, chemotherapy, conventional radiation therapy, stereotactic radiosurgery, and other minimally invasive procedures [20]. In light of these advances and the involvement of multiple care teams, a number of clinical tools and classification systems have been developed to help guide treatment decisions.

Neurologic Oncologic Mechanical and Systemic (NOMS) Decision Framework

The Neurologic Oncologic Mechanical and Systemic (NOMS) decision framework was developed to provide guide treatment of patients with metastatic spine disease through an assessment of four critical elements: neurologic, oncologic, mechanical stability, and systemic disease [21]. Initially published in 2013, the NOMS system is based on a number of integral publications and over 15 years of clinical experience from the multidisciplinary spine team at the Memorial Sloan-Kettering Cancer Center. The goal of the system is to incorporate the four key domains to guide treatment, specifically the use of radiation, systemic therapy, and/or surgical intervention.

The neurologic assessment analyzes the degree of spinal cord compromise, including a *clinical* assessment of myelopathy and radiculopathy. It also involves a *radiographic* assessment of the degree of metastatic epidural spinal cord compression (MESCC). A six-point grading system was designed and subsequently validated by the Spine Oncology Study Group (SOSG) to quantify the degree of MESCC, and is presented later in this chapter [22, 23].

The oncologic assessment refers to the effectiveness of radiation or chemotherapy for local and systemic tumor control. Tumors can be considered radiosensitive or radioresistant based on their response to conventional external beam radiation therapy (CEBRT). For example, lymphoma, myeloma, and germ cell tumors in particular have been shown to be extremely responsive to radiation therapy [24]. Thus, a course of radiotherapy along with the appropriate systemic medical therapy may be the appropriate initial treatment for these tumors, even with some element of neurologic compromise. Solid tumors, however, are not as uniformly radiosensitive. Breast, prostate, and ovarian cancers represent relatively radiosensitive pathologies. On the other hand, renal, thyroid, hepatocellular, colon, non-small-cell lung, sarcoma, and melanoma represent strongly radioresistant tumors [24]. Despite this, classically radioresistant pathologies have exhibited responsiveness to the high concentration of radiation offered by SRS and other high accuracy modalities which spare dosing to normal structures. Chemotherapeutic options are highly individualized to the individual histology, but multidisciplinary discussion of available treatments is critical in the ever-expanding landscape of targeted, immunologic, and other novel anti-cancer drugs.

The mechanical assessment in NOMS is unique, in that it represents a potential independent indication for surgical intervention and/or cement augmentation, regardless of the neurologic or oncologic assessment. The SOSG defines instability as the "loss of spinal integrity as a result of a neoplastic process that is associated with movement-related pain, symptomatic or progressive deformity, and/or neural compromise under physiologic loads." This is therefore dependent on both clinical and radiographic findings. To help guide clinicians in making this diagnosis, the SOSG devised the Spinal Instability Neoplastic Score (SINS), which is covered later in this chapter [25].

The systemic assessment provides an overall outlook through consideration of the patient's diagnosis and prognosis. Before moving forward with a treatment, the patient's ability to tolerate the intervention based on their global tumor burden and other comorbidities must be considered. In other words, the long-term benefit of an invasive, timely, or costly procedure may not be realized in a patient with a short life expectancy.

Furthermore, an aggressive treatment approach may cause more harm than benefit for many patients. A number of prognostic scoring systems have been developed to estimate a patient's expected prognosis and survival, thereby helping care providers determine if a specific intervention (typically surgical) would be worth undertaking [26–30]. These are covered in a separate chapter later in this text. Unfortunately, however, these estimations can be wrongly influenced by physicians' tendency to overestimate survival time, or by continued advancements in the effectiveness of pharmacotherapy. Spine surgeons therefore should most strongly consider whether patients would have an opportunity to adequately recover from the indicated surgery and return to pharmacotherapy to attempt systemic tumor control. Of course, this requires detailed conversations between the patient, family, and multiple care teams.

Although the NOMS decision framework has not undergone a formal prospective validation, it has been shown to be effective and appropriate in guiding treatment decisions for patients with spinal metastases. These treatments include surgical resection [31, 32], traditional radiotherapy [33], and novel methods such as stereotactic radiosurgery [34]. The system continues to be a widely recognized and accepted treatment tool by spinal surgeons and oncologists alike. Pratt and the International Spine Oncology Consortium recently published a similar algorithm to the NOMS framework, that also reflects that need for multidisciplinary efforts and communication [35]. Known as the Mechanical stability, neurological risk, oncological parameters, and preferred treatment (MNOP) algorithm, this framework encompasses the key aspects of the NOMS decision framework, while also expanding recommendations to better involve medical oncologists and cancer rehabilitation specialists.

Spinal Instability Neoplastic Score (SINS)

Published in 2010 by the Spine Oncology Study Group, the Spinal Instability Neoplastic Score (SINS) was developed in order to aid in predicting spine stability of neoplastic lesions [25]. Furthermore, the SINS score serves as the primary determinant of mechanical stability according to the NOMS treatment decision framework. In summary, the SINS score is an 18-point scale based on location of the lesion, pain, type of bone lesion, radiographic spinal alignment, vertebral body collapse, and posterolateral involvement of spinal elements (Table 3.4) [25]. The summation of these scores results in a classification of stable (score 0–6), unstable (score 13–18), or indeterminate (score 7–12). The management of patients with scores in the indeterminate range has remained controversial. In response, Pennington et al. completed a retrospective

Table 3.4 Spinal Instability Neoplastic Score (SINS)

Component	Score
Location	
Junctional (O-C2; C7-T2; T11-L1; L5-S1)	3
Mobile spine (C3-6; L2-4)	2
Semirigid (T3-10)	1
Rigid (S2-S5)	0
Mechanical pain	
Yes	3
No	2
Pain-free lesion	1
Bone lesion	
Lytic	2
Mixed (lytic/blastic)	1
Blastic	0
Radiographic spinal alignment	
Subluxation/translation present	4
Deformity (kyphosis/scoliosis)	2
Normal	0
Vertebral body collapse	
>50% collapse	3
<50% collapse	2
No collapse with >50% body involved	1
None of the above	0
Posterolateral involvement	
Bilateral	3
Unilateral	1
None of the above	0
Total	
Stable	0–6
Indeterminant	7–12
Unstable	13–18

review of 51 consecutive patients with metastatic spine disease evaluated at a single institution over a one-year time period to better delineate the indeterminate range [36]. They found that a SINS score of 10 or greater was associated with a greater than 50% likelihood of undergoing surgical stabilization, whereas patients with a score of 9 or less underwent surgical stabilization in only 11% of cases. They concluded that, although the unique clinical and radiographic criteria must be weighed for each patient, a lesion with a SINS score of 9 or less may not require surgical stabilization

In regard to the effectiveness of SINS, Versteeg et al. performed a retrospective review of patients with spinal metastases treated with either surgery or radiotherapy over the time surrounding the introduction of the SINS classification (2009–2013) [37]. They found that, following the introduction of SINS in 2011, patients in both treatment groups experienced more remarkable improvement in SINS score. They found that, following the introduction of SINS in 2011, the mean score upon presentation was significantly lower for both groups when compared to patients presenting prior to 2011 (10.3 versus 11.2 for the surgical cohort and 7.2 versus 8.4 for the radiotherapy cohort). These findings suggested that SINS may successfully increase awareness of instability and result in earlier referrals for procedural intervention for patients properly indicated. Similarly, SINS has been shown to be reliable and reproducible amongst both orthopaedic surgeons and non-orthopaedic oncology specialists, with Campos et al. reporting an overall interobserver reliability of 0.79, and an intraobserver reliability of 0.96 [38]. Fisher et al. also completed a prospective analysis of 37 radiologists and 30 patients with spinal metastases, finding that radiologists were able to identify 98.7% of patients with an unstable spine according to SINS, thereby appropriately initiating surgical consultation [39].

Hussain et al. published a 2018 validation study of SINS via a prospective cohort analysis of 131 patients who underwent surgical stabilization for spinal metastases [40]. They found that there was a significant positive correlation between increasing SINS and degree of both preoperative pain and preoperative disability (via brief pain inventory walking score, and MD Anderson Symptom Inventory activity and walking scores). Surgical stabilization resulted in significant improvement in nearly all patient-reported outcome measures for both patients with indeterminate and unstable SINS, and these correlations remained significant when neurologic status was controlled for.

Metastatic Epidural Spinal Cord Compression (MESCC)

Compression of the spinal cord by metastatic disease is associated with considerable disability and mortality. As previously mentioned, the Spine Oncology Study Group (SOSG) developed and subsequently validated a six-point grading system to quantify the degree of MESCC [22, 23]. Utilizing axial T2-weighted images at the level of most remarkable compression: Grade 0 is defined as tumor confined to the bone only; Grade 1, tumor extension into the epidural space without deformation of the spinal cord; Grade 2, spinal cord compression by CSF is visible; and Grade 3, spinal cord compression without visible cerebrospinal fluid. These are further subdivided into Grade 1a, epidural impingement without deformation of the thecal sac; Grade 1b, deformation of the thecal sac without spinal cord abutment; and Grade 1c, deformation of the thecal sac with spinal cord abutment, but without compression. Assuming no mechanical instability, conventional radiation therapy should be considered as the initial treatment for grades 0, 1a, and 1b. Surgical decompression should be strong considered for grades 2 and 3 (defined as high-grade ESCC), prior to radiation therapy. The initial management of grade 1c tumors remains controversial, but may present an indication for stereotactic radiosurgery to limit the degree of spinal cord toxicity [41]. Through a prospective survey of 7 members of the Spine Oncology Study Group (SOSG) in regard to imaging for 25 patients, Bilsky et al. determined that the current 6-point ESCC grading scale is both reliable and reproducible [23]. Furthermore, the T2-weighted images were superior indicators of ESCC compared with T1-weighted images with and without Gadolinium.

Ryu et al. subsequently developed a modified version of this scale to also reflect the patient's neurological status in the context of their radiographic degree of spinal cord compression [42]. The neurological grade consists of five grades (A through E), depending on the degree of symptoms. Grade A, no symptoms; grade B, a focal minor symptom (i.e., axial or radicular pain); grade C, functional paresis due to compression of a nerve root or spinal cord with muscle strength of 4 out of 5 or greater; grade D, nonfunctional paresis with muscle strength of 3 out of 5 or less; and grade E, complete paralysis or urinary and rectal incontinence. The team performed a prospective analysis of 62 patients with a total of 85 lesions causing metastatic epidural compression, with grade A, B, or C neurological status. They found that radiosurgery for these patients resulted in mean tumor volume reduction of 65% and neurological function improvement for 81% of patients, thereby supporting the use of their modified system.

Conclusion

The use of high-quality classification and staging systems can help guide treatment of patients with oncological pathology of the spine while respecting the complex and critical anatomy of the spinal cord and column (Fig. 3.1). For many years, this field had lacked standardization, but a recent push for clinical tools to improve decision-making and interdisciplinary communication has resulted in the formation of a number of classification and staging systems. However, the evidence-based development of these tools has been inherently limited by the limited number of patients, wide range of clinical presentations, and oftentimes, limited degree of follow-up. An understanding of the value of and evidence for the available and widely utilized classification systems is therefore critical. The Enneking and

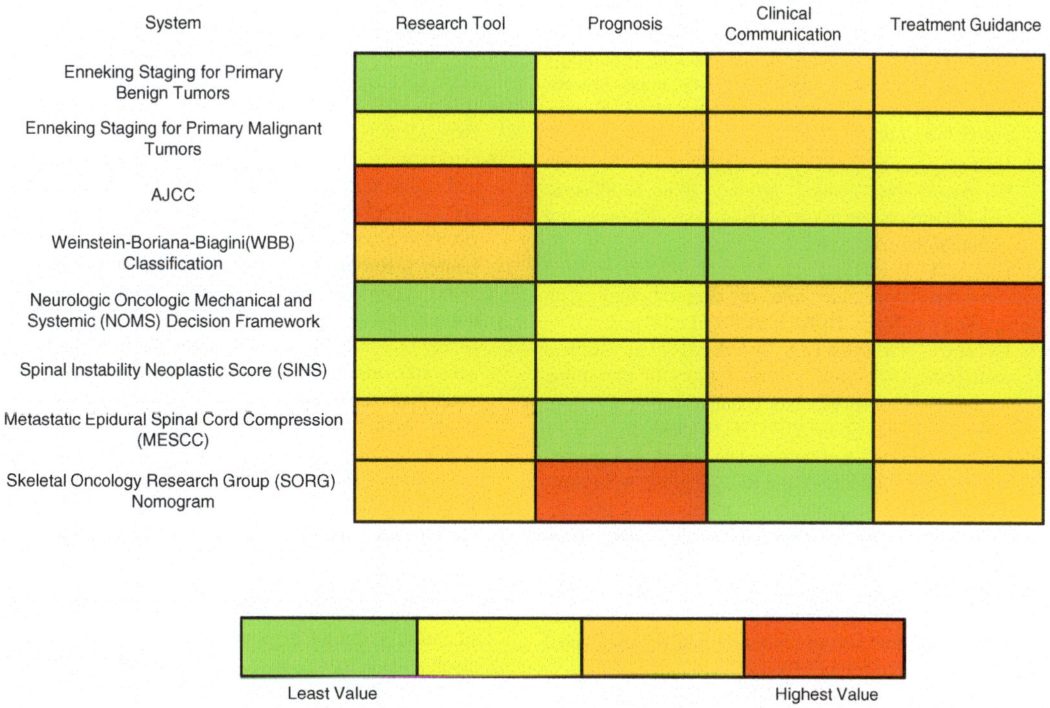

Fig. 3.1 Relative value of classification and staging systems across four key clinical domains

WBB staging systems have proven to be valuable tools in the staging and surgical planning of primary lesions of the spine. Similarly, the NOMS decision framework, utilizing the SINS and ESCC, has served as the cornerstone guiding the management of metastatic lesions to the spine. Ongoing multicenter efforts such as the Epidemiology Process and Outcomes in Spine Oncology (EPOSO) and the Primary Tumor Research and Outcomes Network (PTRON) are collecting comprehensive prospective data that may help to refine our current classification systems. As the understanding of spinal orthopaedic oncology and the value of classification systems within this complex field continue to grow, clinicians will be able to provide a higher quality of care for this expanding population of patients.

References

1. Gospodarowicz M, Benedet L, Hutter RV, Fleming I, Henson DE, Sobin LH. History and international developments in cancer staging. Cancer Prev. 1998;2(6):262–8.
2. Enneking WF, Spanier SS, Goodman MA. A system for the surgical staging of musculoskeletal sarcoma. Clin Orthop Relat Res (1976-2007). 1980;153:106–20.
3. Ragsdale BD, Madewell JE, Sweet DE. Radiologic and pathologic analysis of solitary bone lesions. Part II: periosteal reactions. Radiol Clin N Am. 1981;19(4):749–83.
4. Harrop JS, Schmidt MH, Boriani S, Shaffrey CI. Aggressive "benign" primary spine neoplasms: Osteoblastoma, aneurysmal bone cyst, and giant cell tumor. Spine. 2009;34(22S):S39–47.
5. Dickey ID, Rose PS, Fuchs B, et al. Dedifferentiated chondrosarcoma: the role of chemotherapy with updated outcomes. JBJS. 2004;86(11):2412–8.
6. Fisher CG, Saravanja DD, Dvorak MF, et al. Surgical management of primary bone tumors of the spine: validation of an approach to enhance cure and reduce local recurrence. Spine. 2011;36(10):830–6.
7. Chan P, Boriani S, Fourney DR, et al. An assessment of the reliability of the enneking and weinstein-boriani-biagini classifications for staging of primary spinal tumors by the spine oncology study group. Spine. 2009;34(4):384–91.
8. Tanaka K, Ozaki T. New TNM classification (AJCC eighth edition) of bone and soft tissue sarcomas: JCOG bone and soft tissue tumor study group. Jpn J Clin Oncol. 2018;49(2):103–7.
9. Heck RK Jr, Stacy GS, Flaherty MJ, Montag AG, Peabody TD, Simon MA. A comparison study of staging systems for bone sarcomas. Clin Orthop Relat Res. 2003;415:64–71.
10. Hart RA, Boriani S, Biagini R, Currier B, Weinstein JN. A system for surgical staging and management of spine tumors: a clinical outcome study of giant cell tumors of the spine. Spine. 1997;22(15):1773–82.
11. Fisher CG, Keynan O, Boyd MC, Dvorak MF. The surgical management of primary tumorsof the spine: initial results of an ongoing prospective cohort study. Spine. 2005;30(16):1899–908.
12. Boriani S, Biagini R, Bertoni F, Malaguti MC, Di Fiore M, Zanoni A. En bloc resections of bone tumors of the thoracolumbar spine: a preliminary report on 29 patients. Spine. 1996;21(16):1927–31.
13. Yamazaki T, McLoughlin GS, Patel S, Rhines LD, Fourney DR. Feasibility and safety of en bloc resection for primary spine tumors: A systematic review by the spine oncology study group. In: 50 landmark papers every spine surgeon should know. Boca Raton: CRC Press; 2018. p. 61–4.
14. Amendola L, Cappuccio M, De Iure F, Bandiera S, Gasbarrini A, Boriani S. En bloc resections for primary spinal tumors in 20 years of experience: effectiveness and safety. Spine J. 2014;14(11):2608–17.
15. Portenoy RK. Cancer pain. Epidemiology and syndromes. Cancer. 1989;63(11):2298–307.
16. Perrin RG, Laxton AW. Metastatic spine disease: epidemiology, pathophysiology, and evaluation of patients. Neurosurg Clin N Am. 2004;15(4):365–73.
17. Jacobs WB, Perrin RG. Evaluation and treatment of spinal metastases: an overview. Neurosurg Focus. 2001;11(6):1–11.
18. Wong DA, Fornasier VL, MacNab I. Spinal metastases: the obvious, the occult, and the impostors. Spine. 1990;15(1):1–4.
19. Bilsky MH. New therapeutics in spine metastases. Expert Rev Neurother. 2005;5(6):831–40.
20. Gerszten PC, Mendel E, Yamada Y. Radiotherapy and radiosurgery for metastatic spine disease: what are the options, indications, and outcomes? Spine. 2009;34(22S):S78–92.
21. Laufer I, Rubin DG, Lis E, et al. The NOMS framework: approach to the treatment of spinal metastatic tumors. Oncologist. 2013;18(6):744–51.
22. Bilsky M, Smith M. Surgical approach to epidural spinal cord compression. Hematol Oncol Clin North Am. 2006;20(6):1307–17.
23. Bilsky MH, Laufer I, Fourney DR, et al. Reliability analysis of the epidural spinal cord compression scale. J Neurosurg Spine. 2010;13(3):324–8.
24. Williams JR, Zhang Y, Zhou H, et al. A quantitative overview of radiosensitivity of human tumor cells across histological type and TP53 status. Int J Radiat Biol. 2008;84(4):253–64.
25. Fisher CG, DiPaola CP, Ryken TC, et al. A novel classification system for spinal instability in neoplastic disease: an evidence-based approach and expert consensus from the spine oncology study group. Spine. 2010;35(22):E1221–9.

26. Yamashita T, Siemionow KB, Mroz TE, Podichetty V, Lieberman IH. A prospective analysis of prognostic factors in patients with spinal metastases: use of the revised tokuhashi score. Spine. 2011;36(11):910–7.
27. Ulmar B, Naumann U, Catalkaya S, et al. Prognosis scores of tokuhashi and tomita for patients with spinal metastases of renal cancer. Ann Surg Oncol. 2007;14(2):998–1004.
28. Tokuhashi Y, Matsuzaki H, Oda H, Oshima M, Ryu J. A revised scoring system for preoperative evaluation of metastatic spine tumor prognosis. Spine. 2005;30(19):2186–91.
29. Bauer HC, Wedin R. Survival after surgery for spinal and extremity metastases: prognostication in 241 patients. Acta Orthop Scand. 1995;66(2):143–6.
30. Pereira NRP, Janssen SJ, van Dijk E, et al. Development of a prognostic survival algorithm for patients with metastatic spine disease. JBJS. 2016;98(21):1767–76.
31. Han S, Wang T, Jiang D, et al. Surgery and survival outcomes of 30 patients with neurological deficit due to clear cell renal cell carcinoma spinal metastases. Eur Spine J. 2015;24(8):1786–91.
32. Arrigo RT, Kalanithi P, Cheng I, et al. Predictors of survival after surgical treatment of spinal metastasis. Neurosurgery. 2011;68(3):674–81.
33. Komatsu T, Kunieda E, Oizumi Y, Tamai Y, Akiba T. An analysis of the survival rate after radiotherapy in lung cancer patients with bone metastasis: is there an optimal subgroup to be treated with high-dose radiation therapy? Neoplasma. 2012;59(6):650–7.
34. Sellin JN, Reichardt W, Bishop AJ, et al. Factors affecting survival in 37 consecutive patients undergoing de novo stereotactic radiosurgery for contiguous sites of vertebral body metastasis from renal cell carcinoma. J Neurosurg Spine. 2015;22(1):52–9.
35. Spratt DE, Beeler WH, de Moraes FY, et al. An integrated multidisciplinary algorithm for the management of spinal metastases: an international spine oncology consortium report. Lancet Oncol. 2017;18(12):e720–30.
36. Pennington Z, Ahmed AK, Westbroek EM, et al. SINS score and stability: evaluating the need for stabilization within the uncertain category. World Neurosurg. 2019;128:e1034.
37. Versteeg AL, Van der Velden JM, Verkooijen HM, et al. The effect of introducing the spinal instability neoplastic score in routine clinical practice for patients with spinal metastases. Oncologist. 2016;21(1):95–101.
38. Campos M, Urrutia J, Zamora T, et al. The spine instability neoplastic score: an independent reliability and reproducibility analysis. Spine J. 2014;14(8):1466–9.
39. Fisher CG, Versteeg AL, Schouten R, et al. Reliability of the spinal instability neoplastic scale among radiologists: an assessment of instability secondary to spinal metastases. Am J Roentgenol. 2014;203(4):869–74.
40. Hussain I, Barzilai O, Reiner AS, et al. Patient-reported outcomes after surgical stabilization of spinal tumors: symptom-based validation of the spinal instability neoplastic score (SINS) and surgery. Spine J. 2018;18(2):261–7.
41. Yamada Y, Bilsky MH, Lovelock DM, et al. High-dose, single-fraction image-guided intensity-modulated radiotherapy for metastatic spinal lesions. Int J Radiat Oncol Biol Phys. 2008;71(2):484–90.
42. Ryu S, Rock J, Jain R, et al. Radiosurgical decompression of metastatic epidural compression. Cancer. 2010;116(9):2250–7.

Advanced Imaging Technologies in the Evaluation and Staging of Adult Spine Tumors

4

Anick Nater and Michael G. Fehlings

The clinical management of patients harboring a spinal tumor aims to cure when possible, to minimize morbidity, and to maximize long-term survival. While most symptomatic primary spinal tumors require a systematic evaluation to determine their suitability for total resection, the diagnosis of any spinal primary or secondary neoplasm warrants thorough staging. In fact, clinical management depends on the accurate determination of the local involvement, the detection of nodal spread, and the quantification and qualification (i.e., location and extent) of metastases. This evaluation provides essential baseline information that enables the assessment of focal disease progression, response to treatment, and recurrence of the primary, along with any secondary malignancies at follow-ups, guiding subsequent re-staging, and therapeutic decisions. Evidence of metastatic tumors, especially in the spine, is of high significance as it profoundly influences the course of the disease, prognosis, treatment selection and planning, as well as patient's quality of life.

This chapter articulates around three theme questions. Once an adult patient is diagnosed with a spinal tumor, the following questions need to be taken into consideration:

A. What imaging modalities are currently available and how are they used in the initial characterization of the lesion and assessment of the overall tumor burden?

   What is the current evidence supporting their utilization in general and on a disease-specific basis?

B. What are the special considerations after surgical and/or radiation therapy?

C. What is the evolution of imaging technologies in the evaluation and staging of adult spine tumors?

Introduction

Spinal metastases are much more frequent than primary spinal tumors. A recent population-based analysis revealed that during 2009–2011, the incidence rate of primary benign and malignant spinal neoplasms in adults was 2.35 and 0.70 per 100,000 individuals, respectively, while it was 25.96 per 100,000 people for spinal metastases [1, 2]. However, while lesions in the extradural compartment are far more likely to be metastases, primary tumors are more common than metastases in the intradural and intramedullary compartments [3]. Despite the fact that research has mainly been focused on metastatic disease, the principles of evaluation and staging are essentially the same for all primary tumors regardless of their site of origin.

A. Nater · M. G. Fehlings (✉)
Division of Neurosurgery, Toronto Western Hospital, University Health Network, Toronto, ON, Canada
e-mail: Michael.Fehlings@uhn.ca

K. Singh, M. Colman (eds.), *Surgical Spinal Oncology*,
https://doi.org/10.1007/978-3-030-50722-0_4

The skeletal system is constantly remodeling, balancing between synthesis and degradation. Osteoblasts produce an osteoid matrix that is later mineralized with hydroxyapatite crystals. Primary and secondary tumors interfere with both bone formation and mineralization, as well as bone resorption. Although some primary neoplastic cells, such as osteosarcoma, may produce bone matrix themselves [4], most osteosclerotic activity in primary and skeletal metastases results from indirect osteoblast-stimulated bone synthesis or direct reparative osteoblast-reactive hypermetabolism. On the other hand, osteolysis results from osteoclast-mediated bone degradation. The optimal imaging technique for the diagnosis, evaluation, and staging of spinal tumors therefore depends on the underlying pathophysiology (osteosclerotic, osteolytic, or mixed) and the radiographic appearance of the neoplastic lesion [5].

Although computed tomography (CT) and magnetic resonance imaging (MRI) have become the workhorses of structural imaging, radiographs and CT myelography still have specific clinical values. While ultrasound offers a real-time anatomic insight, nuclear medicine studies depict biochemical events.

Evaluation and Staging of Spinal Tumors

There is no gold standard single method or protocol for evaluating and staging spinal neoplasms. Instead, there are numerous modalities with different advantages and disadvantages, and the choice usually depends on availability, cost, type of spinal tumor, sensitivity, specificity, radiation dose, acquisition time, clinicians' experience and preferences, as well as patient's general condition and her/his relative and absolute contraindications.

Conventional Radiography

Conventional spine radiography using X-rays is widely accessible, rapidly available, and cheap. They are ubiquitous to evaluate patients presenting with neck or back pain in primary and emergency care settings, particularly in patients with a known history of cancer. In neoplastic processes, their ability is limited to demonstrating areas of osteolysis (hypodensity) or osteosclerosis (hyperdensity) [6]. Typical radiographic findings associated with skeletal tumors include vertebral body collapse, pedicle erosion ("wink-owl" sign), paraspinal soft tissue shadow (i.e., paraspinal mass), and osteosclerosis and osteolysis generally sparing the intervertebral disc margins [7]. The pattern of osteolysis may indicate the aggressiveness of the tumor. Generally speaking, benign tumors tend to grow slowly and thus have distinctive margins; they are referred to as "geographic" lesions [8].

The limited ability of radiographs to reveal anatomical defects has been recognized for several decades. Edelstyn et al. [9] reported that between 50% and 75% of the cancellous bone thickness in the beam axis on the lateral view had to be absent to become radiographically apparent, and the defect needed to be even more significant to be visualized on the AP view. Between 17% and 26% of vertebral metastasis fail to exhibit radiologic evidence of disease on spinal radiographs [10, 11]. Because of superimposition effects, the identification of neoplastic processes is more challenging in the skull, spine, and pelvis [12]. Radiologic diagnosis is facilitated when there is cortical involvement and a high level of vertebral mineralization [9]. However, cortical involvement is rather rare in both pathologic [9] and osteoporotic fractures [13]. In addition, vertebral mineralization tends to decrease with age [9]. Moreover, vertebral collapse identified on radiographs were not associated with tumor deposit in 22% of cancer patients [11]. Consequently, radiographs are not a suitable stand-alone technique for adequate evaluation and staging of spinal tumors [6, 12].

Nevertheless, they still offer some clinical advantages. Although there is no universally accepted definition for spinal instability, plain radiographs are commonly obtained to assess overall alignment and mechanical spinal stability in the subacute setting. Moreover, chest X-ray is an easy and cheap screening tool in the context of a metastatic workup. In a prospective study including 40 consecutive patients with skeletal metastases of unknown origin, findings on plain radiographs of the chest led to the diagnosis of lung cancer in 43% of patients [14].

With regards to the field of spinal oncology, plain radiographs are useful in assessing and monitoring (i) spinal stability and deformity (upright, flexion, extension and lateral bending), (ii) global spinal balance (3-foot standing, i.e., weight-bearing full spine, sagittal, and coronal views), (iii) deformities, (iv) arthrodesis (i.e., fusion), (v) spinal alignment, as well as positioning and integrity of the instrumentation and implant system postoperatively, and (vi) although a normal radiograph cannot rule out the presence of a metastasis, an abnormality on X-ray in the appendicular skeleton prompts further evaluation, and therefore, it is useful as a "rule-in" method [12].

Computerized Tomography (CT)

Given its relatively low cost, widespread availability, and exceptional speed, computed tomography (CT) with intravenous (IV) and oral contrast is the favored initial modality for the Tumor, Nodal, and systemic Metastasis (TNM) staging system, which is a recognized standard for classifying the extent of spread of cancer. In fact, for most types of cancers, the TNM system is the preferred method for the initial and subsequent staging [12, 15].

With regards to the skeletal system, CT has the advantage of not involving superimposition of anatomical structures, higher spatial resolution, ability to use windowing to optimize bone and soft-tissue contrast, and ability to acquire whole-body (WB) imaging while minimizing radiation exposure using low-dose technique. Moreover, because data are acquired from a single imaging procedure consisting of multiple contiguous or one helical scan, it is possible to obtain CT axial, sagittal, coronal reformatted images, and even 3D reconstructions, which can be useful for complex resection planning. Given that the volume acquisition has the same value regardless of the direction in which it is measured, these reformatted images have the same quality as the source images [16]. As a result, CT offers significant advantages in the evaluation of spinal tumors, as a result [6]. In fact, CT is considered the best modality for the evaluation of mineralized tissues [17].

In the evaluation of spinal tumors, CT is performed in most cases with a large field of view and no contrast medium, given that the use of IV contrast does not provide relevant additional information. Because it depicts both trabecular and cortical bone with high resolution, CT permits excellent visualization of the bony architecture. It is useful for assessing osteoslerotic, osteolytic, and periosteal reactions, as well as the presence of bony fragment in the spinal canal. Specifically for surgical planning, CT angiography (CTA) may provide enough information regarding the tumor blood supply and its relationship to the surrounding vasculature to avoid performing a conventional angiography [16]. Moreover, in patients who cannot get an MRI (e.g., patients with a pacemaker or who suffer from extreme claustrophobia) or who underwent spinal reconstruction involving metallic devices, the opacification of the cerebrospinal fluid (CSF) in CT myelogram enables identification of structural causes for abnormal CSF distribution, such as in cases of intradural spine lesions or compression of the thecal sac by an extradural mass lesion [18]. Of note, myelography has been associated with a risk of acute neurologic deterioration in patients with severe spinal cord compression causing a high-grade block and should be used with caution in this circumstance [19].

However, CT has limited sensitivity for bone marrow infiltration [12, 20]. This constitutes a significant shortcoming in the assessment of spinal metastases, as they primarily arise in the vertebral bone marrow [16]. In addition, it may be difficult to appreciate cortical alterations in patients with osteoporosis or degenerative changes [7]. Finally, ionizing radiation exposure is always a drawback to keep in mind [20].

CT is the preferred technique for further bony appraisal of suspect scintigraphy or MRI findings, especially when a positive uptake is associated with a normal radiograph [7]. Further, CT is useful for characterizing spatial configuration of the lesion, which is particularly critical in the planning of surgical treatment involving resection and instrumentation. In addition, CT is useful for investigating spinal stability (e.g., SINS classification), ossification processes, and fracture risk [12, 18]. Lastly, it is the best method to assess arthrodesis and spinal alignment along with positioning and integrity of the instrumentation and implant system postoperatively.

Magnetic Resonance Imaging (MRI)

In spinal tumors, when possible, appropriate evaluation of the tumor component of the TNM system virtually always requires that CT is supplemented by magnetic resonance imaging (MRI). To date, MRI is the gold standard for the initial identification and anatomical evaluation of spinal tumors [21].

MRI is currently the modality of choice in the detection and examination of spinal tumors. It enables detailed characterization of the tumor vascularity, bone marrow, and spinal canal involvement. It also delineates the relationship of the tumor with surrounding paraspinal and neurovascular structures, including intrinsic spinal cord signal abnormalities [22]. MRI provides such high soft-tissue and bone marrow contrast, as well as three-dimensional spatial resolution that neoplastic processes in the bone marrow can be observed even when cortical and trabecular bone components are still intact [12]. T1-weighted images (WI), T2-WI, T2-WI fat saturated (typically short tau inversion recovery, i.e., STIR), and postcontrast T1-WI fat-saturated sequences are usually obtained [18]. Vertebral bone marrow changes are best demonstrated on T1-WI [18], whereas the extent and degree of canal compromise and spinal cord compression is generally best appreciated on T2-WI. The epidural spinal cord compression (ESCC) scale [23] is based on axial T2-WI MRI; this grading system is particularly useful in treatment planning. T1-WI with contrast enhancement aids to better delineate epidural extension and the location of tumors relative to the different spinal compartments (extradural, intradural-extramedullary, and intramedullary), which helps in elaborating an appropriate differential diagnosis [22]. It also helps in differentiating enhanced viable tumor from areas of non-enhanced necrosis [16] or simple cystic areas that may be present in some benign tumors, which is particularly useful for biopsy planning, because it optimizes the likelihood of obtaining a diagnostic sample during fine needle aspiration, core needle biopsy, or surgical quick sections. Contrast enhancement is best demonstrated on fat-saturated T1-WI MRI. However, when imaging the cervical or thoracic spine, phase-encoded motion artifacts due to respiration and/or swallowing may lead to inhomogeneous suppression of the fat signal, which may hamper the overall image quality as a result [16]. Furthermore, the application of STIR for intramedullary tumors may be limited by poor signal to noise and greater sensitivity to motion than standard T2-weighted sequences [3].

Diffusion-weighted imaging (DWI) is a quantitative form of MRI based on measurement of the random motion, i.e., diffusion, of biological molecules, mainly water, within a voxel of tissue. Cell membranes (i.e., high cellularity), cellular swelling, blood vessels, and fibrotic tissues typically restrict diffusion, thus exhibiting lower diffusion coefficients and appearing with a relatively high signal intensity in DWI. DWI remains sensitive to T1 and T2 relaxation, and T2 shine-through is a known cause of artifactual high signal on DWI. Therefore, restricted diffusion is reflected by a high signal in DWI confirmed by low signal on apparent diffusion coefficient (ADC) maps, i.e., abnormal diffusion restriction. There is a growing interest for the DWI technique in spine oncology as neoplastic tissues generally consist of densely cellular and highly vascularized structures, and therefore exhibiting restricted diffusion [24]. In particular, tumors infiltrating the bone marrow, such as plasmacytoma/multiple myeloma, can be difficult to detect using traditional MRI sequences; DWI can help differentiate them from hyperplastic or other benign changes [18].

Technical shortcomings of DWI are related to the small size of the spinal cord, the heterogeneous magnetic environment, and inherent motion in and around the spine. Despite these, and despite a lack of definition of the clinical utility of DWI in spine oncology, this technique has gained popularity. For example, DWI is sensitive to ischemic damage and changes in spinal marrow, which can aid in distinguishing benign from malignant insufficiency fractures. The usefulness of DWI in this setting had yet to be defined [25].

As mentioned above for CTA, in the context of surgical planning, MR angiography (MRA) may provide valuable anatomical vascular information that might justify or preclude the need for a conventional angiography [16]. In addition to better imaging of the bone marrow, the fact that MRI does not involve ionizing radiation is another advantage over CT for staging. Furthermore, in patients with poor renal function, the use of gadolinium can be avoided given that T1-WI and STIR sequences provide adequate imaging of the bone marrow [12].

Thanks to recent advancements including fast image acquisition, rolling platform extenders mounted on top of a conventional MRI table, and the implementation of dedicated software, whole-body MRI (WB-MRI) is now feasible in scan times under 1 hour [3].

Nuclear Medicine and Molecular Imaging

Kircher et al. [26] define molecular imaging in oncology as "in vivo characterization and measurement of the key biomolecules and molecularly based events that are fundamental to the malignant state." Molecular imaging technologies are used across numerous fields, including nuclear medicine, radiology, pharmacology, molecular and cell biology, engineering, physics, and mathematics [26]. There are various molecular imaging techniques used in nuclear medicine that provide physiological (i.e., functional) imaging with two- (i.e., planar) or three-dimensional depictions. In nuclear medicine, quantification refers to the ability to reliably quantify activity [27, 28].

Bone Scintigraphy (BS) and Single-Photon Emission Computed Tomography (SPECT)

Bone imaging involves the use of a radionuclide, most often Technetium-99m (99mTc), bound to a bisphosphonate, typically methylene diphosphonate (MDP), forming the radiotracer 99mTc-MDP. The amount of 99mTc-MDP that becomes integrated to hydroxyapatite crystals during bone synthesis is proportional to local blood flow and osteoblastic activity. 99mTc-MDP rapidly localizes to areas of both bone perfusion and synthesis and clears quickly from the background [29].

Whole-body (WB), regional, and three-phase images are different types of planar bone imaging. Planar whole-body images, i.e., bone scintigraphy or bone scan (BS), have been used for several decades. BS permits a rapid survey of the entire skeleton in a single examination, at relatively low costs and with good sensitivity [29]. BS has been used for decades as the primary method for staging, and despite its limitations related to diagnostic specificity, it is still widely use in clinical practice [30]. Because of their greater resolution, regional bone images allow further detailed evaluation of specific body parts. In three-phase bone imaging, the radiotracer is injected as a bolus. The serial images obtained over time serve as an angiographic depiction of regional arterial and venous flow in bones and soft tissues. In addition, there are no contraindications to this imaging modality, and it is a procedure that is well tolerated by patients [29].

Bone scans are highly sensitive but perform relatively poorly in terms of specificity. In fact, benign and malignant primary neoplasms, metastatic tumors, fracture healing, Paget's disease, infectious processes, and inflammatory processes such as active degenerative osteoarthritis are all associated with radionuclide uptake (i.e., a positive or "hot" bone scan). Furthermore, certain conditions are typically associated with "cold" or photopenic, i.e., false-negative, bone scan, such as in tumors that cause active osteolysis (e.g., very aggressive, osteolytic bone tumors where almost no reactive hypermetabolism bone synthesis occurs), in indolent processes that induce little bone healing (e.g., chordoma), in isolated bone-marrow infiltration (e.g., metastasis from renal cell carcinoma, lymphoma, leukemia, or plasmacytoma/multiple myeloma), and in areas where the blood flow is disrupted (bone infarcts) [12, 31]. Observation of diffuse increased bone uptake throughout the skeleton, sometimes in the context of decreased renal activity suggested by the "absent kidney sign" (i.e., no physiologic pooling of radionuclide in the kidneys), may fail to highlight any "hot spots" and may be misinterpreted as a negative scan. This phenomenon is called "superscan." It is typically seen with prostate carcinoma. Radiologic correlation is generally diagnostic [29].

BS is often complemented by SPECT or SPECT/CT imaging. The SPECT technology uses newer gamma cameras and software that allow tomographic acquisitions and thus can provide three-dimensional representations of specific areas. This offers a more precise pathophysiologic assessment and localization of the regions of bone synthesis within the "hot" vertebra. SPECT is particularly useful for areas markedly surrounded by soft tissue, such as the thoracolumbar spine and pelvis. It also helps differentiate malignant lesion from other entities such as degenerative facet joint arthropathy, active pars defect, or other benign processes [7].

Positron-Emission Tomography (PET)

PET computes the three-dimensional distribution of radioactivity emitted by positron emitter labeled radiotracers. The glucose analogue ^{18}F-fluoro-2-deoxy-D-glucose (^{18}F-FDG) is one of the most commonly used radiotracers in oncology, especially for evaluating bone metastases. ^{18}F-FDG accumulates in cells proportionally to their glucose intake; ^{18}F-FDG is thus a marker for elevated glucose metabolism [6].

^{18}F-FDG is not specific to neoplastic cells. However, alterations in glucose metabolism are one of the early events in carcinogenesis. In fact, most neoplasms are metabolically highly active and demonstrate increased expression and activity of glucose transporters in the cell membrane and glycolytic enzyme hexokinase. They also tend to favor the anaerobic glycolytic pathway, adding to their already augmented glucose demands. These combined mechanisms result in tumor cells incorporating and retaining higher levels of ^{18}F-FDG, relative to surrounding non-neoplastic cells [26].

Vertebrae, paraspinal muscles, CSF, epidural fat, leptomeninges, and nerve roots normally show relatively low ^{18}F-FDG uptake and thus consist of the background tissues for evaluating ^{18}F-FDG avidity for spinal tumors. Although the spinal cord is also generally considered a background tissue, focal increase, mostly in the cervical and lumbar segment, has been described as a physiologic variant finding. Additionally, other sources of false-positive results are a shortcoming of ^{18}F-FDG PET. Cancer patients may exhibit marrow hyperplasia as a response to endogenous or exogenous hematopoietic stimulating factors [32]; some therapeutic protocols involve using granulocyte colony-stimulating factor (G-CSF) [6], which stimulates metabolic activity in the bone marrow. The resulting increased uptake of ^{18}F-FDG may be misinterpreted as diffuse neoplastic marrow infiltration. Moreover, in the spine, because of partial volume effects, this bone marrow hyperplasia may also lead to higher ^{18}F-FDG uptake by neighboring structures located within the spinal canal. Consequently, given the variability in physiologic ^{18}F-FDG avidity within the spine, the diagnosis of a spinal tumor requires that evidence from anatomic imaging, such as those provided by CT or MRI, corroborate PET results [32].

Some tumor entities are associated with low-level ^{18}F-FDG uptake. In fact, in PET examination, the ability to detect a lesion depends on several biological and technical factors, including the size, cellularity and overall glycolytic activity of the lesion, background ^{18}F-FDG uptake in surrounding tissues, proper patient preparation, and type of scanner used. For primary bone tumors, ^{18}F-FDG uptake is variable. Although malignant tumors tend to be more ^{18}F-FDG avid than benign tumors, this principle is more consistent for tumors of the same histologic type than for different ones [33]. For instance, the mean ^{18}F-FDG uptake was similar for giant cell tumors than for malignant lymphomas of the bone [34]. Ewing's sarcoma and low-grade osteosarcomas [35], along with low-grade chondrosarcomas and osteochondromas, have been reported to have low ^{18}F-FDG uptake [34]. Similarly, low-grade lung adenocarcinoma, renal cell carcinoma, and neuroendocrine (mucinous) neoplasms are often associated with low ^{18}F-FDG uptake [36]. In addition, osteoblastic metastases usually show lower metabolic activity and are thus often undetected by ^{18}F-FDG [37].

Ultimately, in contrast to CT, MRI, BS, and SPECT that enable the identification of tumors based on structural changes, ^{18}F-FDG PET allows detection and quantitative characterization of neoplasms based on direct physiologic activity even before any morphologic alterations become evident on anatomic imaging studies [38].

Moreover, unlike BS and SPECT, ^{18}F-FDG PET also offers the advantage of detecting neoplastic processes not only in the skeleton but also in multiple organ systems. ^{18}F-FDG-PET can thus be used for complete, whole-body staging and for identifying the site of primary tumor in patients who present with a metastasis but have no prior history of cancer.

There is strong evidence that ^{18}F-FDG uptake correlates with both poor prognosis and poor response to treatment for certain neoplasms, including hepatocellular carcinoma, low-grade lymphoma, and prostate cancer. For example, patients with high ^{18}F-FDG uptake tend to present with higher disease stage and metastatic spread and are less likely to respond to radiotherapy, transarterial chemoembolization, and liver transplantation [36].

Nonetheless, ^{18}F-FDG PET is expensive, lacks spatial resolution for precise localization and characterization of the increased radiotracer uptake, and has limited specificity [38]. Of note, from this point on, PET will refer to ^{18}F-FDG PET unless otherwise specified.

Although Fluorine 18-Sodium Fluoride (^{18}F-NaF) was approved by the FDA in 1972 for the detection of osteogenic activity, it was rapidly replaced by 99mTc, given the better imaging abilities of the latter for gamma cameras in contrast to the high-energy photons of ^{18}F-NaF. Similarly to 99mTc-MDP, ^{18}F-NaF becomes integrated to hydroxyapatite crystals during bone synthesis proportionally to local blood flow and osteoblastic activity. The increased use of combining PET and CT may encourage a renewed interest in ^{18}F-NaF in the form of ^{18}F-NaF PET/CT for clinical use in neoplastic bone imaging [39].

Hybrid Techniques

Hybrid techniques include SPECT/CT, PET/CT, and PET/MRI. They couple the visualization of bone metabolism with anatomical imaging, thanks to the fusion of complementary images. Consequently, the combination of the two techniques enhances the overall diagnostic yield in a synergistic manner since the resulting specificity is superior to either modality used on its own [6]. PET/CT and PET/MRI studies are traditionally generated using the retrospective fusion of data obtained on two separate apparatuses [12], but similarly to SPECT/CT, PET/CT and PET/MRI now exist as a single integrated device [40]. Of note, although simultaneous acquisition improves image quality by eliminating temporal and spatial registration changes, the clinical throughput is more limited, and software solutions and the stability of the scanner are less robust compared to individual PET and MRI systems [41]. In addition, PET/CT and PET/MRI allow estimation of the metabolic tumor volume (MTV) and total lesion glycolysis (TLG) [27]. In PET, quantification is a process that involves measuring the maximum standardized uptake value (SUV_{max}), which corresponds to the single pixel value of the most active voxel of osseous radioactivity concentration in a given lesion [27, 28]. MTV is the sum of the volume of voxels with SUV surpassing a threshold value in a tumor [42], whereas TLG is the product of MTV and the mean SUV of the MTV [43].

Evidence Related to Current Imaging Modalities

To date, there is no standardized protocol related to the characterization and determination of overall tumor burden. Although the decision-making process regarding which combination of techniques to employ in conjuncture with the elected course of action is greatly influenced by the type of primary tumor and ultimately tailored to each individual patient, various studies have attempted to compare current imaging modalities. The vast majority of these studies were performed for metastatic vertebral disease.

It must be emphasized that because systematic and universal biopsy is not feasible or ethical, comparative studies of imaging to detect tumors suffer from lack of a gold standard. For example, many comparative studies of imaging methods use different scanners, protocols, and surrogate parameters as their diagnostic reference standard. In addition, a diverse combination of histopathologic analysis and radiographic confirmation is reported with different imaging techniques. Consequently, it is difficult to generalize the overall body of evidence. We recognize that the inclusion of publications in this section is incomplete; the goal is to present the general trends and ongoing uncertainties so as to highlight the necessity of a multimodal approach.

All MRI studies were performed on a 1.5-Tesla (T) scanner unless specified otherwise. The diagnostic accuracy was typically quantified as (i) the proportion of true positive and true negative in all evaluated cases, i.e., standard accuracy; (ii) the diagnostic odds ratio (DOR), i.e., for instance, the ratio of the odds of a test revealing bone metastases in patients that have bone metastases relative to the odds of the test revealing bone metastases in patients who do not have bone metastases, (iii) the area under receiver operating characteristic (AUROC) curve that is a combined measure of sensitivity and specificity, depicting the average value of sensitivity for all possible values of specificity [44–46].

Primary Spinal Tumors

Yang et al. [47] reported that compared to CT and plain radiograph, although MRI demonstrated a higher sensitivity (92.75% vs. 86.96% vs. 76.81%), specificity (89.86% vs. 88.41% vs. 68.96%), and accuracy (91.30% vs. 86.96% vs. 78.26%) in the diagnosis of primary spinal tumors, respectively, only sensitivity and accuracy were statistically different.

Franzius et al. [48] evaluated 32 and 38 patients with histologically proven osteosarcomas and Ewing's sarcomas, respectively. Of note, the location (i.e., appendicular vs. axial skeleton) of the primary malignancies was not specified. There were a total of 54 bone metastases (49 from Ewing's sarcomas and 5 from osteosarcomas). BS detected all five metastases from osteosarcoma but PET detected none. However, PET was superior in identifying metastases from Ewing's sarcoma (sensitivity: 100% vs. 68%; specificity: 96% vs. 87%; and accuracy: 97% vs. 82%). PET was shown to have higher sensitivity and specificity for spinal metastases than BS in lymphoma [49].

In their review, Lütje et al. [50] concluded that PET complemented with either low-dose WB-CT or WB-MRI was more sensitive than radiographs for the diagnosis and skeletal screening of multiple myeloma. Response therapy was better assessed with PET than WB-MRI. ^{18}F-FDG uptake decreases within hours after effective therapy and persistent positive PET results correlated with earlier relapse, whereas it takes approximately 9–12 months for lesions to resolve on MRI.

Bone Metastasis

The sensitivity of PET has been reported to be higher for osteolytic lesions and lower for osteosclerotic lesions than BS [37, 51]. Therefore, BS usually identifies metastases from breast, prostate, and lung cancers, which often demonstrate mainly osteosclerotic activity. On the other hand, primarily osteolytic metastases, such as renal cell or thyroid carcinoma, as well as plasmacytoma or multiple myeloma, are better detected by PET [52]. PET/CT is more sensitive than BS in detecting bone metastases in patients with cancer with the added advantage of identifying unknown primary tumors and visceral metastases [52]. Moreover, although PET/CT and BS had equal specificity (98%), PET/CT has greater sensitivity (97% vs. 83%) and accuracy (98% vs. 93%) for detecting skeletal metastases in patients with cancer [53].

The number of lesions demonstrated by 99m Tc-MDP bone scan and ^{18}F–NaF PET/CT was equal in 4/37 (11%) of the cases. ^{18}F–NaF PET/CT showed a greater number of pathological foci in 89% of participants. ^{18}F–NaF PET/CT was able to show both lytic and blastic lesions, and small lesions were better visualized due to the advantage of sectional imaging with much better resolution and higher target/background ratio. ^{18}F–NaF PET/CT demonstrated a greater number of metastases in 10/12 (83%) of the patients when compared to ^{18}F–NaF PET/CT. In the other two patients, bone metastasis could be demonstrated only by ^{18}F–NaF PET/CT. The uptake of ^{18}F-FDG was variable in blastic lesions, and cranial bone involvement was missed by ^{18}F–NaF PET/CT in some cases due to physiological bone metabolism.

In detecting bone metastases in cancer patients, a meta-analysis revealed that on both a per-patient and per-lesion basis, while

(i) PET/CT and PET had similar specificity, the sensitivity, and diagnostic accuracy was significantly higher with PET/CT, and
(ii) SPECT and BS had similar sensitivity, the specificity, and diagnostic accuracy was higher with SPECT. Overall, PET and MRI were similarly accurate but significantly better than BS and CT (Table 4.1) [54].

Although both WB-PET/CT and WB-PET/MRI had high diagnostic ability for skeletal metastases, PET/MRI was slightly superior on a per-patient and per-lesion basis for correctly identifying malignant lesions [55]. Another study revealed similar results. When comparing WB-MRI and PET/CT, although WB-MRI detected skeletal metastases with statistically greater sensitivity (94% vs. 78%) and accuracy (91% vs. 78%) than PET/CT, both had relatively equal specificity (76% vs. 80%) [56]. Eiber et al. [57] reported equivalent overall

Table 4.1 Summary evidence for detecting bone metastases

Author, year, type of study	Detecting bone metastases
Yang, 2011, meta-analysis	*Cancer patients* *Per-patient basis* *Pooled sensitivity estimates* PET/CT (93.7%) > MRI (90.6%) = PET (89.7%) > BS (86.0%) = SPECT (82.6%) > CT (72.9%) *Pooled specificity estimates* PET/CT (97.4%) = PET (96.4%) = MRI (95.4%) = CT (94.8%) > SPECT (92.8%) > BS (79.9%) *Pooled DOR estimate* PET/CT > PET = MRI = CT > SPECT > BS) *Per-lesion basis* *Pooled sensitivity estimates* PET/CT (94.2%) > MRI (90.4%) > PET (80.1%) > CT (77.1%) = SPECT (76.8%) > BS (74.5%) *Pooled specificity estimates* PET/CT (97.2%) = PET (96.9%) > SPECT (96.3%) = MRI (96.0%) > BS (92.1%) > CT (83.2%) *Pooled DOR estimate* PET/CT > PET = MRI > SPECT > BS > CT
Liu, 2011, meta-analysis	*Breast cancer* *Per-patient basis* *Pooled sensitivity estimates* MRI (97.1%) > PET (83.3%) = BS (87.0%) *Pooled specificity estimates* MRI (97.0%) = PET (94.5%) > BS (88.1%) *Pooled DOR estimates* MRI > PET = BS *Diagnostic accuracy (summary AUROC)* MRI > PET > BS *Per-lesion basis* *Pooled sensitivity estimates* BS (87.8%) > PET (52.7%) *Pooled specificity estimates* PET (99.6%) > BS (96.1%), *Pooled DOR estimates and diagnostic accuracy (summary AUROC)* PET > BS

(continued)

Table 4.1 (continued)

Shen, 2014, meta-analysis	*Prostate cancer* *Per-patient basis* (*there was not enough data to analyze SPECT) *Pooled sensitivity estimates* MRI (0.95) > choline-PET/CT (0.87) > BS (0.79) *Pooled specificity estimates* choline-PET/CT (0.97) > MRI (0.96) > BS (0.82) *Pooled DOR estimates* MRI (343.16) > choline-PET/CT (150.70) > BS (20.32) *Summary AUROC* MRI (0.9870) > choline-PET/CT (0.9541) > BS (0.8876) *Per-lesion basis* (*there were not enough data to analyze MRI) *Pooled sensitivity estimates* SPECT (0.90) > choline-PET/CT (0.83) > BS (0.59 *Pooled specificity estimates* choline-PET/CT (0.95) > SPECT (0.85) > BS (0.75) *Pooled DOR estimates* choline-PET/CT (99.78) > SPECT (78.16) > BS (6.21 *Summary AUROC* choline-PET/CT (0.9494) > SPECT (0.9381) > BS (0.7736)
Takenaka, 2009, prospective cohort study	*Non-small-cell lung cancer (NSCLC)* *Per-patient basis* *Sensitivity estimate* PET/CT (96.0%), BS (96.0%), WB-MRI with DWI (96.0%), and WB-DWI (96.0%) > WB-MRI without DWI (64.0%) *Specificity estimate* WB-MRI without DWI (90.0%) = WB-MRI with DWI (90.0%) = PET/CT (85.6%) > BS (83.3%) > WB-DWI (78.9%) *Accuracy* WB-MRI with DWI (91.3%) > PET/CT (87.8%) = BS (86.1%) > WB-MRI without DWI (84.3%) = WB-DWI (82.6%) *Per-lesion basis* *Sensitivity estimate* PET/CT (97.0%) > BS (95.5%) = WB-MRI with DWI (95.5%) = WB-DWI (95.5%) > WB-MRI without DWI (73.1%) *Specificity estimate* WB-MRI without DWI (96.4%) = WB-MRI with DWI (96.1%) > PET/CT (95.4%) = BS (95.0%) > WB-DWI (93.7%) *Accuracy* WB-MRI with DWI (96.1%) > PET/CT (95.5%) = BS (95.0%) = WB-MRI without DWI (94.8%) > WB-DWI (93.9%)
Liu, 2017, meta-analysis	*Spinal metastasis* *Per-patient basis* *Sensitivity* MRI (94.1%) = SPECT (90.3%) = PET (89.8%) > BS (80.0%) = CT (79.2%) *Specificity* MRI (94.2%) = CT (92.3%) = BS (92.8%) > SPECT (86.0%) > PET (63.3%) *Diagnostic odds ratio* MRI (151.7) > SPECT (57.2) > BS (36.4) > CT (19.3) = PET (12.5) *Diagnostic ability* (*summary ROC curve could not be calculated for CT because there were only two studies included) MRI (0.9693) > SPECT (0.9525) > BS (0.8968) > PET (0.8295) *Per-lesion basis* *Sensitivity* SPECT (92.3%) = MRI (90.1%) = PET (88.7%) > BS (80.2%) > CT (66.7%) *Specificity* MRI (96.9%) = CT (95.4%) > SPECT (72.0%) = BS (73.5%) = PET (70.9%) *Diagnostic odds ratio* MRI (286.1) > SPECT (43.4) > CT (24.2) = PET (18.8) > BS (8.6) *Diagnostic ability* MRI (0.9887) > BS (0.8297) > SPECT (0.8281) = PET (0.8281) > CT (0.7255)

> Statistically significantly superior

performance for WB-PET/CT and WB-PET/MRI.

In their meta-analysis, Wu et al. [58] highlighted the ongoing uncertainty regarding the superiority of WB-MRI over BS. Indeed, despite showing significantly higher DOR, WB-MRI and BS had comparable sensitivity and specificity (0.84 vs. 0.83 and 0.96 vs. 0.94, respectively) [58]. Another meta-analysis revealed the comparable sensitivity, specificity, and accuracy of WB-DWI and WB-MRI with DWI. The authors suggested that WB-DWI could be used as an independent technique to identify bone metastases [59].

Of note, in their review, Ellmann et al. [6] reported that ^{18}F-fluoride is a promising radionuclide tracer for the evaluation and staging of spinal tumors. This is because it is associated with easier early detection of skeletal metastases, greater bony accumulation compared to 99mTc-MDP and has the advantages of not imposing dietary or physical activity limitations. Lastly, unlike FSG moieties, ^{18}F-fluoride does not contribute to overall increases in blood glucose concentration.

Disease-Specific Studies

SPECT is more sensitive than BS and is also superior in characterizing equivocal lesions in patients with breast cancer with bone metastases [60]. On a per-lesion basis, SPECT was also statistically significantly more sensitive (85% vs. 17%) and accurate (96% vs. 85%) than PET, whereas both modalities had comparable specificity (99% vs. 100%) in the detection of bone metastases from breast cancer. Although PET showed much less sensitivity at identifying osteosclerotic lesions than SPECT (6% and 92%, respectively), PET more readily revealed osteolytic lesions (90% vs. 35%) [61]. Consequently, Uematsu et al. [61] highlighted that PET should not be used as a stand-alone modality.

Liu et al. [62] concluded that for diagnosis of bone metastases in patients with breast cancer, MRI was superior to PET and BS on a per-patient basis, while despite a much lower sensitivity, PET had a higher specificity and accuracy than BS on a per-lesion basis (Table 1). Another meta-analysis reported greater sensitivity, specificity, and accuracy (AUROC) for PET-CT (0.93; 0.99; 0.98) than for BS (0.81; 0.96; 0.94) in detecting bone metastases in patients with breast cancer [63].

In their review, Azad et al. [5] highlighted the low glycolysis rate associated with skeletal metastases from prostate cancer and the scarce number of studies using the conventional ^{18}F-FDG PET as a result. They also reported that although various radiotracer imaging methods, e.g., ^{11}C-choline-PET/CT, ^{18}F-choline-PET/CT, or ^{18}F-fluoride-PET/CT are available to detect bone metastases in patients with metastatic prostate cancer, none have been demonstrated to be superior [5]. Shen et al. [64] performed a meta-analysis comparing choline-PET/CT, MRI, SPECT, and BS in the diagnosis of bone metastases in patients with prostate cancer. While new PET tracers have shown promising results, because of their high accuracy in the detection of bone metastasis in prostate cancer, to date, ^{11}C-choline and ^{18}F-choline are the most frequently used. The authors also reported that MRI showed better diagnostic accuracy than choline-PET/CT and BS ($p < 0.05$), and choline-PET/CT was better than BS ($p < 0.05$). The authors concluded that MRI and choline-PET/CT were more accurate than SPECT and BS for detecting bone metastases in patients with prostate cancer (Supplement Table 4.1).

The SKELETA clinical trial prospectively evaluated the ability of WB-MRI-DWI, ^{18}F-NaF PET/CT, SPECT/CT, and BS to identify bone metastases in 26 breast and 27 prostate high-risk cancer patients. Overall, WB-MRI-DWI and ^{18}F-NaF PET/CT showed similar sensitivity, specificity, and accuracy on both a per-patient and per-lesion basis when the equivocal lesion findings of the imaging were classified suggestive for metastases or for nonmetastatic origin and were superior to SPECT/CT and BS [65].

In their prospective study on 95 patients with small-cell lung cancer (SCLC), among which 30 harbored bone metastases, Lee et al. [66] concluded that PET/CT could replace BS because on a per-patient basis, PET/CT showed 100% sensitivity, specificity, and accuracy as oppose to 37%,

92%, and 75%, respectively, for BS, and on a per-lesion basis, the sensitivity, specificity and accuracy were 86.9%, 100%, and 88.4% for PET/CT and 28.6%, 0%, and 25.3% for BS, respectively. Similarly, a meta-analyses reported higher sensitivity (92% vs. 77% vs. 86%) and specificity (98% vs. 92% vs. 88%) for PET/CT compared to MRI and BS, respectively, for patients with lung cancer [67]. However, Tekenaka et al. [68] prospectively evaluated the sensitivity, specificity, and accuracy of BS, PET/CT, WB-DWI (i.e., precontrast-enhanced DWI in coronal and sagittal planes), WB-MRI without DWI (i.e., pre- and postcontrast-enhanced inphase T1-gradient echo, precontrast-enhanced opposed-phase T1-gradient echo, and precontrast-enhanced STIR turbo spin-echo images in coronal and sagittal planes), and WB-MRI with DWI (i.e., combination of WB-DWI and WB-MRI) in 25 patients with bone metastases from non-small-cell lung cancer (NSCLC). The authors concluded that WB-MRI with DWI is more specific and accurate than BS and PET/CT in detecting bone metastases in patients with NSCLC (Supplement Table 4.1) [68].

A recent systematic review highlighted that despite the heterogeneity of the studies, with the majority lacking independent reference standard, WB-MRI was associated with a higher ability to identify bone lesion in patients with multiple myeloma than PET/CT with a sensitivity ranging from 68% to 100% and from 47% to 100% for WB-MRI and PET/CT, respectively. However, WB-MRI had a lower specificity (37–83% vs. 62–85.7%) [69].

Spinal Metastases

In their recent meta-analysis, Liu et al. [7] compared MRI, CT, PET, BS, and SPECT for the detection of vertebral metastases. The diagnostic odds ratio (DOR) is a measure of effectiveness for diagnostic tests. It is the ratio of the odds of the test revealing a vertebral metastasis in patients that have a vertebral metastasis relative to the odds of the test revealing a vertebral metastasis in patients who do not have a vertebral metastasis. The authors concluded that MRI was the best modality for diagnosing vertebral metastases both on a per-patient and per-lesion basis, while SPECT was the second best modality on a per-lesion basis (Supplement Table 4.1).

Staging

Antoch et al. [70] reported a superior performance in overall TNM staging for PET/CT over WB-MRI with a greater standard accuracy for T-stage (80% vs. 52%) and N-stage (93% vs. 77%), but with comparable ability to differentiate between M0 and M1 disease (94% vs. 93%).

However, Heusch et al. [71] reported that PET/CT and PET/MRI had comparable accuracy for TNM staging in patients with solid tumors.

Special Considerations Posttreatment

After 4–12 weeks from treatment initiation for bone metastasis, successful therapy may be associated with increased osteosclerotic activity, giving rise to the "flare phenomenon" on BS, resulting in the appearance of previously occult lesions as "new" deposits. This phenomenon makes the distinction between disease progression and temporary healing osteoblastic response from successful therapy challenging up to 6 months after treatment has been started [6, 12]. Nonetheless, it was reported that only 52% of treatment responders showed scintigraphic improvement and 62% of nonresponders showed scintigraphic deterioration [72], which could delay the decision to change the therapeutic regimen to a more effective one [5].

Metallic spinal instrumentation impacts image acquisition and reconstruction in CT and MRI scans, degrading the image quality and hindering a thorough assessment of the surrounding structures as a result [73]. By absorbing radiation, metal implants not only impede the planning but also the execution of postoperative percutaneous RT with photons and particularly with protons or heavier ions [74]. While metallic instrumentation causes beam hardening, splay artifacts, scatter effects, and nonlinear partial volume effects along its edges in CT, the resulting inhomogeneous magnetic fields in MRI induce false spatial readouts leading to geometric distortion, signal loss, and pile-up effects, and failure of homogeneous fat suppression [75]. Just as a higher magnetic field strength creates more obtrusive artifacts, so too do CT images obtained using a scanner with more than four channels does accentuate artifacts [73].

The specificities related to CT and MRI scanners, acquisition protocols, and reconstruction algorithms are beyond the scope of this section since most surgeons have no control over these factors. In CT imaging, metal-related artifacts are typically more profound in the soft-tissue window. When instrumentation is present, soft tissues are optimally appraised by interactively changing the window width and level settings. Also, wide window settings are best for reviewing images. Materials with a lower X-ray beam attenuation coefficient, i.e., density, create less artifacts: plastic (with polyetheretherketone (PEEK) being the main plastic material, such as in carbon fiber-reinforced PEEK implants) < titanium < vitallium < stainless steel < cobalt-chrome [73].

Large differences between the magnetic properties of human tissues and metal instrumentation produce more local magnetic field inhomogeneities, which alter the phase and the frequency of local spins, and therefore increase image artifacts. Among others, the composition, the size, and the orientation of instrumentation impact the severity of artifacts. Metal-related artifacts on MRI can be minimized by using non-ferromagnetic or paramagnetic instrumentation, such as carbon fiber-reinforced PEEK and titanium, rather than ferromagnetic implants, such as those made of stainless steel, by opting for the smallest implants and construct (e.g., smaller screws and thinner plates), and by positioning the instrumentation parallel to the direction of the main magnetic field. While fast spin-echo pulse sequence is the most resistant to metal-related artifacts, gradient-recalled echo (GRE) sequence is the least. In addition, fat saturation techniques are particularly sensitive to susceptibility artifact from spinal instrumentation; thus, it is preferable to use STIR when evaluating the instrumented spine. Given that an MRI scan with lower magnetic field strength might not be available, selecting imaging parameters such as small field of view, high-resolution image matrix, thin sections, increased echo train length, and higher gradient strength for small voxel sizes may help decrease the extend of artifacts in MRI images obtained from high-field-strength magnet [73].

Furthermore, scattering effects of ionizing radiation or particles with metallic instrumentation are associated with the risk of over irradiation of neighboring structures, limiting the use of postoperative radiotherapy, as a result. Jackson et al. [76] measured radiation dose across four 3-level constructs in two spinal locations (upper and lower thoracic) in a cadaveric metastatic tumor model. They compared four groups, all of which included the same posterior instrumentation, which consisted of an anterior polyether ether ketone (PEEK) cage, an anterior titanium cage, an anterior bone cement cage (polymethyl methacrylate), and a posterior instrumentation alone group. The distribution of radiation therapy was significantly more uniform with the PEEK construct [76]. Numerous studies support the safety and efficacy of Carbon-Fiber Reinforced PEEK (CFR-PEEK) fixation systems, i.e., rods and screws, with regards to intraoperative complications, stability at weight bearing, and at functional recovery. In addition, their radiolucency and minimal dose alteration allow for more accurate treatment planning and execution, as well as for early local recurrence detection on follow-up imaging [74, 77–79].

Radiation therapy induce well-known changes in the bone marrow depending on the patient age, absorbed dose, size of the radiation field, beam energy, and fractionation, as well as interval between treatment and MRI image acquisition. Although the bone marrow shows no apparent change in the first 2 weeks following a dose of 30 Gy on T1- and T2-WI, STIR reveals an increased signal intensity generally associated with bone marrow edema [18, 80]. However, bone marrow shows an early and transient increase in contrast enhancement at 2 weeks after the initiation of radiation therapy, followed by a marked decrease at 4 weeks [81]. Fatty replacement usually starts at 3 weeks after treatment, reflected as an increasingly heterogeneous signal on T1-WI. In the chronic phase (at 6 weeks), the bone marrow may display two imaging patterns: homogeneous fatty replacement, i.e., homogeneous T1-WI hyperintensity, or a central high T1-WI area surrounded by a band-like intermediate T1 signal (sandwich vertebral body), believed to represent a central fatty core surrounded by red marrow regeneration [18, 80].

Granulation, scar tissue, or epidural fibrosis, particularly within the surgical epidural and perineural spaces, may show enhancement on MRI with contrast from up to 6 weeks to 6 months postoperatively [82], which may be difficult to distinguish from tumor recurrence or progression. Therefore, early imaging following tumor resection helps to establish a postoperative baseline for the patient, but also may maximize the ability to differentiate residual enhancing tumor from postsurgical changes. Also, STIR may ease the assessment of enhancing tissue, especially in the presence of metallic implants and impaired fat suppression [3].

Future Advances

A great deal of interest has focused on creating more efficient software programs to increase diagnostic image quality generated from less robust data sets, lower doses of ionizing radiation, and shorter imaging periods. However, the next generation of advances in imaging for the detection and staging of spinal tumors include continuing to improve existing hardware modalities and investigating new technologies.

High-Field MRI

The size and extent of the spinal cord still represents an important challenge for MR image acquisition in the spine. High magnetic field imaging of the spine is a potential solution. This technology not only improves resolution for sequences requiring rapid-acquisition, e.g., MRA, but 7T MRI offers over four times the baseline signal-to-noise (SNR) in contrast to the conventional 1.5T. Thus, small structures, such as the spinal cord, can be better imaged. Downsides associated with high field imaging include increased specific absorption rate (SAR) and, as mentioned earlier, stronger sensitivity to susceptibility distortions, as observed with metallic implants. Of note, SAR corresponds to the electromagnetic energy, expressed as watts per kilogram, delivered to tissue, which results in tissue heating during an MRI examination.

Optimized and new MRI sequences aim to improve the identification and delineation of lesions, as well as differentiate tumor histologies and grades. For instance, improvement in T2-WI may enhance the visualization of lesions, especially within the spinal cord and CSF space by reducing artifacts from patient motion and CSF pulsation. Furthermore, optimized and new MRI sequences show great promise beyond the initial detection and staging of spinal neoplasms. For instance, they may in the future better help distinguish between residual/recurrent tumor and from posttreatment changes, evaluate responses to treatment, and determine with better accuracy the proximity of key spinal cord tracts, which can be useful for surgical planning and/or prognostication [3].

Diffusion Tensor Imaging

One example of such progress is diffusion tensor imaging (DTI). Although DTI is similar to DWI in that it evaluates the level of water diffusion restriction, it also involves a directional component. It has been used to investigate white matter tracts in the CNS, where the diffusion of water molecules is restricted by myelin sheaths of axons. Therefore, diffusion is typically greater in the direction of the long axis of the white matter fibers, and rather limited in directions perpendicular to the tracts. This property called anisotropy can be both quantified and used to generate three-dimensional images illustrating white matter tracts, i.e., diffusion tensor tractography [18, 83]. In their review, Liu et al. [83] reported that fractional anisotropy may help identify and evaluate spinal cord lesions according to three main relationships between the white matter tracts and spinal cord tumors: (i) displacement of fibers, (ii) fibers crossing the tumor, and (iii) complete encasement of fibers within the tumor.

Displacement of white matter fibers is thought to characterize benign spinal cord tumors and be an indication for total resection. Intramedullary ependymoma tends to be encapsulated, forming a plane of cleavage separating the tumor from the spinal cord and displacing the white matter fibers as a result. Similarly, 75–85% of intra-medullary astrocytomas are low-grade fibrillary or pilocytic and tend to displace the tracts. Conversely, high-grade astocytomas often infiltrate adjacent to neural tissue and thus tend to encase white matter fibers [83].

Dynamic Contrast-Enhanced MRI

Dynamic contrast-enhanced MRI (DCE-MRI) is a non-invasive perfusion imaging technique that involves modeling the kinetic properties of gadolinium as it is absorbed through tissue. It can be used to examine and monitor alterations in bone marrow microcirculation that result from angiogenesis and changes in blood vessel permeability in spinal neoplasms [50]. DCE-MRI uses various measures of tumor vascularity, such as capillary permeability (k trans) and plasma volume (Vp). However, its potential diagnostic utility is debated primarily because of limited field of view and substantial institutional variability in perfusion imaging protocols [21].

Liu et al. [84] examined DTI and DCE-MRI perfusion in 12 patients with intramedullary tumors and 13 with tumor-like in the cervicomedullary junction region and cervical spinal cord. Liu et al. [84] found that neoplasms were associated with significantly lower mean fractional anisotropy values while the mean trace apparent diffusion coefficient and peak height values were significantly larger in contrast to tumor-like lesions. The AUROC curve was the highest for peak height, with a sensitivity of 90.9% and specificity of 80% using a cutoff value of 4.523 for distinguishing tumors and tumor-like lesions. The authors concluded that DTI and DCE-MRI perfusion could help differentiate between intramedullary tumors and TLL in the cervicomedullary junction region and cervical spinal cord [84].

Other potential advantages of DCR-MRI relate to determining patients who would benefit from antiangiogenic drugs, such as bevacizumab, a monoclonal antibody inhibiting vascular endothelial growth factor (VEGF), assessing disease activity, and response to therapy [50]. In fact, DCR-MRI may facilitate the discrimination between viable and necrotic tumor deposits by assessing the degree of ablation of the microvasculature [6]. The development of diverse fast acquisition sequences, including parallel imaging and trigger techniques, shows promise in improving image quality. This will ease the implementation of DTI and DCR-MRI in clinical spinal oncology. For instance, the "field-of-view" optimized and constrained undistorted singe shot (FOCUS) is a recent DWI sequence based on a two-dimensional spatially selective radiofrequency pulse, which employs a reduced field of view in the phase-encoding direction, decreasing distortion as a result [83]. Nonetheless, to date, many of the newer MRI methods, such as perfusion, diffusion, functional, or spectroscopic imaging, still require further development to overcome shortcomings before their utility in spinal oncology can be accepted. In addition, long scan times for these technologies are also an ongoing practical limitation [3, 83].

Newer PET Radiolabeled Molecules

There are several metabolic and tumor-directed PET tracers under investigation. For instance, 3-fluoro-3-deoxy-Lthymidine (^{18}F-FLT) is a marker of DNA synthesis and demonstrates higher uptake in cells with high proliferation rates. Therefore, ^{18}F-FLT may help differentiate hematologic disorders by showing high cycling activity in the bone marrow [50]. In addition, tumor-directed agents are also being used and appraised, such as radiolabeled bombesin analogs, DOTATATE, ^{18}F-FES against the gastrin-releasing peptide receptor (GRPr), somatostatin receptor, and estrogen receptor. Targeted molecular imaging shows potential in detecting, staging, and monitoring response to treatment. Current limitations to the application of this approach include inter- and intra-tumoral heterogeneity, alteration of expression of molecular targets after any treatment, along with issues related to availability and cost effectiveness [21].

Conclusion

To date, there is no gold standard imaging modality or protocol for the evaluation and staging of spinal tumors. For each patient, the choice of the optimal diagnostic and staging imaging method or technique is ensured via a multidisciplinary approach involving the surgeon, radiologist, medical oncologist, and radiation oncologist. The selection of imaging studies is based on availability, cost, type of spinal tumor, sensitivity, specificity, radiation dose, acquisition time, clinicians' experience and preferences, and the patient's general condition and her/his relative and absolute contraindications.

Advances in imaging for the identification and staging of spinal metastasis are directed toward improving hardware design as well as sequence, data acquisition, sampling, processing, and reformatting software so as to enhance sensitivity, specificity, and accuracy. This will facilitate the assessment of various parameters and biomarkers on a morphological, functional, and molecular level. Additional improvements relate to minimizing scan duration, cost, and exposure to ionizing radiation.

References

1. Sohn S, Kim J, Chung CK, Lee NR, Park E, Chang UK, et al. A nationwide epidemiological study of newly diagnosed spine metastasis in the adult Korean population. Spine J. 2016;16(8):937–45.
2. Sohn S, Kim J, Chung CK, Lee NR, Sohn MJ, Kim SH. A nation-wide epidemiological study of newly diagnosed primary spine tumor in the adult Korean population, 2009-2011. J Korean Neurosurg Soc. 2017;60(2):195–204.
3. Vertinsky AT, Krasnokutsky MV, Augustin M, Bammer R. Cutting-edge imaging of the spine. Neuroimaging Clin N Am. 2007;17(1):117–36.
4. Orguc S, Arkun R. Primary tumors of the spine. Semin Musculoskelet Radiol. 2014;18(3):280–99.
5. Azad GK, Cook GJ. Multi-technique imaging of bone metastases: spotlight on PET-CT. Clin Radiol. 2016;71(7):620–31.
6. Ellmann S, Beck M, Kuwert T, Uder M, Bauerle T. Multimodal imaging of bone metastases: from preclinical to clinical applications. J Orthop Translat. 2015;3(4):166–77.
7. Liu T, Wang S, Liu H, Meng B, Zhou F, He F, et al. Detection of vertebral metastases: a meta-analysis comparing MRI, CT, PET, BS and BS with SPECT. J Cancer Res Clin Oncol. 2017;143(3):457–65.
8. Bloomer CW, Ackerman A, Bhatia RG. Imaging for spine tumors and new applications. Top Magn Reson Imaging. 2006;17(2):69–87.
9. Edelstyn GA, Gillespie PJ, Grebbell FS. The radiological demonstration of osseous metastases. Experimental observations. Clin Radiol. 1967;18(2):158–62.
10. Bach F, Larsen BH, Rohde K, Borgesen SE, Gjerris F, Boge-Rasmussen T, et al. Metastatic spinal cord compression. Occurrence, symptoms, clinical presentations and prognosis in 398 patients with spinal cord compression. Acta Neurochir. 1990;107(1–2):37–43.
11. Wong DA, Fornasier VL, MacNab I. Spinal metastases: the obvious, the occult, and the impostors. Spine (Phila Pa 1976). 1990;15(1):1–4.
12. Heindel W, Gubitz R, Vieth V, Weckesser M, Schober O, Schafers M. The diagnostic imaging of bone metastases. Dtsch Arztebl Int. 2014;111(44):741–7.
13. Waterloo S, Ahmed LA, Center JR, Eisman JA, Morseth B, Nguyen ND, et al. Prevalence of vertebral fractures in women and men in the population-based Tromso Study. BMC Musculoskelet Disord. 2012;13:3.
14. Rougraff BT, Kneisl JS, Simon MA. Skeletal metastases of unknown origin. A prospective study of a diagnostic strategy. J Bone Joint Surg Am. 1993;75(9):1276–81.
15. Hicks RJ, Ware RE, Lau EW. PET/CT: will it change the way that we use CT in cancer imaging? Cancer Imaging. 2006;6:S52–62.
16. Rodallec MH, Feydy A, Larousserie F, Anract P, Campagna R, Babinet A, et al. Diagnostic imaging of solitary tumors of the spine: what to do and say. Radiographics. 2008;28(4):1019–41.
17. Ciftdemir M, Kaya M, Selcuk E, Yalniz E. Tumors of the spine. World J Orthop. 2016;7(2):109–16.
18. Chokshi FH, Law M, Gibbs WN. Conventional and advanced imaging of spine oncologic disease, nonoperative post-treatment effects, and unique spinal conditions. Neurosurgery. 2018;82(1):1–23.
19. Mullan J, Evans JP. Neoplastic disease of the spinal extradural space; a review of fifty cases. AMA Arch Surg. 1957;74(6):900–7.
20. Shah LM, Salzman KL. Imaging of spinal metastatic disease. Int J Surg Oncol. 2011;2011:769753.
21. Soliman M, Taunk NK, Simons RE, Osborne JR, Kim MM, Szerlip NJ, et al. Anatomic and functional imaging in the diagnosis of spine metastases and response assessment after spine radiosurgery. Neurosurg Focus. 2017;42(1):E5.
22. Mechri M, Riahi H, Sboui I, Bouaziz M, Vanhoenacker F, Ladeb M. Imaging of malignant primitive tumors of the spine. J Belg Soc Radiol. 2018;102(1):56.
23. Bilsky MH, Laufer I, Fourney DR, Groff M, Schmidt MH, Varga PP, et al. Reliability analysis of the epidural spinal cord compression scale. J Neurosurg Spine. 2010;13(3):324–8.
24. Del Vescovo R, Frauenfelder G, Giurazza F, Piccolo CL, Cazzato RL, Grasso RF, et al. Role of whole-body

diffusion-weighted MRI in detecting bone metastasis. Radiol Med. 2014;119(10):758–66.
25. Tanenbaum LN. Clinical applications of diffusion imaging in the spine. Magn Reson Imaging Clin N Am. 2013;21(2):299–320.
26. Kircher MF, Hricak H, Larson SM. Molecular imaging for personalized cancer care. Mol Oncol. 2012;6(2):182–95.
27. Matsumoto Y, Baba S, Endo M, Setsu N, Iida K, Fukushi JI, et al. Metabolic tumor volume by (18) F-FDG PET/CT can predict the clinical outcome of primary malignant spine/spinal tumors. Biomed Res Int. 2017;2017:8132676.
28. Van den Wyngaert T, Strobel K, Kampen WU, Kuwert T, van der Bruggen W, Mohan HK, et al. The EANM practice guidelines for bone scintigraphy. Eur J Nucl Med Mol Imaging. 2016;43(9):1723–38.
29. Brenner AI, Koshy J, Morey J, Lin C, DiPoce J. The bone scan. Semin Nucl Med. 2012;42(1):11–26.
30. Cook GJ, Azad GK, Goh V. Imaging bone metastases in breast cancer: staging and response assessment. J Nucl Med. 2016;57(Suppl 1):27S–33S.
31. Knoeller SM, Uhl M, Gahr N, Adler CP, Herget GW. Differential diagnosis of primary malignant bone tumors in the spine and sacrum. The radiological and clinical spectrum: minireview. Neoplasma. 2008;55(1):16–22.
32. Batouli A, Braun J, Singh K, Gholamrezanezhad A, Casagranda BU, Alavi A. Diagnosis of non-osseous spinal metastatic disease: the role of PET/CT and PET/MRI. J Neuro-Oncol. 2018;138(2):221–30.
33. Costelloe CM, Chuang HH, Chasen BA, Pan T, Fox PS, Bassett RL, et al. Bone windows for distinguishing malignant from benign primary bone tumors on FDG PET/CT. J Cancer. 2013;4(7):524–30.
34. Schulte M, Brecht-Krauss D, Heymer B, Guhlmann A, Hartwig E, Sarkar MR, et al. Grading of tumors and tumorlike lesions of bone: evaluation by FDG PET. J Nucl Med. 2000;41(10):1695–701.
35. Dimitrakopoulou-Strauss A, Strauss LG, Heichel T, Wu H, Burger C, Bernd L, et al. The role of quantitative (18)F-FDG PET studies for the differentiation of malignant and benign bone lesions. J Nucl Med. 2002;43(4):510–8.
36. Flavell RR, Naeger DM, Aparici CM, Hawkins RA, Pampaloni MH, Behr SC. Malignancies with low fluorodeoxyglucose uptake at PET/CT: pitfalls and prognostic importance: resident and fellow education feature. Radiographics. 2016;36(1):293–4.
37. Cook GJ, Houston S, Rubens R, Maisey MN, Fogelman I. Detection of bone metastases in breast cancer by 18FDG PET: differing metabolic activity in osteoblastic and osteolytic lesions. J Clin Oncol. 1998;16(10):3375–9.
38. Kircher MF, Willmann JK. Molecular body imaging: MR imaging, CT, and US. Part I. Principles. Radiology. 2012;263(3):633–43.
39. Bastawrous S, Bhargava P, Behnia F, Djang DS, Haseley DR. Newer PET application with an old tracer: role of 18F-NaF skeletal PET/CT in oncologic practice. Radiographics. 2014;34(5):1295–316.
40. Jones T, Townsend D. History and future technical innovation in positron emission tomography. J Med Imaging (Bellingham). 2017;4(1):011013.
41. Marner L, Henriksen OM, Lundemann M, Larsen VA, Law I. Clinical PET/MRI in neurooncology: opportunities and challenges from a single-institution perspective. Clin Transl Imaging. 2017;5(2):135–49.
42. Biehl KJ, Kong FM, Dehdashti F, Jin JY, Mutic S, El Naqa I, et al. 18F-FDG PET definition of gross tumor volume for radiotherapy of non-small cell lung cancer: is a single standardized uptake value threshold approach appropriate? J Nucl Med. 2006;47(11):1808–12.
43. Larson SM, Erdi Y, Akhurst T, Mazumdar M, Macapinlac HA, Finn RD, et al. Tumor treatment response based on visual and quantitative changes in global tumor glycolysis using PET-FDG imaging. The visual response score and the change in total lesion glycolysis. Clin Positron Imaging. 1999;2(3):159–71.
44. Park SH, Goo JM, Jo CH. Receiver operating characteristic (ROC) curve: practical review for radiologists. Korean J Radiol. 2004;5(1):11–8.
45. Simundic AM. Measures of diagnostic accuracy: basic definitions. EJIFCC. 2009;19(4):203–11.
46. Glas AS, Lijmer JG, Prins MH, Bonsel GJ, Bossuyt PM. The diagnostic odds ratio: a single indicator of test performance. J Clin Epidemiol. 2003;56(11):1129–35.
47. Yang L, Zhang S, Gu R, Peng C, Wu M. Imaging features of primary spinal osseous tumors and their value in clinical diagnosis. Oncol Lett. 2019;17:1089–93.
48. Franzius C, Sciuk J, Daldrup-Link HE, Jurgens H, Schober O. FDG-PET for detection of osseous metastases from malignant primary bone tumours: comparison with bone scintigraphy. Eur J Nucl Med. 2000;27(9):1305–11.
49. Moog F, Kotzerke J, Reske SN. FDG PET can replace bone scintigraphy in primary staging of malignant lymphoma. J Nucl Med. 1999;40(9):1407–13.
50. Lutje S, de Rooy JW, Croockewit S, Koedam E, Oyen WJ, Raymakers RA. Role of radiography, MRI and FDG-PET/CT in diagnosing, staging and therapeutical evaluation of patients with multiple myeloma. Ann Hematol. 2009;88(12):1161–8.
51. Uchida K, Nakajima H, Miyazaki T, Tsuchida T, Hirai T, Sugita D, et al. (18)F-FDG PET/CT for diagnosis of osteosclerotic and osteolytic vertebral metastatic lesions: comparison with bone scintigraphy. Asian Spine J. 2013;7(2):96–103.
52. Ozulker T, Kucukoz Uzun A, Ozulker F, Ozpacac T. Comparison of (18)F-FDG-PET/CT with (99m) Tc-MDP bone scintigraphy for the detection of bone metastases in cancer patients. Nucl Med Commun. 2010;31(6):597–603.
53. Chang CY, Gill CM, Joseph Simeone F, Taneja AK, Huang AJ, Torriani M, et al. Comparison of the diagnostic accuracy of 99 m-Tc-MDP bone scintigraphy and 18 F-FDG PET/CT for the detection of skeletal metastases. Acta Radiol. 2016;57(1):58–65.
54. Yang HL, Liu T, Wang XM, Xu Y, Deng SM. Diagnosis of bone metastases: a meta-analysis comparing (1)

(8)FDG PET, CT, MRI and bone scintigraphy. Eur Radiol. 2011;21(12):2604–17.
55. Beiderwellen K, Huebner M, Heusch P, Grueneisen J, Ruhlmann V, Nensa F, et al. Whole-body [(1)(8)F] FDG PET/MRI vs. PET/CT in the assessment of bone lesions in oncological patients: initial results. Eur Radiol. 2014;24(8):2023–30.
56. Schmidt GP, Schoenberg SO, Schmid R, Stahl R, Tiling R, Becker CR, et al. Screening for bone metastases: whole-body MRI using a 32-channel system versus dual-modality PET-CT. Eur Radiol. 2007;17(4):939–49.
57. Eiber M, Takei T, Souvatzoglou M, Mayerhoefer ME, Furst S, Gaertner FC, et al. Performance of whole-body integrated 18F-FDG PET/MR in comparison to PET/CT for evaluation of malignant bone lesions. J Nucl Med. 2014;55(2):191–7.
58. Wu Q, Yang R, Zhou F, Hu Y. Comparison of whole-body MRI and skeletal scintigraphy for detection of bone metastatic tumors: a meta-analysis. Surg Oncol. 2013;22(4):261–6.
59. Liu LP, Cui LB, Zhang XX, Cao J, Chang N, Tang X, et al. Diagnostic performance of diffusion-weighted magnetic resonance imaging in bone malignancy: evidence from a meta-analysis. Medicine (Baltimore). 2015;94(45):e1998.
60. Ben-Haim S, Israel O. Breast cancer: role of SPECT and PET in imaging bone metastases. Semin Nucl Med. 2009;39(6):408–15.
61. Uematsu T, Yuen S, Yukisawa S, Aramaki T, Morimoto N, Endo M, et al. Comparison of FDG PET and SPECT for detection of bone metastases in breast cancer. AJR Am J Roentgenol. 2005;184(4):1266–73.
62. Liu T, Cheng T, Xu W, Yan WL, Liu J, Yang HL. A meta-analysis of 18FDG-PET, MRI and bone scintigraphy for diagnosis of bone metastases in patients with breast cancer. Skelet Radiol. 2011;40(5):523–31.
63. Rong J, Wang S, Ding Q, Yun M, Zheng Z, Ye S. Comparison of 18 FDG PET-CT and bone scintigraphy for detection of bone metastases in breast cancer patients. A meta-analysis. Surg Oncol. 2013;22(2):86–91.
64. Shen G, Deng H, Hu S, Jia Z. Comparison of choline-PET/CT, MRI, SPECT, and bone scintigraphy in the diagnosis of bone metastases in patients with prostate cancer: a meta-analysis. Skelet Radiol. 2014;43(11):1503–13.
65. Jambor I, Kuisma A, Ramadan S, Huovinen R, Sandell M, Kajander S, et al. Prospective evaluation of planar bone scintigraphy, SPECT, SPECT/CT, 18F-NaF PET/CT and whole body 1.5T MRI, including DWI, for the detection of bone metastases in high risk breast and prostate cancer patients: SKELETA clinical trial. Acta Oncol. 2016;55(1):59–67.
66. Lee JW, Lee SM, Lee HS, Kim YH, Bae WK. Comparison of diagnostic ability between (99m) Tc-MDP bone scan and (18)F-FDG PET/CT for bone metastasis in patients with small cell lung cancer. Ann Nucl Med. 2012;26(8):627–33.
67. Qu X, Huang X, Yan W, Wu L, Dai K. A meta-analysis of (1)(8)FDG-PET-CT, (1)(8)FDG-PET, MRI and bone scintigraphy for diagnosis of bone metastases in patients with lung cancer. Eur J Radiol. 2012;81(5):1007–15.
68. Takenaka D, Ohno Y, Matsumoto K, Aoyama N, Onishi Y, Koyama H, et al. Detection of bone metastases in non-small cell lung cancer patients: comparison of whole-body diffusion-weighted imaging (DWI), whole-body MR imaging without and with DWI, whole-body FDG-PET/CT, and bone scintigraphy. J Magn Reson Imaging. 2009;30(2):298–308.
69. Gariani J, Westerland O, Natas S, Verma H, Cook G, Goh V. Comparison of whole body magnetic resonance imaging (WBMRI) to whole body computed tomography (WBCT) or (18)F-fluorodeoxyglucose positron emission tomography/CT ((18)F-FDG PET/CT) in patients with myeloma: systematic review of diagnostic performance. Crit Rev Oncol Hematol. 2018;124:66–72.
70. Antoch G, Vogt FM, Freudenberg LS, Nazaradeh F, Goehde SC, Barkhausen J, et al. Whole-body dual-modality PET/CT and whole-body MRI for tumor staging in oncology. JAMA. 2003;290(24):3199–206.
71. Heusch P, Nensa F, Schaarschmidt B, Sivanesapillai R, Beiderwellen K, Gomez B, et al. Diagnostic accuracy of whole-body PET/MRI and whole-body PET/CT for TNM staging in oncology. Eur J Nucl Med Mol Imaging. 2015;42(1):42–8.
72. Coombes RC, Dady P, Parsons C, McCready VR, Ford HT, Gazet JC, et al. Assessment of response of bone metastases to systemic treatment in patients with breast cancer. Cancer. 1983;52(4):610–4.
73. Stradiotti P, Curti A, Castellazzi G, Zerbi A. Metal-related artifacts in instrumented spine. Techniques for reducing artifacts in CT and MRI: state of the art. Eur Spine J. 2009;18(Suppl 1):102–8.
74. Ringel F, Ryang YM, Kirschke JS, Muller BS, Wilkens JJ, Brodard J, et al. Radiolucent carbon fiber-reinforced pedicle screws for treatment of spinal tumors: advantages for radiation planning and follow-up imaging. World Neurosurg. 2017;105:294–301.
75. Do TD, Sutter R, Skornitzke S, Weber MA. CT and MRI techniques for imaging around orthopedic hardware. Rofo. 2018;190(1):31–41.
76. Jackson JB 3rd, Crimaldi AJ, Peindl R, Norton HJ, Anderson WE, Patt JC. Effect of polyether ether ketone on therapeutic radiation to the spine: a pilot study. Spine (Phila Pa 1976). 2017;42(1):E1–7.
77. Tedesco G, Gasbarrini A, Bandiera S, Ghermandi R, Boriani S. Composite PEEK/carbon fiber implants can increase the effectiveness of radiotherapy in the management of spine tumors. J Spine Surg. 2017;3(3):323–9.
78. Boriani S, Tedesco G, Ming L, Ghermandi R, Amichetti M, Fossati P, et al. Carbon-fiber-reinforced PEEK fixation system in the treatment of spine tumors: a preliminary report. Eur Spine J. 2018;27(4):874–81.

79. Nevelsky A, Borzov E, Daniel S, Bar-Deroma R. Perturbation effects of the carbon fiber-PEEK screws on radiotherapy dose distribution. J Appl Clin Med Phys. 2017;18(2):62–8.
80. Ollivier L, Brisse H, Leclère J. Bone marrow imaging: follow-up after treatment in cancer patients. Cancer Imaging. 2002;2(2):90–2.
81. Otake S, Mayr NA, Ueda T, Magnotta VA, Yuh WT. Radiation-induced changes in MR signal intensity and contrast enhancement of lumbosacral vertebrae: do changes occur only inside the radiation therapy field? Radiology. 2002;222(1):179–83.
82. Ortiz AO, de Moura A, Johnson BA. Postsurgical spine: techniques, expected imaging findings, and complications. Semin Ultrasound CT MR. 2018;39(6):630–50.
83. Liu X, Tian W, Chen H, LoStracco TA, Zhang J, Li MY, et al. Advanced neuroimaging in the evaluation of spinal cord tumors and tumor mimics: diffusion tensor and perfusion-weighted imaging. Semin Ultrasound CT MR. 2017;38(2):163–75.
84. Liu X, Tian W, Kolar B, Hu R, Huang Y, Huang J, et al. Advanced MR diffusion tensor imaging and perfusion weighted imaging of intramedullary tumors and tumor like lesions in the cervicomedullary junction region and the cervical spinal cord. J Neuro-Oncol. 2014;116(3):559–66.

5 Modern Multidisciplinary Care in Spine Tumors

Brittany L. Siontis

Trends in Cancer Mortality

The American Cancer Society estimates just over 1.6 million new cancer diagnoses in 2019, compared to over 1.7 million in 2018 [1, 2]. As incidence declines, cancer-specific mortality improves. The annual decrease in cancer death rate in men and women is 1.8% and 1.4%, respectively. Importantly, the cancer death rate has dropped by 27% from 1991 to 2016 translating to over 2.6 million fewer cancer deaths than would have occurred had cancer incidence remained at its peak [1].

The improvement in cancer incidence and mortality is multifactorial. Significant efforts have been made toward early detection. One such effort was the National Lung Screening Trial (NLST), a randomized study comparing annual low-dose chest computed tomography (CT) to chest radiograph as a screening modality in high-risk individuals, which showed a significant relative risk reduction in mortality in lung cancer with early detection [3]. Reduction in tobacco use is also related to decreased cancer incidence, with the Centers for Disease Control and Prevention (CDC) report a decline in current smokers from 20.9% in 2005 to 14% in 2017, with an associated increase in even smokers who have quit [4]. Finally, advances in systemic therapy for local and metastatic disease have largely contributed to decreased cancer mortality. These include widespread use of targeted therapies such as tyrosine kinase inhibitors (TKIs) and monoclonal antibodies, and immunotherapy such as checkpoint inhibitors. It is, therefore, increasingly important to recognize these trends to allow appropriate multidisciplinary decision-making when approaching patients with advanced disease, specifically those with spine involvement which can be associated with a significant burden of cancer morbidity for these patients.

Lung adenocarcinoma is a notable example where multidisciplinary care has led to dramatic improvements in survival. Overall prognosis for lung adenocarcinoma has traditionally been poor, particularly in the metastatic setting in which the 5-year overall survival is less than 10% [5]. However, a subset of patients with advanced non-small-cell lung cancer (NSCLC) harbor activating mutations in epidermal growth factor receptor (EGFR), the receptor tyrosine kinase ROS1, or anaplastic lymphoma kinase (ALK) for which targeted therapies are now available. Recently, the third-generation EGFR-TKI osimertinib was found to be associated with a progression-free survival (PFS) of 18.9 months compared to 10.5 months with first- or second-generation TKI [6]. This benefit was also noted in patients with brain metastases, in which the median PFS of central nervous system (CNS) disease was

B. L. Siontis (✉)
Department of Medical Oncology, Mayo Clinic, Rochester, MN, USA
e-mail: Siontis.brittany@mayo.edu

K. Singh, M. Colman (eds.), *Surgical Spinal Oncology*, https://doi.org/10.1007/978-3-030-50722-0_5

15.2 months for osimertinib compared to 9.6 months with first- or second-generation TKI. Several additional studies of various TKIs including alectinib, ceritinib, and crizotinib have shown improved PFS, many of which had durable responses [7–9]. Spinal metastases remain a major source of morbidity in patients with advanced lung cancer, with over 50% of advanced lung cancer patients with bone metastases found to have spinal involvement. Novel systemic agents may allow for a more aggressive approach to spinal metastases that historically were considered futile. In fact, the presence of activating mutations in patients with spinal metastases was associated with an improved overall survival (HR 0.38, $p = 0.03$) [10]. Thus, nuances in diagnosis and treatment must be weighed when intervention is being considered.

Over the past decade, our understanding of the immune system's role in cancer has evolved, and the use of immunotherapy has contributed to improved survival in several solid tumors. In randomized studies, checkpoint inhibition with anti-PD1/PDL1 antibodies alone or in combination with cytotoxic chemotherapy have consistently shown significant improvement in overall survival in the metastatic setting compared to chemotherapy alone [11, 12]. One-year survival in metastatic melanoma has improved from approximately 25% in the pre-immunotherapy era to a 3-year OS rate of 63% with dual checkpoint blockade [13]. Checkpoint inhibitors alone or in combination with tyrosine kinase inhibitors have also significantly improved PFS and OS in metastatic renal cell carcinoma [14, 15].

Each of the diseases discussed above have a propensity to develop spine metastases, leading to significant morbidity and mortality for patients. Historically, aggressive local therapies were avoided due to the overall poor prognosis of this patient population. However, it is imperative to consider the improved survival in the era of novel systemic therapies when determining whether aggressive intervention in the setting of spinal metastases should be undertaken. A multidisciplinary approach can offer opportunities for meaningful treatment options and prognosis improvements.

Systemic Therapy for Primary Bone Tumors

Primary bone tumors involving the spine may be benign, such as giant cell tumor of bone (GCTB) or malignant, including osteosarcoma, Ewing sarcoma, chondrosarcoma, and chordoma. Management of osteosarcoma and Ewing sarcoma with multi-agent chemotherapy, possibly in combination with surgery and/or radiation therapy, remains the standard of care. Historical clinical trials, primarily in the pediatric population, have clearly demonstrated the role for surgery and/or radiation interdigitated with chemotherapy [16, 17]. Attempts to improve outcomes by intensification of chemotherapy based on percent viable tumor on resected specimen in osteosarcoma were unsuccessful resulting in little change to the treatment paradigm of these tumors [18]. While there have been few advances, the standard approach to management of these tumors continues to require close multidisciplinary collaboration.

Chondrosarcoma, the second most common primary bone tumor after osteosarcoma, most commonly occurs in the pelvis [19, 20]. Surgery has remained the mainstay of treatment because of the tumor's relative insensitivity to chemotherapy and radiation. However, given the tumor's propensity for axial locations, surgical resection can be challenging. Furthermore, the utility of surgical intervention is reduced in the metastatic setting prompting the need for development of more effective systemic treatment options. Mutations in IDH1/2 lead to hypermethylation of DNA and histones resulting in enhanced tumorigenesis [21]. Importantly, more than 50% of conventional chondrosarcomas harbor somatic mutations of IDH, making this an attractive therapeutic target [22, 23]. Ongoing clinical trials are evaluating the role of IDH inhibitors in various solid tumors including chondrosarcoma (NCT02073994, NCT02273739, and NCT02481154). Additional pathways that may serve as therapeutic targets in chondrosarcoma include the hedgehog pathway, SRC pathway, and mTOR pathway. Results of these investigations are promising and if proven efficacious may significantly alter the treatment paradigm and long-term prognosis for chondrosarcoma including opportunities for combined modality approaches.

Chordoma, a malignancy of the notochord remnants, is a primary malignancy of the axial skeleton for which en bloc resection remains standard of care [24]. However, given the location of these tumors, complete resection is often not feasible. Radiation therapy has been known to provide both a therapeutic and palliative advantage when complete surgical resection is not recommended [25–27]. Systemic therapy options for chordoma are limited, with cytotoxic chemotherapy having little efficacy [28]. A phase II study of the multi-kinase inhibitor imatinib in advanced chordoma showed a clinical benefit rate of 64% with duration of 6 months or longer [29]. Additional studies have evaluated the role of other TKIs in advanced chordoma including sunitinib and sorafenib, though these agents have never been compared head-to-head [30, 31]. A subset of chordomas exhibit EGFR mutations, and in these cases lapatinib, an oral EGFR inhibitor, has shown activity [32]. Brachyury, a transcription factor involved in notochord development, has been known to be overexpressed in chordoma [33]. There are ongoing clinical trials evaluating therapeutic strategies that exploit this overexpression, specifically drug therapy in combination with radiation (NCT03595228, NCT02383498).

Giant cell tumor of bone (GCTB) is a rare, benign but locally aggressive skeletal tumor that typically occurs after skeletal maturity in patients in their 20s and 30s [34]. In the United States, GCTB represents 15–20% of all benign bone tumors [34]. GCTB, though generally benign, does represent a spectrum of neoplasia and has unpredictable clinical behavior. Malignant transformation is rare, but in a Swedish population-based registry, malignancy accounted for up to 8% of all diagnoses of GCTB [35]. While complete surgical resection may provide the most durable local control, alternative treatment strategies may provide good disease control with functional advantages, such as joint preservation. GCTB often occurs in the appendicular skeleton, but spinal GCTB are not infrequent and pose a treatment challenge. Spinal tumors are considered to have an overall worse prognosis compared to appendicular tumors with a higher rate of local recurrence, likely due to difficulty in achieving a negative margin resection [36, 37].

Bone remodeling is modulated by production of receptor activator of nuclear factor κB ligand (RANKL) by osteoblasts. Osteoclasts are dependent on RANKL, and in its absence undergo apoptosis. GCTB have high expression of RANKL on neoplastic stromal cells resulting in activation of RANK-positive osteoclast-like giant cells [38, 39]. Denosumab, a human monoclonal antibody against RANKL, blocks interaction between the tumor stromal and osteoclast-like giant cells resulting in loss of both cell types and reversal of osteolysis. Based on its mechanism of action, denosumab was evaluated in patients with locally advanced or recurrent GCTB and shown to halt bone destruction and induce tumor regression in 20/20 patients when administered subcutaneously at a dose of 120 mg every 4 weeks [40]. An international phase II study of denosumab in GCTB is ongoing with interim analysis showing tumor response in 163/169 patients after a median follow-up of 13 months [41]. Patients enrolled in this trial have received denosumab monthly for a minimum of 6 years with some of the patients receiving drug for more than 8 years. Therefore, neoadjuvant denosumab may be used to reconstitute the bony shell and aid in complete surgical resection. Figure 5.1 shows representative MR images for a patient with a spinal/paraspinal GCTB pre-denosumab (A-C) and after 3 months of treatment (D-E). The patient subsequently underwent complete resection. For patients who are deemed inoperable, denosumab offers a reasonable treatment option for control of disease and improvement in symptoms. However, as therapy is administered monthly, treatment-related toxicities including osteonecrosis of the jaw (ONJ) and atypical bone fracture are observed in higher frequency than in patients receiving therapy for osteoporosis. It was recently reported that 6% of patients on long-term denosumab for GCTB developed ONJ while 4% developed atypical bone fracture [42]. This is compared to 1%

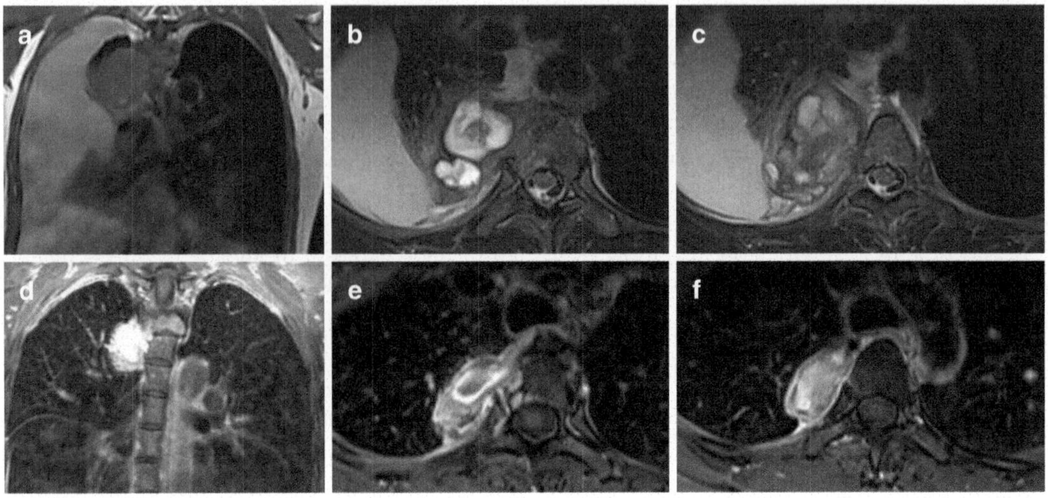

Fig. 5.1 Spinal/paraspinal GCTB before (**a**–**c**) and after (**d**–**f**) 3 months of denosumab. Coronal T1 (**a**); axial T2 (**b**, **c**); T1 gadolinium with fat saturation; coronal (**d**); and axial (**e**, **f**)

incidence in patients receiving therapy for osteoporosis. Thus, close monitoring for toxicity is important when receiving therapy long-term.

Systemic Therapy for Metastatic Disease

Bone metastases are unfortunately increasingly common, particularly in patients with advanced lung, prostate, renal, thyroid, and breast cancer. As both systemic and local treatment modalities continue to improve, the approach to patients with metastatic disease to bone is no longer limited to single modality therapy. Several approaches with combined systemic and local therapy to augment response have provided encouraging results. For example, TKI and immunotherapy have both been shown to enhance tumor response to radiotherapy. Renal cell carcinoma (RCC) is traditionally felt to be relatively radioresistant, with higher doses of radiation needed to achieve response [43]. Multiple TKIs have shown efficacy in metastatic RCC. Interestingly, a retrospective analysis in RCC patients receiving stereotactic radiosurgery for metastatic RCC to the spine noted significantly improved local control rate in patients receiving concurrent front-line TKI therapy [44]. Synergy with combination immunotherapy and radiation therapy has also been reported. Radiation can induce antigen expression, release pro-inflammatory cytokines that recruit immune cells, promote antigen cross-presentation, and induce tumor expression of death receptors [45, 46]. Therefore, combining radiation with immunotherapy may have synergistic effects and is being explored in multiple cancers including lung and others. While this may be an attractive approach to management of local disease, this treatment strategy may also apply to the metastatic setting, particularly in the situation of oligometastatic disease where resection may not be feasible. These are just a few examples that highlight how a multidisciplinary approach may greatly improve long-term outcomes for patients with advanced disease.

While treatment of existing bone metastases often provides palliation to patients, it is important to consider options for prevention of further bone metastases. Bisphosphonates such as zolendronic acid and RANKL inhibitors such as denosumab have been evaluated in this setting in multiple diseases at risk for bone involvement including multiple myeloma, breast cancer, and prostate cancer. Direct comparison of denosumab vs. zolendronic acid in patients with multiple myeloma and bone disease showed that monthly denosumab was noninferior to monthly zolendronic acid for time to first skeletal-related event (HR 0.98, 95% CI 0.85–1.14) [47]. However, in men with castration-resistant prostate cancer, denosumab was superior to zolendronic acid in prevention of skeletal-related events (HR 0.82, 95% CI 0.71–0.95, $p = 0.0002$) [48]. Denosumab was also found to be superior to bisphosphonates in breast cancer patients with bone metastases for reducing skeletal-related events (RR 0.78, 95% CI 0.72–0.85, $p < 0.00001$) [49]. Interestingly, combination of zolendronic acid with hypofractionated radiation therapy for treatment of vertebral metastases in various solid tumors was well tolerated and suggested a reduction in the rate of vertebral collapse with improved pain and adequate tumor control [50]. Together these data inform on the use of preventative agents, as well as potential for combination with radiation to improve disease control and patient symptoms.

Perioperative Drug Safety

As previously highlighted, the efficacy of systemic therapies continues to improve, resulting in improved overall survival even in advanced disease. Therefore, there is a trend toward a more aggressive approach in the management of metastatic disease including utilization of radiation, surgery, vertebral augmentation, and ablative procedures. In patients receiving novel therapies including TKI, immunotherapy, etc., it is important to consider the implications of treatment on bleeding risk and wound healing when surgical interventions are planned as these risks differ from traditional cytotoxic chemotherapy.

Agents that have antiangiogenic activity including bevacizumab or TKI with VEGF inhibition can lead to impaired wound healing and increased bleeding. Several studies have evaluated perioperative complications with the use of these agents to identify the optimal time between treatment and surgical intervention. Withholding systemic treatment in the metastatic setting has implications on overall tumor burden, thus one must be thoughtful about the risks and benefits of the duration of any periprocedural drug holding period.

Bevacizumab has a half-life of 20 days, thus the general consensus is to hold for at least 4 weeks prior to surgery. Oral TKIs with VEGF inhibition have a much shorter half-life and can be held for a shorter period of time in the perioperative setting. Studies in renal cell carcinoma suggest a 3 day washout for sorafenib, 1 week for sunitinib, and 5–7 weeks for bevacizumab [51, 52]. Another case series of TKI and surgery in RCC suggested a washout of 2 weeks [53].

While there are no widely agreed upon guidelines, Table 5.1 outlines general recommendations for holding drugs perioperatively to ensure adequate wound healing and minimize risk of bleeding complications. Of importance, each TKI has its own labeling instructions for the recommended duration for which the drug should be held before and after invasive procedures. It is imperative to discuss timing of surgery with the medical oncologist to determine when the patient should be instructed to hold the drug with attention being given to each patient's individual risk factors in the context of systemic therapy.

There is no clear consensus on the perioperative management of immunotherapy. A single-institution, retrospective analysis showed immune checkpoint inhibitors to be safe in the perioperative setting in multiple diseases and

Table 5.1 Guidelines for perioperative management of systemic therapies

Drug category	Preoperative hold	Postoperative hold
Antiangiogenic agents (pazopanib, sunitinib, bevacizumab, axitinib)	Bevacizumab[a]: 4–6 weeks Other: 1–2 weeks	Bevacizumab[a]: 4 weeks Other: 1–2 weeks
TKI without angiogenesis effect (imatinib)	No hold	Resume when tolerating oral intake
Immunotherapy	No hold	No hold
Cytotoxic chemotherapy	3–4 weeks based on individual patient count recovery	2–4 weeks based on wound healing progress and surgeon clearance

[a]Longer perioperative hold recommended for bevacizumab due to 20-day half-life

various surgical procedures [54]. In that series, the median time from last dose to surgery was 16 days (1–32 days), and the median time from surgery to first dose was 18 days (8–14 days). The wide range exhibited even within a single institution highlights the lack of consensus. As immunotherapy is being evaluated in the neoadjuvant setting, available data regarding safety of these agents in the perioperative setting allow for more informed recommendations. Of interest, immunotherapy has been proposed as a possible intervention to reduce postoperative immunosuppression and thus reduce perioperative tumor growth, supporting the safety of these agents in the perioperative period [55]. Therefore, gaps in therapy are not likely required.

It is important to understand and recognize that patients receiving immunotherapy are at risk of hypophysitis and adrenal insufficiency. The rate of these drug-related toxicities varies by agent and is reported at an incidence rate of <0.1 to 6.4% [56]. Patients may be on long-term hormone replacement including levothyroxine and hydrocortisone. If not appropriately recognized, these patients could suffer adrenal crisis in the postoperative setting.

Conclusion

As systemic therapies improve, overall survival for patients with primary or metastatic spinal tumors also continues to improve. This must be considered in development of treatment plans in the metastatic setting as combined modality approaches should be considered. A multidisciplinary approach is essential to ensure opportunities for meaningful intervention are not missed. Furthermore, close communication between the surgeon and the medical oncologist is imperative to ensure appropriate management of systemic therapies in the perioperative setting.

References

1. Siegel RL, Miller KD, Jemal A. Cancer statistics, 2019. CA Cancer J Clin. 2019;69(1):7–34.
2. Siegel RL, Miller KD, Jemal A. Cancer statistics, 2018. CA Cancer J Clin. 2018;68(1):7–30.
3. National Lung Screening Trial Research T, Aberle DR, Adams AM, Berg CD, Black WC, Clapp JD, et al. Reduced lung-cancer mortality with low-dose computed tomographic screening. N Engl J Med. 2011;365(5):395–409.
4. Wang TW, Asman K, Gentzke AS, Cullen KA, Holder-Hayes E, Reyes-Guzman C, et al. Tobacco product use among adults – United States, 2017. MMWR Morb Mortal Wkly Rep. 2018;67(44):1225–32.
5. Goldstraw P, Chansky K, Crowley J, Rami-Porta R, Asamura H, Eberhardt WE, et al. The IASLC lung cancer staging project: proposals for revision of the TNM stage groupings in the forthcoming (eighth) edition of the TNM classification for lung cancer. J Thorac Oncol. 2016;11(1):39–51.
6. Soria JC, Ohe Y, Vansteenkiste J, Reungwetwattana T, Chewaskulyong B, Lee KH, et al. Osimertinib in untreated EGFR-mutated advanced non-small-cell lung cancer. N Engl J Med. 2018;378(2):113–25.
7. Shaw AT, Ou SH, Bang YJ, Camidge DR, Solomon BJ, Salgia R, et al. Crizotinib in ROS1-rearranged non-small-cell lung cancer. N Engl J Med. 2014;371(21):1963–71.
8. Shaw AT, Kim DW, Mehra R, Tan DS, Felip E, Chow LQ, et al. Ceritinib in ALK-rearranged non-small-cell lung cancer. N Engl J Med. 2014;370(13):1189–97.
9. Peters S, Camidge DR, Shaw AT, Gadgeel S, Ahn JS, Kim DW, et al. Alectinib versus crizotinib in untreated ALK-positive non-small-cell lung cancer. N Engl J Med. 2017;377(9):829–38.
10. Choi BD, Shankar GM, Sivaganesan A, Van Beaver LA, Oh K, Shin JH. Implication of biomarker mutations for predicting survival in patients with metastatic lung cancer to the spine. Spine (Phila Pa 1976). 2018;43(21):E1274–E80.
11. Reck M, Rodriguez-Abreu D, Robinson AG, Hui R, Csoszi T, Fulop A, et al. Pembrolizumab versus chemotherapy for PD-L1-positive non-small-cell lung cancer. N Engl J Med. 2016;375(19):1823–33.
12. Gandhi L, Rodriguez-Abreu D, Gadgeel S, Esteban E, Felip E, De Angelis F, et al. Pembrolizumab plus chemotherapy in metastatic non-small-cell lung cancer. N Engl J Med. 2018;378(22):2078–92.
13. Callahan MK, Kluger H, Postow MA, Segal NH, Lesokhin A, Atkins MB, et al. Nivolumab plus ipilimumab in patients with advanced melanoma: updated survival, response, and safety data in a phase I dose-escalation study. J Clin Oncol. 2018;36(4):391–8.
14. Motzer RJ, Tannir NM, McDermott DF, Aren Frontera O, Melichar B, Choueiri TK, et al. Nivolumab plus ipilimumab versus sunitinib in advanced renal-cell carcinoma. N Engl J Med. 2018;378(14):1277–90.
15. Rini BI, Plimack ER, Stus V, Gafanov R, Hawkins R, Nosov D, et al. Pembrolizumab plus axitinib versus sunitinib for advanced renal-cell carcinoma. N Engl J Med. 2019;380(12):1116–27.
16. Souhami RL, Craft AW, Van der Eijken JW, Nooij M, Spooner D, Bramwell VH, et al. Randomised trial of two regimens of chemotherapy in operable osteosarcoma: a study of the European Osteosarcoma Intergroup. Lancet. 1997;350(9082):911–7.

17. Womer RB, West DC, Krailo MD, Dickman PS, Pawel BR, Grier HE, et al. Randomized controlled trial of interval-compressed chemotherapy for the treatment of localized Ewing sarcoma: a report from the Children's Oncology Group. J Clin Oncol. 2012;30(33):4148–54.
18. Marina NM, Smeland S, Bielack SS, Bernstein M, Jovic G, Krailo MD, et al. Comparison of MAPIE versus MAP in patients with a poor response to preoperative chemotherapy for newly diagnosed high-grade osteosarcoma (EURAMOS-1): an open-label, international, randomised controlled trial. Lancet Oncol. 2016;17(10):1396–408.
19. Samuel AM, Costa J, Lindskog DM. Genetic alterations in chondrosarcomas - keys to targeted therapies? Cell Oncol (Dordr). 2014;37(2):95–105.
20. Mavrogenis AF, Angelini A, Drago G, Merlino B, Ruggieri P. Survival analysis of patients with chondrosarcomas of the pelvis. J Surg Oncol. 2013;108(1):19–27.
21. Ward PS, Patel J, Wise DR, Abdel-Wahab O, Bennett BD, Coller HA, et al. The common feature of leukemia-associated IDH1 and IDH2 mutations is a neomorphic enzyme activity converting alpha-ketoglutarate to 2-hydroxyglutarate. Cancer Cell. 2010;17(3):225–34.
22. Meijer D, de Jong D, Pansuriya TC, van den Akker BE, Picci P, Szuhai K, et al. Genetic characterization of mesenchymal, clear cell, and dedifferentiated chondrosarcoma. Genes Chromosomes Cancer. 2012;51(10):899–909.
23. Schaap FG, French PJ, Bovee JV. Mutations in the isocitrate dehydrogenase genes IDH1 and IDH2 in tumors. Adv Anat Pathol. 2013;20(1):32–8.
24. Boriani S, Bandiera S, Biagini R, Bacchini P, Boriani L, Cappuccio M, et al. Chordoma of the mobile spine: fifty years of experience. Spine (Phila Pa 1976). 2006;31(4):493–503.
25. Chen YL, Liebsch N, Kobayashi W, Goldberg S, Kirsch D, Calkins G, et al. Definitive high-dose photon/proton radiotherapy for unresected mobile spine and sacral chordomas. Spine (Phila Pa 1976). 2013;38(15):E930–6.
26. DeLaney TF, Liebsch NJ, Pedlow FX, Adams J, Dean S, Yeap BY, et al. Phase II study of high-dose photon/proton radiotherapy in the management of spine sarcomas. Int J Radiat Oncol Biol Phys. 2009;74(3):732–9.
27. Indelicato DJ, Rotondo RL, Begosh-Mayne D, Scarborough MT, Gibbs CP, Morris CG, et al. A prospective outcomes study of proton therapy for chordomas and chondrosarcomas of the spine. Int J Radiat Oncol Biol Phys. 2016;95(1):297–303.
28. Stacchiotti S, Casali PG. Systemic therapy options for unresectable and metastatic chordomas. Curr Oncol Rep. 2011;13(4):323–30.
29. Stacchiotti S, Longhi A, Ferraresi V, Grignani G, Comandone A, Stupp R, et al. Phase II study of imatinib in advanced chordoma. J Clin Oncol. 2012;30(9):914–20.
30. George S, Merriam P, Maki RG, Van den Abbeele AD, Yap JT, Akhurst T, et al. Multicenter phase II trial of sunitinib in the treatment of nongastrointestinal stromal tumor sarcomas. J Clin Oncol. 2009;27(19):3154–60.
31. Bompas E, Le Cesne A, Tresch-Bruneel E, Lebellec L, Laurence V, Collard O, et al. Sorafenib in patients with locally advanced and metastatic chordomas: a phase II trial of the French Sarcoma Group (GSF/GETO). Ann Oncol. 2015;26(10):2168–73.
32. Stacchiotti S, Tamborini E, Lo Vullo S, Bozzi F, Messina A, Morosi C, et al. Phase II study on lapatinib in advanced EGFR-positive chordoma. Ann Oncol. 2013;24(7):1931–6.
33. Vujovic S, Henderson S, Presneau N, Odell E, Jacques TS, Tirabosco R, et al. Brachyury, a crucial regulator of notochordal development, is a novel biomarker for chordomas. J Pathol. 2006;209(2):157–65.
34. Larsson SE, Lorentzon R, Boquist L. Giant-cell tumor of bone. A demographic, clinical, and histopathological study of all cases recorded in the Swedish Cancer Registry for the years 1958 through 1968. J Bone Joint Surg Am. 1975;57(2):167–73.
35. Amelio JM, Rockberg J, Hernandez RK, Sobocki P, Stryker S, Bach BA, et al. Population-based study of giant cell tumor of bone in Sweden (1983-2011). Cancer Epidemiol. 2016;42:82–9.
36. Luksanapruksa P, Buchowski JM, Singhatanadgige W, Bumpass DB. Systematic review and meta-analysis of en bloc vertebrectomy compared with intralesional resection for giant cell tumors of the mobile spine. Global Spine J. 2016;6(8):798–803.
37. Harrop JS, Schmidt MH, Boriani S, Shaffrey CI. Aggressive "benign" primary spine neoplasms: osteoblastoma, aneurysmal bone cyst, and giant cell tumor. Spine (Phila Pa 1976). 2009;34(22 Suppl):S39–47.
38. Atkins GJ, Kostakis P, Vincent C, Farrugia AN, Houchins JP, Findlay DM, et al. RANK expression as a cell surface marker of human osteoclast precursors in peripheral blood, bone marrow, and giant cell tumors of bone. J Bone Miner Res. 2006;21(9):1339–49.
39. Roux S, Amazit L, Meduri G, Guiochon-Mantel A, Milgrom E, Mariette X. RANK (receptor activator of nuclear factor kappa B) and RANK ligand are expressed in giant cell tumors of bone. Am J Clin Pathol. 2002;117(2):210–6.
40. Branstetter DG, Nelson SD, Manivel JC, Blay JY, Chawla S, Thomas DM, et al. Denosumab induces tumor reduction and bone formation in patients with giant-cell tumor of bone. Clin Cancer Res. 2012;18(16):4415–24.
41. Chawla S, Henshaw R, Seeger L, Choy E, Blay JY, Ferrari S, et al. Safety and efficacy of denosumab for adults and skeletally mature adolescents with giant cell tumour of bone: interim analysis of an open-label, parallel-group, phase 2 study. Lancet Oncol. 2013;14(9):901–8.
42. Palmerini E, Chawla NS, Ferrari S, Sudan M, Picci P, Marchesi E, et al. Denosumab in advanced/unresect-

able giant-cell tumour of bone (GCTB): for how long? Eur J Cancer. 2017;76:118–24.
43. Balagamwala EH, Angelov L, Koyfman SA, Suh JH, Reddy CA, Djemil T, et al. Single-fraction stereotactic body radiotherapy for spinal metastases from renal cell carcinoma. J Neurosurg Spine. 2012;17(6):556–64.
44. Miller JA, Balagamwala EH, Angelov L, Suh JH, Rini B, Garcia JA, et al. Spine stereotactic radiosurgery with concurrent tyrosine kinase inhibitors for metastatic renal cell carcinoma. J Neurosurg Spine. 2016;25(6):766–74.
45. Kalbasi A, June CH, Haas N, Vapiwala N. Radiation and immunotherapy: a synergistic combination. J Clin Invest. 2013;123(7):2756–63.
46. Tang C, Wang X, Soh H, Seyedin S, Cortez MA, Krishnan S, et al. Combining radiation and immunotherapy: a new systemic therapy for solid tumors? Cancer Immunol Res. 2014;2(9):831–8.
47. Raje N, Terpos E, Willenbacher W, Shimizu K, Garcia-Sanz R, Durie B, et al. Denosumab versus zoledronic acid in bone disease treatment of newly diagnosed multiple myeloma: an international, double-blind, double-dummy, randomised, controlled, phase 3 study. Lancet Oncol. 2018;19(3):370–81.
48. Fizazi K, Carducci M, Smith M, Damiao R, Brown J, Karsh L, et al. Denosumab versus zoledronic acid for treatment of bone metastases in men with castration-resistant prostate cancer: a randomised, double-blind study. Lancet. 2011;377(9768):813–22.
49. Wong MH, Stockler MR, Pavlakis N. Bisphosphonates and other bone agents for breast cancer. Cochrane Database Syst Rev. 2012;2:CD003474.
50. Pichon B, Campion L, Delpon G, Thillays F, Carrie C, Cellier P, et al. High-dose hypofractionated radiation therapy for noncompressive vertebral metastases in combination with zoledronate: a phase 1 study. Int J Radiat Oncol Biol Phys. 2016;96(4):840–7.
51. Pooleri GK, Nair TB, Sanjeevan KV, Thomas A. Neo adjuvant treatment with targeted molecules for renal cell cancer in current clinical practise. Indian J Surg Oncol. 2012;3(2):114–9.
52. Thomas AA, Rini BI, Stephenson AJ, Garcia JA, Fergany A, Krishnamurthi V, et al. Surgical resection of renal cell carcinoma after targeted therapy. J Urol. 2009;182(3):881–6.
53. Harshman LC, Yu RJ, Allen GI, Srinivas S, Gill HS, Chung BI. Surgical outcomes and complications associated with presurgical tyrosine kinase inhibition for advanced renal cell carcinoma (RCC). Urol Oncol. 2013;31(3):379–85.
54. Elias AW, Kasi PM, Stauffer JA, Thiel DD, Colibaseanu DT, Mody K, et al. The feasibility and safety of surgery in patients receiving immune checkpoint inhibitors: a retrospective study. Front Oncol. 2017;7:121.
55. Bakos O, Lawson C, Rouleau S, Tai LH. Combining surgery and immunotherapy: turning an immunosuppressive effect into a therapeutic opportunity. J Immunother Cancer. 2018;6(1):86.
56. Barroso-Sousa R, Barry WT, Garrido-Castro AC, Hodi FS, Min L, Krop IE, et al. Incidence of endocrine dysfunction following the use of different immune checkpoint inhibitor regimens: a systematic review and meta-analysis. JAMA Oncol. 2018;4(2):173–82.

Part II

Primary Spine Tumors in the Mobile Spine

Peter Rose

Modern Care of Benign Tumors of the Spine

6

Oren Zarnett, Nathaniel E. Schaffer, Ilyas S. Aleem, Ahmad Nassr, and Raphaële Charest-Morin

Introduction

Although metastases, myeloma, and lymphoma predominate among neoplastic lesions found in the spine, benign tumors may represent a majority of the remaining ~5% that are primary tumors of the bone. In contrast with the metastatic spine population, benign tumors typically occur in the young and active population. Presentation may vary from an incidental finding to severe pain and neurologic symptoms. Of these benign lesions, the most commonly encountered are aneurysmal bone cysts (ABCs), giant-cell tumors of the bone (GCTs), osteoid osteomas (OOs), osteoblastomas (OBs), hemangiomas, osteochondromas, and Langerhans-cell histiocytosis [1, 2] (Table 6.1).

With appropriate investigation and carefully planned biopsy, the diagnosis can be made. Each histological subtype has its own characteristics. While most benign lesions share the same systemic and local staging, the management of each lesion should be tailored to its histology, anatomic constraints, clinical presentation, and patient characteristics. Similar to the primary malignant bone tumors, the management of all these benign tumors should follow the oncologic principles elaborated by Enneking [3]. Referral to a tertiary center with experience in treating these rare tumors should be sought early in the

Table 6.1 Primary benign bone tumors of the spine

Tumor type	Incidence (%) involving spine (versus appendicular skeleton)	Enneking staging
Aneurysmal bone cyst	15	S2, S3
Giant cell tumor of the bone	10	S3
Osteoid osteoma	20	S1, S2
Osteoblastoma	40	S3
Hemangioma	Most	S1
Osteochondroma	<5	S1, S2

O. Zarnett (✉)
Department of Orthopaedic Surgery, University of British Columbia, Vancouver General Hospital, Vancouver, BC, Canada
e-mail: oren.zarnett@alumni.ubc.ca

N. E. Schaffer
Department of Orthopaedic Surgery, University of Michigan, Ann Arbor, MI, USA
e-mail: naschaff@med.umich.edu

I. S. Aleem
Department of Orthopaedic Surgery, University of Michigan, Ann Arbor, MI, USA

Department of Neurosurgery, University of Michigan, Ann Arbor, MI, USA
e-mail: ialeem@med.umich.edu

A. Nassr
Department of Orthopaedic Surgery, Mayo Clinic, Rochester, MN, USA

R. Charest-Morin
Division Spine, Department of Orthopaedic Surgery, University of British Columbia, Vancouver General Hospital, Vancouver, BC, Canada
e-mail: Raphaele.charestmorin@vch.ca

K. Singh, M. Colman (eds.), *Surgical Spinal Oncology*,
https://doi.org/10.1007/978-3-030-50722-0_6

process, and multidisciplinary management is a key component when treating these tumors. This chapter will provide an overview of the investigation of a solitary spinal lesion, lay the general oncologic principles of treatment, and review the presentation, diagnosis, and alternative treatments of the most commonly encountered primary benign bone tumors of the spine.

General Principles

Evaluation

An isolated spinal lesion mandates a thorough workup, since the management of primary bone tumors differs significantly from the management of the more common metastatic spine disease. An appropriate diagnosis along with local and systemic staging is necessary before treatment of any new lesion can be considered. While some benign bony lesions have a classic appearance and the diagnosis can be made by careful review of imaging, atypical features or uncertainty about the diagnosis usually mandates a tissue diagnosis.

Biopsy planning should either be discussed with, or performed by, an oncologic spine surgeon who will perform the definitive surgery. Especially in the case of a malignant lesion, any tissue plane that is contaminated by the biopsy needs to be excised. It has been demonstrated that biopsy for malignant bone lesions in the spine performed outside of a referral center was associated with increased local recurrence [4, 5]. Careful planning ensures that no structures are excised unnecessarily. In the event of a benign tumor, the biopsy tract is not usually excised, but with an unknown lesion, it should be assumed that the lesion is malignant until proven otherwise, and hence, the general biopsy principles should be applied.

Clinical Studies

Upright radiographs are useful both to characterize the lesion and to determine if there is any secondary instability. Some benign latent lesions may present as "red herrings" and not as the source of the patient's symptoms. Radiographs can help diagnose other common causes of pain. The AP and lateral radiographs should be done in an upright posture as this gives information about potential instability (vertebral body collapse, kyphosis, translation, etc.).

Most lesions, however, will require additional imaging such as a computed tomography (CT) or magnetic resonance imaging (MRI) for both diagnostic and surgical planning purposes. CT is the most accurate method for evaluating the bony anatomy and particular characteristics of the tumor (cortical destruction, calcification, etc.). It delineates the extent of osseous involvement and is the diagnostic study for some bone-based lesions such as osteoid osteoma. Furthermore, it can provide useful information regarding potential instability and allows proper planning for the biopsy. However, in general, CT is not as sensitive as MRI in the early detection of metastatic disease and primary malignant bone tumors.

MRI is the best imaging modality for the evaluation of the epidural space and neural structures. T1-weighted images are helpful for delineating bone marrow architecture, fat content within masses, and subacute hemorrhage. The administration of gadolinium-based contrast material results in enhancement proportional to soft tissue vascularity and is helpful for differentiating cystic lesions from cyst-like solid masses. Most pathologic processes are often highlighted on T2-weighted images due to their increased fluid content.

Nuclear medicine studies (technetium 99 m, SPECT, PET) are sensitive to areas with increased radionuclide uptake. This is observed where there is an increased osteoid reaction to destructive processes in bones. However, these scans (with the exception of SPECT) are limited in their capacity to depict a detailed surgical anatomy when compared with CT or MRI. A bone scan can be used as a screening tool to determine whether a lesion is solitary or multifocal.

Some lesions have classical location. Osteoid osteoma, osteoblastoma, osteochondroma, and ABC are commonly encountered in the posterior elements, whereas GCT, Langerhans-cell histiocytosis, and hemangioma more often affect the vertebral body.

Lastly, as with any new lesion, workup consists of local and systemic staging. Systemic staging is completed with a chest CT scan. While most benign tumors do not require any systemic staging, the more aggressive lesions (giant cell-tumor, osteoblastoma) can present with pulmonary metastasis that should be assessed for at the time of initial presentation.

Staging

The Enneking classification is the most commonly employed staging system for primary bone tumors. Enneking classified primary bone tumors into five categories along a spectrum from a benign latent lesion to an aggressive metastatic sarcoma [3]. Along this spectrum, benign lesions are broken into three categories: latent, active, and aggressive (Table 6.2). The basis of the classification system was to describe the biology of the lesion in order to guide treatment.

Benign latent lesions (S1) are often asymptomatic. They are fully encapsulated, intracompartmental lesions that adhere to fixed boundaries. They have slow growth initially that ultimately plateaus. From a histologic level, they have mature well-differentiated cells. There is a low cell-matrix ratio and there are no surrounding inflammatory changes. A quiescent hemangioma would be an example of a latent lesion.

Benign active lesions (S2) are slow-growing lesions that may cause pain. As the lesion grows, it can cause eccentric remodeling of the nearby cortex without perforating through it. Compared to benign lesions, there are more cells relative to the matrix, but the cells are still well differentiated. There is a small zone of inflammatory cells between the capsule and normal bone. An osteoid osteoma is an example of an active lesion.

Table 6.2 Characteristics of benign lesions classified by the Enneking classification

	Latent (S1)	Active (S2)	Aggressive (3)
Growth	–	+	++
Cell to matrix ratio	+	++	+++
Reactive zone	–	+	++
Adheres to anatomic boundaries	√	√	–

Benign aggressive benign lesions (S3) are often painful, with their growth not limited to cortical boundaries. They sometimes present with an associated soft tissue mass. There is a reactive zone surrounding the lesion and tumor cells may extend beyond the pseudocapsule that surrounds the tumor. The cells are well differentiated with a benign appearance, but the occasional mitotic figure may be present. Giant cell tumor of bone is typically an aggressive lesion.

The Weinstein-Boriani-Biagini (WBB) classification describes a lesion according to its anatomic location as it relates to the spine [6]. On axial presentation, the WBB divides the vertebra into 12 zones. Zone 1 represents the left half of the spinous process followed by the others in a counter-clock-wise manner. Last, a lesion is further classified according to its layer: extraosseus, intraosseus superficial, intraosseus deep, extraosseus extradural, or intradural. The goal of this classification is to describe lesions and to help guide treatment according to the local anatomy.

Understanding the biological behavior of a lesion and its proximity to local critical structures is a prerequisite for formulating a treatment plan. These tumors are best treated in centers with experience in treating these complex and rare lesions. The treatment of an aggressive primary benign bone lesion, either surgical or with alternative treatment options, should be discussed in a multidisciplinary panel as its treatment needs to be individualized.

Principles of Surgical Treatment

The general indications to operate for benign tumors of the spine are mechanical instability, uncontrolled pain, neurologic deficit, and to achieve local control/cure [7, 8]. Depending on the many variables, surgery may entail either an en bloc resection or an intralesional resection. An en bloc resection refers to the removal of the tumor as a single piece. To be complete, the description of an en bloc resection should be accompanied by its margins. A wide margin is defined when there is a healthy cuff of tissue surrounding the tumor. A marginal margin is when the resection is in the reactive layer surrounding the tumors. A margin is intralesional when the tumor has been breached during the surgery or when tumor cells are observed at the periphery of the tumor specimen. In contradistinction, an intralesional curettage can be planned and refers to the resection of the tumor in a piecemeal fashion. The tumor capsule is voluntarily opened, and the tumor is resected. The intralesional resection or curettage can be defined as a gross total if the resection was complete.

The Enneking staging system can provide a rough guide for the margins required when resecting benign tumors of the spine. S1 tumors generally do not require surgical intervention [9]. For S2 tumors, the recurrence rate may be acceptable with intralesional excision [10, 9]. In contrast, intralesional resection of stage 3 tumors is frequently associated with an unacceptable rate of recurrence, and en bloc resection may be preferred [11, 9].

The Enneking principles are widely applied in the treatment of appendicular primary bone tumors, but due to the anatomical complexities of the spine, its application traditionally has been limited. However, with technological advances and a better understanding of the behavior of these tumors, the oncologic principles behind the Enneking staging have gained acceptance in the spinal community. An aggressive bony lesion that extends beyond the cortex (extracompartmental) has drastically different implications for resection if it extends into the spinal canal, anteriorly compromising the vena cava or aorta, or posteriorly into the paraspinal musculature. Wide en bloc resection may be a good option for the latter, but not feasible if it requires sacrificing the spinal cord or major vessels in order to achieve negative margins, especially of the benign nature. In some cases, the morbidity of an en bloc resection may be deemed worse than the recurrence risk of intralesional resection. Hence, a gross total resection might be preferred in some situations.

The location and morphology of the tumor will also dictate surgical planning, and the Weinstein-Boriani-Biagini (WBB) surgical staging system provides a framework with which to make these decisions. As a general principle, an en bloc resection is feasible if enough bone in the posterior ring (formed by the lamina and pedicles) is free of disease to allow clearance of the thecal sac during resection.

Management by Histology

Presentation and treatment are summarized in Table 6.3.

Giant Cell Tumor (GCT)

Introduction

Giant cell tumor of bone is a primary bone tumor that accounts for approximately 5% of all primary bony tumors [12, 13, 14]. It most commonly presents in the second through fourth decade of life. While it is a benign lesion, there is a 2–7.5% rate of pulmonary metastasis that needs consideration during the initial workup [15, 16, 17, 18]. In the appendicular skeleton, it has a predilection for the metaepiphyseal area of long bones; however, approximately 10% of GCTs are found in the spine and sacrum. Spinal GCTs are highly vascular and have a predilection for the thoracic and lumbar spine [19].

There are three main cell types on microscopic examination: giant cells, monocytes, and mononuclear stromal cells [20]. The stromal cells, thought to be of osteoblastic origin, are considered to be the neoplastic cell in GCTs. The H3F3A mutation is found in 92% GCT stromal cells and can be a tool for histopathological diagnosis [20, 21].

Giant cell tumors are primary bone tumors that typically appear as expansile osteolytic lesions [19]. Their appearance is created from thickening of existing trabeculae and cortex in response to the tumor. In keeping with Enneking

Table 6.3 Primary benign spinal lesions

Diagnosis	Age	Presentation	Management/Treatment
Aggressive hemangioma	Any age-increased incidence with age	Mostly asymptomatic, pain and myelopathy are possible	For asymptomatic lesion, no treatment For symptomatic lesion, vertebroplasty/ kypholasty/ embolization/surgery
Osteoid osteoma	Second and third decades	Pain relieved by NSAID Scoliosis Male > female	If pain not controlled, thermal ablation or intralesional resection depending on location
Osteoblastoma	Second and third decade	Dull, localized pain Male > female	Surgical en bloc resection if feasible with acceptable morbidity or intralesional surgery
Osteochondroma	Third decade	Variable Asymptomatic to nerve compression Hereditary multiple exostosis: patients presenting with multiple osteochondromas	Surgical resection if symptomatic
Aneurysmal bone cyst	Second decade	Slow gradual onset of pain. Female > male	Surgical resection with en bloc resection if feasible with acceptable morbidity or intralesional surgery. Alternative with serial embolization has been successful in case series
Giant cell tumor	Second to fourth decades	Insidious pain Female > male	Surgical resection with en bloc resection if feasible with acceptable morbidity. Intralesional surgery is an alternative but increased local recurrence. Denosumab is an option for inoperable tumor and as an neoadjuvant

S2 or S3 lesions, GCTs can form a thin neocortex, or no cortex at all, with an accompanying soft tissue mass. While not pathognomonic, one feature of GCTs is that there can be an eccentric sclerotic margin opposite the side where the lesion is growing. When giant cell tumors are present in the vertebral body, there can be an associated pathological fracture causing vertebral body collapse and sometimes vertebra plana. The differential diagnosis of a GCT includes telangiectatic osteosarcoma, chordoma, brown tumor, and aneurysmal bone cyst.

Treatment

Surgery

Recently, the role of medical treatment has emerged as a treatment option for unresectable GCTs. However, surgery remains the mainstay of treatment for GCTs when an appropriate surgical resection can be performed. Surgical options include intralesional or *en bloc* resection [22]. Mechanical (e.g., PMMA), chemical (e.g., phenol), and thermal (e.g., liquid nitrogen) adjuvants are commonly employed to reduce recurrence rates following intralesional curettage. The application of these adjuncts in the spine is limited due to the vicinity of the neural structures and the risk of iatrogenic injury. While intralesional resection is a commonly employed technique in the appendicular skeleton, it should be used with caution in the spine due to the high recurrence rate. Local recurrence is particularly difficult to manage in the spine due to the complex anatomy.

In a series of 49 patients, Boriani et al. [23] reported a 9% recurrence rate when S3 lesions were treated with *en bloc* resection, and a 62% recurrence rate when treated with intralesional excision. They also reported a 6.3% recurrence rate when S2 lesions were treated with intralesional excision. Differentiating S2 and S3 lesions can be challenging, but typically, S3 lesions are more aggressive, expansile, and have a soft tissue component (see Table 6.2). In a different large international retrospective study with 82 patients, intralesional resection was associated with an increased local recurrence rate when compared to *en bloc* resection [24]. Furthermore, mortality correlated with local recurrence. In 2009, the spine oncology study group (SOSG) recommended that when feasible, an *en bloc* resection should be considered for the treatment of spinal GCT [25]. However, consideration must be given to the anticipated morbidity of an *en bloc* resection in the setting of a benign but aggressive disease.

After surgical resection, the National Comprehensive Cancer Network has recommended the following for surveillance: local and chest surveillance every 6 months for the first 2 years and then yearly thereafter.

Medical Therapy

The hallmark of GCTs is the multinucleated giant cells that express high levels of the receptor of the activator nuclear factor kappa-B ligand (RANKL). Activation of this pathway leads to osteolysis. Denosumab is a monoclonal antibody that specifically inhibits RANKL and it was hypothesized that this medication could halt progression in inoperable GCTs. The first clinical trial funded by AMGEN (the pharmaceutical company producing denosumab) found a clinical response rate of 85% at 6 months [26]. Furthermore, on histopathological reports, over 90% of the multinucleated giant cells had disappeared with this treatment [27]. The second clinical trial with 282 patients reported 75% of clinical response rate, mostly a partial one [28]. These studies led to FDA approval in 2013 for inoperable GCTs (Fig. 6.1). However, when used as the definitive treatment, it may require lifelong therapy. In spine surgery, in addition to its role in unresectable GCTs, it has been used as a neoadjuvant to reduce and calcify the tumor prior to surgery. Further, neoadjuvant therapy has also been shown to reduce intraoperative blood loss [29]. In 2016, the AOSpine Knowledge Forum Tumor (AOSKFT) recommended denosumab either as a stand-alone for treatment of inoperable GCT or as an adjuvant prior to surgical resection [30]. Recommended preoperative duration was 6 months or until maximal tumor reduction/calcification has been observed. While this is a promising medication, there is uncertainty about long-term treatment and its potential adverse events such as osteonecrosis of the jaws and atypical femoral shaft fracture [31]. Furthermore, there is concern for tumor recurrence after denosumab discontinuation. This is supported by the fact that the stromal cells, the neoplastic cells in GCTs, are not eliminated with denosumab. In the axial skeleton, its use has been tempered by increased recurrence rates and the concern from some case reports of malignant transformation following its administration [32, 33, 34, 35]. As with any new treatment, caution is warranted. However, despite its risks and drawbacks, denosumab does have a role in unresectable tumors or for use as a neoadjuvant.

Selective Arterial Embolization

Due to the hypervascular nature of these lesions, preoperative embolization is commonly employed to limit blood loss during intralesional excision and facilitate dissection of segmental arteries during *en bloc* resection of mobile spine GCTs [30, 36, 37, 38]. While surgical management is the first line treatment for giant cell tumors, selective arterial embolization has been employed with some success in some recurrent and unresectable lesions. Serial embolizations are carried out until there is no collateral blood flow to the lesion. Small case series have shown reossification with a low neurologic complication rate [39, 40, 41, 42, 43, 44].

Radiation

Nearly all GCTs are radiosensitive; however, in the past, the use of radiotherapy has been tempered by the risk of secondary malignant transformation [45, 46, 47]. Different sources report the risk of secondary transformation between 11 and 27%; however, the use of megavoltage machines compared to orthovoltage machines has dramatically decreased this risk. Regardless,

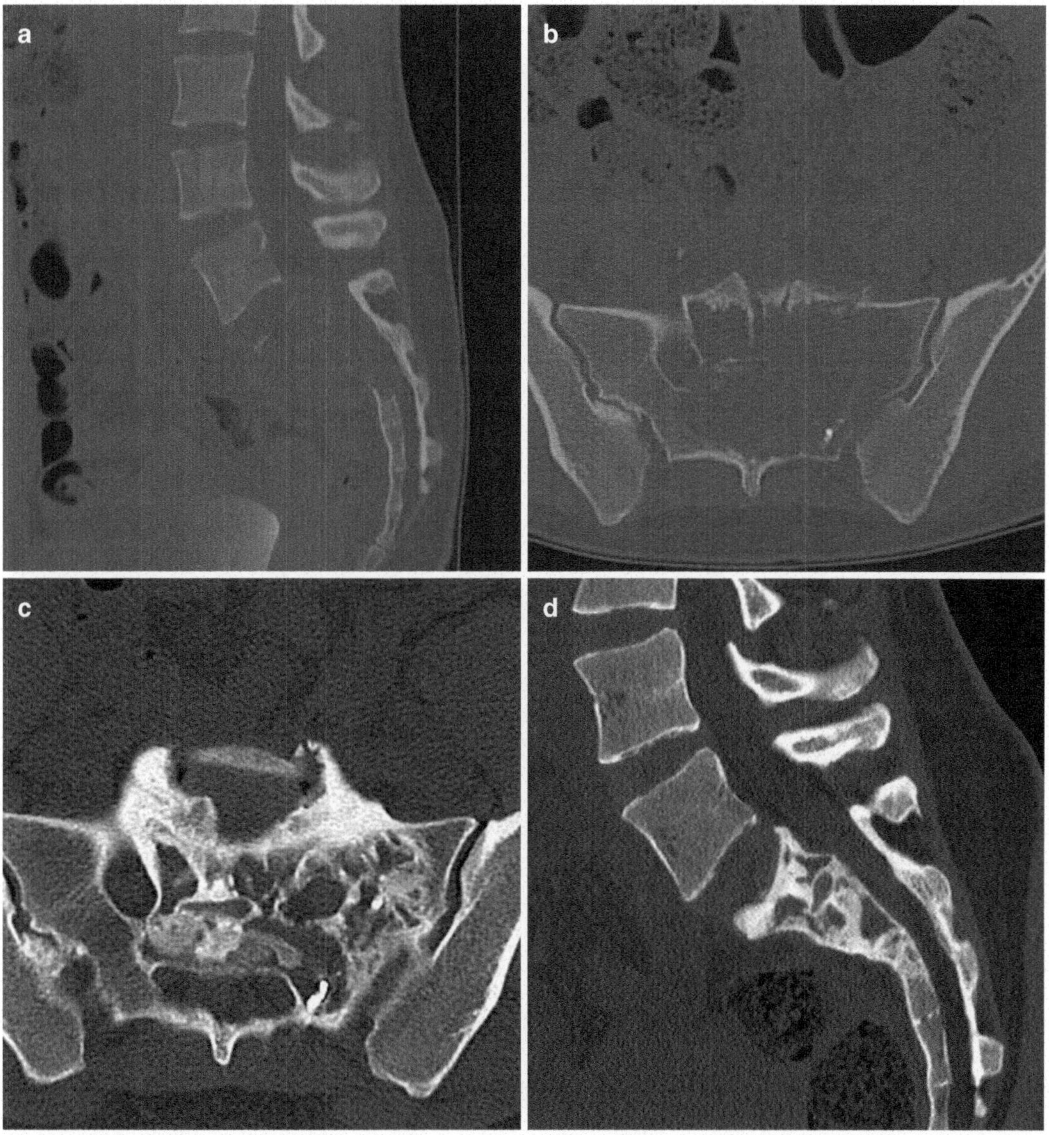

Fig. 6.1 Giant cell tumor involving the sacrum. (**a**, **b**) Pre-denosumab on axial and sagittal CT scan. (**c**, **d**) After 1 year on denosumab on axial and sagittal CT scan

radiation does have a role in metastatic and non-operable GCTs of the spine.

Aneurismal Bone Cyst

Introduction

An aneurysmal bone cyst (ABC) is a benign bone tumor that most commonly presents in the second decade of life [48]. It appears as a lytic, expansile lesion with a predilection for the posterior elements of the spine. It comprises 1.4% of all bone tumors and 15% of primary tumors of the spine. Aneurysmal bone cysts contain a blood-filled sac with an endothelial lining that can be a primary tumor, or secondary to another benign or malignant lesion.

Approximately 75% of aneurysmal bone cysts have a balanced translocation involving the proto-oncogene, *USP6*, found on chromosome 17p13 [20, 49]. The discovery of this genetic alteration has become an important tool for pathologists to diagnose an ABC. The absence of the mutation mandates consideration of an alternate diagnosis or that the ABC may be secondary to another lesion.

Aneurysmal bone cysts can present as active or aggressive lesions according to the Enneking classification. They usually appear as lytic, expansile masses. Further characterization of the lesion with MRI reveals fluid-fluid levels from hemosiderin settling when the patient lies supine for the scan. The differential diagnosis for an ABC includes secondary ABC and telangiectatic osteosarcoma. Care needs to be taken to exclude the latter for any monostotic lytic lesion.

Treatment

Aneurysmal bone cysts are frequently locally aggressive and require treatment both for pain control, stability, and to protect adjacent neural structures.

Surgery

Surgery is considered the mainstay of treatment of ABCs. Intralesional resection is associated with a 25% recurrence rate in the spine due to incomplete resection [50]. While this may be acceptable in the appendicular skeleton, given the risk of local recurrence and potential involvement of neural elements, a more aggressive approach is sometimes warranted. *En bloc* resection and gross total resection have been employed successfully with no recurrences in several large case series [25]. En *bloc* resection, however, may be associated with significant morbidity depending on tumor location and dimension. In 2009, the SOSG recommended an aggressive gross total resection for an ABC. While recurrence is attributable to the completeness of the resection, the growth and anatomic location of the ABC should factor into the surgical approach. When an incomplete resection is performed, adjuvant therapies similar to those employed with GCTs can be considered.

Embolization

Preoperative embolization of hypervascular lesions is routinely employed to reduce intraoperative blood loss and to aid in the dissection of segmental arteries [30]. Prior to embolization, it is important to understand the local vascular anatomy, especially the location of the key feeders of the anterior spinal artery to prevent iatrogenic cord injury.

Recent literature supports the use of selective arterial embolization (SAE) as a stand-alone treatment for ABCs [51, 48, 52]. When SAE is chosen as the definitive treatment, multiple episodes of SAE are anticipated. Embolization has been shown to result in reossification of the lesion and resolution of pain in both the sacrum and mobile spine. Further, patients with nerve root weakness improved following SAE. Several studies have shown SAE to be safe, but contain conflicting reports on its efficacy [53, 54].

In one retrospective study, Terzi et al. showed that SAE was safe but 26% of patients crossed over into another treatment group because of local recurrence/tumor progression [54]. Amendola et al. reported successful outcomes with SAE. However, some patients required up to seven embolization procedures [53]. Especially important in the pediatric population is the cumulative radiation exposure required for angiographic imaging during the procedure, which may be a negative consideration for SAE. Other contraindications include situations where a feeding vessel also branches to the cord or anastomoses with the vertebral artery.

Intralesional Injection

Intralesional injection of doxycycline has been utilized in the armamentarium of treatment options for ABCs [55, 56]. It has been shown to inhibit MMPs, osteoclasts, and induce osteoclast apoptosis. Initial studies restricted its use to non-operable or recurrent cases, but recent studies have expanded its use as a stand-alone treatment for patients with minor or no neurological deficits and with a low spinal instability score (SINS <12) [55]. Following injection, lesions have been shown to reossify with a significant improvement in patients' pain visual analogue scale (VAS) scores. This still represents an emerging treatment and should not be considered as a first-line therapy.

There have been several reports of injection of concentrated bone marrow aspirate in an attempt to induce healing of the lesion with mesenchymal stem cells. There have been several positive results, but this is not yet routine or standard of care [57].

Radiation

Radiation therapy can be effective for treating ABCs, but with the advent of SAE, it is being used less often [58]. It has been used as adjuvant therapy in cases of subtotal resection, but concerns over radiation-induced myelitis and secondary sarcomas have largely impeded its use in most centers. Newer and more accurate radiation techniques have decreased these risks, but a paucity of long-term data combined with good alternatives has limited radiation use to the adjuvant setting in only the most difficult cases [59].

Medical Treatment

Given the surgical challenge of aneurysmal bone cysts, there has been a drive to develop medical management for treatment of these lesions. Given the similar radiographic appearance of ABCs and GCTs, along with the presence of multinucleated giant cells in ABCs, it has been hypothesized that ABCs might have a similar response to that seen for giant cell tumors treated with denosumab [60]. Further, it has been shown that ABCs express RANKL, the target of denosumab, similar to GCTs [61]. There have been various case reports of aneurysmal bone cysts treated with denosumab; however, at present, this use is still off-label for the treatment of ABCs and cannot be recommended for routine use [62].

Osteoid Osteoma/Osteoblastoma

Introduction

Both osteoid osteomas and osteoblastomas are benign osteoid-producing primary bone tumors. Twenty and forty percent of osteoid osteomas and osteoblastomas, respectively, are located in the spine [63, 14]. They occur more frequently in males, and they have a predilection for involving the posterior spinal elements [64]. Osteoid osteomas are small self-limiting entities, while osteoblastomas are more locally aggressive. Given their larger size, osteoblastomas may involve both the vertebral bone and neural elements.

Osteoid osteomas are defined as having a central nidus of less than 15–20 mm in size and typically occur in the second and third decades of life [14]. They often present with night pain that is alleviated by salicylates. The natural history of osteoid osteomas is usually self-limiting. When treated with nonsteroidal anti-inflammatories (NSAIDs), pain lasts for an average of 2.5 years before the lesion burns itself out [65, 66]. In the pediatric population, osteoid osteomas are a common cause of painful scoliosis whose etiology is thought to be secondary to muscle spasm from the lesion on the side of the curve's concavity [67].

In contrast to osteoid osteomas, ostoblastomas are more aggressive and not self-limiting. They can be locally aggressive and cause destructive changes to the surrounding bone and soft tissue [63]. The central nidus is greater than 20 mm, and 10% of patients have a secondary aneurysmal bone cyst. Osteoblastomas are painful and do not respond to NSAIDs as readily as osteoid osteomas [68]. In addition to pain, they can present with neurologic symptoms from compression of nerve roots or adjacent spinal cord. These lesions are benign, but there have been case reports of malignant transformation [64].

Demonstration of a central nidus can be diagnostic if visible on radiographs or CT scan. Further, scintigraphy can show radioactive uptake at the lesion. MRI is helpful for osteoblastomas to help delineate compression and involvement of adjacent neural structures.

Osteoid osteomas contain a central nidus of woven bone with a surrounding fibrovascular stroma. Size is the main differentiating feature between osteoid osteomas and osteoblastomas, as they look similar on histologic examination. While osteoid osteomas and osteoblastomas have different clinical presentations, they share similar structural genetic alterations in the AP-1 transcription factor *FOS* or *FOSB* [20, 69]. Differential diagnosis includes infection, aneurysmal bone cyst, fibrous dysplasia, chondrosarcoma, Ewing sarcoma, and osteosarcoma.

Treatment

Osteoid osteomas typically respond to NSAIDs and this treatment may be used to control pain symptoms. Failure of nonsurgical management due to intractable pain necessitates procedural or surgical treatment. In the pediatric population, the scoliosis associated with osteoid osteomas typically resolves after treatment of the tumor. Nonsurgical management of osteoblastomas is rarely indicated due to their locally aggressive nature.

Surgery

Failure of nonsurgical treatment of osteoid osteomas necessitates further intervention. Following surgery, many studies demonstrate resolution of pain and resolution of scoliosis curve progression. Surgical options include intralesional versus *en bloc* resection. The most important surgical factor is ensuring excision of the nidus [70]. Quraishi et al. showed in a large series that intralesional piecemeal resection resulted in a 7% recurrence rate and that there were no recurrences in their hands with *en bloc* resection. Newer technologies such as intraoperative O-arm and navigation can help ensure the nidus is resected, which can otherwise be a challenge intraoperatively [71, 72, 73] (Fig. 6.2).

Osteoblastomas almost always warrant surgical intervention. Consideration of intralesional excision can be made for S2 lesions; however, *en bloc* resection is the accepted treatment for most S3 tumors to prevent recurrence and on-going compromise of adjacent structures. In a case series of 51 osteoblastomas, all recurrences occurred in S3 lesions (either treated with intralesional or *en bloc* resection), and no recurrences occurred following intralesional resection of S2 lesions [74]. As only 10 S2 lesions were included, it is difficult to draw definitive conclusions based on this study. However, where *en bloc* resection is not possible due to anatomic constraints, a gross total resection can be considered weighing the risk of recurrence rate.

Thermal Ablation

With the morbidity of surgery, and the potential need for spinal instrumentation, both laser and radiofrequency thermal ablation have gained traction in the treatment of osteoid osteomas [75, 30, 76]. Thermal ablation is considered the gold standard in the appendicular skeleton with the local recurrence rate <5%. Percutaneous thermal ablation has been shown to be as effective in reducing pain associated with these lesions [77]. With radiofrequency ablation, a temperature of 90 °C is usually applied for approximately 6 minutes to achieve a satisfactory ablation of the nidus [78, 79]. Thermal necrosis to adjacent structures remains a risk, and it is generally contraindicated when the lesion is within 5 mm of a neural element or if the cortex is absent. Thermal ablation is generally only indicated for small lesions (osteoid osteomas) and not appropriate for osteoblastomas due to their size and aggressive biology. Similar to thermal ablation, cryoablation can be used to treat these lesions. It has the advantage that the edge of the ice ball can be seen on a CT scan, which may be safer to use around neural elements.

Aggressive Hemangiomas

Introduction

Vertebral hemangiomas are common benign vascular tumors that are found in 11% of people at the time of autopsy [80, 81, 14]. The prevalence is likely higher, as one study using CT scans found that they are present in 26% of the population [82]. Hemangiomas are more common in older individuals with a predisposition for females more than males [80]. While most are asymptomatic and do not need any treatment, in about 1% of cases they can be more aggressive, causing pain and occasionally neurologic symptoms from pathological fracture and extraverte-

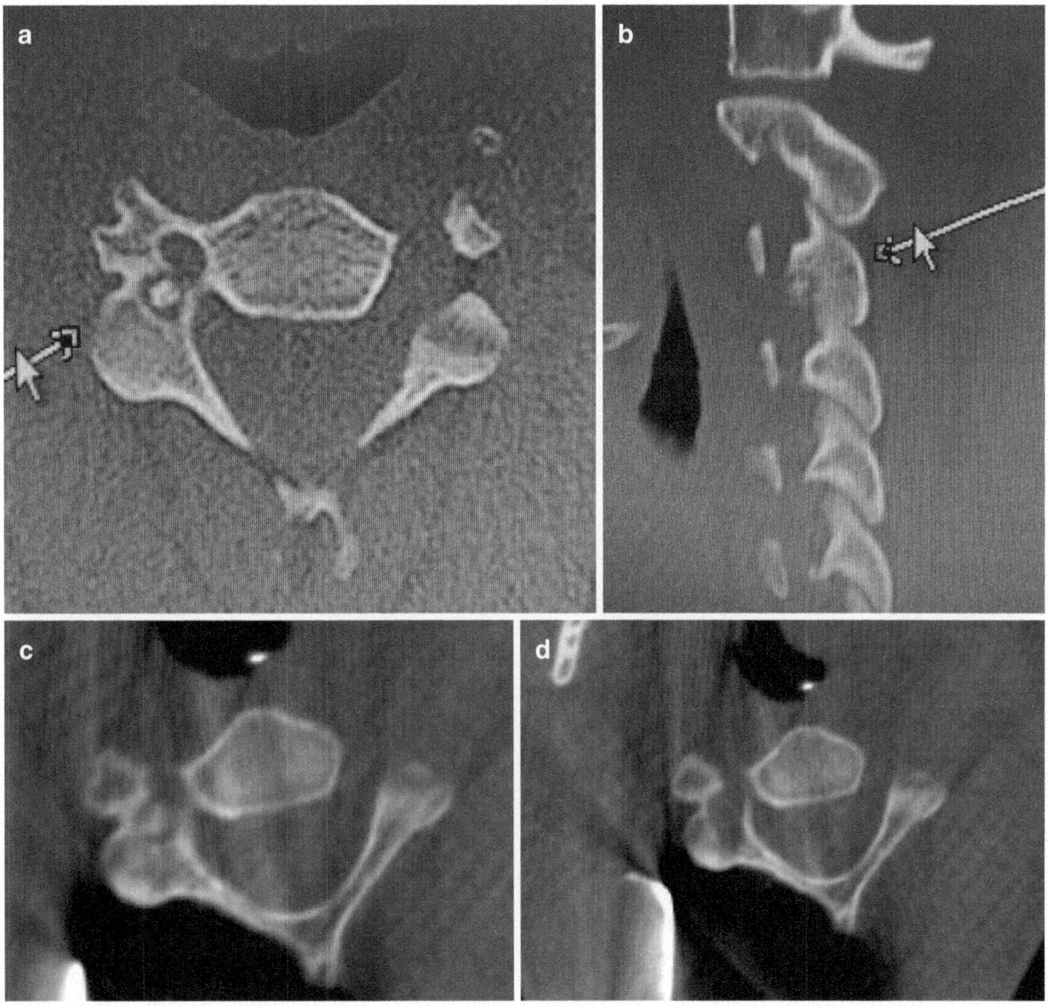

Fig. 6.2 (**a**, **b**) Osteoid osteoma of C3 with close vicinity to the vertebral artery on a sagittal and axial CT scan. (**c**, **d**) Location precluded thermal ablation. Intraoperative operative CT scan images showing axial imaging pre- and post-nidus resection

bral extension compressing nerve roots or the spinal cord.

The main histologic subtypes of vertebral hemangiomas are cavernous, capillary, and mixed. They invade the medullary canal of the vertebral body, giving rise to vertically oriented trabecuale. This gives the “jail cell” and “polka dot” appearance on sagittal/coronal and axial CT slices, respectively. On MRI, vertebral hemangiomas have a high signal intensity on both T1- and T2-weighted images [83]. However, more aggressive lesions have a paucity of adipose tissue and, therefore, may have a less intense T1-weighted signal compared to their more benign counterparts. Fat-suppressed images and STIR sequences have shown some utility in helping to identify more aggressive asymptomatic lesions.

Treatment

Aggressive hemangiomas causing intractable pain and/or cord compression warrant treatment. Various modalities have been reported with success, and at present, there is no gold standard. Treatment modalities include surgery (intralesional versus *en bloc* resection), ethanol ablation, vertebroplasty, radiation, or a combination of the above.

Surgery

Surgery has a role for symptomatic lesions, especially those presenting with neurologic deficits. Preoperative embolization has been shown to reduce intraoperative blood loss and is commonly employed across most centers [84]. There is a wide range of approaches to the surgical management of aggressive vertebral hemangiomas. General principles to consider are compressive neurology requiring decompression, debulking, or excising the tumor to prevent progression to structures in close proximity, and treating any associated instability or fracture with instrumentation. When the lesion warrants surgical attention, both intralesional and *en bloc* resection are options. While some centers advocate for *en* bloc resection, intralesional resection can have very low recurrence rates. In the largest case series of aggressive hemangiomas, there was only a 3% recurrence rate when intralesional resection was employed [85]. Depending on the location of the lesion, the low recurrence rate may justify a less morbid procedure. While there are a wide variety of options to treat aggressive vertebral hemangiomas, the approach needs to be individualized to the lesion and the local anatomy.

Ethanol Injection

Ethanol is commonly used either as an intraoperative adjunct or as an injection by interventional radiology [86, 87]. Ethanol is toxic to the endothelium, causing necrosis. It is a safe procedure; however, since hemangiomas are post-capillary structures, there is a theoretical risk of retrograde flow into segmental arteries with local or systemic toxicity. Doppman et al. recommended slower injection of alcohol when the lesion is at the level of the artery of Adamkiewicz to prevent iatrogenic cord injury. There have been multiple studies that report good outcomes with improvement of pain and neurologic symptoms following ethanol ablation [88, 86]. However, patients can develop secondary pathological fractures following this treatment if the bony architecture cannot support their weight following ablation of the tumor, and consideration is often given to include spinal instrumentation or a kyphoplasty to avoid this complication [87, 89].

Radiation Therapy

Radiotherapy is another modality used in the treatment of symptomatic hemangiomas. It can produce long-term disease control and improvement in pain scores [90, 91]. The use of radiotherapy alone can be effective for slowly progressing neurologic symptoms, but in the setting of myelopathy and cord compression, surgery should be strongly encouraged. With the doses of radiation required for vertebral hemangiomas, the risk of secondary malignancy to out-of-field organs is very low [92]. Radiotherapy can be an effective tool both on its own and as an adjunct to other therapies.

Vertebroplasty/Kyphoplasty

Vertebroplasty/kyphoplasty is another treatment that has a role in vertebral hemangiomas [93]. The exothermic reaction from the cement can cause some thermal necrosis to surrounding tumor cells, but more importantly, it provides structural support to the vertebrae. While it can be used on its own with good pain relief, it is commonly used as an adjunct to radiation, ethanol ablation, or surgical decompression [94, 95, 96].

Osteochondroma

Introduction

Osteochondromas consist of an outgrowth of cortical and medullary bone contiguous with the host bone, are capped by cartilage, and are the most common benign primary tumors of bone. Osteochondromas represent 36% of all benign bone tumors, but they are relatively underrepresented in the spine [97]. Only 1–4% of all osteochondromas occur in the spine [97, 98]. The majority of these lesions appear as solitary growths, but as many as 25% may be associated with multiple hereditary exostosis (MHE), an

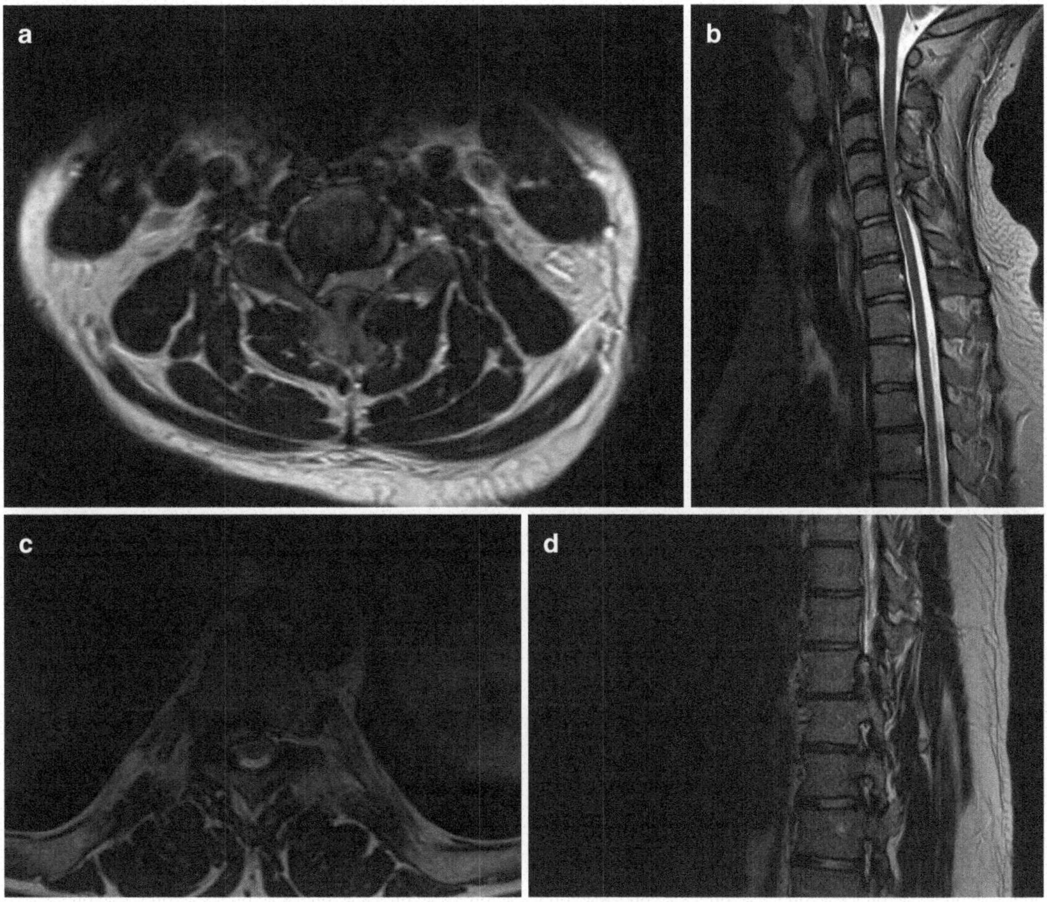

Fig. 6.3 Patient with MHE. (**a**, **b**) Osteochondroma originating from C4 lamina causing cervical myelopathy on axial and sagittal T2 imaging. (c, **d**) Osteochondroma in the foramen of T8 causing radicular pain on axial and sagittal T2 imaging

autosomal dominant heritable disorder in which patients may develop many osteochondromas distributed throughout the skeleton (Fig. 6.3). It is estimated that approximately 9% of patients with MHE develop spinal lesions [97]. Patients with solitary osteochondromas of the spine present at a mean age of 30–33, whereas those patients with MHE are diagnosed with spinal lesions at a mean age of 20–22 [97, 99, 100, 98]. Males are more frequently affected than females at a rate of 1.9–2.4:1 [99, 98].

Within the spine, osteochondromas typically develop at the tips of the spinous and transverse processes, but may also develop in the vertebral body, pedicle, or facet [99, 101]. This is because the lesions are formed by displacement of a fragment of physeal cartilage, which, separated from the physis, continues to expand and undergo enchondral ossification [97, 102, 103].

A CT scan is usually required to make the diagnosis and is the imaging test of choice to identify the pathognomonic features of the contiguous cortex covered by cartilage flaring out from the host bone along with continuity of the underlying medullary bone [97, 104, 101, 105]. MRI is useful for demonstrating neural compression, marrow content, and the cartilage cap [106]. The thickness of the cartilage cap in particular is important to assess on imaging, as the principal differential diagnosis for osteochondroma is secondary chondrosarcoma, and the two can be distinguished by the thickness of the cartilage.

MRI has traditionally been the test of choice to assess the cartilage thickness [107, 108, 109, 110]. Bernard et al. have suggested that MRI-based assessment of malignancy gives a 100% sensitivity and 98% specificity with a cartilage-thickness cutoff of 2 cm [111].

Treatment

Many osteochondromas of the spine can be managed nonsurgically, and indeed, many go unrecognized. There is a small risk of malignant degeneration, which is cited to be 1% for solitary lesions and 10% for lesions associated with MHE [97, 112, 99]. Given the low rate of malignant degeneration, asymptomatic patients need not undergo surgery [97, 113, 106]. However, consideration should be given to following the patient clinically and radiographically to identify secondary malignancy, which should be suspected in tumors with a thick cartilage cap or those that continue to grow after the patient reaches skeletal maturity [99, 100]. The secondary malignancy associated with osetochondromas is typically low grade. As with other benign tumors of the spine, the primary indications for surgery are pain and impingement on neural structures or diagnostic uncertainty despite adequate workup [106].

For osteochondromas, surgery is curative if the cartilage cap is removed but is only indicated for symptomatic lesions [114]. Major neurologic improvement is seen in 70% of patients and some improvement seen in another 18% [97]. If a portion of the cartilage cap remains, recurrence is likely within 6–14 months [97, 115, 116], but the overall recurrence rate is only 4% [99]. After surgery, no oncologic surveillance is mandatory and is based on patient symptoms.

Others

Benign notochordal cell tumors (BNCTs) have been recognized by the WHO classification in 2013, but these tumors are largely underreported [117]. Therefore, the true incidence of benign notochordal cell tumors is unknown. Most of these tumors are incidental findings and are asymptomatic. The alternate diagnosis for these tumors is chordoma. Chordomas and BNCTs show common notochordal histologic and immnophenotypic features (the physaliphorous cell and brachyury gene). Controversies exist as to whether this entity is a precursor of chordoma although absence of malignant transformation has been reported [118–120]. On imaging, typical BNCTs are small (<35 mm), confined to the bone, do not have soft tissue extension, are not lytic, and lack enhancement post gadolinium injection on MRI [121]. Compared to chordoma, histologically, BNCTs lack cellular atypia, mitotic activity, extracellular myxoid matrix, and intratumoral vascularity [121]. Biopsy is suggested when atypical imaging features are encountered, although differentiating between chordoma and BNCTs can be difficult on core biopsy. Importantly, BNCTs should be stable in size on serial scans and therefore, follow-up imaging is mandatory when suspecting this entity. If a presumptuous diagnosis of BNCTs shows enlargement, chordoma should be considered and managed accordingly.

Fibrous Dysplasia

Fibrous dysplasia accounts for 7% of all benign bone tumors. It presents with either a monostotic lesion or a polyostotic presentation and 7–14% of polyostotic lesions are found in the spine [122]. It is characterized by an activating mutation of *GNAS1* (G protein-coupled receptor), resulting in impaired osteoblast differentiation from precursor cells [123]. The primitive bone fails to remodel into lamellar bone and does not realign with mechanical stress. Furthermore, insufficient mineralization is observed. The resultant is immature bone with poor mechanical strength leading to pain, fracture, and deformity. The monostotic presentation is more commonly encountered, and the lesion will typically not grow after skeletal maturity has been reached. The polyostotic lesions are often part of a syndrome such as the McCune Albright syndrome (fibrous dysplasia, café-au-lait spots, endocrinopathy) and Mazabraud syndrome (fibrous dysplasia and intramuscular myxomas). Lesions in the polyostotic presentation will typically continue to enlarge after skeletal maturity, leading to fracture, deformity, and pain. Malignant transformation in fibrous dysplasia is rare, ranging between 0.4 and 4% [124, 125, 126, 127]. X-rays and CT demonstrate a "ground glass" appearance from the fibrous matrix. On MRI, these lesions have low signal intensity on T1- and T2-weighted images [128]. Monostotic lesions are often asymptomatic, found incidentally, and only require clinical observation. Biphosphonates can be used to treat symptomatic lesions with the objective to reduce pain intensity [129]. As with other benign lesions, surgical intervention may be indicated for severe pain, progressive deformity, and secondary neurologic symptoms. The Enneking staging system recommends intralesional resection for symptomatic/active fibrous dysplasia. As with any lesion, careful anatomical consideration should be sought when treating these lesions. Literature is scarce on spinal fibrous dysplasia. The use of vertebroplasty for symptomatic lesions has been reported [130, 131]. Bone grafting can be challenging in fibrous dysplasia with graft resorption and persistence of dysplastic bone [132]. This seems to be especially true in the younger population with polyostotic presentation. Some authors advocate for cortical allograft use in this population [133].

Conclusion

The primary benign tumors of the spine are typically asymptomatic, slow-growing lesions, and occur in relatively young patients. However, they may cause clinical dilemmas when they present with pain, fracture, or neurologic deficit. Evaluation often begins with plain radiographs but usually requires a CT scan, MRI, or both, and biopsy may be required to make the definitive diagnosis. Treatment is primarily observation for the latent lesions. Surgery remains the mainstay of treatment of most aggressive lesions. Depending on the location, tumoral extension, and biological behavior of the tumor, an intralesional resection or an en bloc resection may be the preferred treatment. Due to the complexity and potential morbidity of these surgeries, alternative treatments have emerged. Denosumab is now the first line of treatment for unresectable GCT or when the surgery would be associated with unacceptable morbidity. Thermal ablation is increasingly used for OO with excellent local control rate. The various alternative treatments and the complexity of these tumors support treatment at dedicated tertiary tumor centers with clinical expertise and multidisciplinary panels.

References

1. Flemming DJ, Murphey MD, Carmichael BB, Bernard SA. Primary tumors of the spine. Semin Musculoskelet Radiol. 2000;4(3):299–320.
2. Orguc S, Arkun R. Primary tumors of the spine. Semin Musculoskelet Radiol. 2014;18(3):280–99.
3. Enneking WF. A system of staging musculoskeletal neoplasms. Clin Orthop Relat Res. 1986;204:9–24.
4. Bergh P, Kindblom LG, Gunterberg B, Remotti F, Ryd W, Meis-Kindblom JM. Prognostic factors in chordoma of the sacrum and mobile spine: a study of 39 patients. Cancer. 2000;88(9):2122–34.
5. Yamazaki T, McLoughlin GS, Patel S, Rhines LD, Fourney DR. Feasibility and safety of en bloc resection for primary spine tumors: a systematic review by the Spine Oncology Study Group. Spine. 2009;34(22 Suppl):S31–8.
6. Hart RA, Boriani S, Biagini R, Currier B, Weinstein JN. A system for surgical staging and management of spine tumors. A clinical outcome study of giant cell tumors of the spine. Spine. 1997;22(15):1773–82.
7. Ciftdemir M, Kaya M, Selcuk E, Yalniz E. Tumors of the spine. World J Orthop. 2016;7(2):109–16. PMCID: PMC4757655.
8. Kostuik JP, Errico TJ, Gleason TF, Errico CC. Spinal stabilization of vertebral column tumors. Spine. 1988;13(3):250–6.
9. Boriani S, Weinstein JN, Biagini R. Primary bone tumors of the spine. Terminology and surgical staging. Spine. 1997;22(9):1036–44.
10. Boriani S, Capanna R, Donati D, Levine A, Picci P, Savini R. Osteoblastoma of the spine. Clin Orthop Relat Res. 1992;278:37–45.
11. Bernard SA, Brian PL, Flemming DJ. Primary osseous tumors of the spine. Semin Musculoskelet Radiol. 2013;17(2):203–20.

12. Martin C, McCarthy EF. Giant cell tumor of the sacrum and spine: series of 23 cases and a review of the literature. Iowa Orthop J. 2010;30:69–75.
13. Mendenhall WM, Zlotecki RA, Scarborough MT, Gibbs CP, Mendenhall NP. Giant cell tumor of bone. Am J Clin Oncol. 2006;29(1):96–9.
14. Thakur NA, Daniels AH, Schiller J, Valdes MA, Czerwein JK, Schiller A, et al. Benign tumors of the spine. J Am Acad Orthop Surg. 2012;20(11):715–24.
15. Chan CM, Adler Z, Reith JD, Gibbs CP Jr. Risk factors for pulmonary metastases from giant cell tumor of bone. J Bone Joint Surg Am. 2015;97(5):420–8.
16. Niu X, Zhang Q, Hao L, Ding Y, Li Y, Xu H, Liu W. Giant cell tumor of the extremity: retrospective analysis of 621 Chinese patients from one institution. J Bone Joint Surg Am. 2012;94(5):461–7.
17. Rosario M, Kim HS, Yun JY, Han I. Surveillance for lung metastasis from giant cell tumor of bone. J Surg Oncol. 2017;116(7):907–13.
18. Wang B, Chen W, Xie X, Tu J, Huang G, Zou C, et al. Development and validation of a prognostic index to predict pulmonary metastasis of giant cell tumor of bone. Oncotarget. 2017;8(64):108054–63.
19. Shi LS, Li YQ, Wu WJ, Zhang ZK, Gao F, Latif M. Imaging appearance of giant cell tumour of the spine above the sacrum. Br J Radiol. 2015;88(1051):20140566.
20. Baumhoer D, Amary F, Flanagan AM. An update of molecular pathology of bone tumors. Lessons learned from investigating samples by next generation sequencing. Genes Chromosomes Cancer. 2019;58(2):88–9.
21. Behjati S, Tarpey PS, Presneau N, Scheipl S, Pillay N, Van Loo P, et al. Distinct H3F3A and H3F3B driver mutations define chondroblastoma and giant cell tumor of bone. Nat Genet. 2013;45(12):1479–82.
22. Luksanapruksa P, Buchowski JM, Singhatanadgige W, Bumpass DB. Systematic review and met-analysis of en bloc vertebrectomy compared with intralesional resection for giant cell tumors of the mobile spine. Global Spine J. 2016;6(8):798–803.
23. Boriani S, Bandiera S, Casadei R, Boriani L, Donthimeni R, Gasbarrini A, et al. Giant cell tumor of the mobile spine. A review of 49 cases. Spine. 2012;37(1):E37–45.
24. Charest-Morin R, Fisher CG, Varga PP, Gokaslan ZL, Rhines LD, Reynolds JJ, et al. En bloc resection versus intralesional surgery in the treatment of giant cell tumor of the spine. Spine. 2017;42(18):1383–90.
25. Harrop JS, Schmidt MH, Boriani S, Shaffrey CI. Aggressive "benign" primary spine neoplasms: osteoblastoma, aneurysmal bone cyst, and giant cell tumor. Spine. 2009;34(22 suppl):S39–47.
26. Thomas D, Henshaw R, Skubitz K, Chawla S, Staddon A, Blay JY, et al. Denosumab in patients with giant-cell tumor of bone: an open-label, phase 2 study. Lancet Oncol. 2010;11(3):275–80.
27. Branstetter DG, Nelson SD, Manivel JC, Blay JY, Chawala S, Thomas DM, et al. Denosumab induces tumor reduction and bone formation in patients with giant-cell tumor of bone. Clin Cancer Res. 2012;18(16):4415–24.
28. Rutkowski P, Ferrari S, Grimer RJ, Stalley PD, Dijkstra SP, Pienkowski A, et al. Surgical downstaging in an open-label phase II trial of denosumab in patients with giant cell tumor of bone. Ann Surg Oncol. 2015;22(9):2860–8.
29. Goldschlager T, Dea N, Boyd M, Reynolds J, Patel S, Rhines LD, et al. Giant cell tumors of the spine: has denosumab changed the treatment paradigm? J Neurosurg Spine. 2015;22(5):526–33.
30. Charest-Morin R, Boriani S, Fisher CG, Patel SR, Kawahara N, Mendel E, et al. Benign tumors of the spine: has new chemotherapy and interventional radiology changed the treatment paradigm? Spine. 2016;41(20S):S178–85.
31. Palmerini E, Chawla NS, Ferrari S, Sudan M, Picci P, Marchesi E, et al. Denosumab in advanced/unresectable giant-cell tumour of bone (GCTB): for how long? Eur J Cancer. 2017;76:118–24.
32. Alaqaili SI, Abduljabbar AM, Altaho AJ, Khan AA, Alherabi JA. Malignant sarcomatous transformation of benign giant cell tumor of bone after treatment with denosumab therapy: a literature review and reported cases. Cureus. 2018;10(12):e3792.
33. Chawla S, Blay JY, Rutowski P, Le Cesne A, Reichardt P, et al. Denosumab in patients with giant-cell tumor of bone: a multicenter, open-label, phase 2 study. Lancet. 2019;20:1719–29.
34. Chinder PS, Hindiskere S, Doddarangappa S, Pal U. Evaluation of local recurrence of bone treated by neoadjuvant denosumab. Clin Orthop Surg. 2019;11(3):352–60.
35. Errani C, Tsukamoto S, Leone G, Righi A, Akahane M, et al. Denosumab may increase the risk of local recurrence in patients with giant-cell tumor of bone treated with curettage. J Bone Joint Surg Am. 2018;100:496–504.
36. Jha R, Sharma R, Rastogi R, Khan SA, Jayaswal A, Gamanagatti S. Preoperative embolization of primary bone tumors: a case control study. World J Radiol. 2016;8(4):378–89.
37. Prando A, de Santos LA, Wallace S, Murray JA. Angiography in giant-cell bone tumors. Radiology. 1976;130(2):323–31.
38. Qiao Z, Jia N, He Q. Does preoperative transarterial embolization decrease blood loss during spine surgery? Interv Neuroradiol. 2015;21(1):129–35.
39. Hosalkar HS, Jones KJ, King JJ, Lackman RD. Serial arterial embolization for large sacral giant-cell tumors: mid- to long-term results. Spine. 2007;32(10):1107–15.
40. Lackman RD, Khoury LD, Esmail A, Donthineni-Rao R. The treatment of sacral giant-cell tumours by serial arterial embolization. J Bone Joint Surg Br. 2002;84(6):873–7.
41. Lin PP, Guzel VB, Moura MF, Wallace S, Benjamin RS, Weber KL, et al. Long-term follow-up of patients with giant cell tumor of the sacrum treated with selective arterial embolization. Cancer. 2002;95(6):1317–25.

42. Nakanishi K, Osuga K, Hori S, Hamada K, Hashimoto N, Araki N, et al. Transarterial embolization (TAE) of sacral giant cell tumor (GCT) using spherical permanent embolic material superabsorbent polymer microsphere (SAP-MS). Springerplus. 2013;2:666.
43. Onishi H, Kaya M, Wada T, Nagoya S, Saski M, Yamashita T. Giant cell tumor of the sacrum treated with selective arterial embolization. Int J Clin Oncol. 2010;15(4):416–9.
44. Thangaraj R, Grimer RJ, Carter SR, Stirling AJ, Spilsbury J, Spooner D. Giant cell tumour of the sacrum: a suggested algorithm for treatment. Eur Spine J. 2010;19(7):1189–94.
45. Bell RS, Harwood AR, Goodman SB, Fornasier VL. Supervoltage radiotherapy in the treatment of difficult giant cell tumors of bone. Clin Orthop Relat Res. 1983;174:208–16.
46. Bennett CJ Jr, Marus RB Jr, Million RR, Enneking WF. Radiation therapy for giant cell tumor of bone. Int J Radiat Oncol Biol Phys. 1993;26(2):299–304.
47. Ma Y, Xu W, Yin H, Huang Q, Liu T, Yang X, et al. Therapeutic radiotherapy for giant cell tumor of the spine: a systematic review. Eur Spine J. 2015;24(8):1754–60.
48. Boriani S, Lo SF, Puvanesarajah V, Fisher CG, Varga PP, Rhines LD, et al. Aneurysmal bone cysts of the spine: treatment options and considerations. J Neuro-Oncol. 2014;120(1):171–8.
49. Panoutsakopoulos G, Pandis N, Kyriazoglou I, Gustafson P, Mertens F, Mandahl N. Recurrent t(16;17)(q22;p13) in aneurysmal bone cysts. Genes Chromosomes Cancer. 1999;26(3):265–6.
50. Vergel De Dios AM, Bond JR, Shives TC, McLeod RA, Unni KK. Aneurysmal bone cyst. A clinicopathologic study of 238 cases. Cancer. 1992;69(12):2921–31.
51. Boriani S, De Iure F, Campanacci L, Gasbarrini A, Bandiera S, Biagini R, et al. Aneurysmal bone cyst of the mobile spine: report on 41 cases. Spine. 2001;26(1):27–35.
52. Henrichs MP, Beck L, Gosheger G, Streitbuerger A, Koehler M, Heindel W, et al. Selective arterial embolization of aneurysmal bone cysts of the sacrum: a promising alternative to surgery. Rofo. 2016;188(1):53–9.
53. Amendola L, Simonetti L, Simoes CE, Bandiera S, De Iure F, Boriani S. Aneurysmal bone cyst of the mobile spine: the therapeutic role of embolization. Eur Spine J. 2013;22(3):533–41.
54. Terzi S, Gasbarrini A, Fuiano M, Barbanti Brodano G, Ghermandi R, Bandiera S, et al. Efficacy and safety of selective arterial embolization in the treatment of aneurysmal bone cyst of the mobile spine: a retrospective observational study. Spine. 2017;42(15):1130–8.
55. Liu X, Han SB, Si G, Yang SM, Wang CM, Jiang L, et al. Percutaneous albumin/doxycycline injection versus open surgery for aneurysmal bone cysts in the mobile spine. Eur Spine J. 2019;28(6):1529–36.
56. Lyons KW, Borsinger TM, Pearson AM. Percutaneous doxycycline foam injections, a novel treatment method for vertebral aneurysmal bone cysts. World Neurosurg. 2019;125:3–5.
57. Barbanti-Brodano G, Girolami M, Ghermandi R, Terzi S, Gasbarrini A, Bandiera S, et al. Aneurysmal bone cyst of the spine treated by concentrated bone marrow: clinical cases and review of the literature. Eur Spine J. 2017;26(Suppl 1):158–66.
58. Elsayad K, Kriz J, Seegenschmiedt H, Imhoff D, Heyd R, Eich HT, et al. Radiotherapy for aneurysmal bone cysts. A rare indication. Strahlenther Onkol. 2017;193:332–40.
59. Park HY, Yang SK, Sheppard WL, Hedge V, Zoller SD, Nelson SD, et al. Current management of aneurysmal bone cysts. Curr Rev Musculoskelet Med. 2016;9:435–44.
60. Lange T, Stehling C, Frohlich B, Klingerhofer M, Kunkel P, Schneppenheim R, et al. Denosumab: a potential new and innovative treatment option for aneurysmal bone cysts. Eur Spine J. 2013;22(6):1417–22.
61. Pelle DW, Ringler JW, Peacock JD, Kampfschulte K, Scholten DJ, Davis MM, et al. Targeting RANKL in aneurysmal bone cysts: verification of target and therapeutic response. Transl Res. 2014;164(2):139–48.
62. Alhumaid I, Abu-Zaid A. Denosumab therapy in the management of aneurysmal bone cysts: a comprehensive literature review. Cereus. 2019; https://doi.org/10.7759/cureus.3989.
63. Galgano MA, Goulart CR, Iwenofu H, Chin LS, Lavelle W, Mendel E. Osteoblastomas of the spine: a comprehensive review. Neurosurg Focus. 2016;41(2):E4.
64. Lucas DR, Unni KK, McLeon RA, O'Connor MI, Sim FH. Osteoblastoma: clinicopathologic study of 306 cases. Hum Pathol. 1994;25(2):117–34.
65. Bottner F, Roedl R, Wortler K, Grethen C, Winkelmann W, Linder N. Cyclooxygenase-2 inhibitor for pain management in osteoid osteoma. Clin Orthop Relat Res. 2001;393:258–63.
66. Carpintero-Benitez P, Aguirre MA, Serrano JA, Lluch M. Effect of rofecoxib on pain caused by osteoid osteoma. Orthopedics. 2004;27(11):1188–91.
67. Saifuddin A, White J, Sherazi Z, Shaikh MI, Natali C, Ransford AO. Osteoid osteoma and osteoblastoma of the spine. Factors associated with the presence of scoliosis. Spine. 1998;23(1):47–53.
68. Berry M, Mankin H, Gebhardt M, Rosenberg A, Hornicek F. Osteoblastoma: a 30-year study of 99 cases. J Surg Oncol. 2008;98(3):179–83.
69. Fittall MW, Mifsud W, Pillay N, Ye H, Strobl AC, Verfaillie A, et al. Recurrent rearrangements of FOS and FOSB define osteoblastoma. Nat Commun. 2018;9(1):2150.
70. Quraishi NA, Boriani S, Sabou S, Varga PP, Luzzati A, Gokaslan ZL, et al. A multicenter cohort study of spinal osteoid osteomas: results of surgical treatment and analysis of local recurrence. Spine J. 2017;17(3):401–8.
71. Ando K, Kobayashi K, Machino M, Ota K, Morozumi M, Tanaka S, et al. Computed tomography-based

navigation system-assisted surgery for primary spine tumor. J Clin Neurosci. 2019;63:22–6.
72. Kadhim M, Binitie O, O'Toole P, Grigoriou E, De Mattos CB, Dormans JP. Surgical resection of osteoid osteoma and osteoblastoma of the spine. J Pediatr Orthop B. 2017;26(4):362–9.
73. Kulkarni A, Patel A. Motion preserving surgery: excision of juxta C5-C6 intervertebral disc osteoid osteoma using 3D C-arm based navigation: technical report. SICOT J. 2018;4:56.
74. Boriani S, Amendola L, Bandiera S, Simcoes CE, Alberghini M, et al. Staging and treatment of osteoblastoma in the mobile spine : a review of 51 cases. Eur Spine J. 2012;21:2003–10.
75. Albisinni U, Facchini G, Spinnato P, Gasbarrini A, Bazzocchi A. Spinal osteoid osteoma: efficacy and safety of radiofrequency ablation. Skelet Radiol. 2017;46(8):1087–94.
76. Yu X, Wang B, Yang S, Han S, Jiang L, Liu X, et al. Percutaneous radiofrequency ablation versus open surgical resection for spinal osteoid osteoma. Spine J. 2019;19(3):509–15.
77. Weber MA, Sprengel SD, Omlor GW, Lehner B, Wiedenhofer B, Kauczor HU, et al. Clinical long-term outcome, technical success, and cost analysis of radiofrequency ablation for the treatment of osteoblastomas and spinal osteoid osteomas in comparison to open surgical resection. Skelet Radiol. 2015;44(7):981–93.
78. Rehnitz C, Sprengel SD, Lehner B, Ludwig K, Omlor G, Merle C, et al. CT-guided radiofrequency ablation of osteoid osteoma and osteoblastoma: clinical success and long-term follow up in 77 patients. Eur J Radiol. 2012;81(11):3426–34.
79. Rehnitz C, Sprengel SD, Lehner B, Ludwig K, Omlor G, Merle C, et al. CT-guided radiofrequency ablation of osteoid osteoma: correlation of clinical outcome and imaging features. Diagn Interv Radiol. 2013;19:330–9.
80. Fox MW, Onofrio BM. The natural history and management of symptomatic and asymptomatic vertebral hemangiomas. J Neurosurg. 1993;78(1):36–45.
81. Pastushyn AL, Slin'ko EI, Mirzoyeva GM. Vertebral hemangiomas: diagnosis, management, natural history and clinicopathological correlates in 86 patients. Surg Neurol. 1998;50(6):535–47.
82. Slon V, Stein D, Cohen H, Sella-Tunis T, May H, Hershkovitz I. Vertebral hemangiomas: their demographical characteristics, location along the spine and position within the vertebral body. Eur Spine J. 2015;24(10):2189–95.
83. Nabavizadeh SA, Mamourian A, Schmitt JE, Cloran F, Vossough A, Pukenas B, et al. Utility of fat-suppressed sequences in differentiation of aggressive vs typical asymptomatic haemangioma of the spine. Br J Radiol. 2016;89(1057):20150557.
84. Robinson Y, Sheta R, Salci K, Willander J. Blood loss in surgery for aggressive vertebral haemangioma with and without embolization. Asian Spine J. 2015;9(3):483–91.
85. Goldstein CL, Varga PP, Gokaslan ZL, Boriani S, Luzzati A, Rhines L, et al. Spinal hemangiomas: results of surgical management for local recurrence and mortality in a multicenter study. Spine. 2015;40(9):656–64.
86. Doppman JL, Oldfield EH, Heiss JD. Symptomatic vertebral hemangiomas: treatment by means of direct intralesional injection of ethanol. Radiology. 2000;214(2):341–8.
87. Singh P, Mishra NK, Dash HH, Thyalling RK, Sharma BS, Sakar C, et al. Treatment of vertebral hemangiomas with absolute alcohol (ethanol) embolization, cord decompression, and single level instrumentation: a pilot study. Neurosurgery. 2011;68(1):78–84.
88. Chandra SP, Singh P, Kumar R, Agarwal D, Tandon V, Kale SS, et al. Long-term outcome of treatment of vertebral body hemangiomas with direct ethanol injection and short-segment stabilization. Spine J. 2019;19(1):131–43.
89. Singh PK, Chandra PS, Vaghani G, Savarkar DP, Garg K, Kumar R, et al. Management of pediatric single-level vertebral hemangiomas presenting with myelopathy by three-pronged approach (ethanol embolization, laminectomy, and instrumentation): a single institute experience. Childs Nerv Syst. 2016;32(2):307–14.
90. Missczyk L, Tukiendorf A. Radiotherapy of painful vertebral hemangiomas: the single center retrospective analysis of 137 cases. Int J Radiat Oncol Biol Phys. 2012;82(2):e173–80.
91. Parekh AD, Amdur RJ, Mendenhall WM, Morris CG, Zlotecki RA. Long-term tumor control with radiotherapy for symptomatic hemangioma of a vertebral body. Spine. 2019;44(12):E731–4.
92. Mazonakis M, Tzedakis A, Lyraraki E, Damilakis J. Radiation dose and cancer risk to out-of-field and partially in-field organs from radiotherapy for symptomatic vertebral hemangiomas. Med Phys. 2016;43(4):1841.
93. Moore JM, Poonnoose S, McDonald M. Kyphoplasty as a useful technique for complicated haemangiomas. J Clin Neurosci. 2012;19(9):1291–3.
94. Girardo M, Zenga F, Bruno LL, Rava A, Masse A, Maule M, et al. Treatment of aggressive vertebral hemangiomas with poly vinyl alcohol (PVA) microparticles embolization, PMMA, and short segment stabilization: preliminary results with at least 5 years of follow-up. World Neurosurg. 2019; https://doi.org/10.1016/j.wneu.2019.04.138.
95. Hao J, Hu Z. Percutaneous cement vertebroplasty in the treatment of symptomatic vertebral hemangiomas. Pain Physician. 2012;15(1):43–9.
96. Premat K, Clarencon F, Cormier E, Mahtout J, Bonaccorsi R, Degos V, et al. Long-term outcome of percutaneous alcohol embolization combined with percutaneous vertebroplasty in aggressive vertebral hemangiomas with epidural extension. Eur Radiol. 2017;27(7):2860–7.
97. Albrecht S, Crutchfield JS, SeGall GK. On spinal osteochondromas. J Neurosurg. 1992;77(2):247–52.

98. Roblot P, Alcalay M, Cazenave-Roblot F, Levy P, Bontoux D. Osteochondroma of the thoracic spine. Report of a case and review of the literature. Spine. 1990;15(3):240–3.
99. Gille O, Pointillart V, Vital J-M. Course of spinal solitary osteochondromas. Spine. 2005;30(1):E13–9.
100. Gunay C, Atalar H, Yildiz Y, Saglik Y. Spinal osteochondroma: a report on six patients and a review of the literature. Arch Orthop Trauma Surg. 2010;130(12):1459–65.
101. Malat J, Virapongse C, Levine A. Solitary osteochondroma of the spine. Spine. 1986;11(6):625–8.
102. Murphey MD, Choi JJ, Kransdorf MJ, Flemming DJ, Gannon FH. Imaging of osteochondroma: variants and complications with radiologic-pathologic correlation. Radiographics. 2000;20(5):1407–34.
103. Rodallec MH, Feydy A, Larousserie F, Anract P, Campagna R, Babinet A, et al. Diagnostic imaging of solitary tumors of the spine: what to do and say. Radiographics. 2008;28(4):1019–41.
104. Cooke RS, Cumming WJ, Cowie RA. Osteochondroma of the cervical spine: case report and review of the literature. Br J Neurosurg. 1994;8(3):359–63.
105. Moriwaka F, Hozen H, Nakane K, Sasaki H, Tashiro K, Abe H. Myelopathy due to osteochondroma: MR and CT studies. J Comput Assist Tomogr. 1990;14(1):128–30.
106. Raswan US, Bhat AR, Tanki H, Samoon N, Kirmani AR. A solitary osteochondroma of the cervical spine: a case report and review of literature. Childs Nerv Syst. 2017;33(6):1019–22.
107. Fanney D, Tehranzadeh J, Quencer RM, Nadji M. Case report 415: osteochondroma of the cervical spine. Skelet Radiol. 1987;16(2):170–4.
108. Hudson TM, Hamlin DJ, Enneking WF, Pettersson H. Magnetic resonance imaging of bone and soft tissue tumors: early experience in 31 patients compared with computed tomography. Skelet Radiol. 1985;13(2):134–46.
109. Hudson TM, Springfield DS, Spanier SS, Enneking WF, Hamlin DJ. Benign exostoses and exostotic chondrosarcomas: evaluation of cartilage thickness by CT. Radiology. 1984;152(3):595–9.
110. Rosenthal DI, Schiller AL, Mankin HJ. Chondrosarcoma: correlation of radiological and histological grade. Radiology. 1984;150(1):21–6.
111. Bernard SA, Murphey MD, Flemming DJ, Kransdorf MJ. Improved differentiation of benign osteochondromas from secondary chondrosarcomas with standardized measurement of cartilage cap at CT and MR imaging. Radiology. 2010;255(3):857–65.
112. Chiurco AA. Multiple exostoses of bone with fatal spinal cord compression; report of a case and brief review of the literature. Neurology. 1970;20(3):275–8.
113. Chatzidakis E, Lypiridis S, Kazdaglis G, Chatzikonstadinou K, Papatheodorou G. A rare case of solitary osteochondroma of the dens of the C2 vertebra. Acta Neurochir. 2007;149(6):637–8.
114. Ozturk C, Tezer M, Hamzaoglu A. Solitary osteochondroma of the cervical spine causing spinal cord compression. Acta Orthop Belg. 2007;73(1):133–6.
115. Arasil E, Erdem A, Yüceer N. Osteochondroma of the upper cervical spine. A case report. Spine. 1996;21(4):516–8.
116. Mavrogenis AF, Papagelopoulos PJ, Soucacos PN. Skeletal osteochondromas revisited. Orthopedics. 2008;31(10)
117. Golden LD, Small JE. Benign notocordal lesions of the posterior clivus: retrospective review of prevalence and imaging characteristics. J Neuroimaging. 2014;24:245–9.
118. Yamaguchi T, Suzuki S, Ishiiwa H, Ueda Y. Intraosseous benign notochordal cell tumours: overlooked precursors of classic chordomas? Histopathology. 2004;44:597–602.
119. Yamaguchi T, Watanabe-Ishiiwa H, Suzuki S, Igarashi Y, Ueda Y. Incipient chordoma: a report of two cases of early-stage chordoma arising from benign notorchordal cell tumors. Mod Pathol. 2005;18:1005–10.
120. Yamaguchi T, Yamato M, Saotome K. First histologically confirmed case of classic chordoma arising in a precursor benign notochordal lesion: differential diagnosis of benign and malignant notochordal lesions. Skelet Radiol. 2002;31:413–8.
121. Usher I, Flanagan AM, Choi D. Systematic review of clinical, radiologic, and histologic features of benign notochordal cell tumors: implication for patient management. World Neurosurg. 2019; https://doi.org/10.1016/j.wneu.2019.06.009.
122. Rosenblum B, Overby C, Levine M, Handler M, Sprecher S. Monostotic fibrous dysplasia of the thoracic spine. Spine. 1987;12(9):939–42.
123. Lee SE, Lee EH, Park H, Sung JY, Lee HW, Kang SY, et al. The diagnostic utility of GNAS mutation in patients with fibrous dysplasia: a meta-analysis of 168 sporadic cases. Hum Pathol. 2012;43(8):1234–42.
124. Harris WH, Dudley HR Jr, Barry RJ. The natural history of fibrous dysplasia. An orthopaedic, pathological, and roentgenographic study. Am J Orthop. 1962;44:207–33.
125. Huvos AG, Higinbotham NL, Miller TR. Bone sarcomas arising in fibrous dysplasia. J Bone Joint Surg Am. 1972;54:1047–56.
126. Ruggieri P, Sim FH, Bond JR, Unni KK. Malignancies in fibrous dysplasia. Cancer. 1994;73:1411–24.
127. Yahut SM Jr, Kenan S, Sissons HA, Lewis MM. Malignant transformation of fibrous dysplasia. A case report and review of the literature. Clin Orthop Relat Res. 1988;228:281–9.
128. Zhang Y, Zhang C, Wang S, Wang H, Zhu Y, Hao D. Computed tomography and magnetic resonance imaging manifestations of monostotic fibrous dysplasia. J Clin Imaging Sci. 2018;8:1–6.
129. Majoor BC, Appelman-Dijkstra NM, Fiocco M, van de Sande MA, Dijkstra PS, Hamdy NA. Outcome of long-term bisphosphonate

therapy in McCune Albright syndrome and polyostotic fibrous dysplasia. J Bone Miner Res. 2017;32(2):264–76.
130. Chen G, Yang H, Gan M, Li X, Chen K, Nalajala B, et al. Polyostotic fibrous dysplasia of the thoracic spine: case report and review of the literature. Spine. 2011;36(22):E1485–8.
131. Wu FL, Jiang L, Liu C, Yang SM, Wei F, Dang L, et al. Fibrous dysplasia of the mobile spine: report of 8 cases and review of the literature. Spine. 2013;38(23):2016–22.
132. Leet AI, Boyce AM, Ibrahim KA, Weintroub S, Kushner H, Collins MT. Bone-grafting in polyostotic fibrous dysplasia. J Bone Joint Surg Am. 2016;98:211–9.
133. Enneking WF, Gearen PF. Fibrous dysplasia of the femoral neck. Treatment by cortical bone-grafting. J Bone Joint Surg Am. 1986;68(9):1415–22.

Low-Grade Spinal Malignancies: Chordoma and Chondrosarcoma

7

Gideon Blumstein, Benjamin Kelley, Scott Nelson, Don Young Park, and Francis Hornicek

Chordoma

Epidemiology

Chordomas are rare primary spinal neoplasms, which arise from notochord remnants. Chordomas are typically slow-growing tumors affecting all age groups, with a higher incidence in patients between 50 and 60 years old [1]. The incidence is estimated to range from 1 to 2 cases per 1,000,000 in the United States. More recent data from the NIH SEER database suggest that the incidence may be as high as 8% of all primary bone tumors. The peak incidence of chordoma is between 40 and 60 years of age; however, chordoma affects people of all ages with varying degrees of frequency. Less than 5% of chordomas are found in pediatric patients and typically have a worse prognosis. Most tumors in those under 20 years of age are in the mobile spine (with very few in the sacrum), near equal distribution in those between 21 and 59 years of age and 30% higher incidence of sacral tumors in those over 60 years. There is an overall slightly male predominance of 1.5:1. However, in sacral tumors the male predominance is 2:1 and in skull base tumors, there is no gender difference. With regards to race, chordoma is about four times more likely to affect Caucasians than the African Americans [2].

G. Blumstein · B. Kelley · D. Y. Park (✉)
F. Hornicek
Department of Orthopaedic Surgery, David Geffen School of Medicine at the University of California Los Angeles, Los Angeles, CA, USA
e-mail: dypark@mednet.ucla.edu

S. Nelson
Department of Orthopaedic Surgery, David Geffen School of Medicine at the University of California Los Angeles, Los Angeles, CA, USA

Department of Pathology, David Geffen School of Medicine at the University of California Los Angeles, Los Angeles, CA, USA

Pathology

After multiple myeloma, chordoma is the second most common primary malignancy of the spine. Chordoma is so named because of its resemblance to the histologic structure of embryonic notochord. The most widely accepted theory regarding the pathogenesis of chordoma is that it arises from collections of embryonic notochord structures, which remain trapped within the bony structure of the spinal column. This understanding of chordoma was based on the common location and microscopic morphology it shares with the notochord structures, and more recent evidence to support this theory includes immunohistochemical analysis and molecular phenotyping.

The exact pathways behind the pathogenesis of chordoma are yet to be fully understood but evidence now supports the involvement of genes encoding for transcription factors involved in

K. Singh, M. Colman (eds.), *Surgical Spinal Oncology*,
https://doi.org/10.1007/978-3-030-50722-0_7

embryogenesis (SOX9) and regulation of notochord development (brachyury) [3]. Interestingly, during embryonic development of the vertebral column, the notochord regresses and becomes incorporated into the center of the intravertebral discs, becoming the nucleus pulposis. However, there have been no reported cases of chordoma arising from the intravertebral disc space, only from the bony elements of the spinal column. This may suggest a possible interaction between trapped notochord cells with the local osseous microenvironment, which may contribute to the pathogenesis [4, 5].

Classification

Chordoma is classified into four widely accepted subtypes: conventional, chondroid, poorly differentiated, and dedifferentiated chordoma (Table 7.1).

Conventional chordoma subtype is the most common, comprising about 80% of chordomas [6, 7]. This subtype is relatively slow growing and typically exhibits low-grade behavior. Gross appearance varies from gray to tan with focal areas of necrosis and a soft gelatinous texture (Fig. 7.1). When growing inside bone, conventional chordoma permeates the marrow space and Haversian system, replacing native cells and sur-

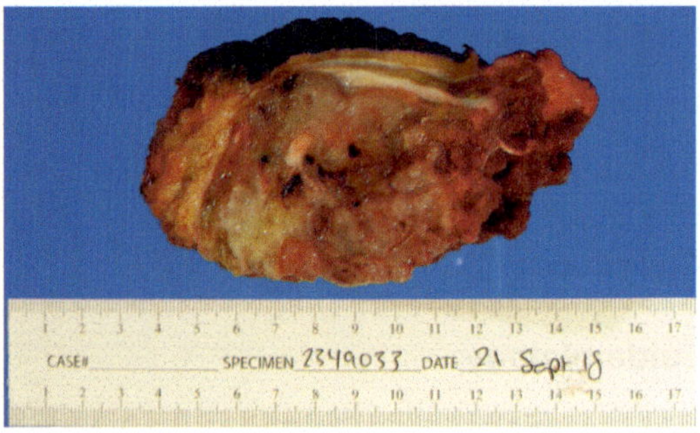

Fig. 7.1 Cross section of sacrococcygeal chordoma specimen showing lobules and sheets of glistening gelatinous grey tumor replacing and expanding the medullary marrow space. At the top portion the posterior cortex, periosteum, and overlying soft tissues are present

Table 7.1 Clinical, histologic, and immunohistochemical features of the four commonly accepted chordoma subtypes

Subtype	General features	Histologic features	Immunohistochemistry
Conventional chordoma	About 97% of all incidence Low-grade, indolent behavior Most common in sacrococcygeal region 70% 5-year survival 40% 10-year survival	Lobulated nests and cords with mucinous or myxoid stroma, high pleomorphism, necrotic regions especially if large, low mitotic figures Physaliphorous cells common Infiltrative within bone but well encapsulated soft tissue components	+ Cytokeratin + T brachyury + S-100 + EMA
Chondroid chordoma	About 2% of all incidence Mostly in skull base, rarely in sacrococcygeal Low-grade, indolent behavior	Biphasic – conventional areas with chondroid component, often well demarcated Chondroid appearance of lacunae but no true hyaline cartilage	No difference in IHC within the two phases + Cytokeratin + T brachyury + S-100 + EMA
Poorly differentiated chordoma	<1% incidence High-grade, more aggressive Younger presentation (mean age 12) Worse prognosis	No physaliphorous cells More mitotic figures Widely observed necrosis	+ Cytokeratin + T brachyury – S-100 – SMARCB1
Dedifferentiated chordoma	About 1% of all incidence Most aggressive, (90% metastasis at presentation) Least common Mostly in sacrococcygeal region Usually seen in recurrence or post radiation but can occur de novo	Biphasic – conventional chordoma areas with adjacent areas with appearance of pleomorphic, spindle cell or osteosarcoma	Dedifferentiated phase – Cytokeratin – T brachyury Conventional phase unchanged IHC

rounding osseous trabeculae. When extending into the soft tissue, these tumors typically form a well-encapsulated soft tissue mass. The microscopic architecture of conventional chordoma is comprised of lobulated nests and cords of cells around mucinous or myxoid stroma (Fig. 7.2a,b). Microscopic appearance shows typical physaliphorous cells with multiple clear cytoplasmic vacuoles, appearing similar to adipocytes. However, due to significant heterogeneity, these cells are not always present and are not considered pathognomonic. Conventional chordoma stains positive for keratin, S-100, and brachyury (Fig. 7.3a,b).

Chondroid chordoma subtype does not differ significantly from conventional chordoma with regards to immunohistochemistry. This subtype is comprised of areas of conventional chordoma, which are often sharply demarcated from other areas where neoplastic cells are spread out within a solid matrix with a similar appearance to hyaline cartilage (these cells mimic the appearance

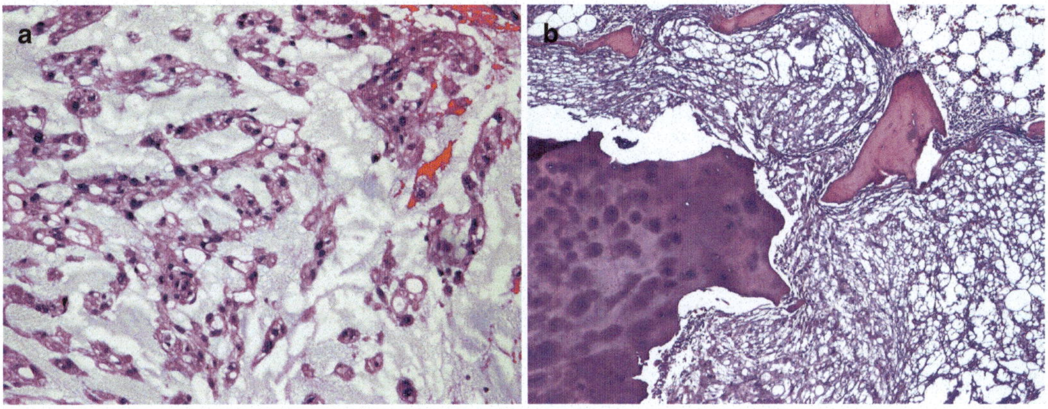

Fig. 7.2 (**a**) Conventional chordoma demonstrating cords of tumor cells within a myxoid matrix. The tumor cells have eosinophilic bubbly or physaliphorous cytoplasm and hyperchromatic nuclei (H&E 100X). (**b**) Chordoma infiltrating hyaline cartilage (left portion) and the bone marrow. Cancellous lamellar bone fragments of the marrow are surrounded by chordoma, with a portion of residual fatty marrow being present in the upper right (H&E 40X)

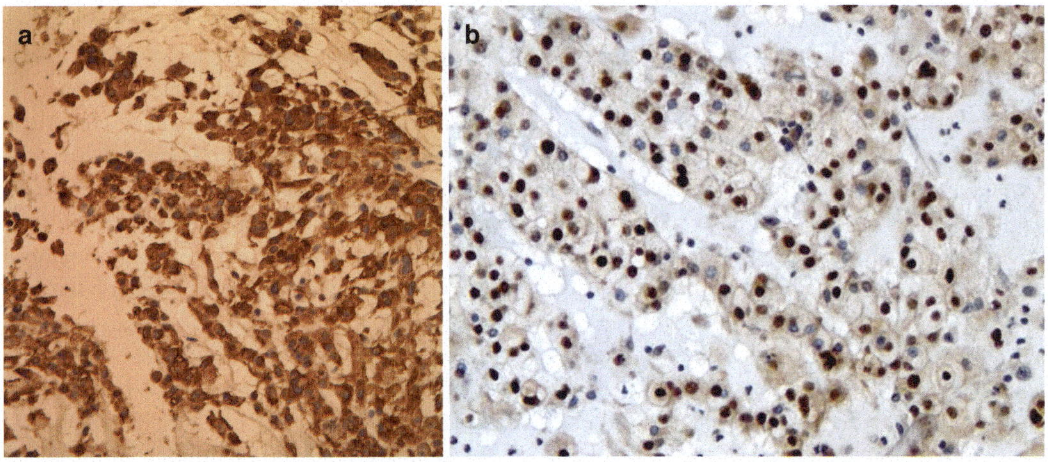

Fig. 7.3 (**a**) Upon immunohistochemical analysis, chordoma cells typically express keratin markers, as well as S-100 and brachyury. Here, chordoma cells demonstrate cytoplasmic positivity for the epithelial marker AE1;AE3 (AE1;AE3, 400X). (**b**) Nuclear positivity for brachyury in chordoma cells is demonstrated (Brachyury 400X)

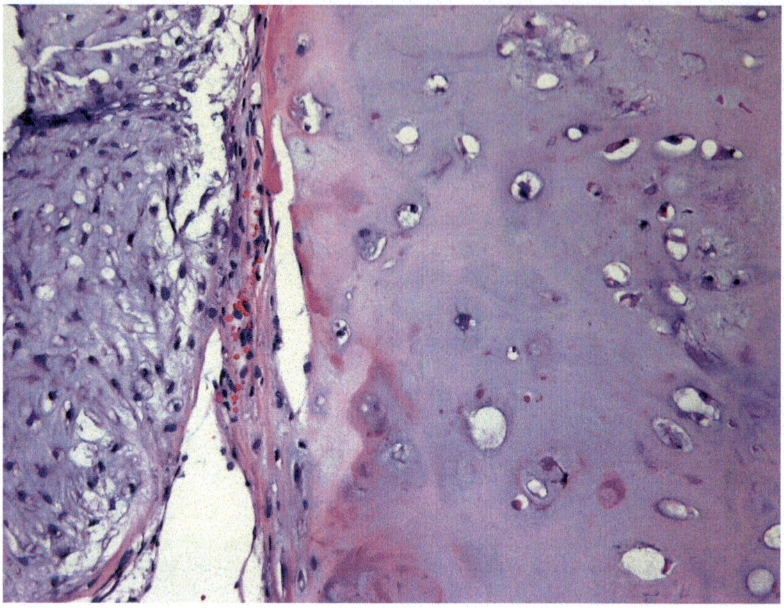

Fig. 7.4 The right half of this photo demonstrates the hyaline cartilage matrix with tumor cells occupying lacunar spaces seen in chondroid chordoma. Directly adjacent on the left side is more typical, conventional-appearing chordoma (H&E 100X)

of chondrocytes in lacunae) [8] (Fig. 7.4). The chondroid areas may be sparse or extensive, and when they are abundant, the tumor is difficult to distinguish morphologically from chondrosarcoma. The neoplastic cells in chondroid chordoma are identical to those found in conventional chordoma; however, the matrix takes on a different appearance. This subtype is found more commonly in the mobile spine than in the sacrococcygeal area. Initially, this subtype was thought to carry a more favorable prognosis; however, more recent studies dispute these findings and reported prognosis and course are similar to conventional chordoma [9].

Recently published work now supports new subtype – poorly differentiated chordoma, with distinct clinical and immunohistochemical features from the three classical varieties. Unlike the other varieties, which exhibit a peak age distribution between 40 and 60 years, poorly differentiated chordoma is found in much younger patients, with a peak distribution of 12 years of age. Another distinctive feature is a higher predilection for the skull base and cervical spine [10, 11]. Poorly differentiated chordoma behaves much more aggressively than conventional or chondroid chordoma, with earlier local recurrence and overall shorter survival. Histologically, poorly differentiated chordoma is remarkable for the absence of physaliferous cells or myxoid stroma (Fig. 7.5). Mitotic figures are more common and necrosis is widely observed. Immunohistochemical analysis shows positive staining for T brachyury and cytokeratin and is notable for the absence of SMARCB1 and S100 in most cases.

Dedifferentiated chordoma is the most aggressive subtype and the least common [12]. As in chondroid chordoma, the dedifferentiated subtype contains areas of conventional chordoma with distinct areas that resemble poorly differentiated spindle cell sarcoma, pleomorphic sarcoma, or osteosarcoma (Fig. 7.6). This subtype comprises about 5% of all chordomas, and is most frequently found in the sacrococcygeal region. The dedifferentiated subtype is most commonly seen in local recurrence or following irradiation of conventional chordoma but may arise from primary tumors. Unlike the other two subtypes, which grow slowly, often over years, dedifferentiated chordoma exhibits high-grade behavior, progresses rapidly, and metastasizes in over 90% of cases. The immunohistochemistry is distinctly different from chondroid and conventional chordoma, with the notable loss of keratin and brachyury.

Benign notochordal cell tumor (BNCT), also known as notochordal hamartoma, is a rare type

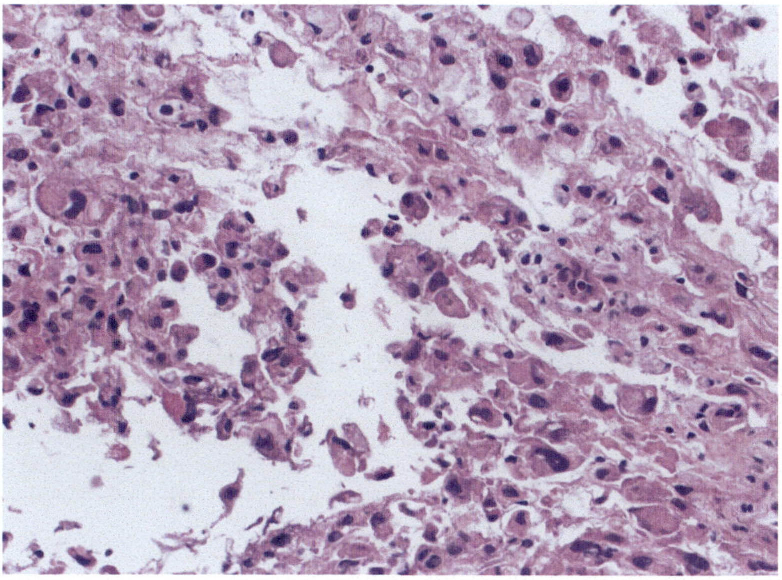

Fig. 7.5 Poorly differentiated chordoma is distinctive from the other subtypes with an absence of physaliferous cells or myxoid stroma. Mitotic figures and cellular necrosis are seen

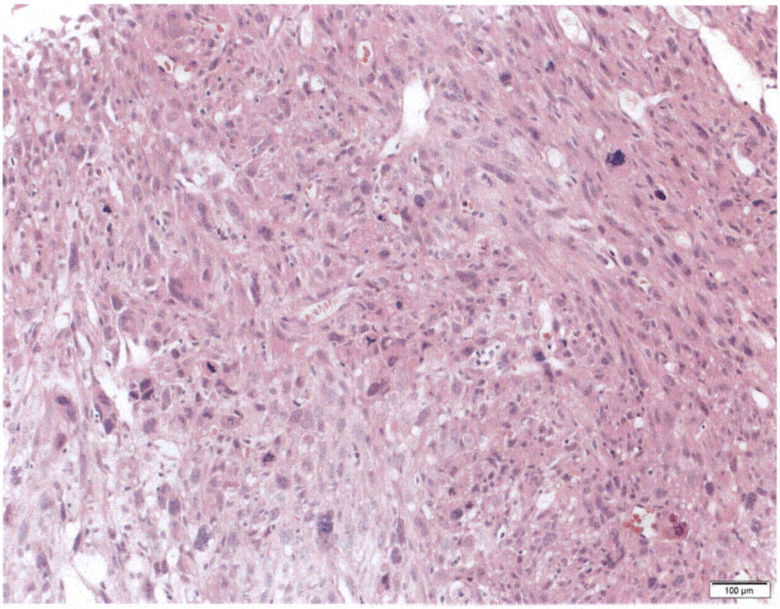

Fig. 7.6 Dedifferentiated chordoma is a histologically high-grade sarcoma. In this example, the tumor is very cellular and is composed of oval to spindled cells arranged in fascicles. Tumor cells are very pleomorphic and mitotic activity, including atypical mitoses are abundant (H&E 200X)

of notochordal tumor, generally considered a benign relative of chordoma. Typically found incidentally in the same sites as chordomas, this entity is usually asymptomatic. Unlike chordoma, it is sclerotic rather than lytic on imaging and does not extend into the soft tissue. However, there have been cases where the two entities coexisted simultaneously either side by side or within the same lesion, giving credence to the theory that they are on a continuum of the same pathological process [13]. Heavy reliance on immunohistochemistry and high-magnification histology may be misleading as both share the same physaliphorous cells and stain positive for T brachyury, S100, and cytokeratins. The diagnosis is made based on the correlation of clinical symptoms, imaging, and certain pathohistologic differences (BNCT are absent of nuclear atypia, necrosis, or intracellular myxoid matrix) (Fig. 7.7a,b).

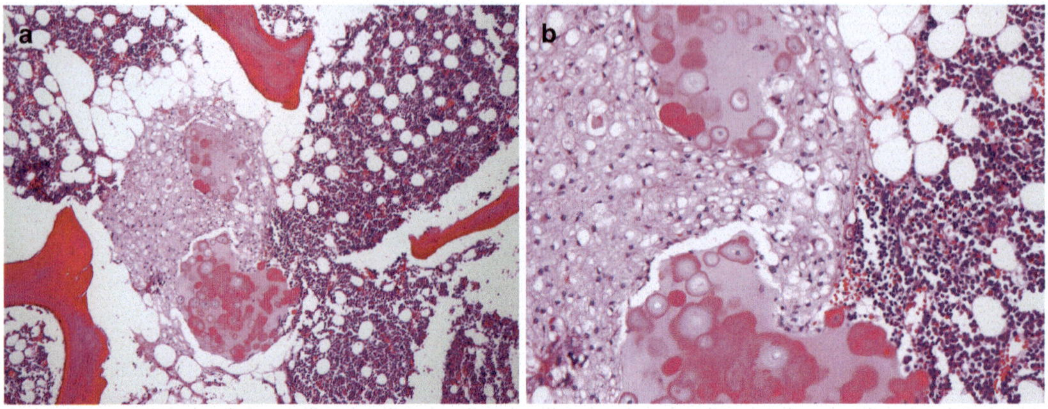

Fig. 7.7 (**a**) This small benign notochordal cell tumor or notochordal hamartoma, is seen to be present within the marrow space of a vertebral body. The tumor nodule is relatively sharply demarcated from the surrounding marrow and is not infiltrative (H&E 40X). (**b**) Higher magnification of the benign notochordal cell tumor demonstrates sheets of bland-appearing epithelioid cells with pink and clear cytoplasm, absent a myxoid background (H&E 100X)

Diagnosis

The most common presenting symptom of patients with chordoma is pain, as well as various neurological symptoms depending on the location of the tumor. Pain is usually reported first, with extremity symptoms including weakness, numbness, and altered sensation due to mass effect. Loss of bowel and/or bladder control is also frequently seen. Due to the slow growth rate of most sacral chordomas and relatively large space of the pelvic cavity, these tumors may be quite large at presentation. In patients with upper cervical tumor location, occipital headaches may be present and in rare cases, dysphagia or dysphonia due to compression of the larynx or esophagus has been reported. Unfortunately, lower back pain is a very common and nonspecific symptom and imaging is typically not obtained until patients have undergone some medical treatment or physical therapy first. For patients with sacral or coccygeal chordoma, this translates to an average time from onset of symptoms to diagnosis of over 2 years and a mean tumor size of 8 cm at time of resection. Any patients with persistent sacral or coccygeal pain should be evaluated with appropriate imaging without delay.

Due to the nonspecific symptoms of chordoma, the first images often obtained are radiographs to evaluate back or neck pain, which typically show lucency or density within the osseous spine with faint calcifications. If chordoma is suspected, it is best evaluated with CT and MRI [14]. CT helps delineate the exact extent of bony involvement and should include fine cuts of 1 mm or less with bone and soft tissue reconstruction. On CT, spine chordoma typically has a lytic component but may have a mixed lytic/sclerotic appearance through the bony regions, with low-density signal in the soft-tissue component due to high water content. MRI with gadolinium contrast is useful to evaluate the soft tissue component of the tumor and relationship with neurological and vascular structures, which is of paramount importance for surgical planning. The typical appearance of chordoma on MRI is high intensity on T2, low-to-medium intensity on T1, and mild or moderate enhancement with gadolinium. CT of the chest, abdomen, and pelvis; bone scan; and PET scans are used for staging purposes and to aid in treatment planning.

Open biopsy must be avoided if chordoma is suspected. A major cause of local recurrence is thought to be local contamination of the operative bed from open biopsies or poorly executed percutaneous biopsy. Ideally, CT-guided biopsy should be performed after discussion with the treating surgeon to plan for a biopsy tract that can be completely excised during surgery without increasing morbidity. Trochar biopsy should be performed to preserve the tumor architecture, which is crucial for correct diagnosis, and to protect the biopsy tract from seeding.

Definitive diagnosis of chordoma requires meticulous care with an oncology team approach, as no histologic or radiographic findings alone are pathognomonic and a full picture must be painted by combining the clinical, radiographic, and histologic features. The differential diagnosis is wide and includes metastatic carcinoma or hematological malignancy (of various types), benign notochordal cell tumors, chondroma, chondroblastoma, osteoma, osteoblastoma, osteosarcoma, giant cell tumors, and aneurysmal bone cysts, to name but a few. Careful consideration of all immunohistochemical, histologic, radiographic, demographic, and clinical features must be considered; over-reliance purely on histology may be dangerous. BNCT, like chordoma is positive for T brachyury, contains physaliphorous cells, and arises at the same sites; however, it is usually asymptomatic and smaller than 2 cm. While the dangers of missing a chordoma diagnosis are obvious, there is significant risk associated with overdiagnosing otherwise benign lesions as chordoma, given the morbidity associated with surgical treatment of chordoma [15].

Staging of chordoma is performed using the MSTS (Enneking) Staging System as well as the American Joint Committee on Cancer TNM system; however, due to the high local recurrence rate, low-stage tumors do not necessarily portent as favorable an outcome as is seen in other bone sarcomas. The use of whole spine MRI is endorsed by some groups to evaluate for regional metastasis; however, strong evidence is lacking due to the rarity of the disease. Likewise, the role of PET CT has remained controversial given the indolent nature of most subtypes of chordoma, though may be of more use in dedifferentiated chordoma [16].

Treatment

Due to the low incidence and high heterogeneity of both disease and treatment, there is significant variability in estimated survival from chordoma. Based on the SEER database, the range of 5-year overall survival is 65–75% and 10-year survival is 32–63%. There has been a trend to improve overall survival over time, attributed to improved imaging and surgical techniques, allowing for more complete en bloc resection (Fig. 7.8a–h). In general, favorable prognostic indicators at presentation are tumor size <4 cm, age <50 years, solitary lesion, and tumor-free margin resection. Certain molecular markers are correlated with alteration in prognosis, including overexpression of PARP1, hTERT, and SOX9 correlated with shorter survival time. SMARBC1 loss was associated with particularly aggressive disease and very short overall survival [17, 18].

To date, no cytotoxic agents have been proven to be effective in chordoma. While significant research is ongoing into molecular-targeted systemic therapy, the mainstay of treatment is surgical resection. Radiation has also played an important role as adjuvant treatment and has been effective as a stand-alone treatment in some studies.

When possible, total en bloc surgical resection with free margins is the treatment of choice in chordoma and offers the best outcomes with regards to relief of symptoms, prevention of local recurrence, and disease-free survival. The rates of local recurrence are reported around 3–8% with free margin en bloc resection compared to 100% with intralesional resection [19]. Unfortunately, due to proximity to vital structures, en bloc resection is often not possible and, in those cases, marginal or intralesional resection may offer significant benefit, relieve symptoms, or prolong symptom-free survival [20]. Extensive preoperative planning is required for successful chordoma surgery and thorough staging should be performed, as metastatic disease is often a contraindication to en bloc resection and would favor palliative surgery or radiation therapy.

If en bloc resection is deemed indicated and feasible, preoperative planning should include detailed plans for approach, resection, and reconstruction, and should include all of the surgical teams involved. Three-dimensional printed models may be helpful in mapping out the surgical plan in detail. Intraoperative navigation may also be helpful in certain cases [21, 22]. Extensive blood loss is not uncommon and a good perioperative plan should include a well-prepared blood

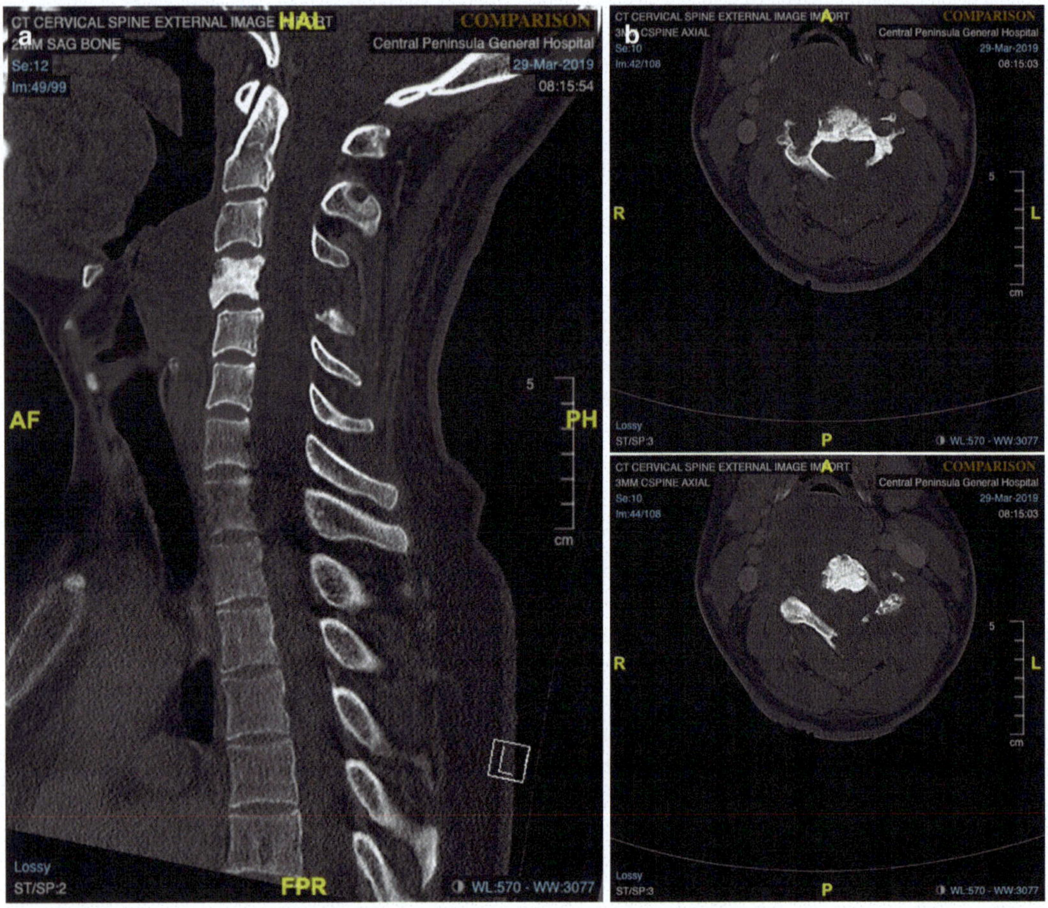

Fig. 7.8 The case is a 33-year-old male with neck pain and dysphagia that has worsened over the past 10 years. He was found to have a large cervical mass and biopsy demonstrated chordoma. (**a**) Sagittal CT image demonstrating the bony changes at C4 with both sclerotic and lytic changes in the vertebral body and posterior elements. There is a large extensive soft tissue mass extending both anteriorly and posteriorly into the spinal canal. (**b**) Axial CT images demonstrating the bony changes with the large soft tissue mass. (**c**) Sagittal MRI images depicting the large soft tissue mass emanating from C4 but extending to C3 and C5 with severe spinal cord compression with spinal cord edema and cord signal change. (**d**) Axial MRI images depicting the tumor encasing the vertebral arteries bilaterally with severe circumferential spinal cord compression. (**e**) AP and lateral fluoroscopic images after bilateral vertebral artery angiogram and coiling procedure. The angiogram demonstrated sufficient collateral flow to allow for bilateral vertebral artery coiling prior to the en bloc resection. Stage 1 of the procedure was the coiling procedure and tracheostomy. Stage 2 was posterior resection of the chordoma with resection of the coiled vertebral arteries, C1 to T2 posterior spinal instrumentation and fusion. Stage 3 was anterior resection with reconstruction using vascularized fibular graft and anterior cervical plating and fusion. (**f**) Intraoperative radiographs of the tumor including the vertebral bodies of C3, C4, and C5 after en bloc resection. (**g**) Postoperative CT 3D reconstructions of the cervical spine after en bloc tumor resection from C3 to C5, anterior strut graft reconstruction with anterior cervical plating, C1 to T2 posterior spinal instrumentation and fusion. (**h**) Postoperative AP and lateral radiographs demonstrating the anterior and posterior reconstruction following en bloc resection

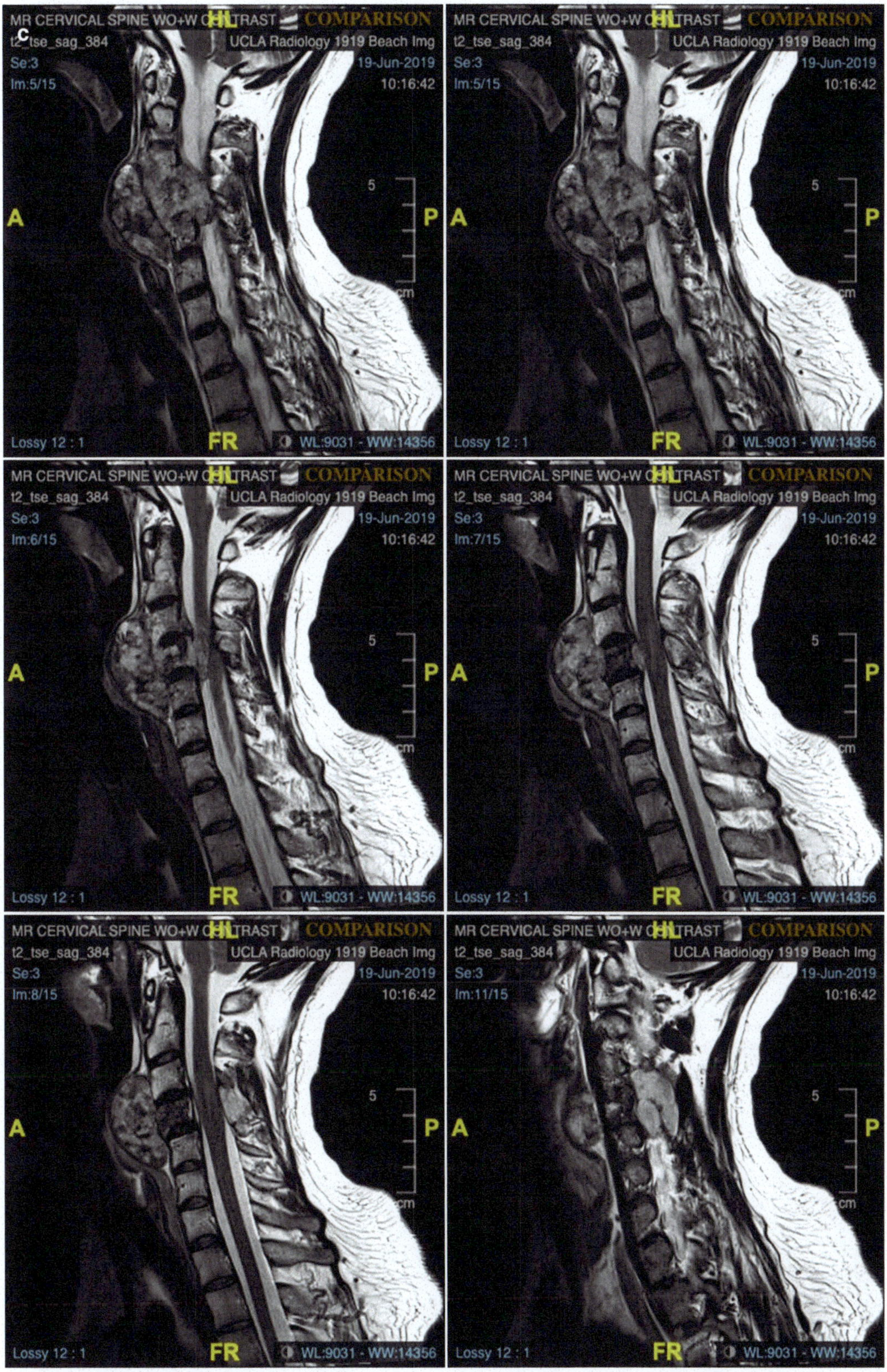

Fig. 7.8 (continued)

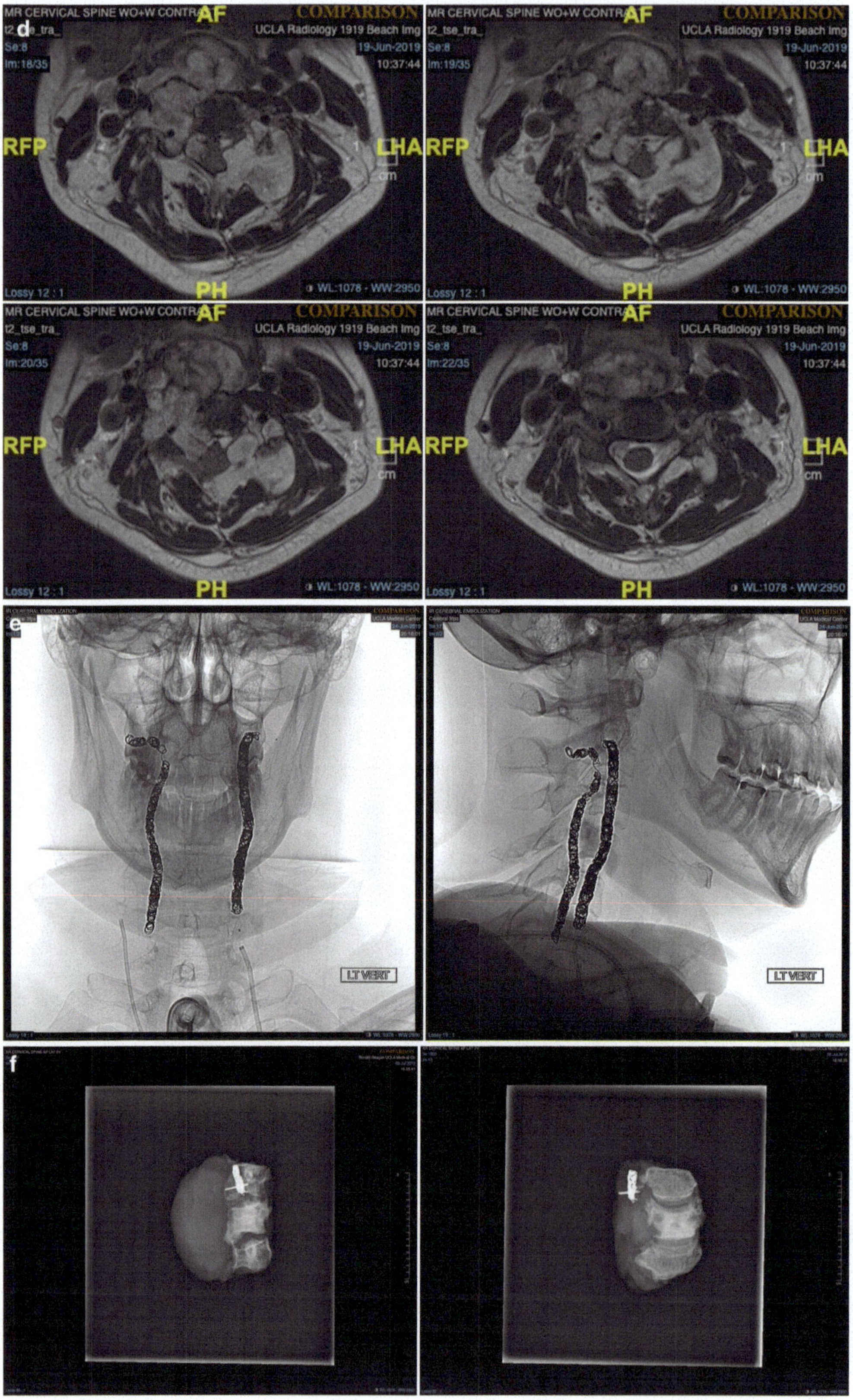

Fig. 7.8 (continued)

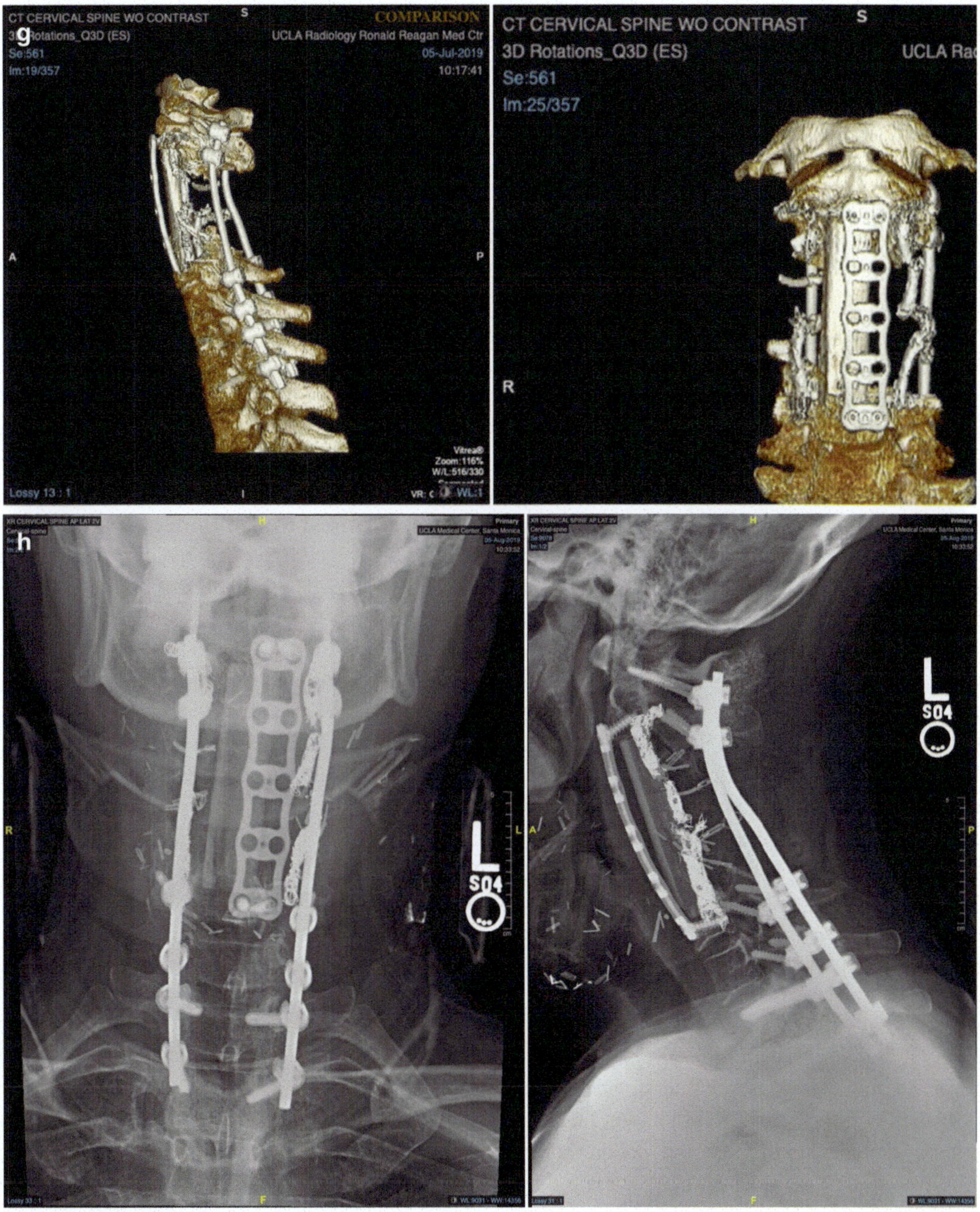

Fig. 7.8 (continued)

bank as well as anesthesia and critical care team to ensure all necessary resources are available to support the patient during and after surgery. In many cases, nerve roots must be sacrificed to perform en bloc resection and a sober and detailed discussion with the patient and family members should be held about the expected deficits and possible complications, including the loss of sensation and motor function, loss of bowel or bladder control, and loss of sexual function. Some patients may not find these acceptable and may favor a more palliative approach [23].

Free-margin en bloc resection of spinal chordomas is only possible in about 50% of cases with local recurrence approaching 100% with incomplete resection. Although chordoma is relatively radioresistant, the ability to accurately deliver higher doses of radiation to the tumor while limiting exposure of adjacent structures has improved. Evidence shows that there is a dose-dependent rate of 5-year local tumor control with 25% control with a dose under 60 Gy and 80% with a dose above 70 Gy [24, 25]. The rate of local control in cases of subtotal resection treated with high-dose radiation (above 70Gy) was equivalent to that achieved with free margin resection. In most studies, early radiation treatment, either preoperative or as adjuvant therapy, has been found to be more effective in controlling local recurrence than salvage radiation for treating recurrence [26]. Additional reported benefits of preoperative radiation include smaller treatment area (lower overall dose), reduced wound seeding, and eliminating possible interference and scatter due to implanted metal if postoperative radiation is used [27].

Stereotactic radiosurgery and particle therapy are favored over traditional photon therapy as these modalities can more accurately deliver high doses of radiation to the tumor with a very sharp drop off of radiation dose to surrounding tissue. Carbon ion therapy has been shown to be more effective than photon or proton therapy in small case series, with the advantage of having even sharper drop off and therefore higher effective doses of radiation than proton therapy, with improved ability to cause double-stranded DNA cleavage. As more carbon ion radiation facilities come available, this therapy may become more widely used in chordoma treatment, but is significantly limited due to availability and significant cost [28]. It is important to note that the limited number of cases and heterogeneity in anatomic location and modes of treatment make proving superiority of a particular method of radiotherapy difficult. Small-scale studies have found lower side effects and improved disease-free survival with heavy ion radiation compared to traditional methods.

While no cytotoxic chemotherapeutic agents have been effective against chordoma, there is extensive work with molecular-targeted therapy. Some of the targets investigated include EGRF, PDGFR-A/B, Her2/Neu, EGFR, c-KIT, VEGFR, and CDK4/6 [29, 30]. To date, no therapy has been shown to be effective under the response evaluation criteria in solid tumors (RECIST); however, there have been some notable effects to certain therapies, including changes in tumor metabolism and appearance on MRI and PET–CT. Small numbers and inevitable limitations in study design lead to a paucity of statistically significant clinical findings; however, extensive research using chordoma cell lines has exposed potential targets, with hope of future success.

Post-Treatment Surveillance

While strong evidence is lacking on the optimal schedule and mode of post-treatment surveillance of chordoma, the Chordoma Global Consensus Group and the European Society for Medical Oncology position recommendation is for local surveillance with an MRI of the region every 3 months for the first year, every 6 months for years 2–4, and yearly from year 5–15. For distant surveillance, the recommendation is for CT of the chest, abdomen, and pelvis with and without contrast and MRI of the whole spine with gadolinium every 6 months for the first year, and then yearly after that point [31].

Prognosis

Significant differences exist in prognosis based on patient age, disease location, and histologic subtype. Further prognostic factors include the adequacy of resection and total radiation dose if treated with radiotherapy. In most studies, the 5-year local recurrence rate for patients with successful total resection with or without radiation therapy is >50%. Recurrence often occurs late (5–10 years) and does not plateau even at 15 years. There is significant variability between the survival rates quoted by different studies; however, the most common range for 5 and 10 year overall survival is 65–75% and 32–63%, respectively. Outcomes are significantly worse following local recurrence or distant metastasis and treatment is seldom curative [32].

Chondrosarcoma

Epidemiology

Chondrosarcomas are a rare heterogeneous group of malignant neoplasms that produce cartilage matrix. After osteosarcoma (and excluding myeloma), chondrosarcoma is the second most common primary malignancy of bone, accounting for 25% of all primary bone tumors with an estimated annual incidence of 1 in 200,000 [33, 34]. The prevalence of chondrosarcoma in the mobile spine is reported between 6.5% and 10%, with 5% occurring in the sacrum [35, 36]. Within the spine, chondrosarcoma can occur in any region, but has a slight predilection for the thoracic region (30%). Chondrosarcoma is twice as common in males than in females. The age distribution of chondrosarcoma is broad, peaking in the fifth and sixth decades, although this varies based on histologic subtype [37]. Nearly 3000 chondrosarcoma cases from the SEER database revealed a mean age of 51 years at the time of diagnosis with a near double male predominance and low rate in the African American population [38]. Pediatric chondrosarcomas represented 10% of the cases, and patients may present at any age. Importantly, this analysis was based on a majority of patients with chondrosarcoma from limbs and may not reflect similar patterns in the spine. Overall, the demographics of chondrosarcoma are similar to that of chordoma.

Pathology

Assuming localized disease, histologic grade is the most important prognostic factor and ranked on a scale of 1 to 3 based on nuclear size, mitotic activity, hyperchromasia, and cellularity, which is characterized by atypical chondrocytes within a hyaline cartilage matrix [39–41]. In 2013, the World Health Organization (WHO) reclassified grade I chondrosarcoma as “atypical cartilaginous tumor” (ACT/CS1) [42, 43] (Fig. 7.9a,b). ACT/CS1 is considered locally aggressive rather than a malignant sarcoma and rarely metastasize [40]. However, this primarily applies to the appendicu-

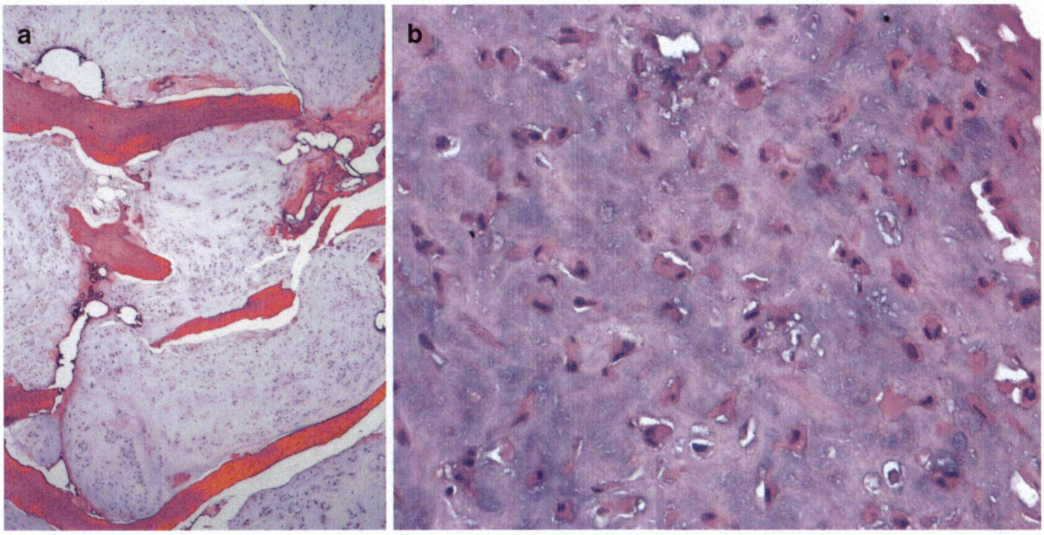

Fig. 7.9 (**a**) The permeative pattern of invasion typical of atypical cartilaginous tumor/chondrosarcoma. Sheets and lobules of malignant cartilage have replaced the marrow, and are completely surrounding cancellous lamellar marrow bone fragments (H&E 20X). (**b**) High magnification of low-grade atypical cartilaginous tumor/chondrosarcoma demonstrating rather monotonous tumor cells within a hyaline cartilage matrix. The individual tumor cells contain small, hyperchromatic nuclei, and abundant eosinophilic cytoplasm. Mitotic activity is typically absent. (H&E 400X)

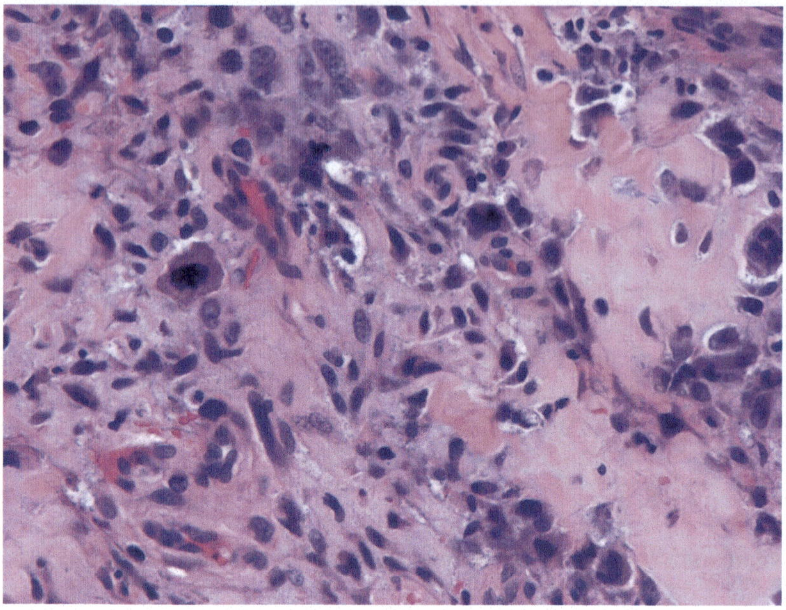

Fig. 7.10 By contrast, this example of high-grade (grade 3) chondrosarcoma displays very pleomorphic anaplastic chondrocytes with obvious mitotic activity (H&E 400X)

lar skeleton, and given that the National Cancer Database from 2002 to 2008 showed inferior survival of Stage IA/IB chondrosarcomas of the spine compared to the appendicular skeleton, spinal variants of grade 1 chondrosarcoma should be treated with caution. Grade 2 chondrosarcomas demonstrate intermediate metastatic potential (10–15%) and survival (10 years, 64–86%) [44, 45]. Grade 3 chondrosarcoma, in turn, faces higher rates of metastases (30–70%) and lower survival (10 years, 30–50%) (Fig. 7.10). However, this grading is subject to interobserver variability, especially between ACT/CS1 and grade 2 chondrosarcoma, highlighting the need for alternative diagnostic molecular markers to help guide treatment decision making [46, 47]. Grade 3 conventional chondrosarcomas are rare as ACT/CS1 and Grade 2 are much more common.

Chondrosarcomas are believed to develop from residual enchondral cartilage "rests," which persist during development after failing to form bone [48]. Chondrosarcomas may arise de novo or occur from the malignant transformation of a benign cartilaginous lesion, osteochondroma, or enchondroma. Osteochondromas are bony projections with a cartilage cap and most commonly located in long bones, but can be found in the spine as well. The autosomal dominant syndrome multiple hereditary exostoses (MHE) are characterized by two or more osteochondromas in the skeleton and caused by a germline mutation of tumor suppressor gene *EXT1* or *EXT2*. Enchondromas are benign cartilage tumors in the medullary canal. While transformation of a solitary enchondroma is rare, the overall rate of malignant transformation reaches 50% (lifetime; all sites) in patients with multiple enchondromas (enchondromatosis) from Ollier's disease or Maffucci syndrome, which are caused by somatic mutations in the *IDH1* or *IDH2* genes [49].

The molecular drivers in chondrosarcoma vary based on pathologic subtype and are best studied in central conventional chondrosarcoma [50]. Mutations in *isocitrate dehydrogenase 1* and *2* (*IDH1* and *IDH2*) are found in nearly all of enchondromas and most of primary central chondrosarcomas. Notably, this mutation is not found in chordoma, making it a useful diagnostic molecular marker. *IDH1* or *IDH2* mutations increase the oncometabolite D2-hydroxyglutarate (D2HG) which promotes tumorigenesis by inducing multiple epigenetic changes, affecting differentiation, and promoting chondrogenic differentiation of mesenchymal stem cells [51]. The physiologic process of enchondral ossification is tightly regulated by the Indian hedgehog (IHH) and parathyroid hormone-like hormone (PTHLH) signaling pathways. IHH pathway expression is high in enchondromas and central chondrosarcomas, maintaining tumor cells in a low differentiated proliferative state. In addition, IHH gene mutations have been identified in 18% of chondrosarcomas with exome sequencing [52]. Clinical trials targeting the IHH pathway have been unsuccessful thus far, however. Collagen type-II alpha1 (COL2A1) mutations have also been identified in 40% of central chondrosarcomas; however, the mutation's role as a driver or malignant transformation is unknown [53].

As in other cancer types, mutations in the p53 and pRb pathway are common. In both peripheral and central chondrosarcoma, these appear to be particularly important in the transition from low-to-high grade as the combined incidence of mutation in these pathways is 96% [54]. In patients with MHE, the absence of *EXT* gene products drives the formation of aberrant osteochondromas but has not been identified as sufficient for transformation to chondrosarcoma. Rather, a second alteration, most commonly in the p53 or pRb pathway is responsible for transformation from osteochondroma to peripheral chondrosarcoma [55]. Regarding the rare subtypes, mesenchymal chondrosarcoma has been characterized as having a specific gene fusion between *HEY1* and *NCOA2* though the mechanism of tumorigenesis is unknown [56].

Classification

As with other spinal tumors, chondrosarcoma can be classified based on location utilizing the Weinstein, Boariani, Biagini (WBB) classification system. Within vertebra, chondrosarcomas can be found in the body, posterior elements, or both [35]. Conventional chondrosarcoma most commonly is located in the vertebral body, whereas peripheral chondrosarcomas more commonly arise from the posterior elements. Sacral chondrosarcomas tend to be eccentrically located, often involving the sacroiliac joints [57].

Chondrosarcomas can also be divided into different subtypes reflecting different cell signaling pathways involved in tumorigenesis [43] (Table 7.2).

Conventional chondrosarcoma accounts for 85% of all subtypes (in all locations) and is categorized based on the lesion's location within the bone as central, peripheral, or periosteal. Central chondrosarcomas are the most common (75%) form, and arise de novo from the medullary canal or transformation of an enchondroma [46]. Peripheral chondrosarcomas, by definition, arise from secondary transformation of an osteochondroma cartilage cap. In both central and peripheral subtypes, progression toward chondrosarcoma is associated with molecular defects in apoptosis and prosurvival pathways. Deregulation of p53 and pRb pathways is observed in most high-grade conventional chondrosarcomas [48, 52].

Rare subtypes account for the remaining 15% of all chondrosarcomas (all sites) and include dedifferentiated chondrosarcoma, mesenchymal chondrosarcoma, clear cell chondrosarcoma, myxoid chondrosarcoma, and periosteal chondrosarcoma. Dedifferentiated chondrosarcoma is characterized by a juxtaposed cartilage tumor with a high-grade noncartilage sarcoma [54] (Fig. 7.11). Dedifferentiated tumors present in older patients, are associated with soft tissue masses, and have a poor prognosis, even in the absence of metastases [35, 46, 55, 56].

Mesenchymal chondrosarcomas are highly malignant and are histologically identified by areas of cartilage combined with areas of undifferentiated small round cells [46] (Fig. 7.12a,b). Mesenchymal tumors occur in younger patients, affect extraskeletal soft tissue, have a poor prognosis, and may recur locally or remotely at long-term follow-up [41, 49]. Clear cell chondrosarcoma is a low-grade subtype characterized by chondrocytes with abundant clear cytoplasm. These tumors are associated with elevated alkaline phosphatase and are low-grade but require long-term surveillance. Periosteal chondrosarcoma (previously termed juxtacortical) arises on the surface of bones, affects young patients, and has a good prognosis despite high histologic grade. Myxoid

Table 7.2 Characteristics of chondrosarcoma subtypes

	Conventional central chondrosarcoma	Conventional peripheral chondrosarcoma	Periosteal (juxtacortical) chondrosarcoma	Mesenchymal chondrosarcoma	Clear cell chondrosarcoma	Dedifferentiated chondrosarcoma
Percent incidence	75%	10%	1%	2%	2%	10%
Precursor lesion	Enchondroma	Osteochondroma	None	None	None	Conventional chondrosarcoma
Associated syndrome	Ollier's disease (enchondromatosis); Maffucci syndrome (enchondromatosis with hemangiomas)	Multiple hereditary osteochondromas (HMO)	None	None	None	None
Most common age range	50's–60's	40's	40's	50's–60's	Any age, peak 30's–50's	Any age, peak 30's–50's
Common locations	Throughout axial and appendicular skeleton	Shoulder girdle, pelvis	Distal humerus, distal femur	Axial skeleton, extra-skeletal (meninges)	Femoral and humeral epiphyses	Pelvis, femur
Frequent histologic grade	Low grade: ACT/CS1 or Grade II	Low grade: ACT/CS1 or Grade II	High grade	High grade	Low grade	High grade
Prognosis	Good if low grade	Good if low grade	Good (despite high grade histology)	Poor	Good	Poor
Chemotherapy sensitivity	Low	Low	Low	Possibly sensitive	Low	Low
Radiation therapy Sensitivity	Low	Low	Low	Sensitive	Low	Low

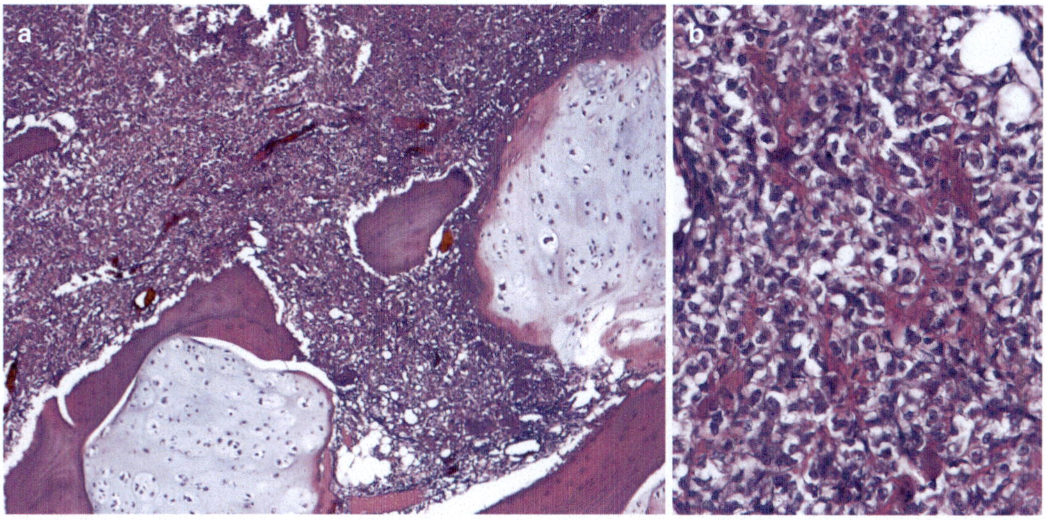

Fig. 7.11 (**a**) Dedifferentiated chondrosarcoma is demonstrated here. Two nodules of low-grade chondrosarcoma are present in the left lower and upper right portion. The dedifferentiated component is directly adjacent to these nodules, and has the appearance of conventional, high-grade osteosarcoma in this example. (H&E 40X). (**b**) Higher magnification of the dedifferentiated component shows sheets of epithelioid cells which are elaborating mineralized immature woven bone (osteoid) in the manner of osteosarcoma (H&E 200X)

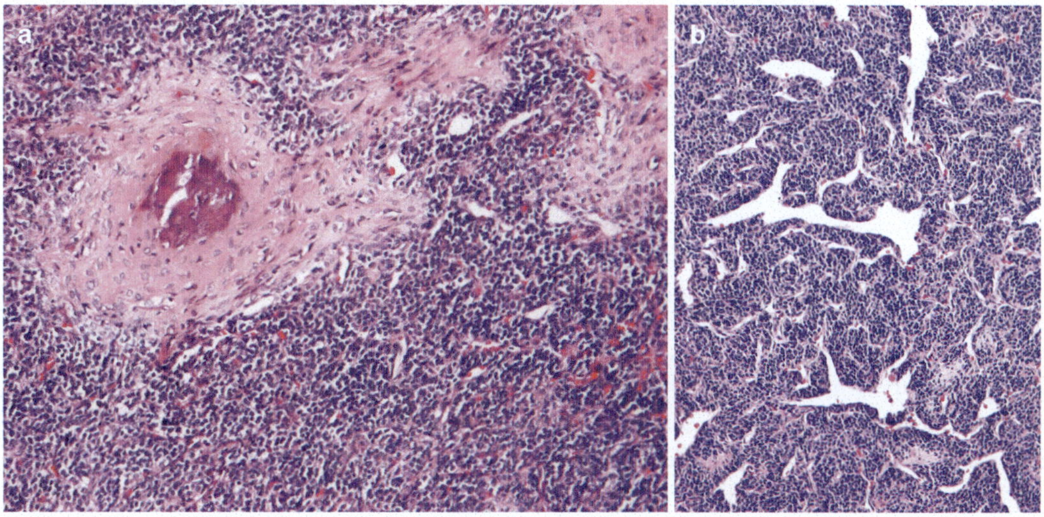

Fig. 7.12 (**a**) As seen here, mesenchymal chondrosarcoma is characterized by nodules of hyaline cartilage juxtaposed with a very cellular small blue round cell component (H&E 100X). (**b**) Gaping, staghorn-shaped vascular structured, also known as a pericytomatous vascular pattern, are typically present in the small blue round cell component of mesenchymal chondrosarcoma (H&E 100X)

chondrosarcoma are now typically considered variants of intermediate or high-grade conventional sarcoma and should be not be confused with extraskeletal myxoid chondrosarcoma (EMC) which is a separate soft tissue sarcoma entity [41, 49].

Diagnosis, Screening, and Staging

The clinical presentation of patients with spinal chondrosarcoma that resembles other spinal tumors is nonspecific and based on tumor location. As the vast majority of tumors are low grade, these masses grow insidiously and time to presentation varies widely as result from 1 week to 20 years. The most common presenting symptom is local pain (80%), as is nocturnal back pain unresponsive to rest [36, 53]. Patients with spinal chondrosarcoma have a high rate of neurological deficit at the time of presentation (24–50%) [46, 49, 56]. Symptoms may include radiculopathy, neurogenic claudication, weakness, abnormal tone, sensory deficits, bowel or bladder incontinence, and gait abnormalities. A palpable mass may also be present (34–40%) [46, 56].

Plain radiographs obtained to first evaluate nonspecific symptoms may demonstrate a lucent or dense lesion, which should prompt advanced cross-sectional imaging. Computed tomography (CT) and magnetic resonance (MR) are the preferred imaging modalities to distinguish chondrosarcoma from other spinal masses as well as to ascertain the tumor's relationship to adjacent structures. Although the wide range of pathologic subtypes leads to variability in the imaging appearance of chondrosarcoma, conventional primary tumor types accounting for 85% of cases are well described. Classically, chondrosarcoma demonstrates lytic bone destruction with "ring and arc" calcifications identifiable on plain radiographs and CT [46, 56]. As most chondrosarcomas have high water content, lesions are often attenuated on CT. Associated lobulated soft tissue components of nonmineralized hyaline cartilage have a high water content, identifiable as low density on CT, low-intermediate signal on T1-weighted MR, and high signal on T2-weighted MR. Peripheral or septal enhancement, or fluid levels may be present on gadolinium-enhanced images [57]. On MR, the high water content of chondrosarcoma lesions is demonstrated as T2-weighted high signal intensity and useful to lesion margins. The imaging features of the various histologic subtypes are variable and not typically used for subtype diagnosis. Mimicking lesions include giant cell tumors, plasmacytomas, and metastases. Imaging of the entire axial spine as well as consideration of whole-body positron emission tomographic (PET) scanning to evaluate for metastatic disease has been advocated, but there is no established guideline for the use of PET in the diagnostic and staging evaluation.

Biopsy is essential to establish definitive diagnosis. This is especially true in chondrosarcoma, which may represent a heterogeneous variety of subtypes. CT-guided fine-needle or core needle biopsy of the most aggressive-appearing areas has been demonstrated to have improved survival and local control compared to open biopsy. Mutation analysis of *IDH1* and *IDH2* may be useful in distinguishing chondrosarcoma from chondroblastic osteosarcoma [58]. Interobserver variability remains problematic in establishing histologic grade and subtype. In addition, the concordance between biopsy diagnosis and diagnosis after definitive surgery has been reported as low as 66% likely reflecting the effect of sampling error [56]. This underscores the importance of embracing a multidisciplinary approach correlating imaging findings with biopsy results.

As with other sarcomas, chondrosarcoma most commonly metastasizes to the lungs, followed by other osseous site, liver, and regional lymph nodes. For patients with intermediate- and high-grade chondrosarcoma, the rates of metastatic disease are much higher than ACT/CS1 (<10%) and require chest CT screening [46, 49]. Given the low rate of metastases in patients with ACT/CS1, imaging of the lungs is not routinely recommended. As with other bone sarcomas, the staging systems utilized for chondrosarcoma are the Enneking Staging System and the tumor, node, metastasis (TNM) staging system developed by the American Joint Committee on Cancer (AJCC).

Treatment

In the absence of reliably effective adjuvant therapies, surgical excision of conventional chondrosarcoma remains the mainstay of treatment as the only reliable chance for long-term disease-free survival. The lack of effective nonsurgical therapies has been the most limiting factor in improving disease-specific survival rates.

The specific surgical strategy may include intralesional curettage with or without adjuvant or wide resection [59]. For intermediate and high-grade chondrosarcoma or aggressive subtypes, wide en bloc excision is recommended to achieve tumor-free margins [46] (Fig. 7.13a–e). For low-grade lesions, wide local excision is also the preferred treatment as higher rates of metastasis and local recurrence have been noted with marginal excision. Multiple studies have documented 100% recurrence rates of patients treated with intralesional excision [59, 60]. In the spine, however, the intimate relationship of neurovascular structures and need for stabilization may make intralesional curettage the only option available. Specifically, Boriani et al.

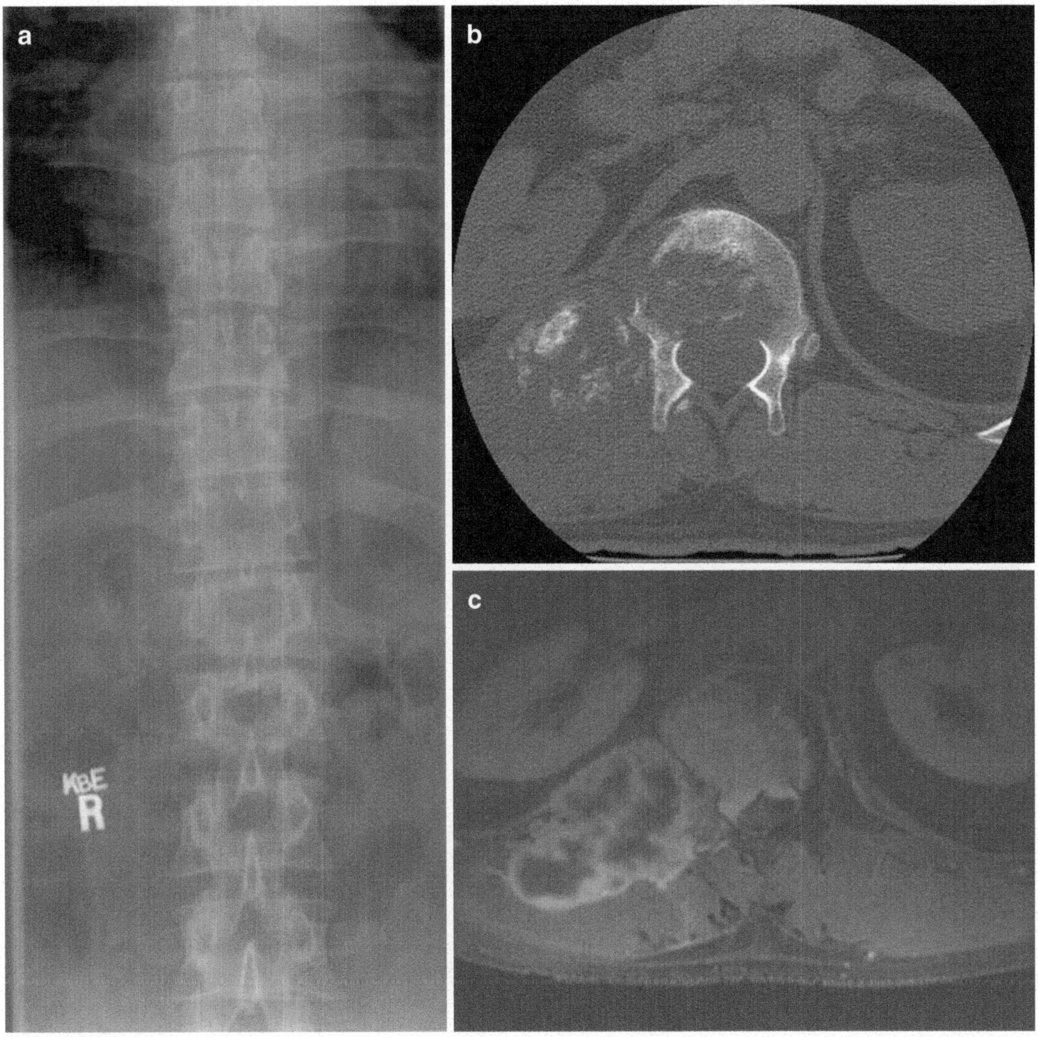

Fig. 7.13 The case is a 30-year-old male with right-sided back pain and a right-sided T12 tumor extending into the right T12 rib. (**a**) AP radiograph of the thoracic spine demonstrating a lytic and destructive lesion on the right side contributing to a T12 vertebral body deformity with "ring and arc" calcifications seen affecting the right T12 rib. (**b**) Axial CT image demonstrating lytic bony destruction of the T12 vertebral body and the calcified mass on the right side affecting the T12 rib and costovertebral articulation. (**c**) Axial MRI image demonstrating the tumor involving the vertebral body and extending into the right rib invading the paraspinal musculature and retroperitoneal space. There is significant spinal cord compression seen ventrally with displacement of the spinal cord to the left. (**d**) Clinical picture of the resected tumor including the T12 vertebral body and surrounding ribs after surgical resection using Tomita saws. The surgery consisted of two stages with the first stage using the posterior approach and the second stage utilizing the lateral approach. (**e**) Postoperative AP and lateral radiographs demonstrating the anterior and posterior reconstruction following en bloc resection

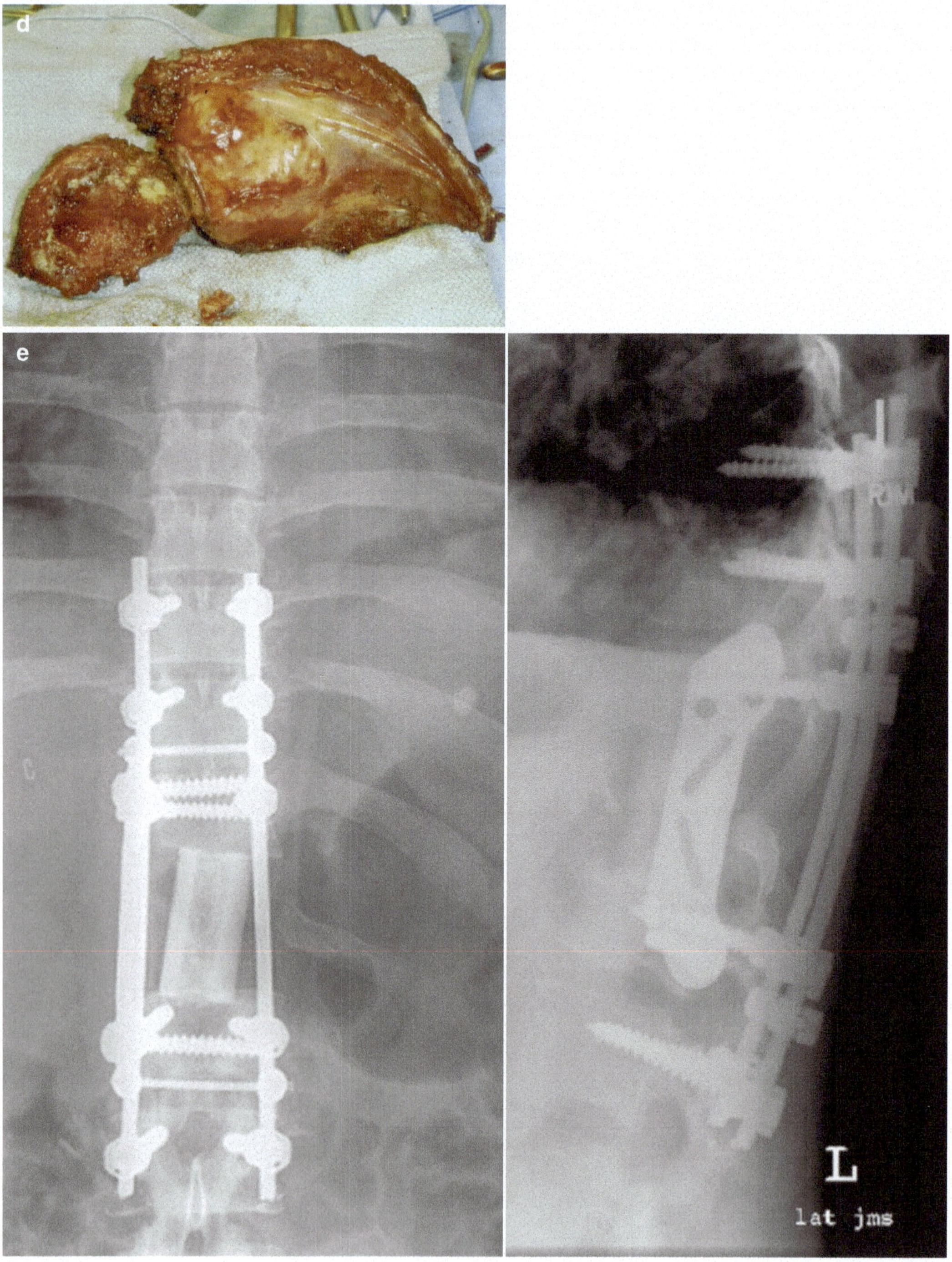

Fig. 7.13 (continued)

proposed the criteria directing treatment toward curettage to include circumferential spinal canal involvement, the need for cord ligation to complete en bloc resection, and the potential for cord ischemia from spinal segmental artery ligation [36].

While en bloc resection has improved clinical results in chondrosarcoma, these patients are at high risk for major complications and require adequate preoperative counseling, optimization, and multidisciplinary care. Recent surgical techniques to improve outcomes include the use of staged procedures, aortic balloon pumps, intraoperative navigation, and the use of vascularized muscle flaps to repair soft tissue defects [34, 46, 61]. Surgical adjuvants include phenol, cryotherapy, heat ablation, and intraoperative radiation to target microscopically invaded dura [62].

Radiation therapy for spinal chondrosarcoma has been given in preoperative, adjuvant, and definitive settings, in cases deemed unresectable or for palliation [63]. In the absence of surgical excision, radiation offers inferior local control; however, tumor-free margins may be difficult to achieve in the spine without significant morbidity. Modalities available include external beam radiotherapy with photons or charged particles including protons and cobalt, and intraoperative plaque brachytherapy [64].

Improvements in three-dimensional treatment planning with intensity-modulated radiation therapy (IMRT) has enabled safe delivery of higher radiation doses to the tumor while excluding adjacent structures including the spinal cord. Importantly, the Spine Oncology Study group (SOSG) expert opinion now recommends 60–65Gy equivalent adjuvant radiation therapy for chondrosarcoma following incomplete resection or lacking tumor-free margins to improve local control [65]. In addition to conventional photon irradiation, alternative radiation modalities have been utilized including stereotactic radiosurgery (SRS) and radiation with protons and carbon ions [64]. The long-term results for these modalities have not been established for spinal chondrosarcoma, however.

Data on these treatments for spinal chondrosarcoma are very limited with no randomized controlled trials; however, results have been promising in skull base chondrosarcoma where en bloc surgical resection is less common. Compared to radiation for chordoma, lower doses in the range of 70 cobalt gray equivalents (CGE) are recommended for chondrosarcoma gross disease [64, 66].

While external beam radiotherapy is generally well tolerated, there are site-specific toxicities reported including hypothyroidism, pharyngitis, fistulas, insufficiency fractures, and wound dehiscence [60, 64]. One study reported sacral insufficiency fractures in 47% of patients treated with pre- and postoperative radiotherapy doses of 50 Gy and 20 Gy, respectively [67]. SRS also has reported complications including acute spinal cord myelopathy and late vocal cord paralysis [68].

Metastatic disease remains a significant concern as over 30% of patients with intermediate- to high-grade chondrosarcoma die of metastases. Histologically, these pulmonary metastases are almost always identical to the primary tumor. Chemotherapy is ineffective for chondrosarcoma, with the exception of mesenchymal and dedifferentiated subtypes, for which adjuvant chemotherapy has been shown to have a survival benefit [46]. In particular, the limited evidence available suggests that mesenchymal chondrosarcomas demonstrate sensitivity to doxorubicin-based combination chemotherapy [69]. Resistance to chemotherapy in conventional chondrosarcoma is multifactorial. Conventional chemotherapeutic agents targeting actively dividing cells may not be effective against the slow-growing chondrosarcoma tumor cells [46, 70]. Chondrosarcoma cells also express the multidrug-resistance 1 gene P-glycoprotein and express a high level of Bcl-2 genes in the anti-apoptotic and prosurvival pathways [71]. The tumor architecture of high extracellular matrix and poor vascularity may also limit chemotherapy penetration physically.

Drugs in phase-II trial include the c-SRC tyrosine kinase inhibitor, dasatinib; the serine/threonine kinase Akt inhibitor, perifosine; and the proapoptotic agonist of Apo2L/ tumor necrosis factor receptor apoptosis-inducing ligand (TRAIL) [72–7]. The high molecular weight melanoma-associated antigen CSPG4 has been identified as a biomarker of poor prognosis and is a potential future target for immunotherapy [8]. Other potential targets include alterations in the pathways related to the IDH enzyme which is effected in Maffuci's syndrome, the p16 and p53 malignant transformation of enchondroma, the altered expression of *EXT* in MHE, and pathways involving IHH and PTHLH [46].

Post-Treatment Surveillance

There is no prospective data to support a specific post-treatment surveillance protocol for chondrosarcoma. The National Comprehensive Cancer Network (NCCN) consensus guidelines recommend physical examination, serology including complete blood count, and local imaging every 3 months for 2 years, 4 months for year 3, 6 months for years 4 and 5, and then annually.

References

1. Sebro R, DeLaney T, Hornicek F, Schwab J, Choy E, Nielsen GP, Rosenthal DI. Differences in sex distribution, anatomic location and MR imaging appearance of pediatric compared to adult chordomas. BMC Med Imaging. 2016;16(1):53. https://doi.org/10.1186/s12880-016-0149-5.
2. Walcott BP, Nahed BV, Mohyeldin A, Coumans JV, Kahle KT, Ferreira MJ. Chordoma: current concepts, management, and future directions. Lancet Oncol. 2012;13(2):e69–76. https://doi.org/10.1016/S1470-2045(11)70337-0.
3. Vujovic S, Henderson S, Presneau N, Odell E, Jacques TS, Tirabosco R, Boshoff C, Flanagan AM. Brachyury, a crucial regulator of notochordal development, is a novel biomarker for chordomas. J Pathol. 2006;209(2):157–65. https://doi.org/10.1002/path.1969.
4. Ghaly M, Seelemann C, Jahani-Asl A. A focused compound screen highlights the significance of epidermal growth factor receptor signalling in chordoma pathogenesis. J Pathol. 2016;240(4):381–3. https://doi.org/10.1002/path.4780.
5. Hoch BL, Nielsen GP, Liebsch NJ, Rosenberg AE. Base of skull chordomas in children and adolescents: a clinicopathologic study of 73 cases. Am J Surg Pathol. 2006;30(7):811–8. https://doi.org/10.1097/01.pas.0000209828.39477.ab.
6. Camidge DR, Herbst RS, Gordon MS, Eckhardt SG, Kurzrock R, Durbin B, Ing J, Tohnya TM, Sager J, Ashkenazi A, Bray G, Mendelson D. A phase I safety and pharmacokinetic study of the death receptor 5 agonistic antibody PRO95780 in patients with advanced malignancies. Clin Cancer Res. 2010;16(4):1256–63. https://doi.org/10.1158/1078-0432.CCR-09-1267.
7. Herbst RS, Eckhardt SG, Kurzrock R, Ebbinghaus S, O'Dwyer PJ, Gordon MS, Novotny W, Goldwasser MA, Tohnya TM, Lum BL, Ashkenazi A, Jubb AM, Mendelson DS. Phase I dose-escalation study of recombinant human Apo2L/TRAIL, a dual proapoptotic receptor agonist, in patients with advanced cancer. J Clin Oncol. 2010;28(17):2839–46. https://doi.org/10.1200/JCO.2009.25.1991.
8. Schoenfeld AJ, Wang X, Wang Y, Hornicek FJ, Nielsen GP, Duan Z, Ferrone S, Schwab JH. CSPG4 as a prognostic biomarker in chordoma. Spine J. 2016;16(6):722–7. https://doi.org/10.1016/j.spinee.2015.11.059.
9. Fernando RI, Litzinger M, Trono P, Hamilton DH, Schlom J, Palena C. The T-box transcription factor Brachyury promotes epithelial-mesenchymal transition in human tumor cells. J Clin Invest. 2010;120(2):533–44. https://doi.org/10.1172/JCI38379.
10. Rosenberg AE, Brown GA, Bhan AK, Lee JM. Chondroid chordoma--a variant of chordoma. A morphologic and immunohistochemical study. Am J Clin Pathol. 1994;101(1):36–41. https://doi.org/10.1093/ajcp/101.1.36.
11. Shih AR, Cote GM, Chebib I, Choy E, DeLaney T, Deshpande V, Hornicek FJ, Miao R, Schwab JH, Nielsen GP, Chen YL. Clinicopathologic characteristics of poorly differentiated chordoma. Mod Pathol. 2018;31(8):1237–45. https://doi.org/10.1038/s41379-018-0002-1.
12. Boriani S, Chevalley F, Weinstein JN, Biagini R, Campanacci L, De Iure F, Piccill P. Chordoma of the spine above the sacrum. Treatment and outcome in 21 cases. Spine (Phila Pa 1976). 1996;21(13):1569–77.
13. Arain A, Hornicek FJ, Schwab JH, Chebib I, Damron TA. Chordoma arising from benign multifocal notochordal tumors. Skelet Radiol. 2017;46(12):1745–52. https://doi.org/10.1007/s00256-017-2727-1.
14. Rodallec MH, Feydy A, Larousserie F, Anract P, Campagna R, Babinet A, Zins M, Drape JL. Diagnostic imaging of solitary tumors of the spine: what to do and say. Radiographics. 2008;28(4):1019–41. https://doi.org/10.1148/rg.284075156.
15. Ropper AE, Cahill KS, Hanna JW, McCarthy EF, Gokaslan ZL, Chi JH. Primary vertebral tumors: a review of epidemiologic, histological and imaging findings, part II: locally aggressive and malignant tumors. Neurosurgery. 2012;70(1):211–9; discussion 219. https://doi.org/10.1227/NEU.0b013e31822d5f17.
16. Stacchiotti S, Sommer J. Building a global consensus approach to chordoma: a position paper from the medical and patient community. Lancet Oncol. 2015;16(e):71–83. https://doi.org/10.1016/S1470-2045(14)71190-8.
17. Houdek MT, Rose PS, Hevesi M, Schwab JH, Griffin AM, Healey JH, Petersen IA, DeLaney TF, Chung PW, Yaszemski MJ, Wunder JS, Hornicek FJ, Boland PJ, Sim FH, Ferguson PC, Other Members of the Sacral Tumor Society. Low dose radiotherapy is associated with local complications but not disease control in sacral chordoma. J Surg Oncol. 2019;119(7):856–63. https://doi.org/10.1002/jso.25399.
18. Rotondo RL, Folkert W, Liebsch NJ, Chen YL, Pedlow FX, Schwab JH, Rosenberg AE, Nielsen GP, Szymonifka J, Ferreira AE, Hornicek FJ, DeLaney TF. High-dose proton-based radiation therapy in the management of spine chordomas: outcomes and clini-

copathological prognostic factors. J Neurosurg Spine. 2015;23(6):788–97. https://doi.org/10.3171/2015.3.SPINE14716.
19. Ji T, Guo W, Yang R, Tang X, Wang Y, Huang L. What are the conditional survival and functional outcomes after surgical treatment of 115 patients with sacral chordoma? Clin Orthop Relat Res. 2017;475(3):620–30. https://doi.org/10.1007/s11999-016-4773-8.
20. Zou MX, Huang W, Wang XB, Li J, Lv GH, Deng YW. Prognostic factors in spinal chordoma: a systematic review. Clin Neurol Neurosurg. 2015;139:110–8. https://doi.org/10.1016/j.clineuro.2015.09.012.
21. Imai R, Kamada T, Araki N, Working Group for Bone and Soft Tissue Sarcomas. Carbon ion radiation therapy for unresectable sacral chordoma: an analysis of 188 cases. Int J Radiat Oncol Biol Phys. 2016;95(1):322–7. https://doi.org/10.1016/j.ijrobp.2016.02.012.
22. Shalaby A, Presneau N, Ye H, Halai D, Berisha F, Idowu B, Leithner A, Liegl B, Briggs TR, Bacsi K, Kindblom LG, Athanasou N, Amary MF, Hogendoorn PC, Tirabosco R, Flanagan AM. The role of epidermal growth factor receptor in chordoma pathogenesis: a potential therapeutic target. J Pathol. 2011;223(3):336–46. https://doi.org/10.1002/path.2818.
23. Liu T, Shen JK, Choy E, Zhang Y, Mankin HJ, Hornicek FJ, Duan Z. CDK4 expression in chordoma: a potential therapeutic target. J Orthop Res. 2018;36(6):1581–9. https://doi.org/10.1002/jor.23819.
24. Chen H, Garbutt CC, Spentzos D, Choy E, Hornicek FJ, Duan Z. Expression and therapeutic potential of SOX9 in chordoma. Clin Cancer Res. 2017;23(17):5176–86. https://doi.org/10.1158/1078-0432.CCR-17-0177.
25. Young VA, Curtis KM, Temple HT, Eismont FJ, DeLaney TF, Hornicek FJ. Characteristics and patterns of metastatic disease from chordoma. Sarcoma. 2015;2015:517657. https://doi.org/10.1155/2015/517657.
26. Gokaslan ZL, Zadnik PL, Sciubba DM, Germscheid N, Goodwin CR, Wolinsky JP, Bettegowda C, Groves ML, Luzzati A, Rhines LD, Fisher CG, Varga PP, Dekutoski MB, Clarke MJ, Fehlings MG, Quraishi NA, Chou D, Reynolds JJ, Williams RP, Kawahara N, Boriani S. Mobile spine chordoma: results of 166 patients from the AOSpine knowledge forum tumor database. J Neurosurg Spine. 2016;24(4):644–51. https://doi.org/10.3171/2015.7.SPINE15201.
27. Radaelli S, Stacchiotti S, Ruggieri P, Donati D, Casali PG, Palmerini E, Collini P, Gambarotti M, Porcu L, Boriani S, Gronchi A, Picci P. Sacral chordoma: long-term outcome of a large series of patients surgically treated at two reference centers. Spine (Phila Pa 1976). 2016;41(12):1049–57. https://doi.org/10.1097/BRS.0000000000001604.
28. Kayani B, Hanna SA, Sewell MD, Saifuddin A, Molloy S, Briggs TW. A review of the surgical management of sacral chordoma. Eur J Surg Oncol. 2014;40(11):1412–20. https://doi.org/10.1016/j.ejso.2014.04.008.
29. Gatfield ER, Noble DJ, Barnett GC, Early NY, Hoole ACF, Kirkby NF, Jefferies SJ, Burnet NG. Tumour volume and dose influence outcome after surgery and high-dose photon radiotherapy for chordoma and chondrosarcoma of the skull base and spine. Clin Oncol (R Coll Radiol). 2018;30(4):243–53. https://doi.org/10.1016/j.clon.2018.01.002.
30. Chen YL, Liebsch N, Kobayashi W, Goldberg S, Kirsch D, Calkins G, Childs S, Schwab J, Hornicek F, DeLaney T. Definitive high-dose photon/proton radiotherapy for unresected mobile spine and sacral chordomas. Spine (Phila Pa 1976). 2013;38(15):E930–6. https://doi.org/10.1097/BRS.0b013e318296e7d7.
31. Freeman JL, Kaufmann AB, Everson RG, DeMonte F, Raza SM. Evidence-based optimization of post-treatment surveillance for skull base chordomas based on local and distant disease progression. Operative Neurosurg. 2019;16(1):27–36. https://doi.org/10.1093/ons/opy073.
32. Stacchiotti S, Gronchi A, Fossati P, Akiyama T, Alapetite C, Baumann M, Blay JY, Bolle S, Poriani S, Bruzzi P, Papanna R, Caraceni A, Casadei R, Colia V, Debus J, other members of the Chordoma Global Consensus Group. Best practices for the management of local-regional recurrent Chordoma: a position paper by the Chordoma Global Consensus Group. Ann Oncol. 2017;28(6):1230–42. https://doi.org/10.1093/annonc/mdx054.
33. Dorfman HD, Czerniak B. Bone cancers. Cancer. 1995;75(1 Suppl):203–10. https://doi.org/10.1002/1097-0142(19950101)75:1+<203::aid-cncr2820751308>3.0.co;2-v.
34. Biermann JS, Chow W, Reed DR, Lucas D, Adkins DR, Agulnik M, Benjamin RS, Brigman B, Budd GT, Curry WT, Didwania A, Fabbri N, Hornicek FJ, Kuechle JB, Lindskog D, Mayerson J, McGarry SV, Million L, Morris CD, Movva S, O'Donnell RJ, Randall RL, Rose P, Santana VM, Satcher RL, Schwartz H, Siegel HJ, Thornton K, Villalobos V, Bergman MA, Scavone JL. NCCN guidelines insights: bone Cancer, version 2.2017. J Natl Compr Cancer Netw. 2017;15(2):155–67.
35. Arshi A, Sharim J, Park DY, Park HY, Bernthal NM, Yazdanshenas H, Shamie AN. Chondrosarcoma of the osseous spine: an analysis of epidemiology, patient outcomes, and prognostic factors using the SEER registry from 1973 to 2012. Spine (Phila Pa 1976). 2017;42(9):644–52. https://doi.org/10.1097/BRS.0000000000001870.
36. Boriani S, Weinstein JN, Biagini R. Primary bone tumors of the spine. Terminology and surgical staging. Spine (Phila Pa 1976). 1997;22(9):1036–44. https://doi.org/10.1097/00007632-199705010-00020.
37. Fisher CG, Versteeg AL, Dea N, Boriani S, Varga PP, Dekutoski MB, Luzzati A, Gokaslan ZL, Williams RP, Reynolds JJ, Fehlings MG, Germscheid NM,

Bettegowda C, Rhines LD. Surgical Management of Spinal Chondrosarcomas. Spine (Phila Pa 1976). 2016;41(8):678–85. https://doi.org/10.1097/BRS.0000000000001485.
38. Giuffrida AY, Burgueno JE, Koniaris LG, Gutierrez JC, Duncan R, Scully SP. Chondrosarcoma in the United States (1973 to 2003): an analysis of 2890 cases from the SEER database. J Bone Joint Surg Am. 2009;91(5):1063–72. https://doi.org/10.2106/JBJS.H.00416.
39. Evans HL, Ayala AG, Romsdahl MM. Prognostic factors in chondrosarcoma of bone: a clinicopathologic analysis with emphasis on histologic grading. Cancer. 1977;40(2):818–31. https://doi.org/10.1002/1097-0142(197708)40:2<818::aid-cncr2820400234>3.0.co;2-b.
40. Fiorenza F, Abudu A, Grimer RJ, Carter SR, Tillman RM, Ayoub K, Mangham DC, Davies AM. Risk factors for survival and local control in chondrosarcoma of bone. J Bone Joint Surg Br. 2002;84(1):93–9.
41. Gelderblom H, Hogendoorn PC, Dijkstra SD, van Rijswijk CS, Krol AD, Taminiau AH, Bovee JV. The clinical approach towards chondrosarcoma. Oncologist. 2008;13(3):320–9. https://doi.org/10.1634/theoncologist.2007-0237.
42. Fletcher CDM, World Health Organization, International Agency for Research on Cancer. WHO classification of tumours of soft tissue and bone. In: World Health Organization classification of tumours. 4th ed. Geneva: World Health Organization; 2013.
43. Angelini A, Guerra G, Mavrogenis AF, Pala E, Picci P, Ruggieri P. Clinical outcome of central conventional chondrosarcoma. J Surg Oncol. 2012;106(8):929–37. https://doi.org/10.1002/jso.23173.
44. Eefting D, Schrage YM, Geirnaerdt MJ, Le Cessie S, Taminiau AH, Bovee JV, Hogendoorn PC, Tc EBN. Assessment of interobserver variability and histologic parameters to improve reliability in classification and grading of central cartilaginous tumors. Am J Surg Pathol. 2009;33(1):50–7. https://doi.org/10.1097/PAS.0b013e31817eec2b.
45. de Andrea CE, Kroon HM, Wolterbeek R, Romeo S, Rosenberg AE, De Young BR, Liegl B, Inwards CY, Hauben E, McCarthy EF, Idoate M, Athanasou NA, Jones KB, Hogendoorn PC, Bovee JV. Interobserver reliability in the histopathological diagnosis of cartilaginous tumors in patients with multiple osteochondromas. Mod Pathol. 2012;25(9):1275–83. https://doi.org/10.1038/modpathol.2012.78.
46. Harsh GR, Vaz-Guimaraes F. Chordomas and chondrosarcomas of the skull base and spine. London: Academic Press; 2018.
47. Bovee JV, Hogendoorn PC, Wunder JS, Alman BA. Cartilage tumours and bone development: molecular pathology and possible therapeutic targets. Nat Rev Cancer. 2010;10(7):481–8. https://doi.org/10.1038/nrc2869.
48. Pansuriya TC, van Eijk R, d'Adamo P, van Ruler MA, Kuijjer ML, Oosting J, Cleton-Jansen AM, van Oosterwijk JG, Verbeke SL, Meijer D, van Wezel T, Nord KH, Sangiorgi L, Toker B, Liegl-Atzwanger B, San-Julian M, Sciot R, Limaye N, Kindblom LG, Daugaard S, Godfraind C, Boon LM, Vikkula M, Kurek KC, Szuhai K, French PJ, Bovee JV. Somatic mosaic IDH1 and IDH2 mutations are associated with enchondroma and spindle cell hemangioma in Ollier disease and Maffucci syndrome. Nat Genet. 2011;43(12):1256–61. https://doi.org/10.1038/ng.1004.
49. Chow WA. Chondrosarcoma: biology, genetics, and epigenetics. F1000Res. 2018;7 https://doi.org/10.12688/f1000research.15953.1.
50. Tarpey PS, Behjati S, Cooke SL, Van Loo P, Wedge DC, Pillay N, Marshall J, O'Meara S, Davies H, Nik-Zainal S, Beare D, Butler A, Gamble J, Hardy C, Hinton J, Jia MM, Jayakumar A, Jones D, Latimer C, Maddison M, Martin S, McLaren S, Menzies A, Mudie L, Raine K, Teague JW, Tubio JM, Halai D, Tirabosco R, Amary F, Campbell PJ, Stratton MR, Flanagan AM, Futreal PA. Frequent mutation of the major cartilage collagen gene COL2A1 in chondrosarcoma. Nat Genet. 2013;45(8):923–6. https://doi.org/10.1038/ng.2668.
51. Schrage YM, Briaire-de Bruijn IH, de Miranda NF, van Oosterwijk J, Taminiau AH, van Wezel T, Hogendoorn PC, Bovee JV. Kinome profiling of chondrosarcoma reveals SRC-pathway activity and dasatinib as option for treatment. Cancer Res. 2009;69(15):6216–22. https://doi.org/10.1158/0008-5472.CAN-08-4801.
52. Wang L, Motoi T, Khanin R, Olshen A, Mertens F, Bridge J, Dal Cin P, Antonescu CR, Singer S, Hameed M, Bovee JV, Hogendoorn PC, Socci N, Ladanyi M. Identification of a novel, recurrent HEY1-NCOA2 fusion in mesenchymal chondrosarcoma based on a genome-wide screen of exon-level expression data. Genes Chromosomes Cancer. 2012;51(2):127–39. https://doi.org/10.1002/gcc.20937.
53. Stuckey RM, Marco RA. Chondrosarcoma of the mobile spine and sacrum. Sarcoma. 2011;2011:274281. https://doi.org/10.1155/2011/274281.
54. Hameetman L, Kok P, Eilers PH, Cleton-Jansen AM, Hogendoorn PC, Bovee JV. The use of Bcl-2 and PTHLH immunohistochemistry in the diagnosis of peripheral chondrosarcoma in a clinicopathological setting. Virchows Arch. 2005;446(4):430–7. https://doi.org/10.1007/s00428-005-1208-4.
55. Grimer RJ, Gosheger G, Taminiau A, Biau D, Matejovsky Z, Kollender Y, San-Julian M, Gherlinzoni F, Ferrari C. Dedifferentiated chondrosarcoma: prognostic factors and outcome from a European group. Eur J Cancer. 2007;43(14):2060–5. https://doi.org/10.1016/j.ejca.2007.06.016.
56. Lin PP. Bone sarcoma: MD Anderson cancer care series. New York: Springer; 2012.
57. Mechri M, Riahi H, Sboui I, Bouaziz M, Vanhoenacker F, Ladeb M. Imaging of malignant primitive tumors of the spine. J Belg Soc Radiol. 2018;102(1):56. https://doi.org/10.5334/jbsr.1410.

58. Kerr DA, Lopez HU, Deshpande V, Hornicek FJ, Duan Z, Zhang Y, Rosenberg AE, Borger DR, Nielsen GP. Molecular distinction of chondrosarcoma from chondroblastic osteosarcoma through IDH1/2 mutations. Am J Surg Pathol. 2013;37(6):787–95. https://doi.org/10.1097/PAS.0b013e31827ab703.
59. Zoccali C, Baldi J, Attala D, Rossi B, Anelli V, Annovazzi A, Ferraresi V. Intralesional vs. extralesional procedures for low-grade central chondrosarcoma: a systematic review of the literature. Arch Orthop Trauma Surg. 2018;138(7):929–37. https://doi.org/10.1007/s00402-018-2930-0.
60. Schoenfeld AJ, Hornicek FJ, Pedlow FX, Kobayashi W, Raskin KA, Springfield D, DeLaney TF, Nielsen GP, Mankin HJ, Schwab JH. Chondrosarcoma of the mobile spine: a review of 21 cases treated at a single center. Spine (Phila Pa 1976). 2012;37(2):119–26. https://doi.org/10.1097/BRS.0b013e31823d2143.
61. Brown MJ, Kor DJ, Curry TB, Warner MA, Rodrigues ES, Rose SH, Dekutoski MB, Moriarty JP, Long KH, Rose PS. Sacral tumor resection: the effect of surgical staging on patient outcomes, resource management, and hospital cost. Spine (Phila Pa 1976). 2011;36(19):1570–8. https://doi.org/10.1097/BRS.0b013e3181f6137d.
62. DeLaney TF, Chen GT, Mauceri TC, Munro JJ, Hornicek FJ, Pedlow FX, Suit HD. Intraoperative dural irradiation by customized 192iridium and 90yttrium brachytherapy plaques. Int J Radiat Oncol Biol Phys. 2003;57(1):239–45. https://doi.org/10.1016/s0360-3016(03)00505-4.
63. De Amorim BK, DeLaney T. Chordomas and chondrosarcomas-the role of radiation therapy. J Surg Oncol. 2016;114(5):564–9. https://doi.org/10.1002/jso.24368.
64. DeLaney TF, Liebsch NJ, Pedlow FX, Adams J, Weyman EA, Yeap BY, Depauw N, Nielsen GP, Harmon DC, Yoon SS, Chen YL, Schwab JH, Hornicek FJ. Long-term results of phase II study of high dose photon/proton radiotherapy in the management of spine chordomas, chondrosarcomas, and other sarcomas. J Surg Oncol. 2014;110(2):115–22. https://doi.org/10.1002/jso.23617.
65. Boriani S, Saravanja D, Yamada Y, Varga PP, Biagini R, Fisher CG. Challenges of local recurrence and cure in low grade malignant tumors of the spine. Spine (Phila Pa 1976). 2009;34(22 Suppl):S48–57. https://doi.org/10.1097/BRS.0b013e3181b969ac.
66. Holliday EB, Mitra HS, Somerson JS, Rhines LD, Mahajan A, Brown PD, Grosshans DR. Postoperative proton therapy for chordomas and chondrosarcomas of the spine: adjuvant versus salvage radiation therapy. Spine (Phila Pa 1976). 2015;40(8):544–9. https://doi.org/10.1097/BRS.0000000000000804.
67. Osler P, Bredella MA, Hess KA, Janssen SJ, Park CJ, Chen YL, DeLaney TF, Hornicek FJ, Schwab JH. Sacral insufficiency fractures are common after high-dose radiation for sacral chordomas treated with or without surgery. Clin Orthop Relat Res. 2016;474(3):766–72. https://doi.org/10.1007/s11999-015-4566-5.
68. Yamada Y, Laufer I, Cox BW, Lovelock DM, Maki RG, Zatcky JM, Boland PJ, Bilsky MH. Preliminary results of high-dose single-fraction radiotherapy for the management of chordomas of the spine and sacrum. Neurosurgery. 2013;73(4):673–80; discussion 680. https://doi.org/10.1227/NEU.0000000000000083.
69. Nooij MA, Whelan J, Bramwell VH, Taminiau AT, Cannon S, Hogendoorn PC, Pringle J, Uscinska BM, Weeden S, Kirkpatrick A, Glabbeke M, Craft AW, European Osteosarcoma I. Doxorubicin and cisplatin chemotherapy in high-grade spindle cell sarcomas of the bone, other than osteosarcoma or malignant fibrous histiocytoma: a European Osteosarcoma Intergroup Study. Eur J Cancer. 2005;41(2):225–30. https://doi.org/10.1016/j.ejca.2004.08.026.
70. Boehme KA, Schleicher SB, Traub F, Rolauffs B. Chondrosarcoma: a rare misfortune in aging human cartilage? The role of stem and progenitor cells in proliferation, malignant degeneration and therapeutic resistance. Int J Mol Sci. 2018;19(1) https://doi.org/10.3390/ijms19010311.
71. Terek RM. Recent advances in the basic science of chondrosarcoma. Orthop Clin North Am. 2006;37(1):9–14. https://doi.org/10.1016/j.ocl.2005.09.001.
72. Schuetze SM, Bolejack V, Choy E, Ganjoo KN, Staddon AP, Chow WA, Tawbi HA, Samuels BL, Patel SR, von Mehren M, D'Amato G, Leu KM, Loeb DM, Forscher CA, Milhem MM, Rushing DA, Lucas DR, Chugh R, Reinke DK, Baker LH. Phase 2 study of dasatinib in patients with alveolar soft part sarcoma, chondrosarcoma, chordoma, epithelioid sarcoma, or solitary fibrous tumor. Cancer. 2017;123(1):90–7. https://doi.org/10.1002/cncr.30379.

High-Grade Primary Spinal Malignancies

8

Marco Girolami, Riccardo Ghermandi, and Alessandro Gasbarrini

Introduction

Primary spine tumors are rare entities representing only 10% of spinal tumors with a prevalence of 2.5–8.5 cases/100,000 persons/year. The spinal location of these high-grade tumors in particular makes treatment challenging with high rates of local recurrence compared to appendicular skeleton location. This is despite the tremendous advancements that have occurred by applying modern oncologic principles to the spine [1–3]. Due to their rapid progression rate, pain as a presenting symptom is frequently accompanied by early neurologic compromise or pathological fracture.

This chapter provides an overview of primary high-grade malignant tumors of the spine and also outlines treatment strategies.

Overview of Primary Bone and Soft Tissue Tumors

Many primary bone and soft tissue tumors can involve the spine (Table 8.1). Although some primary malignancies such as Ewing sarcoma and osteosarcoma are traditionally considered high grade, most diseases fall along a spectrum of variable grading depending on the individual tumor histologic analysis. For example, tumors such as chondrosarcoma or chordoma are traditionally considered low grade, but may present in undifferentiated or dedifferentiated high-grade forms.

Clinical Presentation

The rapid progression rate of these diseases explains pain as the most common and almost constant presenting symptom. Pain typically results from periosteal stretching, epidural involvement (the so-called biological pain), and/or by a pathological fracture ("mechanical pain"). The first is a dull ache, constantly present and worsened at night that does not relieve with recumbency, which is the specific finding of biologic pain. Mechanical pain presents more commonly with ambulation and activity.

Neurological deficit can be an early finding caused by extracompartmental epidural extension of the tumor with compression of the neurologic structures (spinal cord, cauda equina, and/or spinal nerves) or by a pathological fracture. These scenarios can occur alone but most frequently present with a combination of the two.

M. Girolami (✉) · R. Ghermandi · A. Gasbarrini
Department of Oncologic and Degenerative Spine Surgery, IRCCS Istituto Ortopedico Rizzoli, Bologna, Italy

K. Singh, M. Colman (eds.), *Surgical Spinal Oncology*,
https://doi.org/10.1007/978-3-030-50722-0_8

Table 8.1 Primary bone and soft tissue tumor overview

Bone tumors	Soft tissue tumors
Osteogenic tumors Low-grade central osteosarcoma Conventional osteosarcoma *Chondroblastic* *Fibroblastic* *Osteoblastic* Teleangectatic osteosarcoma Small cell osteosarcoma Secondary osteosarcoma Parosteal osteosarcoma Periosteal osteosarcoma High-grade surface osteosarcoma	*Adipocytic tumors* Liposarcoma *Myxoid* *Pleomorphic* *Dedifferentiated*
Cartilage tumors Chondrosarcoma *Grade II, grade III* Dedifferentiated chondrosarcoma Mesenchymal chondrosarcoma Clear cell chondrosarcoma	*(Myo-)/fibroblastic tumors* Fibrosarcoma *Adult* *Myxofibrosarcoma* *Low-grade fibromyxoid fibrosarcoma* *Sclerosing epithelioid fibrosarcoma*
Fibrogenic tumors Fibrosarcoma of the bone	*Fibrohistiocytic soft tissue tumors* Pleomorphic malignant fibrous histiocytoma/undifferentiated high grade pleomorphic sarcoma Giant cell malignant fibrous histiocytoma/undifferentiated pleomorphic sarcoma with giant cells Inflammatory malignant fibrous histiocytoma/undifferentiated pleomorphic sarcoma with prominent inflammation
Fibrohistiocytic bone tumors	*Smooth muscle tumors* Leiomyosarcoma
Osteoclastic giant cell rich tumors Malignant transformation of giant cell tumor of bone	
Ewing sarcoma/primitive neuroectodermal tumors	*Pericytic (perivascular) tumors*
Notochordal tumors Chordoma *Conventional* *Chondroid* *Dedifferentiated* *Undifferentiated*	*Skeletal muscle tumors* Rhabdomyosarcoma *Embryonal (including botryoid, anaplastic)* *Alveolar (including solid, anaplastic)* *Pleomorphic* *Spindle cells/sclerosing*
Vascular tumors Epithelioid hemangioendothelioma Angiosarcoma	*Vascular tumors* Epithelioid hemangioendothelioma Angiosarcoma of soft tissue
	Chondro-osseous tumors Extraskeletal mesenchymal chondrosarcoma Extraskeletal osteosarcoma
Myogenic Leiomyosarcoma of the bone	*Nerve sheath tumors* Malignant peripheral nerve sheath tumor (MPNST) Epithelioid malignant peripheral nerve sheath tumor Malignant triton tumor

Table 8.1 (continued)

Bone tumors	Soft tissue tumors
Lipogenic tumors Liposarcoma of the bone	*Tumors of uncertain differentiation* Synovial sarcoma Epithelioid sarcoma Alveolar soft-part sarcoma Clear cell sarcoma of soft tissue Extraskeletal myxoid chondrosarcoma Extraskeletal Ewing sarcoma Desmoplastic small round cell tumor Extra-renal rhabdoid tumor Intimal sarcoma
Undifferentiated sarcomas U. High-grade pleomorphic sarcoma of the bone	*Undifferentiated/unclassified sarcomas* U. Spindle cell sarcoma U. Pleomorphic sarcoma U. Round cell sarcoma U. Epithelioid sarcoma

Differential Diagnosis

Despite their rarity, primary bone tumors must always be kept in mind as a potential diagnosis, especially when evaluating isolated lesions (especially in young patients, or in adults without history of oncologic disease). Diagnostic workup must include full imaging and laboratory studies, and usually a biopsy.

Differential diagnosis includes the following:

- Metastasis
- Plasmocytoma
- Lymphoma
- Bone infection
- Primary benign aggressive tumors (Enneking stage III)
- Primary low-grade malignancies (Enneking stage IA-B)

Imaging Studies

Plain radiographs are often the first exam in emergency care setting, especially in case of acute onset of symptoms. These may allow detection of a fracture and might raise the suspect of a tumor in case of the "winking owl sign" (absence of a pedicle on anteroposterior view) indicating the presence of a lytic lesion.

Computed tomography (CT) scan of the spine is a more sensitive and specific modality in detecting and characterizing bone destruction, reaction of the host bone, and calcification of tumor matrix (if any). In fact, high-grade tumors usually grow breaching the cortex and extending outside the compartment of origin producing bulky masses in the soft tissues (moth-eaten pattern). In certain diseases (i.e., Ewing sarcoma), progression rate is so rapid that the tumor can produce multiple small permeative lytic lesions in the bone, passing through the cortex (thus, extending outside the compartment) while maintaining its primary shape (permeative pattern, Fig. 8.1).

Tumor matrix can exhibit peculiar calcification patterns such as the osteoid pattern (typical of osteogenic tumors, Fig. 8.2), or the popcorn and ring and arcs patterns (typical of chondrogenic tumors).

Magnetic resonance imaging (MRI) is the imaging technique of choice to determine the extracompartmental extension of these lesions and their relationships with neurologic structures (spinal cord, cauda equina, and nerve roots).

Metabolic exams, such as positron emission tomography (PET) scan with ^{18}fluoro-deoxyglucose (^{18}FDG) or bone scintigraphy, are fundamental to determine the activity of the index lesion and rule out presence of other hypermeta-

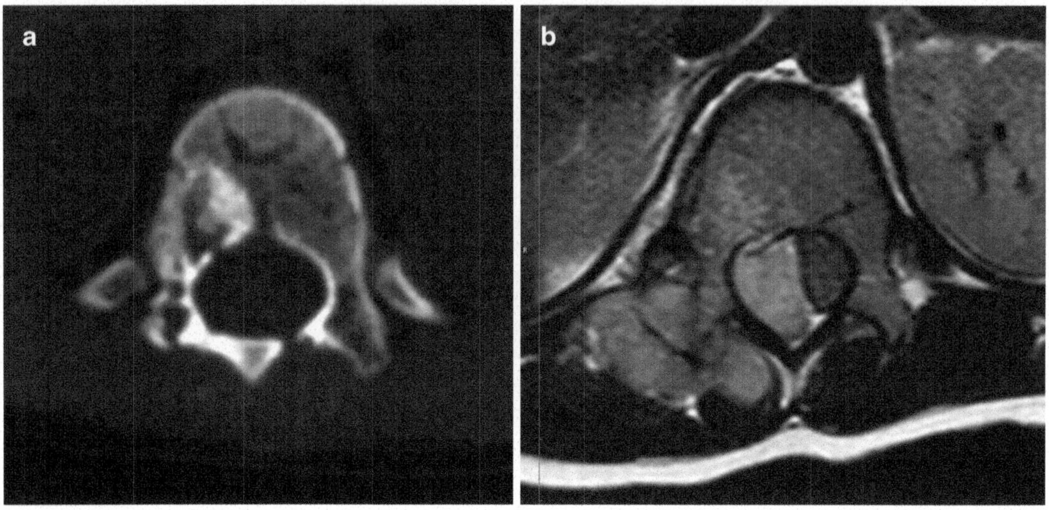

Fig. 8.1 Permeative pattern

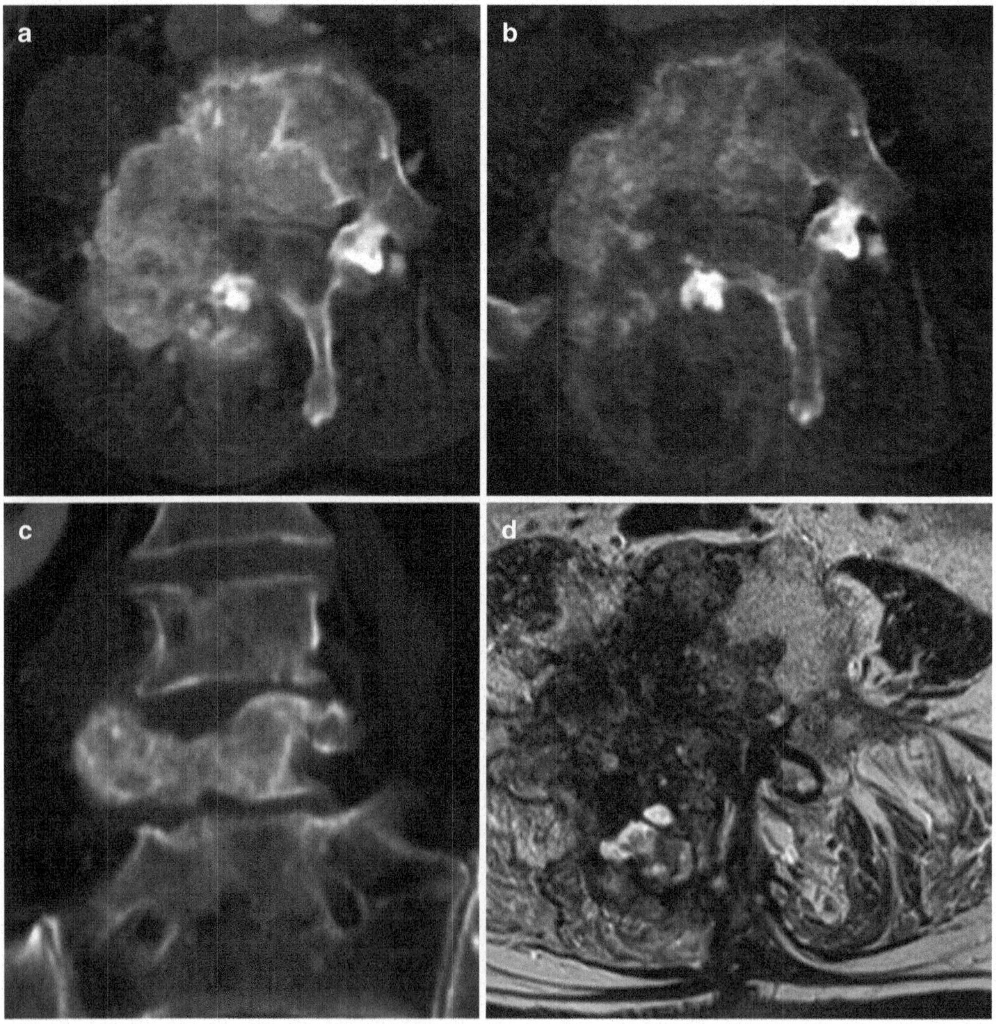

Fig. 8.2 Osteoid pattern of calcification of the tumor matrix, before (A) and after (B) preoperative chemotherapy

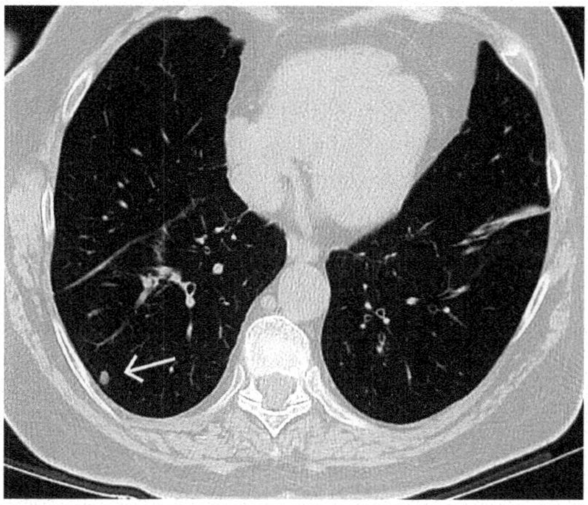

Fig. 8.3 Lung metastasis from osteosarcoma

bolic processes such as synchronous primary tumor or distant metastases. When considering a primary high-grade bone tumor, it is important to mention the possibility of skip metastases, which are foci of disease which in comparison to the main lesion can occur upstream or downstream in the same bone or across a joint in a neighboring bone. In many cases, these are a dedifferentiated form of the same tumor.

Musculoskeletal sarcomas often metastasize to the lungs and liver, thus high-resolution CT scan of the chest and abdomen are mandatory to complete staging (Fig. 8.3).

Laboratory Workup

First-line evaluation should include the following:

- Complete blood count
- Complete blood chemistry including calcium level
- Immunoelectrophoresis of serum proteins
- C-reactive protein (CRP), erythrocyte sedimentation rate (ESR)
- Lactate dehydrogenase (LDH), alkaline phosphatase (ALP)
- Parathyroid hormone (PTH)
- Tumor markers (carcinoembryonic antigen – CEA, CA19-9, CA15-3, CA125, prostate specific antigen – PSA)

Additional exams include evaluation of liver and kidney function (creatinine clearance) and cardiac echo, which are required prior to start chemotherapy.

Biopsy

The gold standard for diagnosis is obtaining a sample of the tumor tissue through the pedicle under CT guidance in order to minimize tissue contamination and allowing for the biopsy tract to be included in the final resected specimen.

In addition, in selected cases, spanning percutaneous stabilization with pedicle screws can be added to restore weight-bearing capacity and in an attempt to prevent pathological fracture (and resulting tumor cell seeding with hematoma), and/or allow administration of neoadjuvant therapies without violating oncology principles. This strategy also may prevent or reverse minor neurologic compromise by means of ligamentotaxis.

Biopsy of cervical spine tumors requires separate discussion, since posteriorly located lesions can be reached by percutaneous image-guided techniques while tumors in the vertebral bodies typically cannot. This is because in the cervical spine, posterior transpedicular techniques are limited by the high obliquity of cervical spine pedicles (up to 45°), which forces an extremely lateral access making the biopsy tract difficult to include in the resection. Additionally, the small dimensions of the pedicles may not always allow an 11–13 gauge trocar to pass. Likewise, biopsy tracts from anterior percutaneous technique (passing through the visceral and the neurovascular bundles of the neck) are unresectable by definition since the approach uses a mobile tissue plane. Furthermore, surgeons should consider that the opportunity to perform en bloc resections with Enneking Appropriate (wide/marginal *tumor-free*) margins in the cervical spine (see § *Surgical planning*) is limited (when compared with the same local extent in the thoracolumbar spine) and burdened by higher rates of complications, thus feasibility should be carefully evaluated before performing the biopsy.

Due to such considerations, a rationale approach to lesions located in the vertebral body of the cervical spine could be incisional biopsy through a standard Smith-Robinson anterior approach and frozen-section histological diagnosis. According to this approach, if pathological findings of metastatic or otherwise incurable lesions are found, one can consider proceeding with intralesional extracapsular debulking. However, if high-grade features are found or the tumor requires a wide margin, obtaining meticulous hemostasis and layer-by-layer closure for further treatment planning is advisable.

Staging

Primary musculoskeletal (bone and soft tissue) tumors are staged according to the surgical staging system introduced by Enneking in 1980 [4]. This classification divides tumors into benign and malignant tumors according to their histopathology and further subdivides them in three stages for each group (Table 8.2). Specifically, malignant tumors are graded A or B according to whether the tumor is intra- or extracompartmental in stages I and II, and whether it is low or high grade in stage III, respectively. According to Enneking, a compartment is defined as an anatomical space bounded by natural barriers to tumor extension (i.e., cortical bone, fascia and fascial septa, articular cartilage, joint capsules, tendons, and tendons sheath).

This chapter focuses on management and care of Enneking stage II(A/B) and IIIB primary musculoskeletal tumors.

Table 8.2 Surgical staging system (Enneking)

Benign	
Stage 1	Latent or inactive
Stage 2	Active
Stage 3	Aggressive
Malignant	
Stage I (low-grade)	A – Intracompartmental
	B – Extracompartmental
Stage II (high-grade)	A – Intracompartmental
	B – Extracompartmental
Stage III (with regional or distant metastases)	A – Low-grade
	B – High-grade

Multidisciplinary Management

Multidisciplinary approach is the standard modality by which such aggressive diseases are managed in most centers. These teams include oncologists, radiotherapists, orthopedic surgeons, pathologists, plastic surgeons, and others. The authors suggest multidisciplinary inclusion of the access surgeons (general, vascular, or thoracic) when approaching the relevant spinal locations of these tumors.

For most high-grade tumors, the first step of treatment is generally neoadjuvant chemotherapy. When effective, this modality limits systemic micrometastases and may produce shrinkage of the tumor mass (Fig. 8.4) and/or calcification of the peripheral shell of the tumor easing subsequent resection (Fig. 8.5).

Local control of the disease can be achieved through radiation therapy (RT), surgery, or a combination of the two. Radiation therapy is complicated by several factors including the relative radioresistance of mesenchymal tumors to conventional radiation therapy techniques and the proximity of delicate neurological and visceral structures that limit the amount of radiation that can be delivered. These challenges have been partly overcome by improved techniques of radiation delivery such as intensity-modulated radiation therapies (IMRT) and stereotactic techniques. Moreover, new sources of radiation, such as proton and carbon-ion radiation therapy, have been used to allow delivery of curative radiation protocol to the tumor with little delivery to the surrounding healthy tissues. However, no radiotherapy modality can be effective in case of mechanical instability, such as with pathological fractures. Lastly, it must be considered that RT has the potential for causing tumor dedifferentiation. This latter particularly occurs when RT fails in achieving local control in low-grade tumors (i.e., chordoma, chondrosarcoma grade 2), which then progress locally with dedifferentiated high-grade areas.

On the other hand, surgery is not always benign. Enneking-appropriate oncologic resection may demand inclusion of viscera and/or neurovascular structures, causing morbidity and

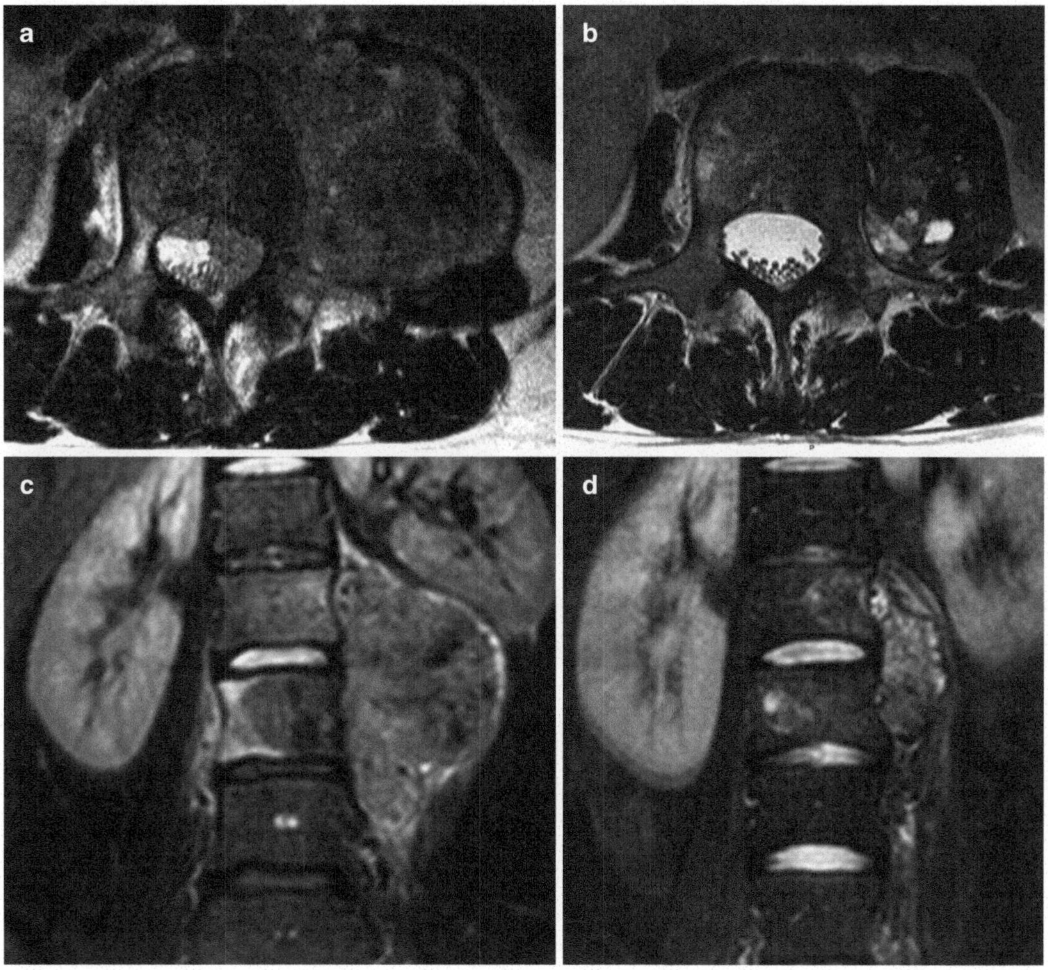

Fig. 8.4 Preoperative chemotherapy produces shrinkage of the tumor mass

perioperative complications. At its worst, aggressive surgery may come with complications but not necessarily the improved local control rates to justify the effort. Therefore, thorough discussion of the case as part of a multidisciplinary team to identifying a shared plan to combine surgery, radiation, and chemotherapy likely provides the best results in terms of systemic/local control and function.

Surgical Planning

The surgical margin is defined as the quantity and quality of the tissues surrounding the tumor after its surgical removal. It can be intralesional (if excision is performed violating the pseudocapsule and entering the tumor), marginal (if resection is performed along the perilesional reactive tissues), wide (if resection is performed in healthy tissues), or radical (if the whole compartment of origin bounded by its natural barriers). Given the anatomical constraints of the bony ring which constitutes part of each human vertebra, it is impossible to achieve truly radical margins of resection in the spine. Therefore, the use of this term is discouraged in spinal oncology.

The Enneking surgical staging system dictates which margin of resection needs to be chosen according to the stage of the tumor (oncologic appropriateness). For example, wide margins are required in cases of stage II A-B tumors, and

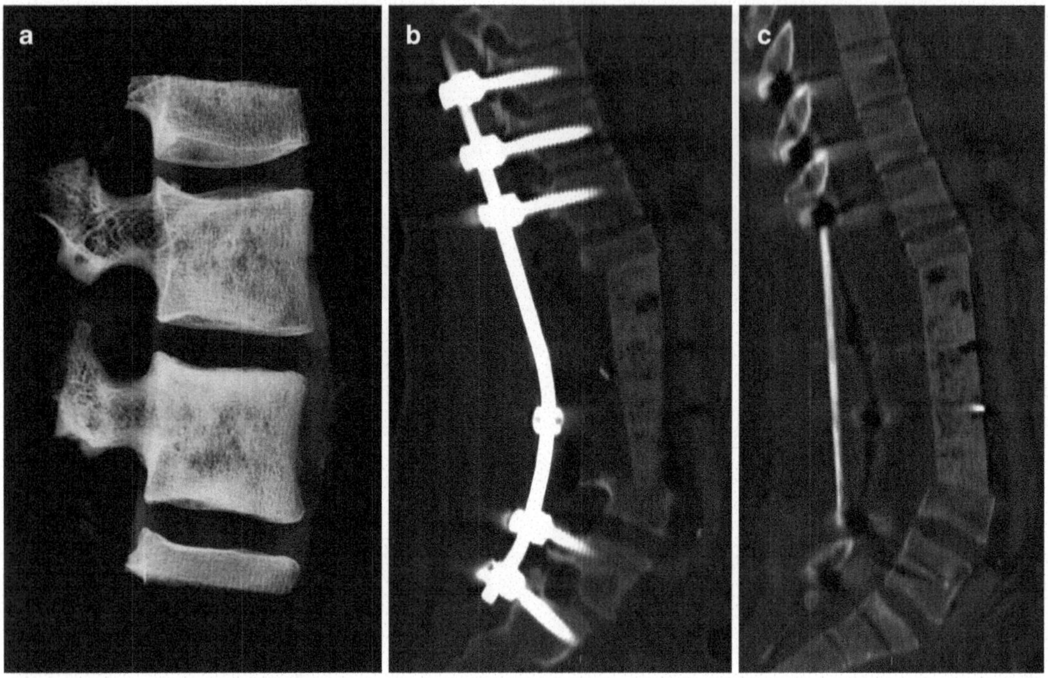

Fig. 8.5 Resected specimen and reconstruction

from an oncological point of view, the successful execution of such surgical procedures is termed "Enneking Appropriate" (EA) (or "Enneking inappropriate" – EI, if not). "Wide en bloc resection" specifically means tumor removal in a single piece with a wide layer of healthy tissue covering it (Fig. 8.6).

In order to achieve this goal, it might be necessary to consider the possible sacrifice of functionally relevant structures (such as spinal nerves).

In case of extensive epidural involvement, there is no healthy tissue margin between the dura and the tumor, thus the margin cannot be better than marginal. In such cases, inclusion of part of the dura in the resected specimen is an option to achieve a wide margin. The drawback of this decision, apart from the need for dural reconstruction and the potential for complications (such as a cerebrospinal fluid fistula, infection, wound dehiscence, meningitis) is that the subdural space might get contaminated, and an eventual recurrence can occur intradurally.

Planning of the resections can be guided by the Weinstein-Boriani-Biagini (WBB) surgical staging system based on local tumor extension [5]. According to the WBB staging system, 11 different subtypes are proposed requiring a single or a combination of approaches (Fig. 8.7).

Aggressiveness of the surgery must take into consideration the likelihood of complications, since occurrence of postoperative complications will postpone postoperative treatments (radiation and chemotherapy). Figures 8.8, 8.9, and 8.10 demonstrate a case of a WBB type 3a resection involving combined anterior and posterior approaches with anterior hemi-sagittal bone cuts, posterior partial laminectomy, and tumor removal through combined approach.

Since surgery is often combined with radiation therapy, radiolucent reconstructive implants (i.e., structural bone allografts, or carbon fiber modular systems) should be prioritized over metallic implants to decrease artifacts on postoperative imaging and preserve radiation plans. Recently, the introduction of carbon-fiber rein-

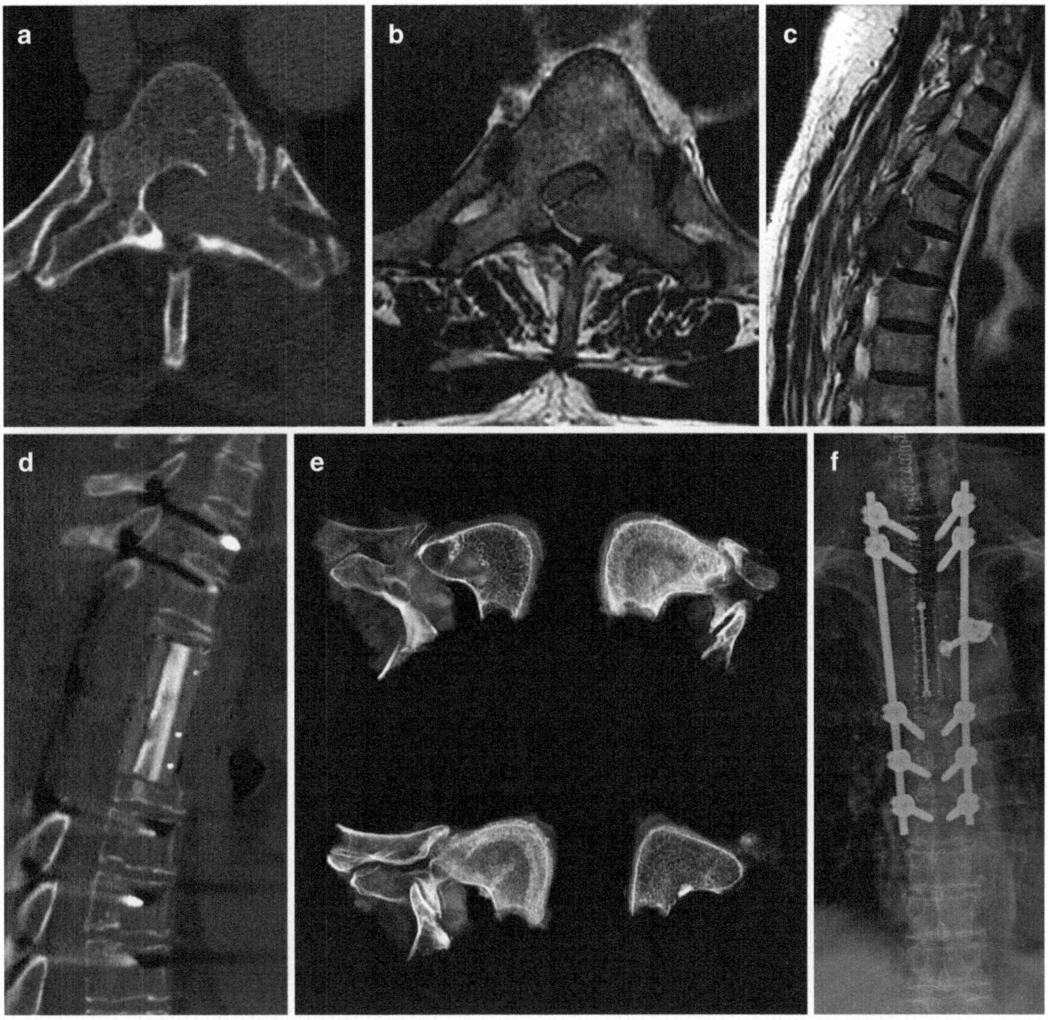

Fig. 8.6 Enneking-appropriate (EA) en bloc resection with wide/marginal margin

forced PEEK (CFR/PEEK) instrumentations has been used with promising results in order to allow optimal combination of surgical resection and high-voltage radiation therapy [6].

Histopathological Examination on Surgical Specimen

Surgical specimens must be submitted to pathology for diagnosis confirmation, margin, and tumor tissue necrosis evaluation. This latter parameter is of extreme importance since it provides information regarding efficacy of preoperative chemotherapy treatments on that specific patient, thus is used to guide selection of the most effective drugs for subsequent treatments. Moreover, it has been proven to be predictive of overall survival.

Follow-Up Protocol

These patients must be accurately monitored after discharge. Follow up protocol must be adapted to any single case and needs to take into account sev-

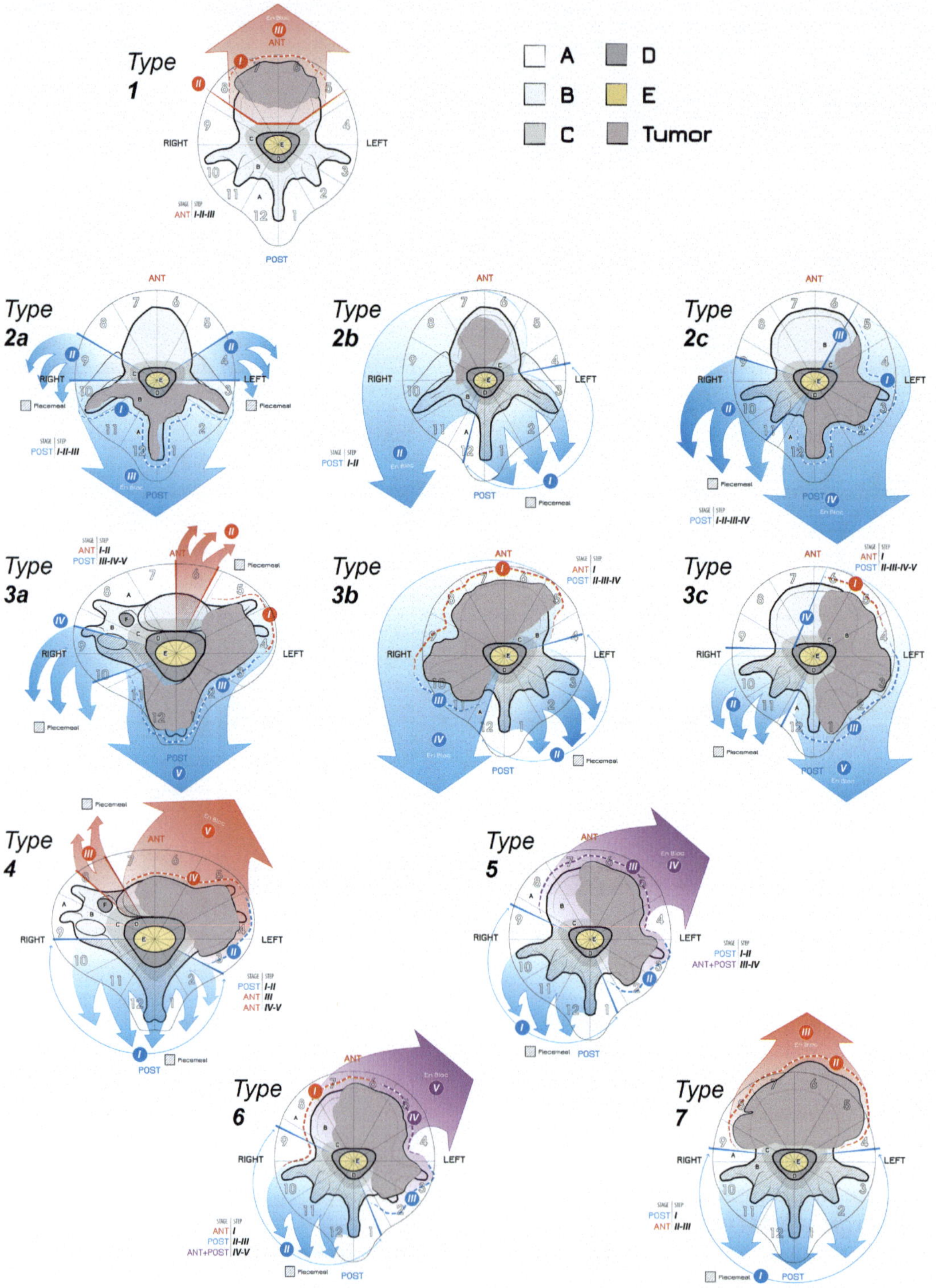

Fig. 8.7 WBB-based subtypes of en bloc resections

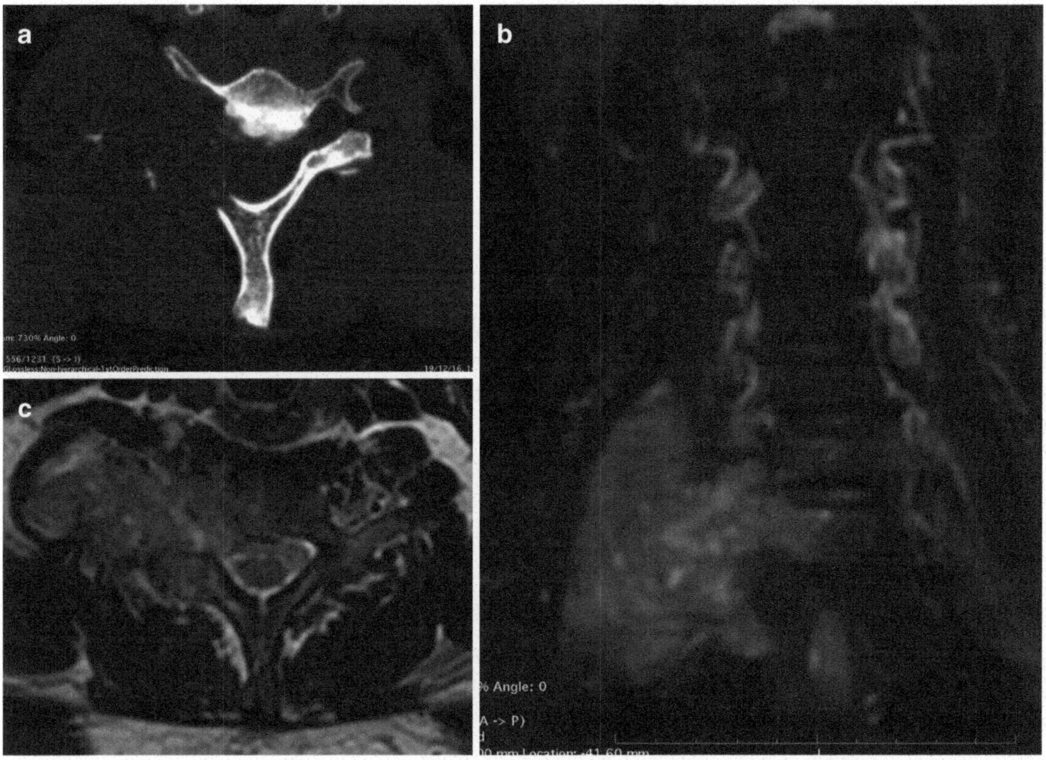

Fig. 8.8 A 45-year-old man with C7 epithelioid sclerosing fibrosarcoma

eral factors including the index disease, the margin achieved with the surgical treatment, comorbidities, and the efficacy of the radiation therapy. As a rule of a thumb, the authors suggest clinical and imaging evaluation every 3 months for the first year, every 4 months for following 2 years, every 6 months for subsequent 2 years, and lastly yearly for 5 more years. MRI can be considered the imaging technique of choice to evaluate for local recurrence. Full-standing radiographs are used to evaluate mechanical stability of the reconstruction. Any worrisome or equivocal finding can be ruled out with CT scan. This latter exam may be helpful at 9–12 months postoperatively to evaluate bone fusion.

Surgeons must be aware that oncologic follow-up includes yearly repetition of CT scans of the chest to rule out pulmonary metastases. This can be taken into consideration opportunistically when planning postoperative imaging studies to evaluate the resection site in case of thoracic tumors.

Controversies

1. *Acute onset of a progressive neurological deficit from an undiagnosed solitary spinal tumor: what to do?*

There is no absolute rule, and every case must be carefully evaluated using all the available data elements. Supportive care should be provided (i.e., corticosteroids, bed rest). In case of progression despite these measures, decompression and stabilization with radiolucent instrumentation can be a viable option. Depending on the local extension of the tumor, decompression could be carried out in a healthy part of the vertebrae, thus avoiding violation of the pseudocapsule. Emergency en bloc resection is discouraged. These complex clinical scenarios represent a difficult situation even for experienced spine tumor surgeons.

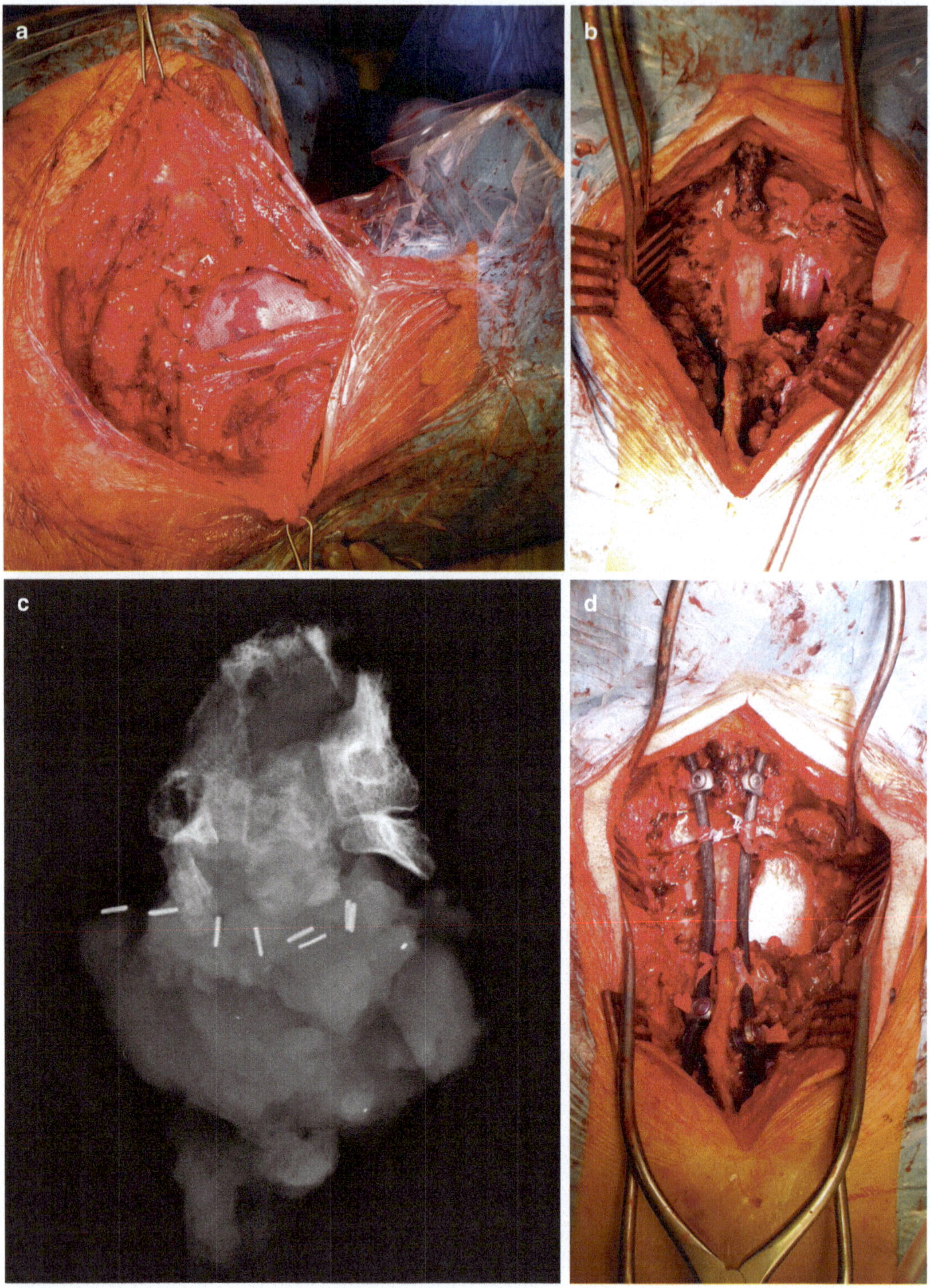

Fig. 8.9 Intraoperative pictures: double approach (A + P) sagittal resection

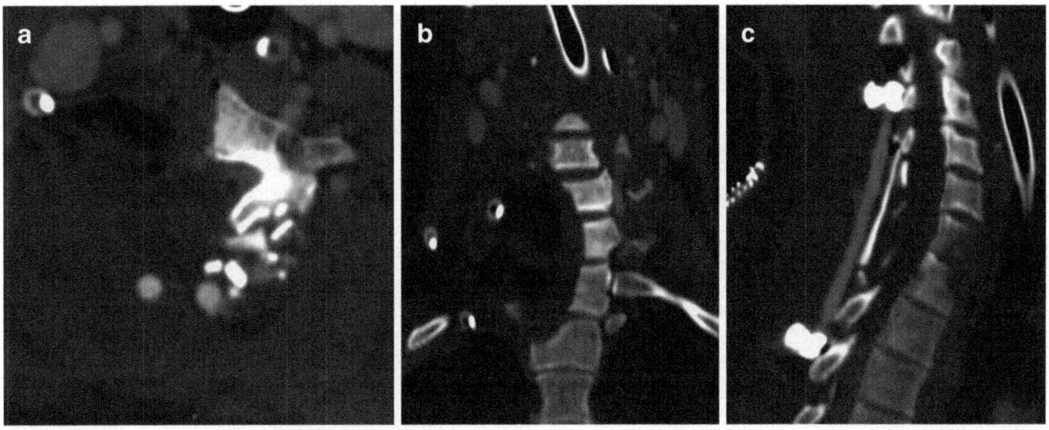

Fig. 8.10 Postoperative CT scan proving the result of the performed resection

2. *Pathological fracture under chemotherapy: timing of surgery?*

In case of a tumor fracture that occurs while the patient is under chemotherapy, one can assume that (1) it is poorly responding to the drug, or (2) excessive bone destruction had already occurred before treatment, or (3) patient compliance in limiting activities is poor. In all of these cases, the occurrence of fracture may cause early discontinuation of the preoperative chemotherapy in favor of undergoing surgery.

In order to decrease the likelihood of this event, the Spine Instability Neoplastic Score (SINS) can be used to estimate the risk of pathological fracture and identify patients with mechanical instability [7]. In the event that the SINS risk is significant (and no other contraindications exist), minimally invasive stabilization techniques can be used to bridge the affected level, neutralizing forces acting on the tumor and providing indirect decompression by means of ligamentotaxis.

3. *Can margin contamination be accepted in order to allow a resection to be performed through a posterior-only procedure, thus avoiding a more complex procedure with multiple approaches?*

The gold standard for the treatment of high-grade primary disease is a multimodal approach that includes chemotherapy plus a combination of surgery and radiation therapy. Within the various surgical approaches, en bloc resection with wide/marginal tumor-free margins has been proven to provide the best local control rates and overall survival. However, such gold standard is not always feasible given the local extension of the tumor. In these selected cases where EA resection is not feasible and margin violation is unavoidable (Fig. 8.11), decrease of the surgical aggressiveness and extent might be considered. In particular, avoidance of extensive anterior approaches often required for oncology surgery has been shown to decrease the overall morbidity of the surgery and thus the risk of complications. This is particularly important since additional unplanned treatments are likely to postpone the initiation of adjuvant radiation and chemotherapy.

There is no strong evidence to support contaminated en bloc resection over piecemeal excision, although the authors discourage a piecemeal approach in general. In our experience, the likelihood of gross residual disease with these two techniques is different, and marginal contamination is far preferable to piecemeal excision.

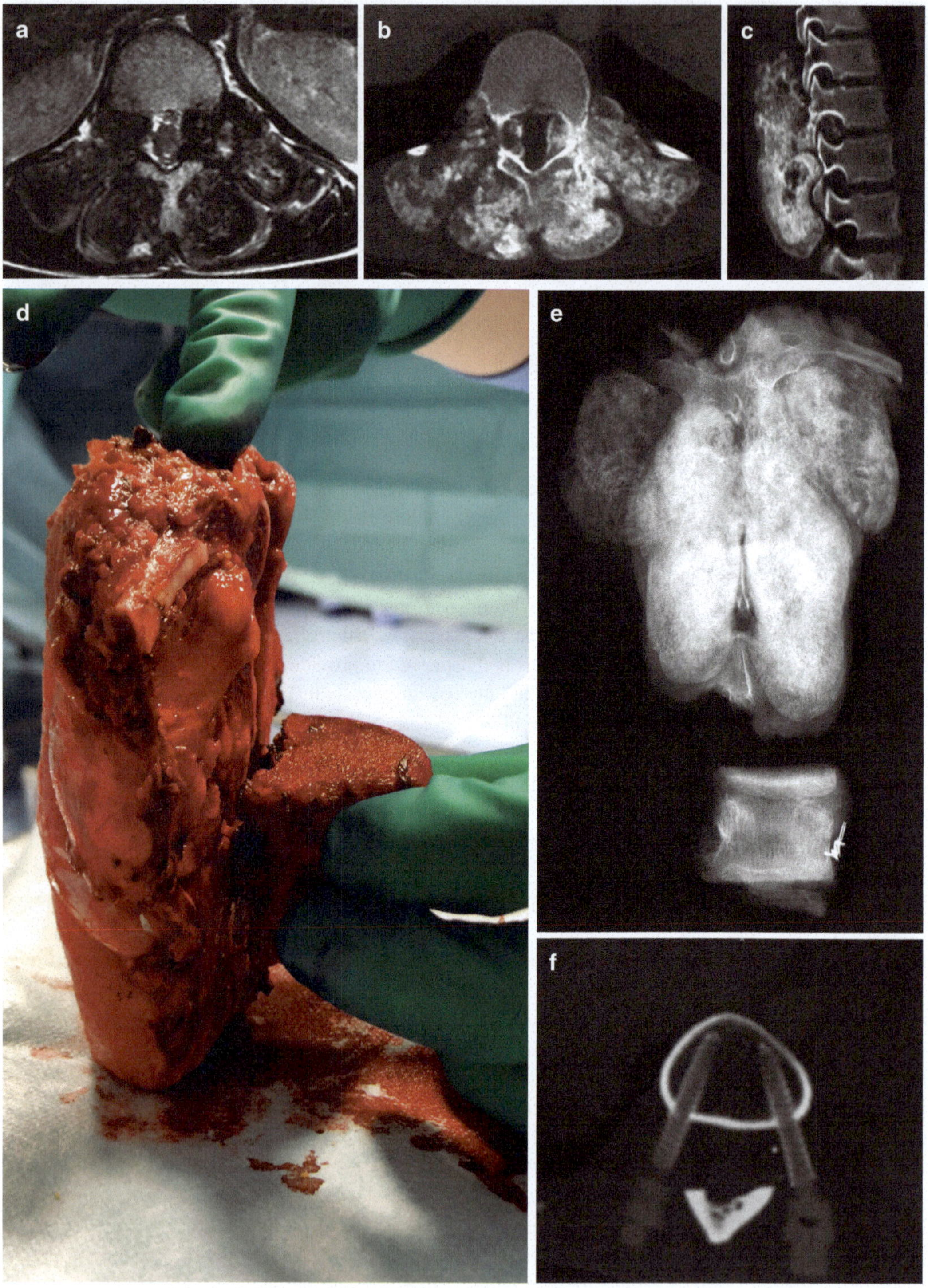

Fig. 8.11 A 13-year-old boy with T11 osteoblastic osteosarcoma

Conclusion

Primary high-grade malignancies of the spine constitute a challenging clinical scenario. Key features of successful treatment include proper diagnosis and staging, multidisciplinary treatment planning, liberal use of adjuvants which typically include both chemotherapy and radiotherapy, and Enneking-appropriate surgical resection for local and systemic control. Additional points to optimize success include the following:

- Primary malignancy should be included on any differential diagnosis of an aggressive solitary spinal lesion, despite its rarity.
- The ultimate patient outcome can be determined very early in treatment, so early referral to a tertiary high-volume oncology center is advisable from the pre-biopsy outset.
- Multidisciplinary approach is keystone of treatment.
- EA en bloc resection with wide/marginal *tumor-free* margin is the gold standard for primary high-grade malignancies.
- Improvements in radiation therapy techniques do not justify mediocre, incomplete, or suboptimal resection technique.
- Radiolucent reconstructive implants optimize adjuvant radiation therapy and postoperative imaging.

Acknowledgment The authors acknowledge the invaluable contribution of Carlo Piovani for case presentations and original artwork.

References

1. Charest-Morin R, Dirks MS, Patel S, et al. Ewing sarcoma of the spine: prognostic variables for survival and local control in surgically treated patients. Spine (Phila Pa 1976). 2018;43(9):622–9. https://doi.org/10.1097/BRS.0000000000002386.
2. Chou D, Bilsky MH, Luzzati A, et al. Malignant peripheral nerve sheath tumors of the spine: results of surgical management from a multicenter study. J Neurosurg Spine. 2017;26(3):291–8. https://doi.org/10.3171/2016.8.SPINE151548.
3. Schwab J, Gasbarrini A, Bandiera S, et al. Osteosarcoma of the mobile spine. Spine (Phila Pa 1976). 2012;37(6):E381–6. https://doi.org/10.1097/BRS.0b013e31822fb1a7.
4. Enneking WF, Spanier SS, Goodman MA. A system for the surgical staging of musculoskeletal sarcoma. 1980. Clin Orthop Relat Res. 2003;415:4–18. https://doi.org/10.1097/01.blo.0000093891.12372.0f.
5. Boriani S. *En bloc* resection in the spine: a procedure of surgical oncology. J Spine Surg. 2018;4(3):668–76. https://doi.org/10.21037/jss.2018.09.02.
6. Pipola V, Boriani S, Ghermandi R, et al. Composite peek/carbon fiber pre-shaped rods and sublaminar bands for posterior stabilization of cervicothoracic junction: a novel technique. J Clin Neurosci. 2020;72:429–33. https://doi.org/10.1016/j.jocn.2019.12.035.
7. Fisher CG, Schouten R, Versteeg AL, et al. Reliability of the Spinal Instability Neoplastic Score (SINS) among radiation oncologists: an assessment of instability secondary to spinal metastases. Radiat Oncol. 2014;9:69. https://doi.org/10.1186/1748-717X-9-69.

Extradural Spine Tumor Mimics

9

Ilyas M. Eli, Lubdha M. Shah, and Andrew T. Dailey

Introduction

Tumors invading the spine are uncommon and constitute a small percentage of all central nervous system tumors. Diagnosis is based on a detailed history of patients who present with axial back pain, radiculopathy, or myelopathy supplemented by correlation with imaging findings that demonstrate a lesion along the spinal axis. As part of the differential diagnosis, surgeons should also consider nonneoplastic spine tumor mimics that can present as a spinal mass. Imaging features of neoplastic lesions can be hard to differentiate from those of nonneoplastic lesions, which is why a patient history and physical examination in addition to multimodality imaging can help with the diagnosis. Proper diagnosis allows for optimal treatment and patient satisfaction and sometimes avoids the wrong surgical approach. Lesions resembling spine tumors can be subdivided into infectious, degenerative, metabolic, inflammatory, hemorrhagic, and other extradural mimics of spine tumors (Table 9.1).

I. M. Eli · A. T. Dailey (✉)
Department of Neurological Surgery, Clinical Neurosciences Center, University of Utah, Salt Lake City, UT, USA
e-mail: neuropub@hsc.utah.edu

L. M. Shah
Department of Radiology, University of Utah, Salt Lake City, UT, USA

K. Singh, M. Colman (eds.), *Surgical Spinal Oncology*,
https://doi.org/10.1007/978-3-030-50722-0_9

The goal of this chapter is to discuss presentation, imaging characteristics (Table 9.2), and treatment options for lesions that commonly mimic extradural spine tumors.

Infectious Mimickers

Osteomyelitis/Discitis

Vertebral osteomyelitis and discitis are presentations of an infectious process involving the vertebral body, intervertebral disc, and/or paraspinal muscles [51]. This process usually results from hematogenous spread or from direct inoculation due to surgery or trauma. Osteomyelitis and discitis can occur individually or in combination. Vertebral osteomyelitis mostly affects the lumbar spine (58%), followed by the thoracic spine (30%) and, less commonly, the cervical spine (11%) [22]. Osteomyelitis/discitis starts along the cartilaginous subchondral endplates, which are colonized by septic emboli. Uncontrolled osteomyelitis and discitis can lead to expansion of the infection to the paraspinal muscles and epidural space. The incidence of vertebral osteomyelitis has increased to 5.4 cases per 100,000 people in 2013 from 2.9 per 100,000 in 1998 [31]. The increased incidence is thought to be related to the increasing population of elderly individuals with chronic diseases, a larger population of immunocompromised patients, more

Table 9.1 Mimics of spine tumor

Tumor type	Examples
Infectious	Vertebral osteomyelitis/discitis Spinal epidural abscess Spinal tuberculosis
Degenerative	Disc extrusion Synovial cyst
Metabolic bone disease	Brown tumor Paget disease
Inflammatory	Inflammatory pseudotumor Rheumatoid arthritis Vertebral sarcoid
Hemorrhagic	Spinal epidural hematoma Hemorrhagic synovial cyst
Others	Vertebral hemangioma Bone island Epidural lipomatosis

illicit intravenous drug use, more cases of spine surgery, and improvement in detection on imaging [7]. The most common pathogenic cause is *Staphylococcus aureus*, which accounts for 32–67% of isolated organisms [50]. Less common organisms include *Escherichia coli* in patients with recurrent urinary tract infections, *Pseudomonas aeruginosa* in patients with nosocomial infections and intravenous drug use, *Streptococcus pneumoniae* in diabetics, and *Salmonella* sp. in patients with sickle cell disease or absent spleens [43].

Patients harboring infection present with symptoms of malaise, diaphoresis, weight loss, fever, and back pain. These symptoms are often

Table 9.2 Imaging summary of spine tumor mimics

Pathology	Degree of enhancement T1	T2	STIR	T1 + C	Other characteristics
Osteomyelitis/discitis	Hypointense	Hyperintense	Hyperintense	Subchondral endplate enhancement	Vertebral height loss, discal edema, paraspinal swelling
Epidural abscess	Hypointense	Hyperintense	Hyperintense	Peripheral enhancement	Epidural phlegmon
Tuberculosis	Hypointense	Hypo-/hyperintense	Hypo-/hyperintense	Marrow enhancement	Kyphotic spinal deformity, calcified paraspinal mass
Hemangioma	Hyperintense	Hyperintense	Hypo-/hyperintense (depending on the degree of vascularity)	Avid	Vertically aligned trabeculae
Bone island	Hypointense	Hypointense	Hypointense	None	Sclerotic islands, calcified islands
Epidural lipomatosis	Hyperintense	Iso-/hyperintense	Hypointense	None	Fat in the dorsal epidural space
Epidural hematoma	Variable	Variable	Variable	Heterogeneous	
Synovial cyst	Hypointense	Hyperintense	Hyperintense	Peripheral	Rounded lesion extending from a degenerative facet joint
Disc herniation	Hypointense	Iso-/hyperintense	Iso-/hyperintense	Peripheral	Peripheral enhancement
Brown tumor	Hypointense	Variable	Variable	Heterogeneous	Expansile and lytic lesion
Paget disease	Heterogeneously hyperintense	Heterogeneously hypointense	Heterogeneously hypointense	Heterogeneous	Sclerotic cortex, disorganized trabeculae, vertebral body expansion
Inflammatory pseudotumor	Hypointense	Variable	Variable	None to minimal	Retro-odontoid lesion

attributed to degenerative causes, which can cause a delay in diagnosis. Less common neurological presentations may include radiculopathy, myelopathy or paresis, and sensory changes, which are found in up to 34% of patients [44]. Symptoms can be correlated to laboratory values of elevated white blood cell (WBC) count, erythrocyte sedimentation rate (ESR), and C-reactive protein (CRP) level. Leukocytosis and positive blood cultures can aid in the diagnosis of systemic infection, which can offer evidence of a pyogenic spondylodiscitis.

Imaging modalities that can be used in the diagnosis of spinal infection include computed tomography (CT) scans and magnetic resonance imaging (MRI). CT imaging shows findings of paraspinal swelling, endplate bone erosion, and epidural soft tissue and can be followed sequentially to assess osseous erosion, which may correlate with instability. With MRI, the disc spaces and the vertebral body may show height loss, are hypointense on T1-weighted images, and have variable but hyperintense signal on T2-weighted images. There may be increased intradiscal height when there is increased fluid (Fig. 9.1). Typically, there is peripheral discal enhancement. Short-TI inversion recovery (STIR) sequences are sensitive to bone marrow edema and are helpful in detecting subtle/early infection. Fat-saturated T1-weighted images are helpful to increase the conspicuity of endplate, epidural, and paraspinal enhancement. Paraspinal involvement, including the psoas and spinal erectae muscles, can be seen as regional fullness that is T1 isointense and T2 hyperintense. Diffusion-weighted imaging (DWI) is helpful for increasing the conspicuity of epidural extension of tumor (Fig. 9.2).

Spine tumors can mimic spine infections radiographically, but the overall clinical, laboratory, and imaging picture will generally support the accurate diagnosis of spine infections. The key imaging feature of discitis–osteomyelitis is that the infection is centered on the subchondral endplate and involves the adjacent endplates, crossing the disc space. Treatment involves isolation of the bacteria involved via blood cultures, and if needed, imaging-guided biopsy of the disc space or any other abnormal tissue. Then, treatment with appropriate antibiotics can be initiated for 6–12 weeks, initially with intravenous antibiotics followed by a period of oral antibiotic treatment. The presence of hardware often requires longer treatment, sometimes resulting in lifelong suppression with oral agents. Surgery may be indicated if there is neurological injury, spinal

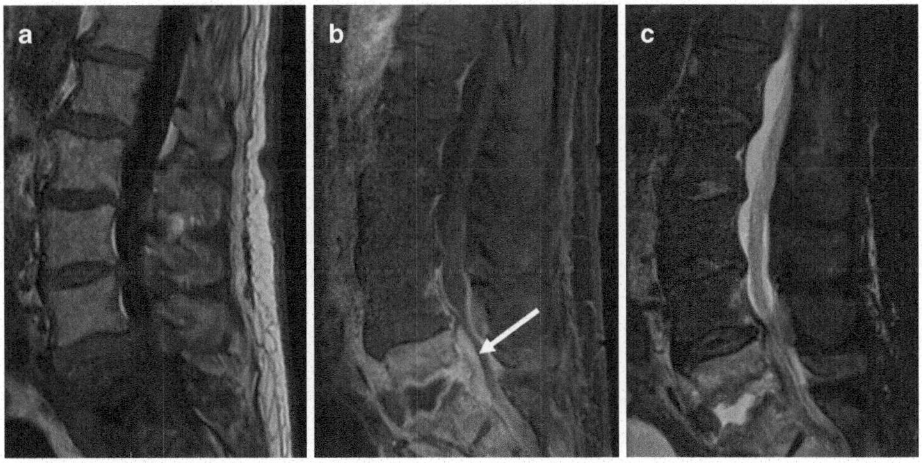

Fig. 9.1 Osteomyelitis/discitis of the lumbar spine. (**a**) Sagittal T1-weighted MRI shows homogenous hypointense signal in the L5 and S1 vertebral bodies. (**b**) Sagittal T1-weighted MRI with contrast and fat saturation shows homogenous enhancement of the L5 and S1 vertebral bodies and their endplates. There is also enhancing epidural phlegmon (arrow). (**c**) Sagittal STIR shows homogenous hyperintense signal in the L5 and S1 vertebral bodies and fluid signal in the intervertebral disc space

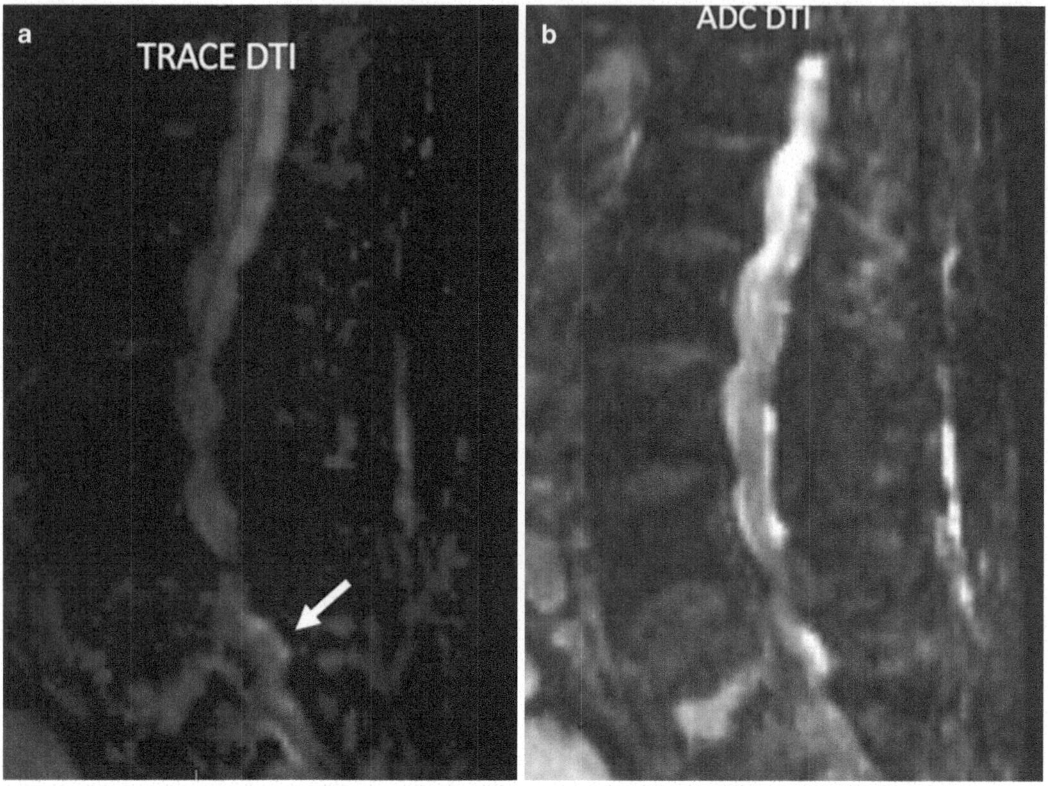

Fig. 9.2 Osteomyelitis/discitis of the lumbar spine. Sagittal diffusion tensor imaging (DTI) trace (**a**) and correlative apparent diffusion coefficient (ADC) map (**b**) show bright signal in the epidural abscess (arrow) and marrow edema in the involved vertebral bodies

cord compression, spinal instability, progressive kyphosis, severe pain, or failed medical management.

Spinal Epidural Abscess

Spinal epidural abscesses (SEAs) are commonly associated with osteomyelitis/discitis but can also occur in isolation. The most common pathogen is *S. aureus*. A SEA is formed as a result of the persistent collection of purulent infection in the epidural space between the dura and ligamentous structures via hematogenous spread or local seeding. A spontaneous SEA most commonly occurs as a sequela of spondylodiscitis spreading via epidural veins [63]. Iatrogenic causes are related to spine surgery, epidural anesthesia, or spine injections. SEAs are most prevalent in the lumbar spine (48%) and are less commonly found in the thoracic (31%) and cervical spine (24%) [27]. SEAs can be multisegmental because of spread within the epidural space and less often can be present in noncontiguous levels [63]. Up to 50% of patients with a SEA have a delay in diagnosis from their initial presentation to definitive diagnosis. The differential diagnosis includes extradural metastasis and epidural hematoma. Common symptoms include back pain, fever, and neurological deficits, a triad that should prompt spinal imaging. Neurological symptoms such as weakness, sensory changes, radiculopathy, and bowel/bladder dysfunction are present in up to 50% of cases.

MRI is the first-line imaging modality for the diagnosis of SEA, which will appear as T1 hypointense and T2 hyperintense (Fig. 9.3). Contrast-enhanced T1-weighted imaging can delineate the extent of the SEA. Fat saturation on these contrast-enhanced T1-weighted sequences

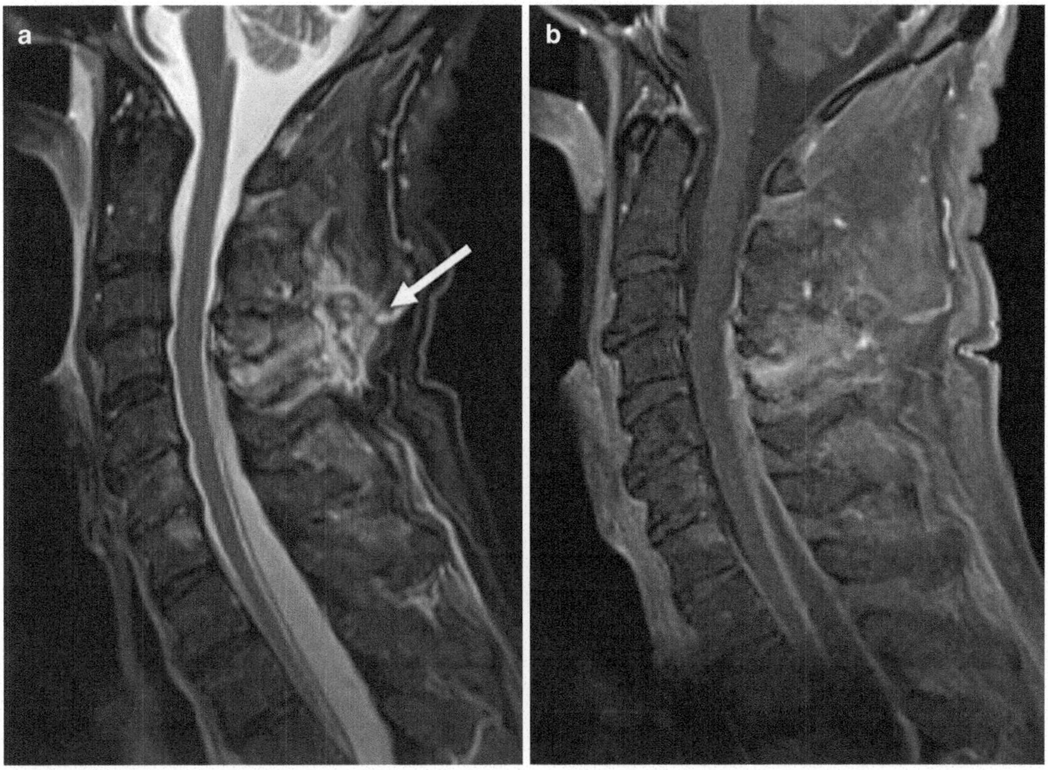

Fig. 9.3 Epidural abscess in the cervical spine. (**a**) Sagittal STIR shows a hyperintense epidural collection in the posterior spinal canal, anteriorly displacing the spinal cord. Interspinous edema is noted at the C4–C5 level (arrow). (**b**) Sagittal T1 with contrast enhancement and fat saturation shows peripherally enhancing epidural collection in the posterior cervical spine

is particularly helpful in increasing the conspicuity of SEA by suppressing the epidural fat. Epidural phlegmon will show heterogeneous ill-defined enhancement, whereas an epidural abscess will demonstrate peripheral enhancement and central T1 hypointensity. Abscesses contain necrotic tissue, pathogens, and neutrophils that cause restriction of the water molecules, resulting in the hyperintense signal on DWI [48]. Although DWI can help delineate a SEA, an epidural hematoma can also show reduced diffusion depending on the age of the blood products (Fig. 9.4). The clinical history and correlation with conventional MRI sequences are critical in differentiating SEA from other diagnoses such as extradural lymphoma, which will show T2 hypointensity, avid homogeneous enhancement, and diffusion restriction.

Although there is a trend toward medical treatment with antibiotics alone in neurologically intact patients with SEA, operative management should always be considered, particularly in cervical and thoracic SEA because of the risk of neurological injury. Risk factors for failure of medical management alone include methicillin-resistant *S. aureus* infection, neurological deficit, elevated WBC over 12,500/mm [3], and/or CRP >115 mg/L. [4]

Spinal Tuberculosis

Tuberculosis affects close to one third of the world's population but with symptoms occurring in only 5–15% of individuals [66]. Skeletal tuberculosis is even rarer, affecting only 10% of those

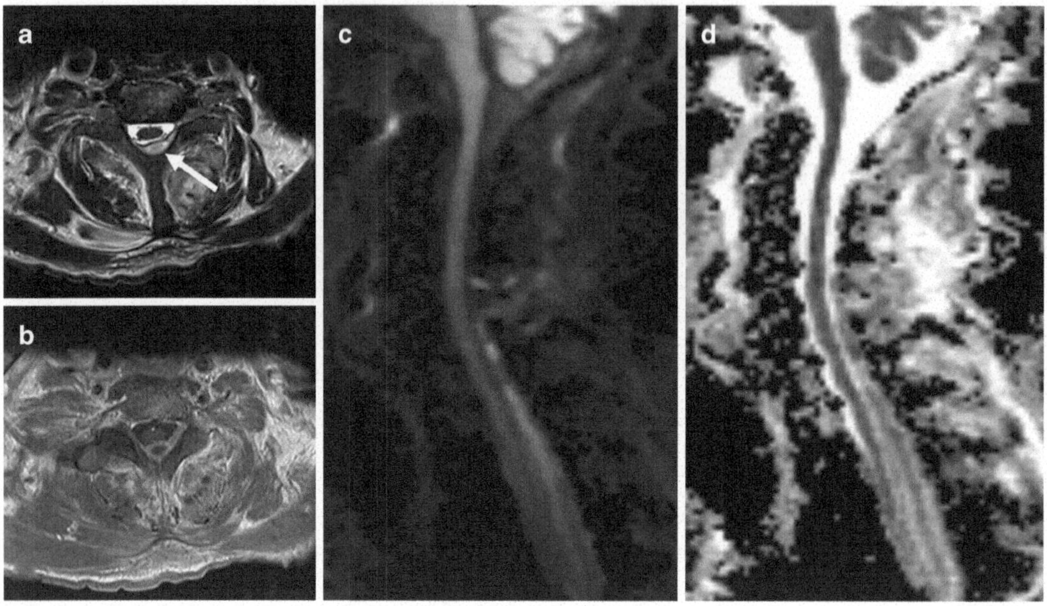

Fig. 9.4 Epidural abscess in the cervical spine. Axial T2-weighted MRI (**a**) shows a heterogeneously hypointense epidural collection in the posterior spinal canal (arrow), which demonstrates peripheral enhancement on the postcontrast T1-weighted image (**b**). Sagittal DTI trace image (**c**) and correlative ADC map (**d**) illustrate heterogeneous restricted diffusion in this collection

patients with active disease, although the spine is the most common skeletal segment involved. Spinal involvement of tuberculosis is a chronic phenomenon, with only a minority of patients having systemic symptoms [19]. Spinal tuberculosis can be very difficult to diagnose and can often be mistaken for spinal metastasis given its vertebral involvement with associated disc and epidural changes. The differential diagnosis includes pyogenic vertebral osteomyelitis, sarcoidosis, lymphoma, and metastatic disease; however, history, clinical, laboratory, and radiographic findings can clue physicians in to the diagnosis without the need for a biopsy, even though that may be necessary in some cases. Spinal tuberculosis should be part of the differential diagnosis in patients who are found to have spinal lesions in the setting of chronic illness, immunosuppression, travel to or residence in areas with endemic tuberculosis, autoimmune disease, drug use, incarceration, low income or poverty, or patients with unstable housing.

Presenting symptoms for spinal tuberculosis may include active pulmonary tuberculosis and systemic symptoms such as weight loss, body aches, malaise, fevers, and night sweats. These symptoms are present in 20–38% of patients with spinal tuberculosis [6, 19]. The most common presenting symptom of spinal tuberculosis is axial back pain, which may be, in part, due to spinal deformity. Spinal tuberculosis causes neurological symptoms less commonly. In addition to clinical examination, further workup includes laboratory tests such as the ESR, CRP, WBC, tuberculosis skin test, and interferon-γ release assay (blood test that detects interferon-γ release from T lymphocytes when exposed to tuberculosis antigens).

The spinal features of tuberculosis include neurological deficit, chronic kyphotic spinal deformity, and cold abscesses. Cold abscesses are the presence of slow-growing purulence emerging from an involved vertebral segment without any inflammation. A paravertebral cold abscess is a diagnostic feature of spinal tuberculosis observed in 50% of cases. These abscesses are often insidious and can be associated with caseous granuloma formation. Approximately 10–20% of affected patients have neurological symptoms depending on the part of the spine involved, with symptoms including radiculopathy, myelopathy, and sensory changes [39]. As the disease progresses, symptoms of myelopathy and paraplegia/tetraplegia can result from significant spinal cord compression caused by cold abscesses, tuberculous caseous lesions, dural fibrosis, granuloma formation, or spinal instability. In the late stages, collapse of the anterior vertebral body frequently occurs, resulting in a kyphotic deformity. The deformity can manifest as a knuckle deformity because of the collapse of a single vertebral body, a gibbus deformity if two or three vertebral bodies collapse, or a global rounded kyphotic deformity resulting from the involvement of multiple vertebral bodies [32]. The deformity features differ between children and adults. In children, the deformity can worsen if it occurs during the growth phases, whereas in adults, it depends on the number of vertebral bodies involved [55, 56].

Imaging plays an important role in the diagnosis and should include chest X-ray and multimodality spinal imaging. Spinal radiographs show the kyphotic deformity with the associated vertebral height loss and spinal angulation. CT can provide more detailed evaluation of the osseous involvement and any calcified paraspinal mass (Fig. 9.5). On MRI, the vertebral marrow of the involved spinal segment will show T1 hypointensity, T2 hyperintensity, and STIR hyperintensity (Fig. 9.6). A characteristic imaging feature of spinal tuberculosis is involvement of multiple vertebral segments with sparing of the disc spaces, much like involvement from metastatic disease. DWI sequences can show diffusion restriction in active disease and absence of diffusion restriction in chronic disease form [45]. After contrast administration, the involved vertebral segment will demonstrate diffuse enhancement of the vertebral body and subligamentous tissues. There may be epidural phlegmon and abscess, which can result in spinal cord compression or displacement. Fludeoxyglucose F18 (FDG-18) positron emission tomography imaging, which can show decreased uptake with treatment, can be useful in monitoring disease response to treatment over time [59].

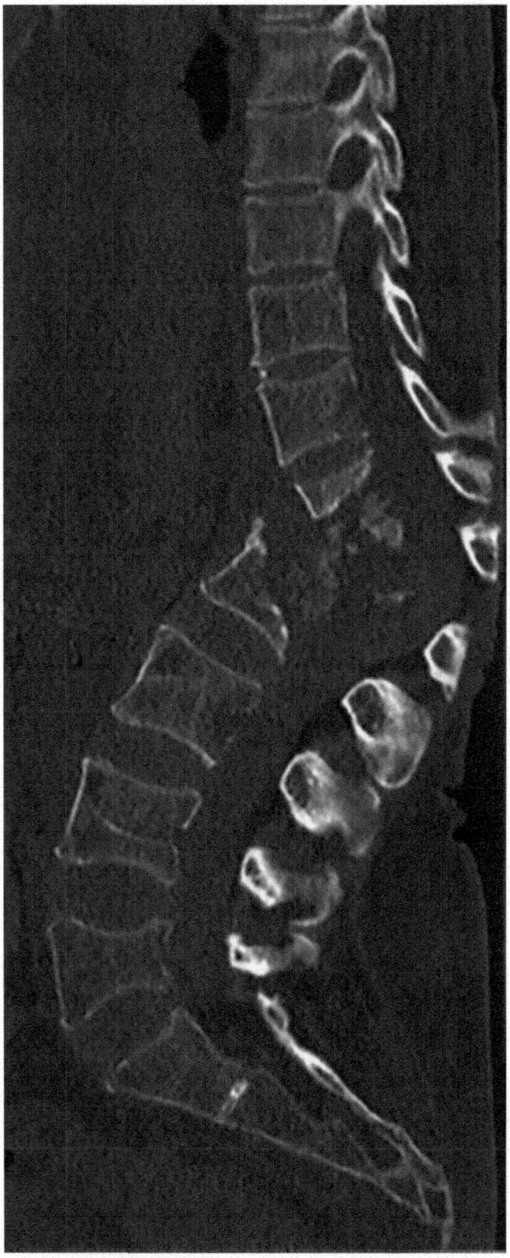

Fig. 9.5 Spinal tuberculosis. Sagittal CT of the thoracolumbar spine demonstrates osseous destructive changes with resulting kyphotic deformity secondary to tuberculosis infection in the spine

Treatment includes first-line drug treatment with isoniazid, rifampin, ethambutol, and pyrazinamide. Surgical treatment is reserved for debridement of large cold abscesses, spinal cord

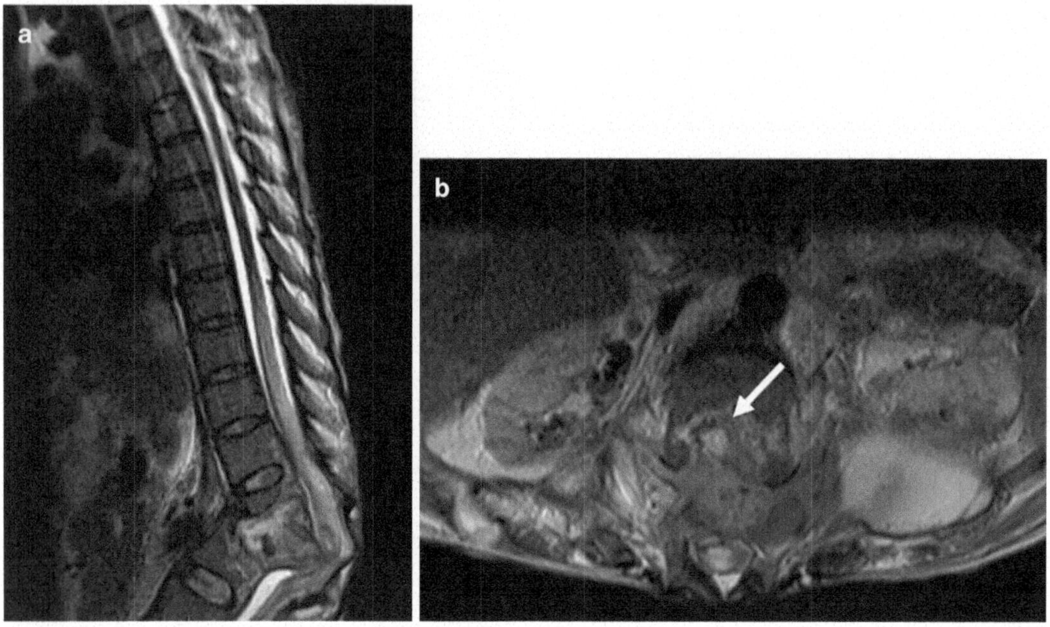

Fig. 9.6 Spinal tuberculosis. (**a**) Sagittal T2-weighted MRI of the thoracolumbar spine demonstrates a kyphotic deformity secondary to tuberculosis infection in the spine. (**b**) Axial T2-weighted image demonstrates the intramedullary hyperintensity (arrow), which may be due to edema and/or gliosis

compression, stabilizing of spinal instability, and correction of spinal deformity.

Hemorrhagic Mimickers

Epidural Hematoma

Spontaneous spinal epidural hematoma is an uncommon finding along the spinal axis and often can be mistaken for a neoplasm occupying the epidural space. Its incidence is just 0.1 per 100,000 per year. Spinal epidural hematoma manifests as an abrupt onset of symptoms ranging from axial pain to neurological symptom of paralysis, and it can occur secondary to trauma, surgery, coagulopathy, underlying arteriovenous malformation, or epidural injection or idiopathically. Anticoagulation use is linked to 17–30% of all cases of spinal epidural hematoma [12], but a majority of spinal epidural hematomas are idiopathic in nature with no identifiable cause (40–60% of cases) [16]. The etiology of the epidural hemorrhage has been postulated to be a rupture of epidural veins, which are valveless and prone to rupture when under increased pressure from sudden Valsalva maneuvers. The dorsal epidural space is a more common location than the ventral epidural space because the ventral epidural plexus is smaller than the dorsal epidural space and is theorized to have more structural support from the posterior longitudinal ligament [71].

The differential diagnosis for lesions in the epidural space includes lymphoma, abscess, metastasis, and lipomatosis. CT will show the hyperattenuation of epidural blood in the acute setting. MRI can not only help determine the age of the epidural blood products but also delineate the extent of the hematoma and effect on adjacent structures, such as spinal cord compression (Table 9.3). In the acute setting, an epidural hematoma will present as a T1-isointense, T2-hyperintense lesion. In the early subacute phase, blood product signal intensities will evolve

Table 9.3 Epidural blood characteristic on MRI

	T1	T2
Hyperacute	Isointense	Hyperintense
Acute	Isointense	Hypointense
Subacute (early/late)	Hyperintense	Hypo-/hyperintense
Chronic	Hypointense	Hypointense

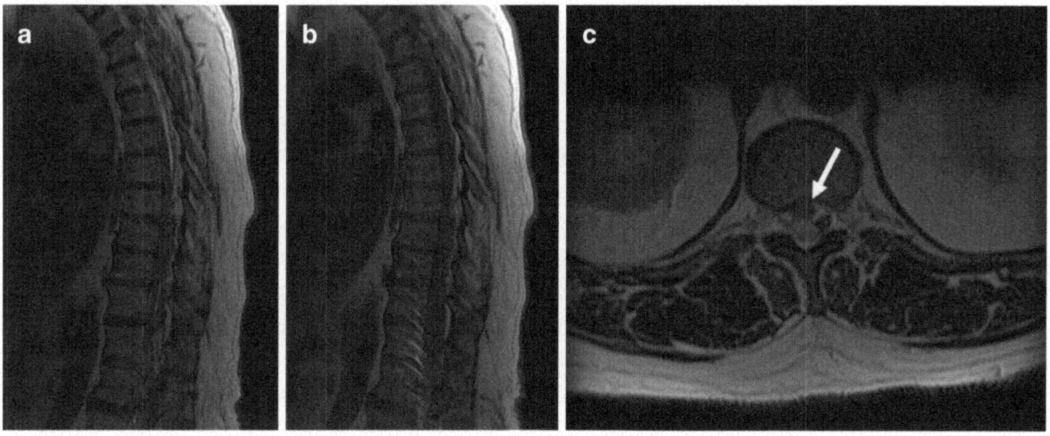

Fig. 9.7 Spontaneous epidural hematoma. Sagittal T2 (**a**) and T1 (**b**) images of the thoracolumbar spine show an epidural collection in the posterior spinal canal with heterogeneous signal intensity due to acute and subacute blood products. (**c**) Axial T2-weighted image demonstrates anterior displacement of the spinal cord (arrow) due to this collection

and appear T1 hyperintense and T2 hypointense, while in the late subacute phase, the epidural hematoma will be hyperintense on both T1- and T2-weighted MRI sequences (Fig. 9.7). After contrast administration, the epidural hematoma may show irregular heterogeneous enhancement. Fat suppression sequences can be used to distinguish hematoma from epidural lipomatosis. DWI can show heterogeneous reduced diffusivity in epidural hematoma, typically subacute in age. Epidural metastases are usually extensions of vertebral osseous metastatic deposits and will demonstrate the imaging characteristics of the native lesion. Fat-suppressed T1-weighted postcontrast imaging will be helpful to show the effect on the adjacent neural structures. As mentioned above, isolated epidural lymphoma will show diffuse contrast enhancement and T2 hypointensity because of the increased cellularity. Lymphoma involving the epidural space can also be seen in the setting of more systemic disease with vertebral and paraspinal involvement.

Treatment of spinal epidural hematoma depends on the magnitude of the symptoms. Neurological deficits warrant surgical intervention in the form of decompression and evacuation of hematoma of the spinal segments involved. Hemilaminectomy, laminectomy, or skip laminectomies with epidural irrigation can be used to evacuate the hematoma. Underlying coagulopathy should be corrected, and anticoagulation should be reversed before surgery to prevent further bleeding complication. Steroids can help with spinal cord edema. In patients who are managed conservatively, serial MRI scans can be used to monitor resolution of the hematoma over time [16].

Degenerative Mimickers

Disc Extrusions

Disc herniation is a common radiographic finding in patients with back pain and radicular symptoms. With a disc herniation, the nucleus pulposus breaches the annulus fibrosus and migrates past the intervertebral disc space. Disc herniations usually occur in the posterolateral aspect where the annulus fibrosus is the thinnest without structural support from the surrounding ligaments. Disc herniations can be classified as protrusion, extrusions, and sequestrations [13]. In the extradural spinal canal, a disc herniation can compress nerve roots and/or the spinal cord. Disc herniations have a proclivity for the lumbar spine, followed by the cervical spine, with the least common occurrence in the thoracic spine. The majority of disc extrusions are degenerative in nature, although herniation can also occur secondary to trauma. The incidence of disc herniation is 5–20 cases per 1000 adults annually, with a female-to-male ratio of 1:2 [17].

When a soft-tissue lesion is encountered in the epidural space, the differential diagnosis is led by disc herniation because it is statistically the most common cause. The differential diagnosis also includes osteophyte, epidural abscess, nerve sheath tumor, and epidural metastasis. Large disc extrusions can sometimes mimic the appearance of epidural tumors. MRI is the best modality to characterize disc herniations, which will appear isointense on T1-weighted imaging. Depending on the degree of water and/or hemorrhage content, the herniated disc material may appear hyper- to hypointense on T2-weighted imaging (Fig. 9.8). A very helpful imaging feature of disc herniations is the pattern of enhancement; a disc will demonstrate peripheral enhancement on contrasted scan. This imaging appearance can be particularly helpful when there is a sequestration, that is, when a disc fragment breaks away from the parent disc and migrates distally in the epidural space. This may be confused for a nerve sheath tumor or other neoplastic process; however, the peripheral enhancement should strongly suggest that the lesion is disc material. Epidural metastases are usually extensions of osseous metastasis that are well delineated on MRI. An adjacent compressed nerve may show T2 hyperintensity and enlargement because of edema and enhancement due to inflammation. CT myelography will show an extradural filling defect and will be helpful to show an osteophytic component.

Treatment of symptomatic disc herniation always starts with conservative management because >85% of disc herniations resolve within 8–12 weeks [65]. Conservative management consists of physical therapy and over-the-counter nonsteroidal anti-inflammatory drugs followed by spinal injections and selective nerve root blocks. Patients who fail conservative management can undergo surgery for symptom relief.

Synovial Cysts

Synovial cysts are cystic lesions of the synovial sheath that protrude from a defect in the facet joint capsule. The herniation of synovial material into the epidural space is thought to be due to

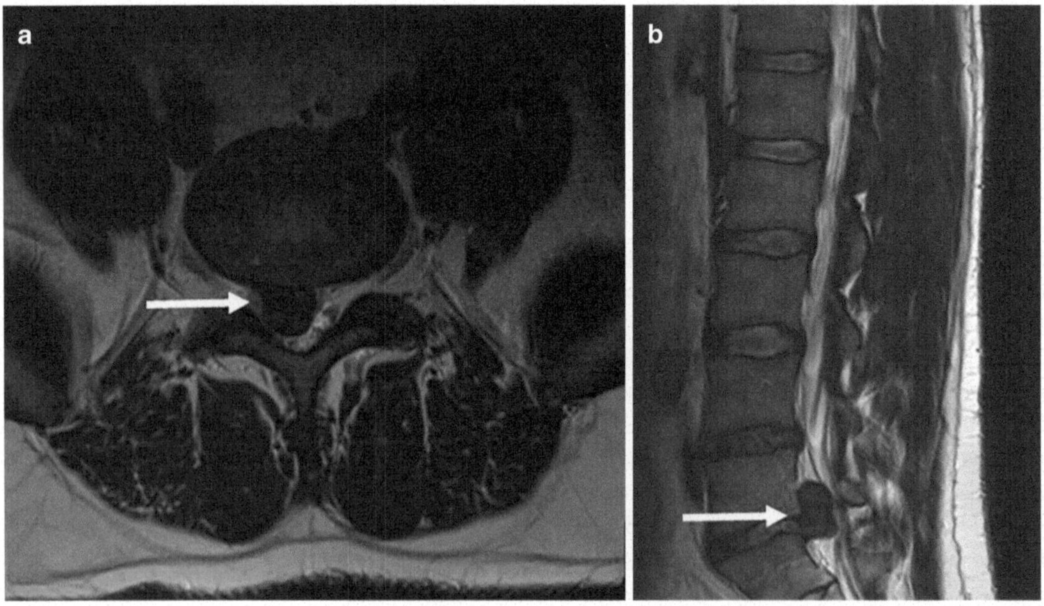

Fig. 9.8 Spontaneous epidural hematoma. (**a**) Axial T2-weighted MRI of the lumbar spine shows a large right central disc extrusion (arrow) that impinges on the central canal and right subarticular zone. (**b**) Sagittal T2-weighted image of the lumbar spine demonstrates cranial extension of this large disc extrusion (arrow) at L5-S1

osteoarthritis, degeneration, spondylolisthesis, and segmental motion. The most common location for synovial cysts is the lumbar spine, but these cysts are also, less commonly, found in the cervical and thoracic spine [8, 11]. The L4–5 level is the most common location, given the location of most spinal instability or joint hypermobility [67]. The cysts are located in the dorsolateral epidural space, and they are typically contiguous with the degenerated facet joint. The most common symptoms for synovial cysts are axial back pain, radiculopathy when there is adjacent nerve irritation/impingement, and neurogenic claudication when there is contribution to spinal stenosis. Rarely, depending on the size of the synovial cyst, patients can present with symptoms of cauda equina [3]. Asymptomatic synovial cysts can also be found incidentally on imaging of the spine, often projecting posteriorly into the paraspinal soft tissue. Hemorrhage within the synovial cyst can also occur (possibly because of trauma) and can exacerbate neurological symptoms [68].

The differential diagnosis of epidural lesions that are rounded in the dorsolateral aspect of the spinal canal includes nerve sheath tumor, epidural abscess, and rarely, epidural metastasis and disc herniation. Synovial cysts should be a leading consideration if the posterolateral epidural lesion is contiguous with a degenerated facet joint. CT will show the facet degeneration with sclerosis, joint space narrowing (with or without vacuum phenomenon), and subchondral cystic change. MRI will show a rounded T1-hypointense lesion extending from a degenerated facet joint. The facet joint often shows an effusion, and the synovial cyst will demonstrate variable T2 signal intensity depending on the degree of internal proteinaceous debris. Synovial cysts typically show a T2-hypointense rim, and this rim enhances with contrast administration (Fig. 9.9).

The treatment of synovial cysts ranges from nonsurgical management (such as percutaneous image-guided cyst aspiration or rupture with steroid injection) to surgical resection. Conservative management in the form of observation in mildly symptomatic lesions has been reported in the literature with complete resolution of cyst [30]. Steroid injection with cyst rupture and aspiration can have good patient outcomes [47]. Surgery in symptomatic patients (neurogenic claudication and cauda equina) involves laminectomy, hemilaminectomy, or decompression and instrumented fusion of the segments involved.

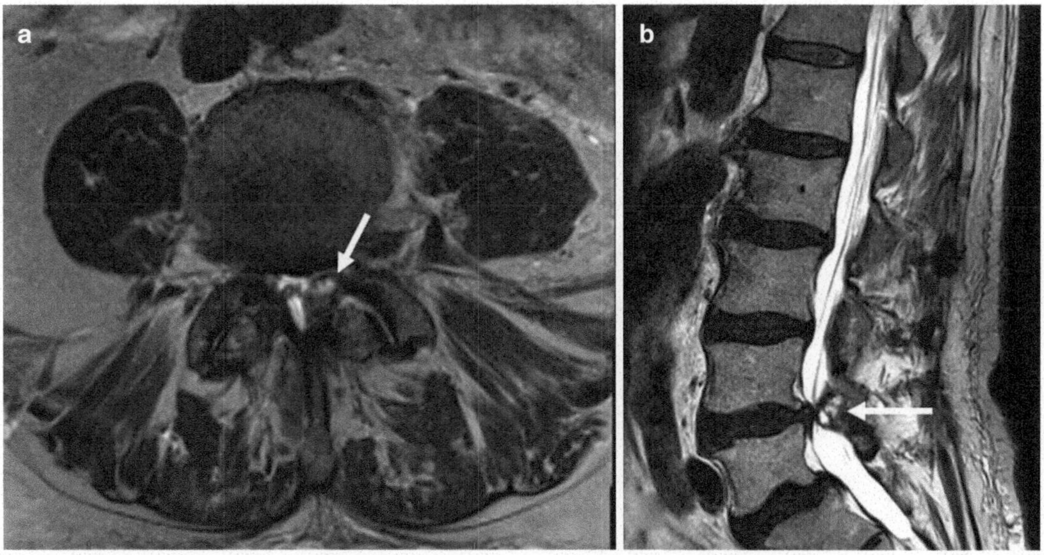

Fig. 9.9 Synovial cyst. (**a**) Axial T2-weighted MRI of the lumbar spine shows a cystic lesion (arrow) extending anteromedially from the left degenerated facet joint. This synovial cyst impinges on the left subarticular zone. (**b**) Sagittal T2-weighted MRI demonstrates the thick T2-hypointense rim of this synovial cyst (arrow), which may be due to mineralization

Metabolic Bone Disease

Brown Tumor

Brown tumor (also called an osteoclastoma) is another uncommon nonneoplastic lesion that occurs in the spine secondary to a reactive process due to bone resorption. Brown tumors can occur in primary or secondary hyperparathyroidism [38]. Because primary hyperparathyroidism is rare, brown tumors are more commonly seen in secondary hyperparathyroidism in the setting of long-term hemodialysis due to renal osteodystrophy. Renal osteodystrophy results in changes in bone metabolism from prolonged chronic renal dysfunction. It is a general term to describe disorders of calcium and phosphate metabolism and their systemic sequelae. Renal impairment results in retention of phosphate and decreased calcitriol synthesis, which results in decreased serum calcium and secondary hyperparathyroidism. Secondary hyperparathyroidism, in turn, results in extensive bone marrow fibrosis and increased bone resorption [34]. Furthermore, renal impairment and chronic dialysis result in osteomalacia, which is typical in the setting of renal dialysis secondary to aluminum toxicity [46]. The reactive process in the spine results in selective areas undergoing more resorption than others, which results in accumulation of connective tissue cells, giant cells, and osteoid deposition. Additionally, hemosiderin deposition from hemorrhage can displace the bone marrow and result in formation of the brown tumor [29].

Brown tumors are typically nonencapsulated and vascular lesions, which demonstrate multinucleated giant cells on histology. Patients can manifest with symptoms of low back pain and can sometimes present with neurological symptoms of radiculopathy, myelopathy, and cauda equina. Brown tumor lesions can also be detected in asymptomatic patients. When a spinal lytic lesion is encountered on imaging, clinical history and laboratory tests are essential for the diagnosis. Laboratory findings include elevated calcium, alkaline phosphatase, and low serum levels of phosphate [25]. A parathyroid assay will demonstrate elevated serum parathyroid hormone levels. In cases where the diagnosis is unclear, a biopsy of the spinal lesion can provide insight into the diagnosis. Additionally, brown tumor and giant cell tumors can be difficult to discern; however, the overall clinical and radiographic findings are useful in the differentiating between both entities.

The differential diagnosis for an expansile and lytic spinal lesion centered in the vertebral body, like brown tumor, includes plasmacytoma, metastasis, lymphoma, and giant cell tumors. CT will show a well-defined lytic lesion, typically solitary. On MRI, the lesion demonstrates T1 hypointensity and T2 hyperintensity or hypointensity, depending on the presence of hemorrhage (Figs. 9.10 and 9.11).

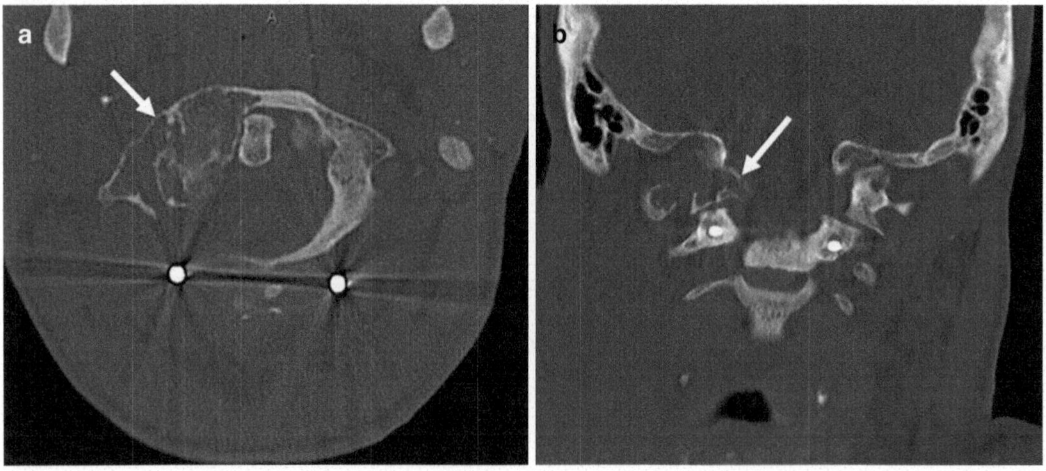

Fig. 9.10 Brown tumor. Axial (**a**) and sagittal (**b**) CT of the craniocervical junction demonstrates a lytic, expansile bone lesion (arrow) centered in the right lateral mass. This is a brown tumor in a patient with hyperparathyroidism related to renal osteodystrophy

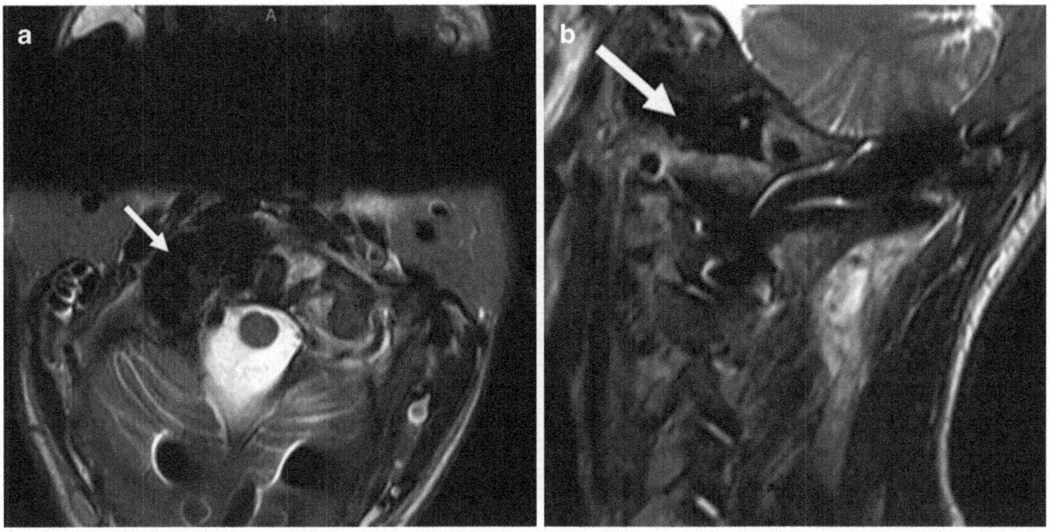

Fig. 9.11 Brown tumor. Axial (**a**) and sagittal (**b**) T2-weighted MRIs of the craniocervical junction demonstrating a homogeneously hypointense brown tumor (arrow) in the C1 lateral mass

The main treatment for brown tumors is to address the underlying disorder of hyperparathyroidism via a surgical parathyroidectomy. In patients with neurological symptoms, resection and decompression can provide the best clinical outcome. Surgery can be a decompression via laminectomy but usually requires a more extensive decompression with circumferential stabilization and fusion, but poor bone quality can often lead to failure of instrumentation in patients on chronic dialysis [35].

Paget Disease

Paget disease (PD), also known as osteitis deformans, is a metabolic disease of bone that results from changes in bone resorption and remodeling. After osteoporosis, it is the second most common primary metabolic bone disease [26]. The pathophysiology is not completely understood, but PD is thought to be due to abnormal pathological remodeling and bone formation that lead to fractures and deformity. The disease has three phases. The first phase involves excessive osteoclastic bone resorption, which is followed by a secondary phase of compensatory osteoblastic activity resulting in disorganized and abnormal bone depositions. The third phase is an inactive sclerotic phase that results in normal or decreased bone activity [10]. PD is linked to genetic factors, although viral and zoonotic causes have been postulated. Patients present with symptoms after the sixth decade of life, and there is a slight predilection toward males [49]. Serum alkaline phosphatase levels are typically elevated. The most common location for PD is the pelvis, followed by the spine (commonly the lumbar segment), but other bones such as the femur, skull, and sternum can also be affected [26]. The most common presenting symptom is bone pain, which occurs at rest and at night. PD in the spine can cause symptoms of low back pain and symptoms related to spinal stenosis. Spinal stenosis is caused by expansion of the vertebral body posteriorly and overgrowth of the facet joints. PD can also result in extraosseous extension involving the anterior and posterior longitudinal ligaments and ligamentum flavum. During the lytic phase, PD can also result in compression fractures in the lumbar spine. Facet arthropathy can also occur in PD, which can result in spondylolisthesis.

The differential diagnosis includes osteoblastic neoplasm, hemangioma, hyperthyroidism, hyperparathyroidism, and vitamin D deficiency. On imaging, PD affects the vertebral body and

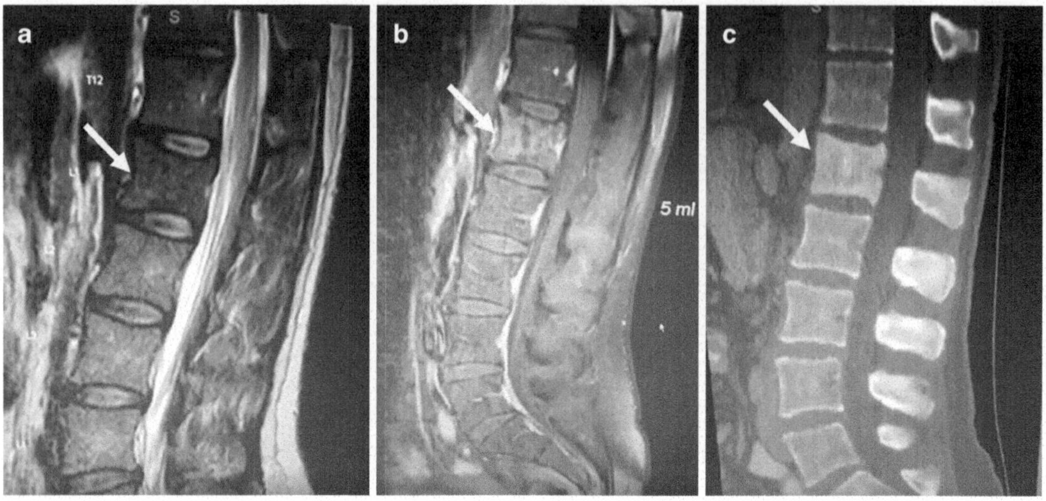

Fig. 9.12 Paget disease. (**a**) Sagittal T2-weighted image shows a mildly expanded L1 vertebral body with heterogeneous hypointensity (arrow). (**b**) Sagittal T1-weighted, contrast-enhanced, fat-saturated image reveals heterogeneous enhancement (arrow) of the L1 level affected by Paget's disease. (**c**) Sagittal CT demonstrates diffuse sclerosis (arrow) in that L1 vertebral body as well as mild expansion

neural arch, which are typically enlarged with trabecular coarsening and cortical thickening. CT scans show sclerotic cortex with disorganized trabeculae and vertebral body expansion (Fig. 9.12). On MRI, the involved vertebral body and/or posterior elements demonstrate T1- and T2-hypointense cortex. The expanded vertebral body and posterior elements may show spinal stenosis and neuroforaminal stenosis. During the active phase, contrast-enhanced T1-weighted images may show heterogeneous enhancement. The extent of PD involvement in the skeletal system can be evaluated using a radionuclide bone scan of the skeletal system, which will demonstrate uptake of the tracer at the sites of increased bone remodeling in the active phase.

Treatment of PD is with antiresorptive medication to decrease the metabolic activity in symptomatic patients. The antiresorptive medications of choice are bisphosphonates, which decrease bone turnover. Calcitonin also inhibits bone turnover and can be used in patients who have contraindications to bisphosphonates. For patients who do not respond to medical treatment, surgical spine decompression can be attempted for severe spinal stenosis and neuroforaminal stenosis. Vertebroplasty can be considered in severely symptomatic patients with vertebral collapse [62].

Inflammatory Mimickers

Inflammatory Pseudotumor

Nonneoplastic lesions can occur behind the odontoid and are termed retro-odontoid pseudotumor (ROP). Such lesions are thought to be the result of craniocervical motion resulting in reactive inflammation followed by the formation of granulation tissue. The most common etiology for ROP is rheumatoid arthritis and atlantoaxial instability. The prevalence of rheumatoid arthritis with atlantoaxial instability can range from 10% to 86% [60]. In atlantoaxial instability, the ROP formation is triggered by chronic mechanical stress, which results in an inflammatory response. The consequent transverse ligament tears and attempted repairs result in hypervascularization with granulation tissue formation with the overall result of formation of an inflammatory mass originating from the transverse ligament [5, 9]. In rheumatoid arthritis, formation of ROP is due to

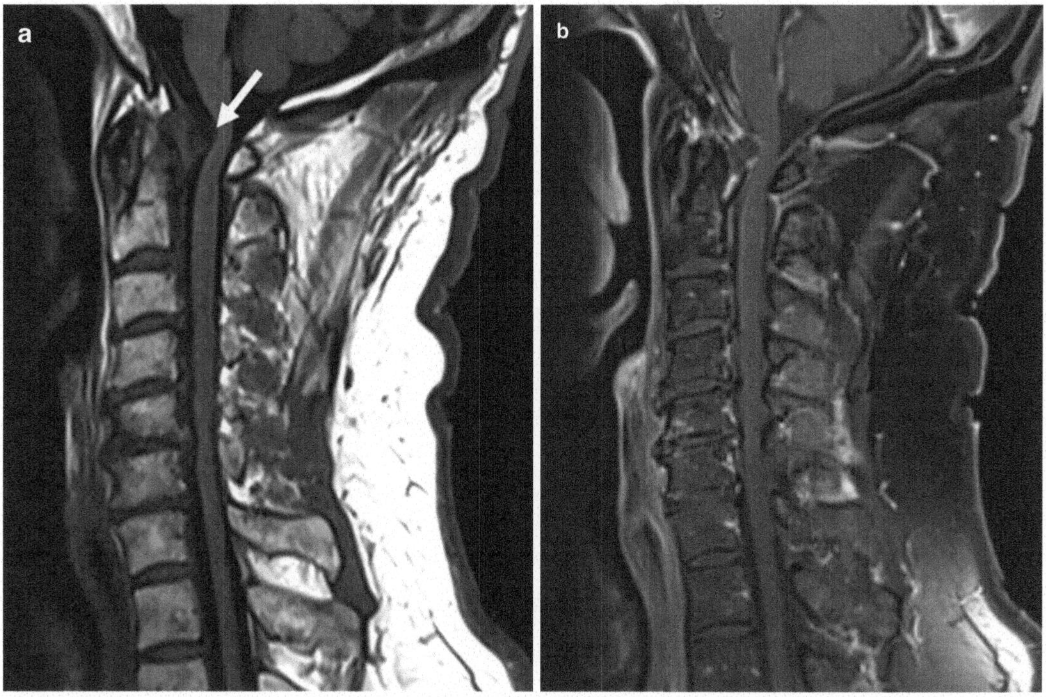

Fig. 9.13 Retro-odontoid pseudotumor. Sagittal MRI of the cervical spine demonstrates (**a**) isointense mass in the retro-odontoid space on T1-weighted sequences and (**b**) mild heterogeneous enhancement on the T1-weighted, contrast-enhanced, fat-saturated image. There is mild mass effect on and posterior displacement of the cervicomedullary junction (arrow)

pannus formation from inflammation of the synovial membrane, which results in chronic inflammation, ligament laxity, and bony erosion around the C1–2 joint [70]. Other rare causes of ROP can include psoriatic arthritis, gout, calcium pyrophosphate deposition disease, hemodialysis-associated amyloidosis, pigmented villonodular synovitis, retro-odontoid synovial cyst, odontoid fractures, and ossification of the posterior longitudinal ligament.

Patient presentation can range from being asymptomatic with incidental discovery of ROP on imaging to myelopathic symptoms related to ROP causing wide-ranging cord compression with or without cord signal change. Other symptoms include neck pain and radiculopathy. Patients who are asymptomatic initially can present with neurological symptoms after having an episode of trauma (e.g., ground-level fall, motor vehicle accident), which can result in an isolated injury to the cord from the ROP facilitated through the trauma [28].

Differential diagnosis of a retro-odontoid mass should include noninflammatory pathologies, such as meningioma, metastatic tumor, chordoma, and osteochondroma. Imaging features that can assist in the diagnosis include retro-odontoid soft tissue with or without mineralization and bone erosion on CT. MRI is complementary, demonstrating the compressive effects of the ROP on the spinal cord/cervicomedullary junction. The ROP is T1 hypointense to isointense and heterogeneously T2 hypointense (Fig. 9.13). Flexion–extension X-rays or flexion–extension CT of the cervical spine can provide functional information to reveal instability, which can be occipitocervical or atlantoaxial; this information can be critical in determining the optimal surgical intervention.

Treatment options for ROP include observation with serial imaging in patients who are asymptomatic. In symptomatic patients, surgical treatment is recommended. The indications for surgical treatment include worsening neck pain, worsening instability, and symptoms of myelopathy. Surgical resection of the ROP via a transoral approach is an option that can have the benefit of enabling histopathological analysis, but the risks of an anterior approach include palatal dehiscence, oral edema, and need for external orthosis or posterior cervical fusion [64]. Endoscopic transnasal, transclival odontoidectomy has also been described in the literature for patients with irreducible basilar invagination. Alternatively, there is evidence in the literature that supports regression or even resolution of the ROP with posterior cervical surgical stabilization [24]. Posterior fixation via C1–2 posterior fusion is recommended for patients with atlantoaxial instability. In patients who have evidence of craniocervical instability, occiput-to-C2 fusion can be performed [69]. Furthermore, depending on the amount of ROP causing spinal cord compression, a C1 decompressive laminectomy can be also performed during the posterior fusion.

Other Spine Tumor Mimickers

Extradural Hemangioma

Extradural hemangiomas are typically located in the vertebral body and are benign incidental findings that are frequently seen on spine imaging. They have a reported incidence of 11% based on autopsy results [57]. The most common location for vertebral hemangiomas is the thoracic spine, followed by the lumbar spine, but they can be seen throughout the spinal axis. Histologically, vertebral hemangiomas are considered malformations of the microcirculation rather than vascular neoplasms. The classification is based on the predominant type of vascular channel: capillary, cavernous, arteriovenous, and venous malformations [52]. In these lesions, thin-walled, endothelial-lined blood vessels form between nonvascular structures, such as fat, muscle, or bone [53]. The small vessels penetrate the bone marrow and form around bony trabeculae, resulting in secondary remodeling of bone trabeculae and adipose tissue involution [20]. The imaging appearance is affected by the degree of vascular versus other elements.

In most cases, vertebral hemangiomas are quiescent lesions and passive in nature, but in rare cases, they can be classified as aggressive. The aggressive form of vertebral hemangioma refers to a lesion that expands further past the vertebral body, often with a soft-tissue component, and encroaches into the epidural, paravertebral, and posterior elements. Aggressive vertebral hemangiomas can result in symptoms related to spinal cord compression due to bony expansion, epidural extension, or vertebral body fracture with retropulsion.

The imaging features of vertebral hemangiomas are characteristic, which enables easy diagnosis. The lesion is localized to the vertebral body and will infrequently extend into the posterior elements. On sagittal and axial CT images, vertebral hemangiomas demonstrate a "honeycomb" or "white polka-dot" appearance due to the prominent vertically aligned trabeculae. This pattern can also be seen on MRI. Vertebral hemangiomas are T1 and T2 hyperintense but hypointense on STIR images (Fig. 9.14) [2]. Because of their vascularity, they show robust enhancement and retain a high signal on fat-suppressed sequences. "Atypical" hemangiomas have greater vascular elements and can appear heterogeneously T1 hypointense and STIR hyperintense, which can be misinterpreted as vertebral metastasis. It is important to look for the internal prominent trabeculae, which may be better seen on a correlative CT. Differentiating aggressive vertebral hemangiomas may require a biopsy. The differential diagnosis of vertebral hemangiomas includes focal fatty marrow changes, Paget disease, and post-spinal radiation changes. Focal fatty marrow changes will lack the prominent internal trabeculae. Paget disease will show an enlarged vertebral body, which is expanded and has an irregular, disorganized trabecular pattern. The fatty marrow changes of radiation treatment will fit a discrete radiation field and will lack the vertical trabeculae pattern.

The primary treatment for vertebral hemangiomas is observation because most are incidental

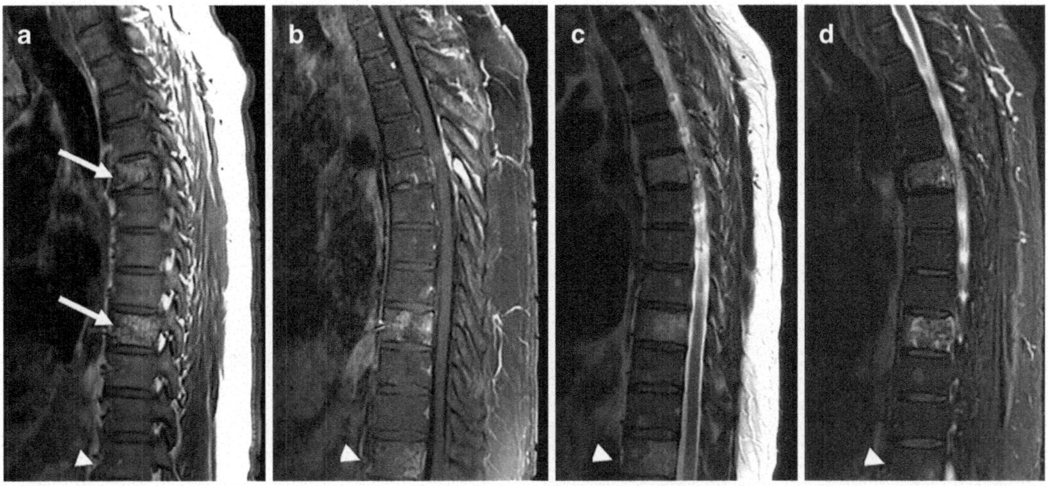

Fig. 9.14 Vertebral hemangioma. (**a**) Sagittal T1-weighted MRI of the thoracic spine demonstrates heterogeneously hyperintense lesions involving two thoracic vertebral bodies. There are prominent internal trabeculations. (**b**) These vertebral hemangiomas show variable enhancement on sagittal T1-weighted, contrast-enhanced, fat-saturated MRI. Sagittal T2 (**c**) and STIR (**d**) images show heterogeneous hyperintensity in these osseous hemangiomas. The most inferior vertebral lesions are predominantly hypointense on T1 (arrowhead), show heterogeneous enhancement and T2 hyperintensity, and demonstrate STIR hypointensity due to varying degrees of fat and vascular elements

findings and patients are asymptomatic. Lesions may rarely fracture and become symptomatic, presenting with back pain, and can be treated conservatively with a brace for pain management. Vertebroplasty can be performed for vertebral body collapse. Aggressive hemangiomas can be treated appropriately for their level of spinal canal compromise and nerve root impingement. Radiation is used for patients with mild and slowly progressing symptoms. Surgery is indicated for patients with myelopathy and weakness due to epidural invasion causing significant spinal cord compression. Surgery can entail decompression or vertebral corpectomy and fusion [37]. There is no overall consensus for best management of aggressive vertebral hemangiomas, which will require individual management on a case-by-case basis [20].

Bone Islands

Bone islands are also known as enostoses, sclerotic islands, or calcified islands. They are thought to be a localized excess of cortical bone formation within cancellous bone adjacent to bony trabeculae. The formation of bone islands is thought to be congenital or developmental in nature and due to failed resorption during the endochondral ossification phase [23]. These lesions are incidental and do not cause symptoms but can be misdiagnosed as sclerotic metastasis or osteoid osteoma. Because they occur during development, they can be discovered in patients in any age group. They are typically stable and do not demonstrate growth.

Their differential diagnosis includes vertebral metastasis and osteoid osteoma. Radiographically, bone islands have a round, ovoid, or oblong shape. They are frequently detected as homogenous hyperdense, variable-sized lesions on CT scans and X-ray (Fig. 9.15) [58]. Bone islands can be a single focal finding or can occur in multiple areas and can have the appearance of "thorny radiation" blending within the trabeculae. MRI shows T1 and T2 hypointensity with no enhancement on T1 sequences with contrast. A nuclear bone scan can demonstrate some uptake and can be used to differentiate bone islands from isolated tumor metastasis. An osteoid osteoma is

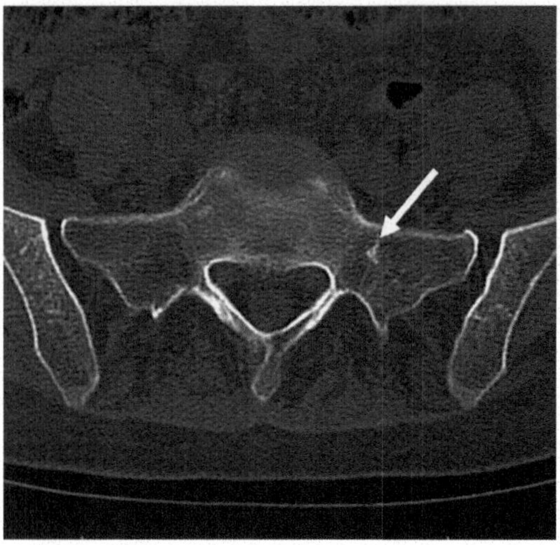

Fig. 9.15 Bone island. Axial CT of the sacrum demonstrates a spiculated lesion in the left sacral ala, which is characteristic of a bone island

typically a solitary lesion in the posterior elements with central sclerosis and radiolucent halo and causes symptoms of axial pain.

Bone islands require no treatment or observation because they are essentially an incidental normal variant.

Lipomatosis

Spinal epidural lipomatosis (SEL) is a rare benign lesion that occurs because of proliferation of adipose tissue within the epidural space. The associations linked to SEL include prolonged use of exogenous steroids, endogenous steroid production, Cushing syndrome, and obesity; there are also idiopathic cases (17% of cases) [18]. Chronic exogenous steroid use is common in many medical conditions such as organ transplantation, rheumatoid arthritis, sarcoidosis, Crohn's disease, lupus erythematosus, and polyarteritis nodosa [41]. In exogenous steroid use and endogenous steroid production, the cause of SEL is thought to be due to hypertrophy of adipose tissue. Obesity is thought to be a predisposing factor rather than a cause, where obese patients are thought to be in a pseudo-Cushing state. Overall, the pathophysiology of SEL is currently unknown. SEL is often an incidental finding on imaging in asymptomatic patients. Rarely, SEL can become symptomatic in patients when it causes spinal cord compression or nerve root impingement. Symptoms can manifest as radiculopathy, myelopathy, neurogenic claudication, plegia, or cauda equina syndrome. Symptoms can also occur in the setting of compression fractures due to osteoporosis from chronic steroid use [1].

The most common locations for symptomatic SEL are the thoracic spine in 58–61% of cases and lumbar spine for 39–42% of cases [15]. Cervical spine involvement is rare but has been reported in the literature. Both CT and MRI demonstrate the presence of contiguous fat in the dorsal epidural space with ventral displacement of the thecal sac. On CT, this prominent fat is hypoattenuating and can anteriorly displace the thecal sac. There are no associated osseous abnormalities. Similarly, MRI will show prominent fat in the dorsal epidural space that is T1 and T2 hyperintense (Fig. 9.16). Fat suppression sequences (such as STIR) will confirm fat tissue and exclude blood products, which would be seen in an epidural hematoma. Epidural hematoma may have T1 hyperintensity due to subacute blood products despite fat suppression. The differential diagnosis for SEL also includes spinal angiolipoma, which will show heterogeneous enhancement on T1-weighted imaging with contrast sequences. An epidural metastasis will extend from vertebral lesions and typically will have a low T1 signal intensity and enhancement. An epidural abscess typically will have associated vertebral osteomyelitis/discitis, is T1 hypointense and T2 hyperintense, and has rim enhancement. Diagnostic criteria that can be used to diagnose SEL include MRI findings of segmental spinal cord compression, epidural fat that is >7 mm in thickness, and patient body mass index >27.5 [42].

Management of SEL can be either conservative or surgical. Nonsurgical management involves eliminating the use of steroids or reducing the dosage. If obesity is the only identifiable cause, then weight reduction can aid in treating SEL [40]. Endogenous steroid production can be elucidated by a thorough endocrinological

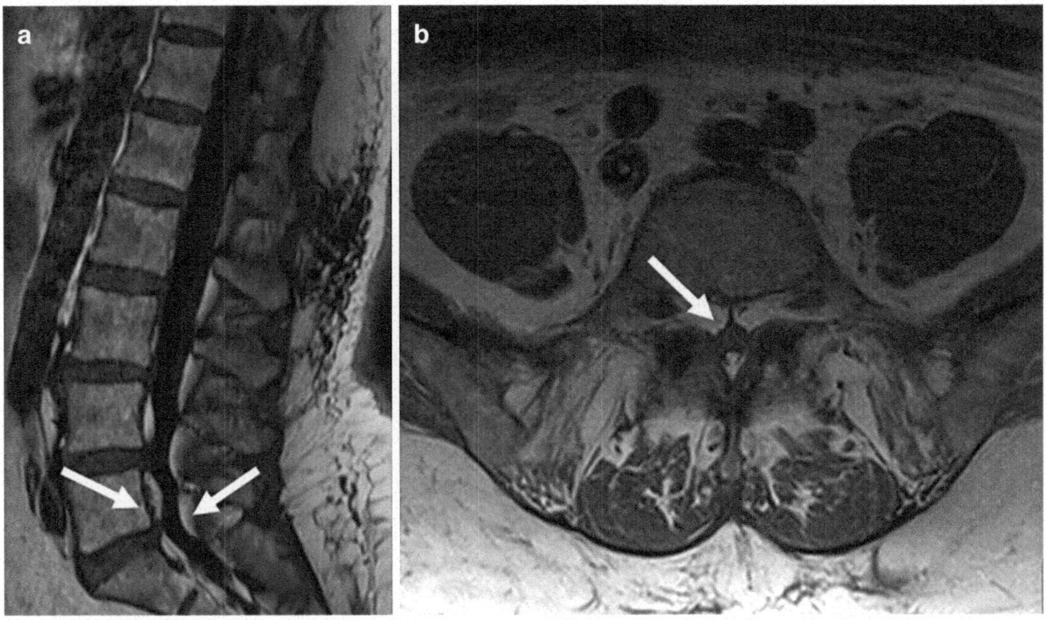

Fig. 9.16 Spinal epidural lipomatosis. Sagittal (**a**) and axial (**b**) T1-weighted MRI of the lumbar spine demonstrates prominent epidural fat circumferentially narrowing the thecal sac (arrow)

workup, and treatment of the underlying cause can aid with reduction or resolution of SEL. In symptomatic patients who fail conservative management, surgical decompression can be offered to resolve neurologic symptoms [14].

Other Tumor Mimics

Additional other rare conditions that should be considered in the differential for spinal tumors mimics include rheumatologic diseases and osseous manifestation of sarcoid.

Rheumatic arthritis (RA) results in chronic inflammation that affects joints, ligaments, multi-organs, and bones. RA can affect the spine, resulting in osseous changes that can be mistaken for a neoplastic process [21]. In the cervical spine, RA can manifest as tumor-like by forming a pannus from inflamed and thickened synovium. In the subaxial spine, RA causes arthritic changes resulting in subluxation and bony erosion. Imaging and laboratory tests are useful in diagnosis. MR imaging will demonstrate pannus formation in the cervical spine, and CT imaging will demonstrate bony erosion. Laboratory tests that are helpful for diagnosis include rheumatoid factor, cyclic citrullinated peptide antibody, erythrocyte sedimentation rate, C-reactive protein, and autoantibodies [36].

Sarcoidosis is a systemic disease characterized by the formation of noncaseating granulomas in different organs, but most commonly in lymph nodes, skin, and lungs [61]. Estimated osseous involvement of patients with sarcoidosis ranges from 1% to 13%; however, sarcoid involving the spine is very rare and only noted in case reports [33, 72]. Vertebral sarcoid can involve the spinal axis most commonly in the thoracic and upper lumbar spine and less commonly in the cervical spine. CT scan demonstrates tumor-like lytic, mixed lytic, and sclerotic lesions. MRI demonstrates granulomatous infiltration of the marrow. Additionally, paravertebral ossification can also occur [54]. Vertebral sarcoid is a very rare finding, but should be included in the differential diagnosis for neoplastic mimics.

Disclosure The authors report no conflict of interest concerning the materials or methods used in this study or the findings specified in this chapter.
Funding There were no external sources of financial support for this chapter.

References

1. Andress HJ, Schurmann M, Heuck A, Schmand J, Lob G. A rare case of osteoporotic spine fracture associated with epidural lipomatosis causing paraplegia following long-term cortisone therapy. Arch Orthop Trauma Surg. 2000;120:484–6.
2. Baudrez V, Galant C, Vande Berg BC. Benign vertebral hemangioma: MR-histological correlation. Skelet Radiol. 2001;30:442–6.
3. Baum JA, Hanley EN Jr. Intraspinal synovial cyst simulating spinal stenosis. A case report. Spine (Phila Pa 1976). 1986;11:487–9.
4. Boody BS, Tarazona DA, Vaccaro AR. Evaluation and management of pyogenic and tubercular spine infections. Curr Rev Musculoskelet Med. 2018;11:643–52.
5. Buttiens A, Vandevenne J, Van Cauter S. Retro-odontoid pseudotumor in a patient with atlanto-occipital assimilation. J Belg Soc Radiol. 2018;102:62.
6. Cormican L, Hammal R, Messenger J, Milburn HJ. Current difficulties in the diagnosis and management of spinal tuberculosis. Postgrad Med J. 2006;82:46–51.
7. Corrah TW, Enoch DA, Aliyu SH, Lever AM. Bacteraemia and subsequent vertebral osteomyelitis: a retrospective review of 125 patients. QJM. 2011;104:201–7.
8. Costa F, Menghetti C, Cardia A, Fornari M, Ortolina A. Cervical synovial cyst: case report and review of literature. Eur Spine J. 2010;19(Suppl 2):S100–2.
9. Crockard HA, Sett P, Geddes JF, Stevens JM, Kendall BE, Pringle JA. Damaged ligaments at the craniocervical junction presenting as an extradural tumour: a differential diagnosis in the elderly. J Neurol Neurosurg Psychiatry. 1991;54:817–21.
10. Dell'Atti C, Cassar-Pullicino VN, Lalam RK, Tins BJ, Tyrrell PN. The spine in Paget's disease. Skelet Radiol. 2007;36:609–26.
11. Doherty PF, Sherman BA, Stein C, White R. Bilateral synovial cysts of the thoracic spine: a case report. Surg Neurol. 1993;39:279–81.
12. Dziedzic T, Kunert P, Krych P, Marchel A. Management and neurological outcome of spontaneous spinal epidural hematoma. J Clin Neurosci. 2015;22:726–9.
13. Fardon DF, Williams AL, Dohring EJ, Murtagh FR, Gabriel Rothman SL, Sze GK. Lumbar disc nomenclature: version 2.0: recommendations of the combined task forces of the North American Spine Society, the American Society of Spine Radiology and the American Society of Neuroradiology. Spine J. 2014;14:2525–45.
14. Ferlic PW, Mannion AF, Jeszenszky D, Porchet F, Fekete TF, Kleinstuck F, et al. Patient-reported outcome of surgical treatment for lumbar spinal epidural lipomatosis. Spine J. 2016;16:1333–41.
15. Fessler RG, Johnson DL, Brown FD, Erickson RK, Reid SA, Kranzler L. Epidural lipomatosis in steroid-treated patients. Spine (Phila Pa 1976). 1992;17:183–8.
16. Figueroa J, DeVine JG. Spontaneous spinal epidural hematoma: literature review. J Spine Surg. 2017;3:58–63.
17. Fjeld OR, Grovle L, Helgeland J, Smastuen MC, Solberg TK, Zwart JA, et al. Complications, reoperations, readmissions, and length of hospital stay in 34 639 surgical cases of lumbar disc herniation. Bone Joint J. 2019;101-B:470–7.
18. Fogel GR, Cunningham PY 3rd, Esses SI. Spinal epidural lipomatosis: case reports, literature review and meta-analysis. Spine J. 2005;5:202–11.
19. Garg RK, Somvanshi DS. Spinal tuberculosis: a review. J Spinal Cord Med. 2011;34:440–54.
20. Gaudino S, Martucci M, Colantonio R, Lozupone E, Visconti E, Leone A, et al. A systematic approach to vertebral hemangioma. Skelet Radiol. 2015;44:25–36.
21. Gillick JL, Wainwright J, Das K. Rheumatoid arthritis and the cervical spine: a review on the role of surgery. Int J Rheumatol. 2015;2015:252456.
22. Gouliouris T, Aliyu SH, Brown NM. Spondylodiscitis: update on diagnosis and management. J Antimicrob Chemother. 2010;65(Suppl 3):iii11–24.
23. Greenspan A. Bone island (enostosis): current concept—a review. Skelet Radiol. 1995;24:111–5.
24. Grob D, Wursch R, Grauer W, Sturzenegger J, Dvorak J. Atlantoaxial fusion and retrodental pannus in rheumatoid arthritis. Spine (Phila Pa 1976). 1997;22:1580–3; discussion 1584.
25. Haddad FH, Malkawi OM, Sharbaji AA, Jbara IF, Rihani HR. Primary hyperparathyroidism. A rare cause of spinal cord compression. Saudi Med J. 2007;28:783–6.
26. Hadjipavlou AG, Gaitanis LN, Katonis PG, Lander P. Paget's disease of the spine and its management. Eur Spine J. 2001;10:370–84.
27. Hadjipavlou AG, Mader JT, Necessary JT, Muffoletto AJ. Hematogenous pyogenic spinal infections and their surgical management. Spine (Phila Pa 1976). 2000;25:1668–79.
28. Hamard M, Martin SP, Boudabbous S. Retroodontoid pseudotumor related to development of myelopathy secondary to atlantoaxial instability on os odontoideum. Case Rep Radiol. 2018;2018:1658129.
29. Hong WS, Sung MS, Chun KA, Kim JY, Park SW, Lee KH, et al. Emphasis on the MR imaging findings of brown tumor: a report of five cases. Skelet Radiol. 2011;40:205–13.
30. Houten JK, Sanderson SP, Cooper PR. Spontaneous regression of symptomatic lumbar synovial cysts. Report of three cases. J Neurosurg. 2003;99:235–8.
31. Issa K, Diebo BG, Faloon M, Naziri Q, Pourtaheri S, Paulino CB, et al. The epidemiology of vertebral

osteomyelitis in the United States from 1998 to 2013. Clin Spine Surg. 2018;31:E102–8.
32. Jain AK, Aggarwal PK, Arora A, Singh S. Behaviour of the kyphotic angle in spinal tuberculosis. Int Orthop. 2004;28:110–4.
33. James DG, Neville E, Carstairs LS. Bone and joint sarcoidosis. Semin Arthritis Rheum. 1976;6:53–81.
34. Jevtic V. Imaging of renal osteodystrophy. Eur J Radiol. 2003;46:85–95.
35. Jia Q, Gao X, Zhou Z, Lan B, Zhao J, Liu T, et al. Urgent surgery for spinal instability or neurological impairment caused by spinal brown tumors occurring in the context of end-stage renal disease. J Neurosurg Spine. 2019:1–8.
36. Jurik AG. Imaging the spine in arthritis-a pictorial review. Insights Imaging. 2011;2:177–91.
37. Kato S, Kawahara N, Murakami H, Demura S, Yoshioka K, Okayama T, et al. Surgical management of aggressive vertebral hemangiomas causing spinal cord compression: long-term clinical follow-up of five cases. J Orthop Sci. 2010;15:350–6.
38. Khalatbari MR, Moharamzad Y. Brown tumor of the spine in patients with primary hyperparathyroidism. Spine (Phila Pa 1976). 2014;39:E1073–9.
39. Khanna K, Sabharwal S. Spinal tuberculosis: a comprehensive review for the modern spine surgeon. Spine J. 2019;19:1858–70.
40. Kniprath K, Farooque M. Drastic weight reduction decrease in epidural fat and concomitant improvement of neurogenic claudicatory symptoms of spinal epidural lipomatosis. Pain Med. 2017;18:1204–6.
41. Koch CA, Doppman JL, Patronas NJ, Nieman LK, Chrousos GP. Do glucocorticoids cause spinal epidural lipomatosis? When endocrinology and spinal surgery meet. Trends Endocrinol Metab. 2000;11:86–90.
42. Kumar K, Nath RK, Nair CP, Tchang SP. Symptomatic epidural lipomatosis secondary to obesity. Case report J Neurosurg. 1996;85:348–50.
43. Kumar Y, Gupta N, Chhabra A, Fukuda T, Soni N, Hayashi D. Magnetic resonance imaging of bacterial and tuberculous spondylodiscitis with associated complications and non-infectious spinal pathology mimicking infections: a pictorial review. BMC Musculoskelet Disord. 2017;18:244.
44. Lee Y, Kim BJ, Kim SH, Lee SH, Kim WH, Jin SW. Comparative analysis of spontaneous infectious spondylitis : pyogenic versus tuberculous. J Korean Neurosurg Soc. 2018;61:81–8.
45. Madhok R, Sachdeva P. Evaluation of apparent diffusion coefficient values in spinal tuberculosis by MRI. J Clin Diagn Res. 2016;10:TC19–23.
46. Malluche HH, Monier-Faugere MC. Risk of adynamic bone disease in dialyzed patients. Kidney Int Suppl. 1992;38:S62–7.
47. Martha JF, Swaim B, Wang DA, Kim DH, Hill J, Bode R, et al. Outcome of percutaneous rupture of lumbar synovial cysts: a case series of 101 patients. Spine J. 2009;9:899–904.
48. Moritani T, Kim J, Capizzano AA, Kirby P, Kademian J, Sato Y. Pyogenic and non-pyogenic spinal infections: emphasis on diffusion-weighted imaging for the detection of abscesses and pus collections. Br J Radiol. 2014;87:20140011.
49. Muschitz C, Feichtinger X, Haschka J, Kocijan R. Diagnosis and treatment of Paget's disease of bone: a clinical practice guideline. Wien Med Wochenschr. 2017;167:18–24.
50. Mylona E, Samarkos M, Kakalou E, Fanourgiakis P, Skoutelis A. Pyogenic vertebral osteomyelitis: a systematic review of clinical characteristics. Semin Arthritis Rheum. 2009;39:10–7.
51. Nickerson EK, Sinha R. Vertebral osteomyelitis in adults: an update. Br Med Bull. 2016; 117:121–38.
52. Nigro L, Donnarumma P. Vertebral hemangiomas: common lesions with still many unknown aspects. J Spine Surg. 2017;3:309–11.
53. Orguc S, Arkun R. Primary tumors of the spine. Semin Musculoskelet Radiol. 2014;18:280–99.
54. Packer CD, Mileti LM. Vertebral sarcoidosis mimicking lytic osseous metastases: development 16 years after apparent resolution of thoracic sarcoidosis. J Clin Rheumatol. 2005;11:105–8.
55. Rajasekaran S. The natural history of post-tubercular kyphosis in children. Radiological signs which predict late increase in deformity. J Bone Joint Surg Br. 2001;83:954–62.
56. Rajasekaran S, Kanna RM, Shetty AP. Pathophysiology and treatment of spinal tuberculosis. JBJS Rev. 2014;2
57. Ross JS, Masaryk TJ, Modic MT, Carter JR, Mapstone T, Dengel FH. Vertebral hemangiomas: MR imaging. Radiology. 1987;165:165–9.
58. Sala F, Dapoto A, Morzenti C, Firetto MC, Valle C, Tomasoni A, et al. Bone islands incidentally detected on computed tomography: frequency of enostosis and differentiation from untreated osteoblastic metastases based on CT attenuation value. Br J Radiol. 2019;92:20190249.
59. Sanchez-Montalva A, Barios M, Salvador F, Villar A, Tortola T, Molina-Morant D, et al. Usefulness of FDG PET/CT in the management of tuberculosis. PLoS One. 2019;14:e0221516.
60. Shi J, Ermann J, Weissman BN, Smith SE, Mandell JC. Thinking beyond pannus: a review of retro-odontoid pseudotumor due to rheumatoid and non-rheumatoid etiologies. Skelet Radiol. 2019;48:1511–23.
61. Soto-Gomez N, Peters JI, Nambiar AM. Diagnosis and management of sarcoidosis. Am Fam Physician. 2016;93:840–8.
62. Tancioni F, Di Ieva A, Levi D, Aimar E, Debernardi A, Colombo P, et al. Spinal decompression and vertebroplasty in Paget's disease of the spine. Surg Neurol. 2006;66:189–91; discussion 191.
63. Torgovnick J, Sethi N, Wyss J. Spinal epidural abscess: clinical presentation, management and outcome (curry WT, Hoh BL, Hanjani SA, et al. Surg Neurol 2005;63:364–71). Surg Neurol. 2005;64:279.

64. Vougioukas VI, Hubbe U, Schipper J, Spetzger U. Navigated transoral approach to the cranial base and the craniocervical junction: technical note. Neurosurgery. 2003;52:247–50; discussion 251.
65. Weinstein JN, Lurie JD, Tosteson TD, Skinner JS, Hanscom B, Tosteson AN, et al. Surgical vs nonoperative treatment for lumbar disk herniation: the Spine Patient Outcomes Research Trial (SPORT) observational cohort. JAMA. 2006;296:2451–9.
66. World Health Organization, Global Tuberculosis Programme. Global tuberculosis control: WHO report. Geneva: Global Tuberculosis Programme.
67. Xu R, McGirt MJ, Parker SL, Bydon M, Olivi A, Wolinsky JP, et al. Factors associated with recurrent back pain and cyst recurrence after surgical resection of one hundred ninety-five spinal synovial cysts: analysis of one hundred sixty-seven consecutive cases. Spine (Phila Pa 1976). 2010;35:1044–53.
68. Xu R, Solakoglu C, Maleki Z, McGirt MJ, Gokaslan ZL, Bydon A. Hemorrhagic synovial cyst: the possible role of initial trauma and subsequent microtrauma in its pathogenesis: case report. Neurosurgery. 2011;68:E858–65; discussion E865.
69. Yamaguchi I, Shibuya S, Arima N, Oka S, Kanda Y, Yamamoto T. Remarkable reduction or disappearance of retroodontoid pseudotumors after occipitocervical fusion. Report of three cases. J Neurosurg Spine. 2006;5:156–60.
70. Yu SH, Choi HJ, Cho WH, Cha SH, Han IH. Retroodontoid pseudotumor without atlantoaxial subluxation or rheumatic arthritis. Korean J Neurotrauma. 2016;12:180–4.
71. Zhong W, Chen H, You C, Li J, Liu Y, Huang S. Spontaneous spinal epidural hematoma. J Clin Neurosci. 2011;18:1490–4.
72. Zubairi AB, Sheerani M, Haque AS, Ahsan H, Fatima K. Osseous spinal sarcoidosis: an unusual but important entity to remember. BMJ Case Rep. 2010;2010:bcr1220092518.

10 Special Anatomical Zone: Sacral and Spinopelvic Tumors

Jean-Paul Wolinsky and Luis G. Fernandez III

Sacral Tumors

To begin our discussion, we include a figure summarizing the frequency and distribution through the spine of spinal tumors from a single surgeon's experience (Fig. 10.1). These data may deviate from population frequencies due to the referral patterns inherent to tertiary care centers in which these cases occurred.

Chordoma

Chordomas serve as a model tumor to begin discussion of surgical management of primary sacral malignancies. Chordomas are relatively rare lesions with a frequency of 0.2–0.5 per 100,000 persons per year; however, they constitute 3–4% of primary bone tumors and 20–34% of primary sacral malignancies [1–3]. Within the craniospinal axis, chordomas are reported to have a predilection for the sacrococcygeal region (45–50%) followed by the spheno-occipital (35–39%) and vertebral areas (15%); however, more recent epidemiologic analyses by SEER suggest a roughly equal distribution of cranial, spinal, and sacral chordomas [4]. Demographically, patients are most commonly white (87.7%) and male (60.1%), with ~74% diagnosed from the fourth decade and beyond. Median survival is ~4.7 years from time of diagnosis; however, 43.8% and 19.8% of patients are alive at 10 and 20 years from diagnosis, respectively [4]. Mortality due to sacral chordomas is often due to local compression of neurologic structures with subsequent complications of paresis including complicated UTIs and decubitus ulcers which may become infected leading to sepsis.

Optimal first-line treatment for chordomas is en bloc resection with wide negative margins; this has been consistently shown to improve disease-free survival and overall survival and decrease rates of local recurrence with acceptable functional outcomes [5–9] (Fig. 10.2). Furthermore, great care should be taken to ensure the tumor capsule remains intact as violation of the capsule has been shown to drastically increase local recurrence to as high as 64% [10, 11]. Locally recurrent chordomas are much more challenging to treat surgically due to indeterminate tumor margins, scarring, and tendency toward more aggressive behavior. Tumor characteristics associated with unfavorable outcomes include recurrent tumor, massive tumor size, and tumor extension into organs and critical vascular/neurologic structures preventing en bloc resection [12].

Chemotherapy is ineffective and these tumors are radio-resistant; in a series by Boriani et al., chordoma patients treated with radiation monotherapy or intralesional resection had a 100%

J.-P. Wolinsky · L. G. Fernandez III (✉)
Department of Neurological Surgery, Northwestern Memorial Hospital, Chicago, IL, USA
e-mail: Jean-Paul.Wolinsky@northwestern.edu; Luis.Fernandez1@northwestern.edu

K. Singh, M. Colman (eds.), *Surgical Spinal Oncology*, https://doi.org/10.1007/978-3-030-50722-0_10

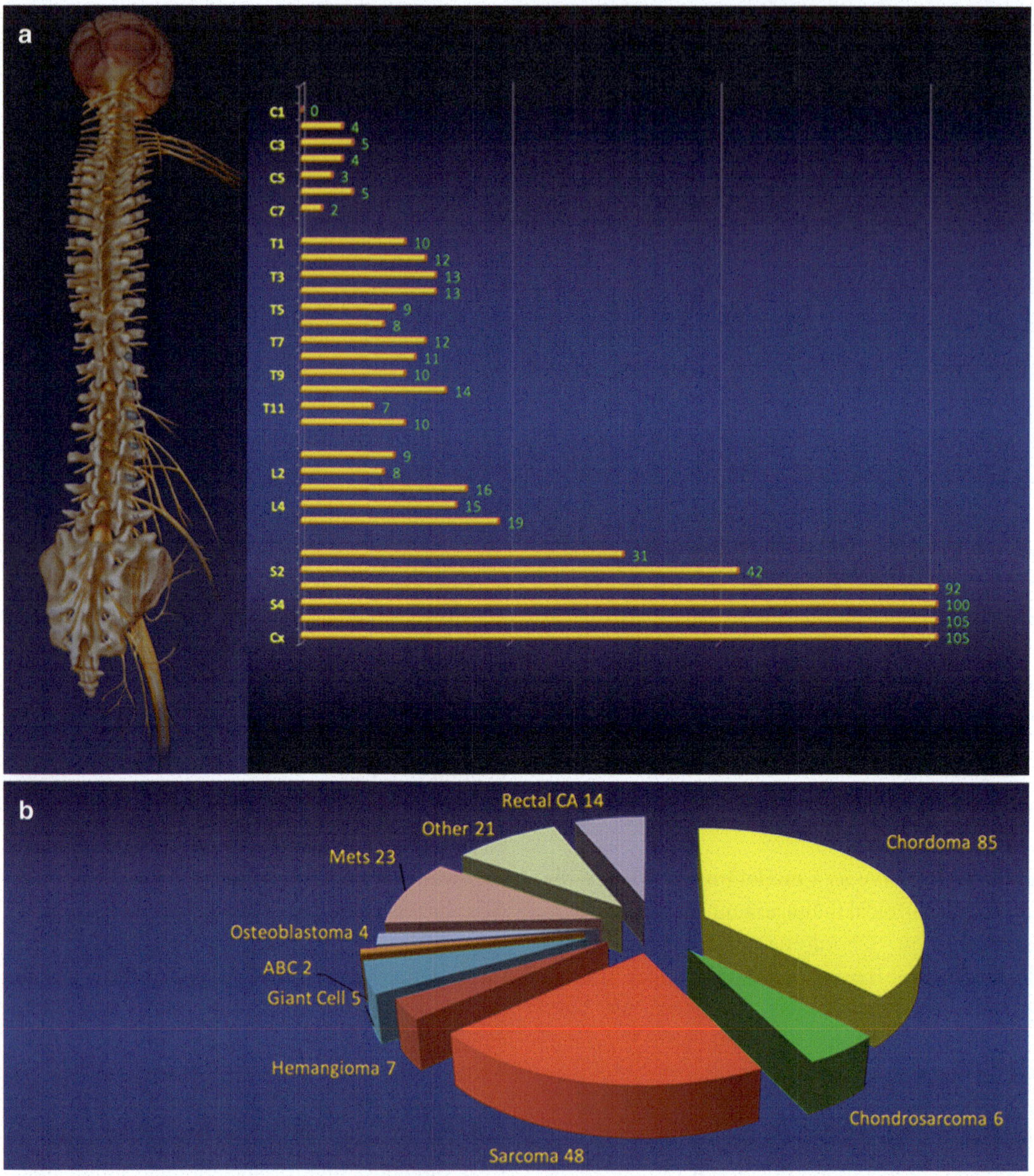

Fig. 10.1 A single surgeon's experience with spinal tumors (**a**). Distribution by spinal level (**b**). Frequency of tumor type

local recurrence rate in 17–20 months versus 20% recurrence at 56–94 months when en bloc resection with margins was obtained [6]. However, adjuvant radiation may be used following en bloc resection to eliminate residual tumor cells near the resection cavity; furthermore, in patients with subtotal resections adjuvant radiation improved disease-free survival from 8 months to 2.12 years [13]. If marginal or intralesional resection is the only feasible surgical outcome, high-dose adjuvant radiation may be employed to improve the probability of durable treatment response.

Chondrosarcoma

Following chordoma, chondrosarcoma is the second-most common primary malignant tumor of the spine accounting for approximately 7–12%

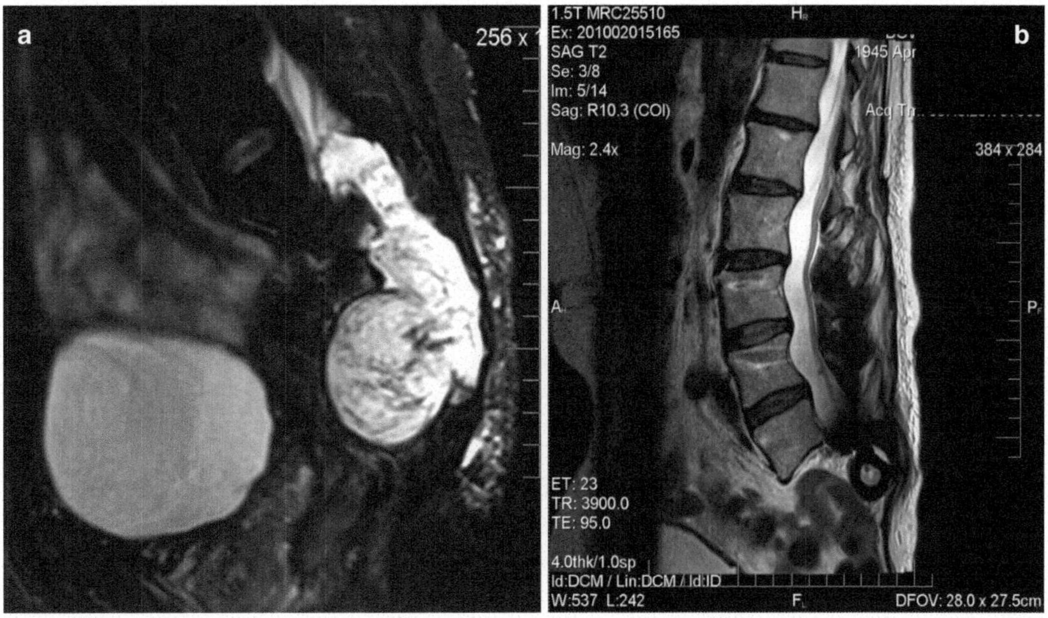

Fig. 10.2 Sacral chordoma (**a**). Pre-resection (**b**). Resection cavity post-total sacrectomy

of these lesions; however, only 10% of chondrosarcomas are found in the spine [3]. Furthermore, less than 1% of chondrosarcomas are sacral, with the majority found in the thoracic (41%) and lumbar spine (43%) [13–15]. These tumors typically arise from the posterior elements and cause symptoms due to local mass effect on surrounding neurologic structures; they are rarely metastatic [13, 15]. Regarding natural history and behavior, chondrosarcomas closely approximate chordomas found at the same spinal level; morbidity and mortality are related to local invasion and compression of organs, neurologic, and vascular structures.

Optimal treatment of chondrosarcomas is similar to that of chordomas, requiring en bloc resection with wide negative margins; adjuvant radiation therapy has also been shown to increase disease-free survival [13]. The frequency of spinal chondrosarcomas is exceedingly low and consequently much of the clinical literature comprises case series and reports; based on several of these studies, long-term overall survival at 10 months following en bloc surgical resection has been reported to be between 35–60% for primary chondrosarcomas versus <10% for metastatic chondrosarcomas, with median survivals reported between 40.2–70.8 months in non-metastatic chondrosarcomas [16, 17]. Chondrosarcoma and osteosarcoma of the pelvis commonly invade the sacrum through the sacroiliac joint. Consequently surgical removal of these lesions often requires a more extensive surgical resection via hemipelvectomy with concurrent hemisacrectomy via iliac and sagittal sacral osteotomies respectively; traditionally radical external hemipelvectomy with removal of the ipsilateral lower extremity was performed for these lesions [18, 19]. Currently, limb sparing internal hemipelvectomy is indicated for patients in whom 1 of 3 anatomic areas is spared of tumor: namely the iliac wing, periacetabular region or the pubic and ischial rami [20]. In patients undergoing internal hemipelvectomy in which the acetabulum is outside of the surgical margin, better functional outcomes have been reported as compared to those in whom the acetabulum was resected [21]. Surgical decision making with regard to extent of resection of the sacrum, ilium, SI joint, acetabulum and surrounding tissues is complex and must be determined on a case by case basis taking into account tumor histology, presence of metastatic disease, functionality of the affected limb(s), patient factors and extent of tumor invasion.

Osteosarcoma

Osteosarcoma is a rare but important spinal tumor, comprising 3.6–14.5% of all primary spinal malignancies [22]. Spinal osteosarcomas have a predilection for the lumbosacral spine with 60–70% of these lesions found in this distribution, most commonly arising in the vertebral body [23]. They have a bimodal distribution with one peak during adolescence and early adulthood and the second in the geriatric population [24]. The large majority of patients with osteosarcoma have no known risk factors; however, 1% of patients with Paget's disease are known to develop osteosarcomas [25, 26]. These neoplasms often present insidiously with progressively worsening pain that may awaken patients from sleep; furthermore, approximately two-thirds of patients present with neurologic deficit [27]. On plain film X-rays, they appear as blastic lesions.

Osteosarcoma is often treated with a multimodal approach of neoadjuvant/adjuvant chemotherapy and en bloc surgical excision with or without adjuvant radiation therapy. Local recurrence rates are estimated at ~20% following en bloc resection with rates as high as 60% if treated with an intralesional excision [28, 29]. The utility of radiotherapy is limited by the radioresistant nature of osteosarcomas and the relatively low radiation tolerance of the presacral organs. Despite the constraints radiotherapy plays a role in sterilizing the reactive zone surrounding the tumor, particularly in areas where marginal dissection planes are required. One series demonstrated that 5-year survival was significantly improved from 27% in patients treated with surgery alone to 43% in patients treated with combined surgery and radiation therapy [30]. In a meta-analysis of patients with primary spinal osteosarcoma with positive or inadequate tumor margins following initial resection, adjuvant chemotherapy and re-operation showed a clinically significant improvement in overall survival, while radiosurgery trended toward significance ($p = 0.06$) with regard to improvement in overall survival [31]. Chemotherapeutic agents which have shown high response rates in meta-analyses include adriamycin (43%), ifosfamide (33%), methotrexate (32%), and cisplatin (26%); 5-year PFS was 58% and OS was 70% in patients treated with combination of methotrexate, adriamycin, and cisplatin or ifosfamide [32].

Much like other malignant primary tumors of the sacrum, en bloc surgical resection remains the first-line therapeutic option for treatment of osteosarcoma; unfortunately, this tumor is highly aggressive with suboptimal outcomes even in patients in which en bloc resection is achieved. Surgeons should be well versed in multimodal approaches to maximize favorable outcomes in patients with this malignancy.

Osteoblastoma/Osteoid Osteoma

Both osteoid osteomas and osteoblastomas are benign spinal tumors which comprise a relatively small fraction of primary sacral tumors. Approximately 2% of spinal osteoid osteomas are found within the sacrum versus 17% of spinal osteoblastomas [33]. Interestingly, although these tumors typically involve the posterior elements of the non-sacral spine, they are classically described as arising within the vertebral bodies when found in the sacrum. Radiographically, they are characterized by a radiolucent defect surrounded by a thick margin of sclerotic bone with possible intralesional calcification on plain films and CT. Osteoblastomas may be distinguished from osteoid osteomas on imaging by its ill-defined margins and occasional association with an epidural soft tissue mass. Both tumors most often present with localized back pain that is worse at night. Osteoblastomas may present with a dull backache that is typically less well localized than in osteoid osteomas. Characteristically, pain associated with these tumors is relieved with salicylates [34]. Management of these lesions is surgical with lower rates of recurrence seen with en bloc resection versus subtotal resection; percutaneous ablation is also commonly used for treatment of osteoid osteomas 34 [34]. Recurrence rates following surgical resection were 17% at 8.4 years; PFS was 87% and 74% at 5 and 10 years, respectively whereas recurrence rates of up to 16% with percutaneous ablation have been reported with osteoid osteoma [35–37].

Giant Cell Tumor

Readers are referred to Chap. 6 for a general discussion of the treatement of axial giant cell tumors. Giant cell tumors arise infrequently in the spine, with only 3–7% of giant cell tumors found there; however, when they do arise in the spine, they have a predilection for the sacrum [23]. Demographically they are seen most often in patients aged 15–40 years and are seen more frequently in women with a 2:1 female-to-male ratio [23, 38]. Despite a histologically benign appearance, these lesions are locally invasive, with high rates of recurrence and can cause significant pain, neurologic symptoms due to mass effect, and destruction of bony elements of the spine due to high concentration of osteoclastic giant cells in these tumors. Pain is typically the presenting symptom with other patients experiencing bowel and bladder dysfunction or other neurologic symptoms due to compression of the sacral nerve roots. These lesions may rarely metastasize in up to 2% of patients, most commonly to the lungs; less than 2% of these lesions may undergo spontaneous malignant transformation [39, 40].

Giant cell tumors differ from chordomas in that they are typically eccentrically located in the anterior spinal elements whereas chordomas tend to be more centrally located. Furthermore, giant cell tumors are radiographically characterized as heterogeneous on CT and MRI due to the presence of hypodense areas of necrosis on CT, hemorrhage corresponding to variable age-dependent signal intensity on T1- and T2-weighted sequences, fluid–fluid levels, and cystic components [23]. T2-weighted sequences of these tumors are characterized by large areas of intralesional hypointensity due to areas of hemorrhage and fibrosis; they are highly vascular on angiographic studies [23].

Management of giant cell tumors involves a combination of neoadjuvant chemotherapy followed by en bloc surgical resection providing the most effective local control and prevention of recurrence. Denosumab is a RANKL monoclonal antibody which inhibits the RANK-RANKL pathway thereby inhibiting osteoclast-like giant cells differentiation and activation has also been used with success in treating some giant cell tumors [41]. Treatment with denosumab ultimately leads to tumor sclerosis, calcification and bony septation; this can present technical challenges if resection follows denosumab treatment as focal areas of sclerosis between the tumor and surrounding neurovascular structures may develop complicating dissection and blurring tumor boundaries [42]. Sambri et al recently published a study comparing patients with sacral and pelvic giant cell tumors, divided into a medical group treated with continuous denosumab and a surgical group treated with neoadjuvant denosumab followed by either total resection or local curettage [43]. The surgical group was further subdivided into those who continued adjuvant denosumab post-op and those in which denosumab therapy was terminated [43]. Results of this study showed no recurrence in the group in which en bloc resection was achieved or those in whom denosumab was continued, whereas 62% of those treated with lesional curettage developed recurrence at a mean of 10 months after cessation of adjuvant denosumab and 33% of the medical group recurred with cessation of denosumab at <8 months [43]. Interestingly, in a small series of 9 patients, serial embolization alone was used to achieve local control in 7 of 9 without progression at a mean follow-up of 8.86 years (median 7.8 years) with good functional outcomes [44]. Embolization may be a useful first-line option in patients in which surgical resection would result in unacceptably high morbidity and or mortality; furthermore, due to the highly vascular nature of these lesions, pre-operative embolization may help prevent blood loss and facilitate excision. Intralesional curettage has proven to be an ineffective method for control of these lesions with local recurrence rates between 43 and 49%; radiotherapy with doses between 40 and 70 Gy has likewise proven to be a suboptimal treatment modality with recurrence rates between 15 and 49% reported in the literature [45, 46]. However, more recently Ruka et al reported improved rates of local control with megavoltage irradiation in a single center series of patients with giant cell tumors, ~20% of which were located in the sacrum or pelvis, who were not surgical candidates due to medical comorbidities, unfavorable anatomic constraints, recurrent tumor and/or an unacceptably high risk of severe disfiguration. 47 Rates of local PFS after megavoltage irradiation of ~ 50Gy in patients with sacral or pelvic lesions was 70.5% at 5 years as compared to 88% in patients with peripheral bone lesions [47]. Furthermore, a well-documented risk of radiation-induced malignant sarcomatous degeneration has been reported to be as high as 3–11% [45, 46, 48].

Teratoma

Teratomas can arise in the spinal canal or more commonly in the sacrococcygeal region; sacrococcygeal teratomas are the most common childhood germ cell tumor with an incidence of approximately 1 per 40,000 live births [49]. These tumors are more frequently seen in females (75–80%) and the majority (70%) are detected by time of birth, either antenatally or in the immediate post-natal period [50, 51]. In adults, these lesions most often present with a mass noted since childhood and/or symptoms secondary to local mass effect. When these tumors arise in the sacrococcygeal region they are often divided into two distributions—pre- and post-sacral; however, combined pre- and post-sacral teratomas are occasionally observed.

Most sacrococcygeal teratomas are benign; however, between 20 and 30% are malignant, and roughly 5–15% are metastatic at the time of diagnosis [52, 53]. Malignant and benign teratomas are diagnosed by histologic exam; however, there are several clinical, biochemical, and radiographic features that are characteristic of each. First and foremost, benign teratomas are more commonly found distal to the coccyx versus malignant teratomas which more commonly arise in the presacral space [54]. Radiographically, benign teratomas are often cystic, without lytic bone changes; this contrasts with malignant teratomas, which are locally invasive. Consequently, benign sacrococcygeal teratomas are often asymptomatic whereas malignant variants often present with urinary/fecal incontinence as well as symptoms secondary to invasion of local pelvic vascular and lymphatic structures. Biochemical markers, such as α-FP and, less commonly, β-HCG, are reliably elevated in malignant teratomas; however, since α-FP is elevated in healthy children at birth with a steady decline over the first year of life, it has very low specificity for distinguishing between benign and malignant teratomas during this interval [55, 56].

Prognosis for benign/mature and malignant teratomas with or without metastatic disease is excellent. Benign, mature teratomas treated solely by en bloc radical resection with coccygeal amputation are largely curable; recurrence occurred in only 11% of patients in a multicenter review [57]. Benign teratomas treated with en bloc resection are not typically treated with adjuvant chemotherapy nor radiation due to the efficacy of surgical resection alone and diminishing benefit of these adjunctive therapies in these lesions. Malignant teratomas, on the other hand, respond robustly to chemotherapy with platinum-based, nitrogen mustard, topoisomerase inhibitors, and other agents. Several chemotherapy regimens have been established including PEB therapy combining cisplatin, etoposide, and bleomycin used by the Children's Cancer Group/Pediatric Oncology Group; JEB therapy combining carboplatin, etoposide, and bleomycin developed by the United Kingdom Children's Cancer Study Group (UKCCSG); and the PEI regimen developed by the German Association of Pediatric Oncology which combines cisplatin, etoposide, and bleomycin [58, 59]. Although survival rates are less favorable for malignant teratomas than benign teratomas, long-term overall survival rates of 80–90% have been achieved in multiple patient subgroups with these more aggressive lesions [46, 48]. The mean recurrence rate for benign teratomas ranges between 0 and 26% with a mean value of 12.9% whereas recurrence rates for immature/malignant teratomas range between 4 and 55% with a mean recurrence rate almost double that of benign teratomas at 20.2% [49, 50, 60–68]. Combined data of mortality following recurrence for all sacrococcygeal teratomas are 35%; however, the mortality rate is higher in patients with recurrence of malignant teratomas at ~55% [69].

The greatest risks for recurrence include incomplete resection at time of initial surgery and rupture of the solid tumor capsule with seeding of tumor cells in the resection bed. Therefore, total en bloc resection should be attempted when feasible to prevent recurrence and decrease the probability of mortality due to the more aggressive behavior of recurrent lesions.

Metastatic Lesions to the Sacrum

Metastatic disease to the sacrum encompasses a wide variety of various primary malignancies; most commonly breast, lung, prostate, thyroid, and renal tumors metastasize to the sacrum while melanoma, myeloma, and lymphoma comprise a significant minority of sacral metastases [23, 70–73]. Spinal metastases are present in ~70% of patient with cancer and symptomatic spinal metastases are present in up to 10% of all cancer patients at some point during their illness and sacral metastases comprise only a small fraction of these [74–78]. They are spread most often by hematogenous dissemination and frequently appear many years after treatment of the primary tumor; however, they may also arise due to direct extension from pelvic primary malignancies such as rectal adenocarcinoma. Clinical presentation varies depending on which local neural, vascular, soft tissue, and osseous structures are compressed due to tumor expansion; unfortunately, sacral metastases are typically diagnosed at advanced stages after they have already extensively invaded the majority of surrounding structures. Widespread spinal metastases and extraspinal involvement are seen in 43–53% and 61–68% of patients with sacral metastases, respectively [79, 80].

Primary treatment modalities for sacral metastases include radiotherapy and surgery with the goal of palliation and pain control; radiotherapy is the first-line treatment for radiosensitive sacral metastases in the absence of acute neurologic compromise and/or biomechanical pelvic instability [81, 82]. Select patients with severe pain or with loss of ambulatory capacity may be considered for surgical intervention; however, in the presence of active systemic disease, surgery is very rarely indicated. Occasionally, patients with locally advanced rectal adenocarcinoma may benefit from sacrectomy in cases in which the tumor is adherent to or invading the sacrum, has not metastasized to distant sites, and in which resection may increase the probability of cure.

Overall metastatic lesions to the sacrum are often best managed with a combination of radiation and occasionally chemotherapy. Surgery occasionally has a role in instances of biomechanical instability, intractable pain, and locally advanced disease in select subsets of patients in the absence of widely metastatic disease.

Sacrectomy Classification by Functional Outcomes and Biomechanical Stability

Sacrectomy can be classified based on level of neural preservation, functional outcome, level of osteotomies, and biomechanical stability (Table 10.1). Major functional considerations following sacrectomy include bowel/bladder function, sexual function, ambulatory capacity, and pelvic stability. Preservation of S3 and above with osteotomy through S2–3 constitutes a low sacral amputation; preservation of S2 and above with osteotomy through S1–2, a mid-sacral amputation; preservation of S1 and above with osteotomy through S1, a high sacral amputation and osteotomy through L5–S1 with sacrifice of S1 nerve roots and below qualifies as a total sacrectomy. Although beyond the scope of this chapter, a hemicorporectomy is distinguished by sacrifice of

Table 10.1 Neurologic function and pelvic stability after sacrectomy by level of neural preservation

Sacrectomy classification	Sacral amputation sub classification	Neural level preserved	Number of roots preserved	Independent ambulation	Bowel continence	Bladder continence	Sexual function	Pelvic instability
Subtotal sacrectomy	Low	S3	Both	Yes	Yes	Yes	Yes	No
	Mid	S2	Both	Yes	Partial	Partial	Partial	No
	High	S1	Both	Yes	No	No	No	No
Total sacrectomy	Total	L5	Both	Yes	No	No	No	Yes

at least L5 and below. Low, mid, and high sacral amputations are considered subtotal sacrectomies, which do not result in pelvic instability and thus do not require pelvic reconstruction; conversely, total sacrectomy and beyond may, but does not always, necessitate lumbo-pelvic reconstruction. Preservation of the S2 nerve roots bilaterally and S3 unilaterally is required for approximately normal bowel, bladder, and sexual function in roughly two-thirds of patients; sacrifice of L5 roots will prevent ambulation [83, 84].

Biomechanics of Lumbopelvic Reconstruction

The sacroiliac (SI) joints are the bridge between the spine, pelvis and lower extremities and consequently are mechanically constrained to maintain spinopelvic integrity. The wedge shaped sacrum prevents caudal migration of the spinal elements cranial to the SI joints, both transmitting and absorbing compressive forces from the spine and pelvis through the SI joints much like a keystone in arch construction [85]. The SI joints must also resist rotational forces, limiting translation to 0.7 mm and 2° of motion which is facilitated by the large surface area of the joint [86, 87]. Much of the resistance to shear loads at the joint is mediated through muscles and ligaments which cross and attach near the joint. For example, the transversus abdominis and muscles of the pelvic floor increase the compression load across the SI joint which augments resistance to shear forces [88]. In addition to the joint itself, the sacrospinous, sacrotuberous, sacroiliac, and iliolumbar ligaments distribute forces across the SI joint and contribute to overall spinopelvic stability. The posterior sacroiliac ligaments provide greatest resistance to sacral extension, while the sacrotuberous, sacrospinous, interosseous and anterior sacroiliac ligaments resist sacral flexion. Resistance to axial rotation is primarily mediated through the anterior and interosseous sacroiliac ligaments while lateral side bending is resisted by the iliolumbar ligaments [89]. Kiapour et al published a review of the biomechanics of the sacroiliac joint with excellent data from several cadaveric studies demonstrating the effects of transecting the aforementioned ligaments, particularly as it related to spinopelvic stability and the SI joint [89]. The sacrospinous and sacrotuberous ligaments are typically transected in lower sacral amputations; however the posterior ligamentous complex is preserved which greatly contributes to overall spinopelvic stability. Gunterberg et al and Stener et al found that sacroiliac stability is not significantly impacted in high sacrectomies provided at least half of the SI joint (at least the upper 50% of the S1 segment) is preserved [90, 91]. In a series by Bergh et al, 33% of patients with high sacrectomies at or above the S1–2 osseous level developed fatigue fractures, however of these only one patient (5.6%) had intractable pain and permanent disability [11]. Furthermore in a retrospective series by Fourney et al, 29 patients underwent en bloc resection of primary sacral tumors, 7 of whom were treated with high sacrectomy without internal fixation and none of which developed delayed instability or fatigue fracture [92]. Total sacrectomy leads to complete dissociation of the spine and pelvis, however there is controversy regarding spinopelvic reconstruction following total sacrectomy. Some authors forego spinopelvic reconstruction in these patients due to concerns regarding increased risk of infection and hardware failure [93, 94, 111]. Furthermore Wuisman et al reported successful mobilization of 5 patients after total sacrectomy without reconstruction at greater than 8 weeks [111]. These patients were noted to have caudal migration of the lumbar spine between the ilia with spinal stability attributed to formation of muscle and scar tissue between the pelvis and spine serving as a suspensory mechanism or "biologic sling" [111]. Gunterberg et al stated that the pelvic ring is considered stable so long as 50% of S1 is left intact, despite a 50% reduction in strength of the pelvic ring as the residual strength is sufficient for load bearing with standing [90]. However if significant portions of the iliac wings are taken during total sacrectomy vertical and rotational spinopelvic instability may result with poor functional outcome. Wuisman et al proposed a scoring system to quantify iliac resection dividing the resections borders into 4 zones with more lateral removal at zones 3 or 4 warranting reconstruction [111]. Other groups favor spinopelvic reconstruction following total sacrectomy for early mobilization [92]. No randomized control trial comparing total sacrectomies with spinopelvic reconstruction versus without has been published at the time of this writing. Consequently no head to head comparisons can be drawn regarding post-operative complications and functional outcomes in total sacretomies with spinopelvic reconstruction versus without. However a review of the literature by Kiatisevi et al in 2016 tabulated functional outcomes and post-operative complications from reports from multiple studies and institutions in patients who underwent total sacrectomy both with and without spinopelvic reconstruction [93–108, 111]. In one of the larger series of 43 patients by Bederman et al, 89.7% of patient were able to ambulate following total sacrectomy with reconstruction, 30.8% of whom were able to ambulate independently, 59% with help and 10.3% were unable to ambulate [103]. Another series of 16 patients by Kiatisevi et al who did not undergo reconstruction following total sacrectomy showed 80.8% of patients were able to ambulate post-operatively (31% without assistance, 31% with a cane and 18.8% with a walker) while 19.2% were non ambulatory (6.3% wheelchair bound and 12.5% bed bound) [102]. Post-operative wound complications in the groups undergoing reconstruction following total sacrectomy ranged between 22 and 50% with most series averaging between 30–40% for post-operative wound complications [84, 95–100, 102–107, 111]. Wound dehiscence in a series of total sacrectomies without reconstruction by Kiatisevi et al was 81.3% [102]. Post-operative deep wound infections have been reported as 25–42% of patients who underwent total sacrectomy without reconstruction as compared to 0–50% in patients who had reconstruction [84, 96, 101, 103, 107, 108, 111]. Subtotal sacrectomy does not typically require reconstruction provided at least 50% of S1 is left intact as mentioned previously [90]. There are two cadaveric studies which re-examined the biomechanical implications of high partial sacrectomy on spinopelvic stability, which suggested that reconstruction should be considered when a partial transverse sacrectomy above the S1 nerve root is performed [109, 110]. Less torsional stiffness was noted with a series of partial S1 transverse sacrectomies and unilateral SI joint resection compared to those carried out below S1 [110]. Furthermore, in the cadaveric series by Hugate et al, partial transverse sacrectomy with an average resection of 25% of the SI joints was associated with lower vertical load failure rate secondary to rotation in the sagittal plane at the lumbosacral junction with subsequent paramedian sacral fractures [109]. The authors attributed these differences as compared to Gunterberg's study to differences in their respective models; in the Gunterberg model they suggest that potting the base of pelvis in epoxy resin redistributed loading forces to the rami rather than at the hip (natural loading position) with decreased moment across the iliac wings altering load distribution across the SI joint [90, 109]. The authors proposed that the epoxy resin base prevented significant splaying or angulation of the iliac wings subsuming the role of the sacrum during physiologic load bearing [109].

Anatomic considerations

Prior to surgical resection of sacral tumors, careful consideration of the surrounding anatomy is critical. Sacral tumors may abut, encase or frankly invade surrounding viscera, joints and neurovascular structures that can complicate their removal and augment the risk of intraoperative and post-operative complications. Lumbar nerve roots and the lumbosacral trunk passing ventral to the sacrum may be secondarily involved by the tumor along with sacral nerve roots as they enter and exit the sacral foramina. The sacral sympathetic trunk which is continuous with the lumbar sympathetic trunk travels caudally against the ventral surface of the sacrum and converge at the coccyx, giving off branches to the superior hypogastric plexus which outputs to the inferior hypogastric plexus; furthermore the parasympathetic outputs arise from the S2–S4 nerve roots forming the pelvic splanchnic nerves. Damage to the parasympathetics can lead to erectile dysfunction and incontinence; sympathetic damage may alter male fertility due to its role in the transport of spermatozoa to the seminal vesicles and coordination of reflexes involved in ejaculation [112].

Pre-op

Treatment of sacral tumors is fundamentally based on the pathology of the tumor in question; therefore, a tissue diagnosis and thorough imaging of the neuraxis and body with MRI brain, cervical, thoracic and lumbar spine, CT chest/abdomen/pelvis, PET, and bone scan is essential to an initial evaluation. Biopsy is directed at the most accessible lesion and should be performed through a posterior trans-sacral route (Fig. 10.3); ventral approaches for biopsy including transrectal and transvaginal biopsy carry the risk of seeding the tumor cells into new body compartments along the biopsy tract, lowering the probability of total resection of neoplastic tissue and potentially necessitating additional ventral dissection to remove disseminated tumor [11, 113, 114]. It is important to mark the percutaneous trans-sacral biopsy tract at the skin, as it will be excised during surgical resection of the primary mass.

Operative Technique

The following describes an overview of the surgical technique for resection of primary sacral tumors. The descriptions that follow are a guide and should be tailored as befits the needs of each individual case. Total sacrectomy as defined above often can be accomplished with a single-stage posterior approach; however, there are instances in which a two-stage approach may be indicated [115, 116]. Patients who have undergone prior lumbosacral or pelvic surgery as well as those who have had prior radiation treatments may have significant scarring of the soft tissue elements to surrounding vessels and/or the rectum. In situations such as these, beginning with an anterior approach establishes control of major vessels including the internal iliacs as well as the middle sacral arteries and veins. Additionally, an anterior approach may be indicated in patients, in which a myocutaneous rectus flap is desired to cover large posterior soft tissue defects following tumor resection. The rectus flap can be mobilized with inferior epigastric vascular pedicles and

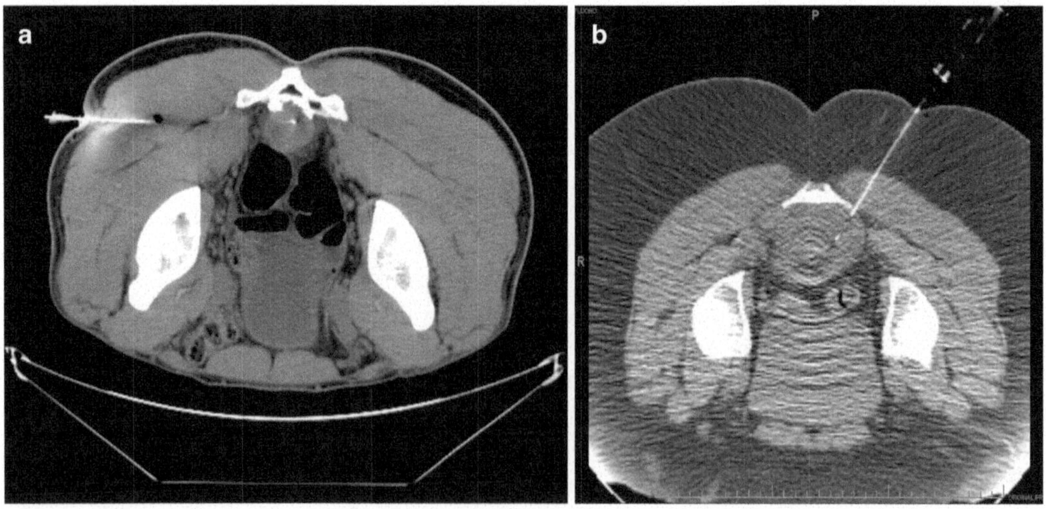

Fig. 10.3 Sacral biopsy trajectory to obtain tissue diagnosis prior to surgery. Comparison of poorly planned biopsy versus optimal trajectory (**a**). Poor biopsy trajectory. Note that this biopsy tract could not reasonably be incorporated into an en bloc resection, as it is too far lateral. Tumor will be seeded through the tract increasing the likelihood of recurrence depending on the tumor type (**b**). Optimal biopsy tract. It can be easily incorporated into future resection

placed in the pelvis, so it may subsequently be used for closure during the second stage of the operation.

Prep

Prior to surgery, the rectum should be irrigated with saline and Betadine until the effluent is clear. This is done in the event of rectal perforation during tumor resection to minimize contamination with bowel flora and feculent material.

Anterior Approach

The patient is positioned supine on a standard operating table for a midline laparotomy.

A standard midline vertical incision is made through the avascular plane of the linea alba, taking care to preserve the inferior epigastric arteries. The incision should be planned such that healthy rectus myocutaneous flap(s) may be harvested for closure of posterior tissue defects following tumor resection during stage II.

The internal iliac arteries and veins are identified, ligated, and sharply divided.

The middle sacral artery and vein are identified, ligated, and sharply divided.

A complete L5–S1 diskectomy is performed.

The myocutaneous flap is then harvested with vascular supply from the preserved inferior epigastric arteries. The flap is placed deep in the pelvis to facilitate retrieval through the posterior sacral defect for closure during stage II following tumor resection (Fig. 10.4).

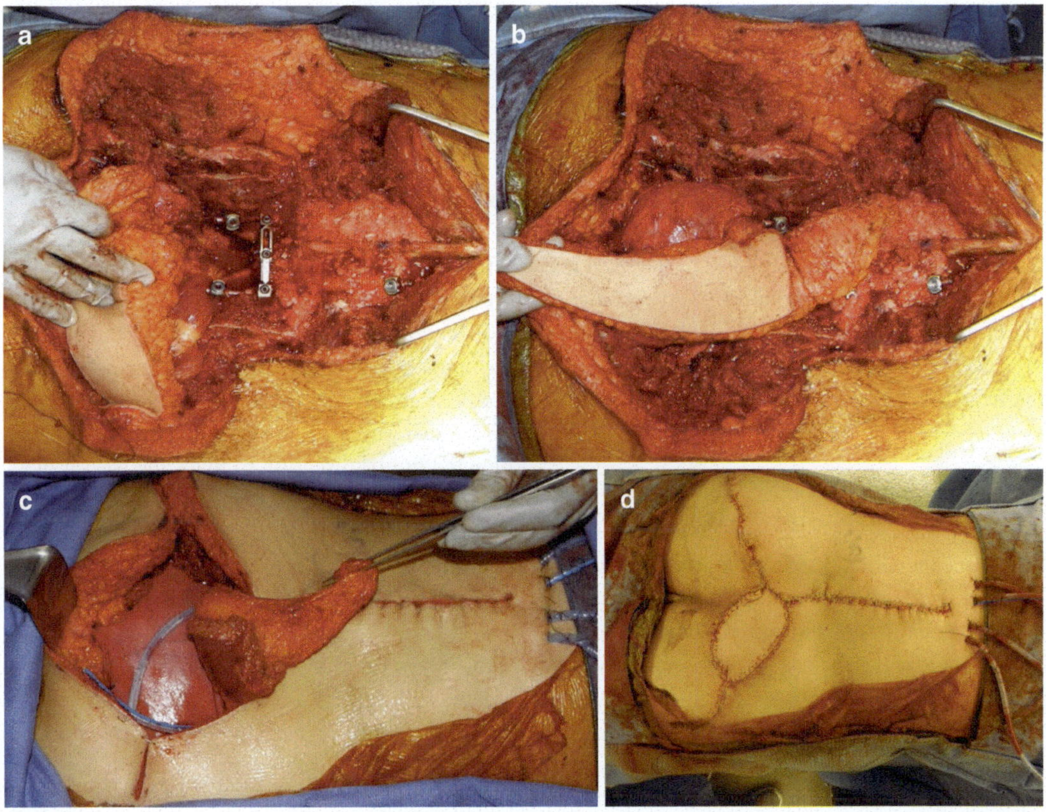

Fig. 10.4 (**a**) Delivery of myocutaneous rectus flap through posterior tissue defect. (**b**) Second view of rotated myocutaneous flap. (**c**) Closure of rostral and lateral margins of tissue defect with myocutaneous flap positioned centrally for closure of sacral defect. (**d**) Final closure with incorporation of rectus flap

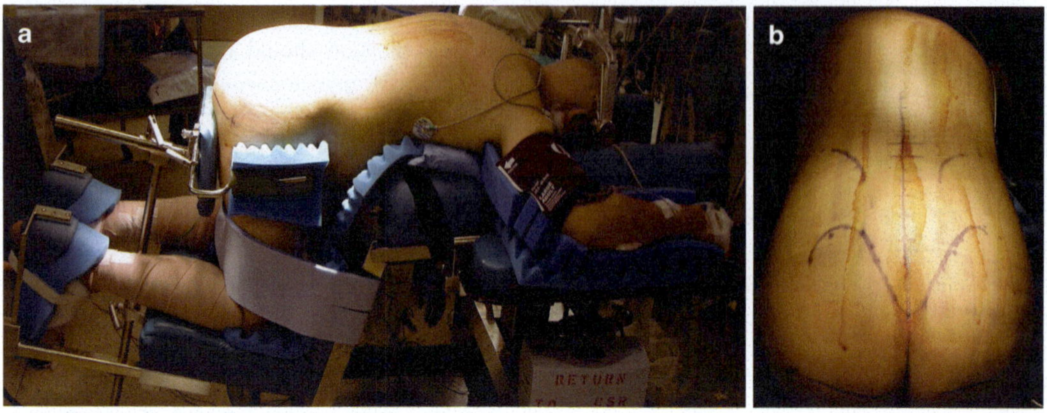

Fig. 10.5 (**a**) The patient is positioned prone in the Andrews table with head placed in three-point fixation with a Mayfield clamp. (**b**) The patient is marked and prepped prior to incision. Care is taken to ensure patient is midline and there is no lateral rotation on the surgical table

Posterior Approach

Positioning

The patient is positioned prone on the Andrews table (Fig. 10.5).

The head is pinned in 3-point fixation using a Mayfield with sitting adapter and suspended over the table (Fig. 10.5). This eliminates facial pressure. It is critically important to avoid Trendelenburg or lateral rotation of the bed during the operation as this could lead to a cervical injury as the patient's head is fixed relative to the body and the table. The table may be raised or lowered provided the relationship between the head and body is maintained.

Incision

A midline incision is made with an elliptical skin incision made around the biopsy tract; the skin, subcutaneous tissue, and muscle of the underlying tract must be excised with the specimen as tumor cells have invariably been seeded here (Figs. 10.6 and 10.8).

The margins of the posterior incision depend on whether total sacrectomy or subtotal sacrectomy is planned. For total sacrectomy, the incision should be carried far enough rostrally to expose L3–L5; if subtotal sacrectomy is planned, exposure to L5 is sufficient. The caudal aspect of the incision must be extended such that the anococcygeal ligament can be divided to permit delivery of the sacrum and coccyx through the posterior tissue defect. The incision is carried through the subcutaneous tissue and lumbosacral fascia.

Principle Dissection

After the fascia is incised, it is dissected off the paraspinous muscles laterally. The fascia is then elevated off the iliac crest, following the avascular plane that extends from each iliac crest bilaterally. A transverse incision is then made in the fascia just superior to the rostral extent of the planned tumor resection to mark the rostral margin of the en bloc resection. A self-retaining retractor is then introduced to retract the fascia laterally.

The paraspinous muscles are then elevated off the spinous processes, lamina, facets, and transverse processes of the spin using a subperiosteal technique; as above L3–L5 must be exposed if total sacrectomy is planned versus L5 alone if subtotal sacrectomy is intended. The paraspinous muscles are then cut transversely at the same level at which the fascia was incised. The paraspinous muscles are then mobilized lat-

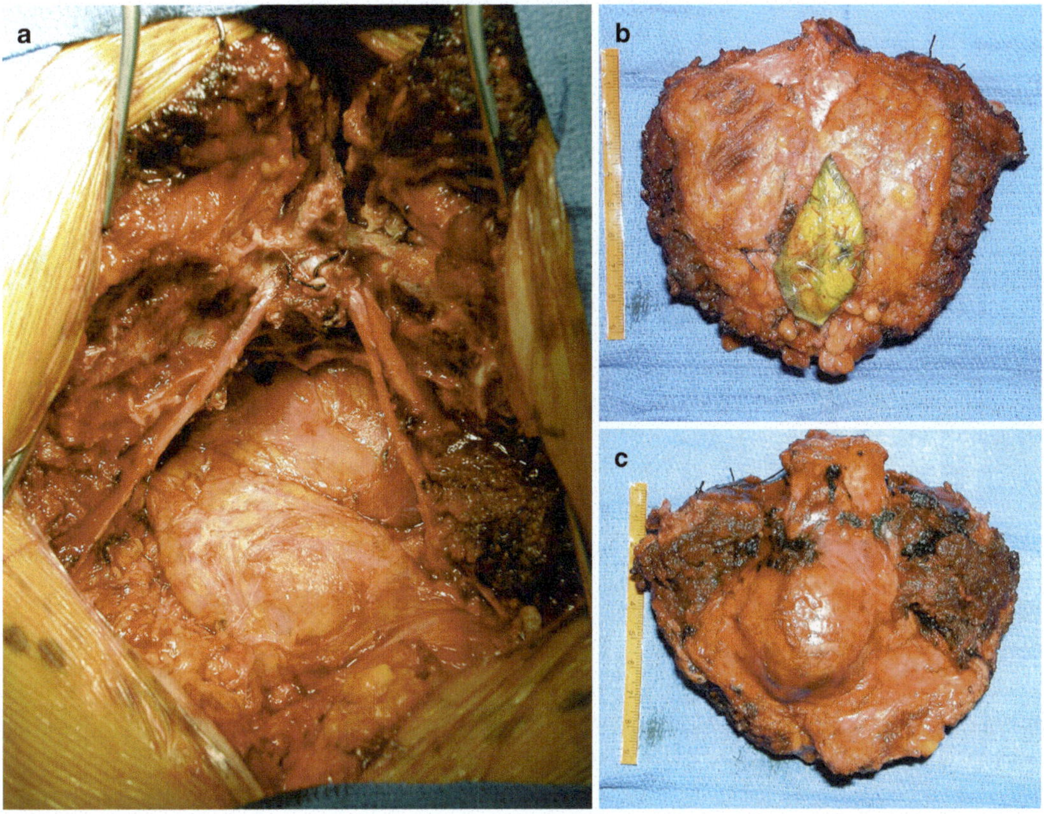

Fig. 10.6 Mid-sacrectomy for chordoma (**a**). Chordoma in situ (**b**). Dorsal aspect of specimen with elliptical skin incision incorporating biopsy into specimen (**c**). Ventral aspect of specimen

erally off the ilium using a subperiosteal technique; the muscles can then be retracted rostrally.

Next, the gluteal muscles inserting on the lateral aspect of the ilium are dissected, and the sciatic notch is identified. To maintain exposure, a self-retaining retractor is introduced.

A laminectomy is performed at the level of the most caudal nerve root to be preserved; subsequently, this nerve root is identified and traced laterally. The laminectomy is then extended laterally to the dorsal foramen of the sacrum and the dorsal nerve root there is released. This is important as failure to release the dorsal nerve root can result in traction injury during mobilization of the sacrum.

Following release of the dorsal nerve root from the foramen, lateral osteotomies are performed with a high-speed diamond burr following a line between the dorsal foramen proximally and the sciatic notch distally. The bone should be drilled until the ventral periosteum is identified; the ventral periosteum can then be removed with a Kerrison punch at which point the ventral nerve root should be visualized.

Following the lateral osteotomies, attention is turned toward the nerve roots to be sacrificed which are identified, ligated with size 0 silk suture, and sharply divided. A midline osteotomy is then performed with the high-speed diamond burr connecting the lateral osteotomies through the vertebral body.

Now, the caudal ligaments and muscles anchoring the distal sacrum and coccyx within the pelvis must be divided. Attention is turned to the most distal nerve root to be spared, identifying and tracing it to where it joins the sciatic nerve within the sciatic notch. The sacrotuberous and sacrospinous ligaments as well as the piriformis and gluteal muscles can now be divided with

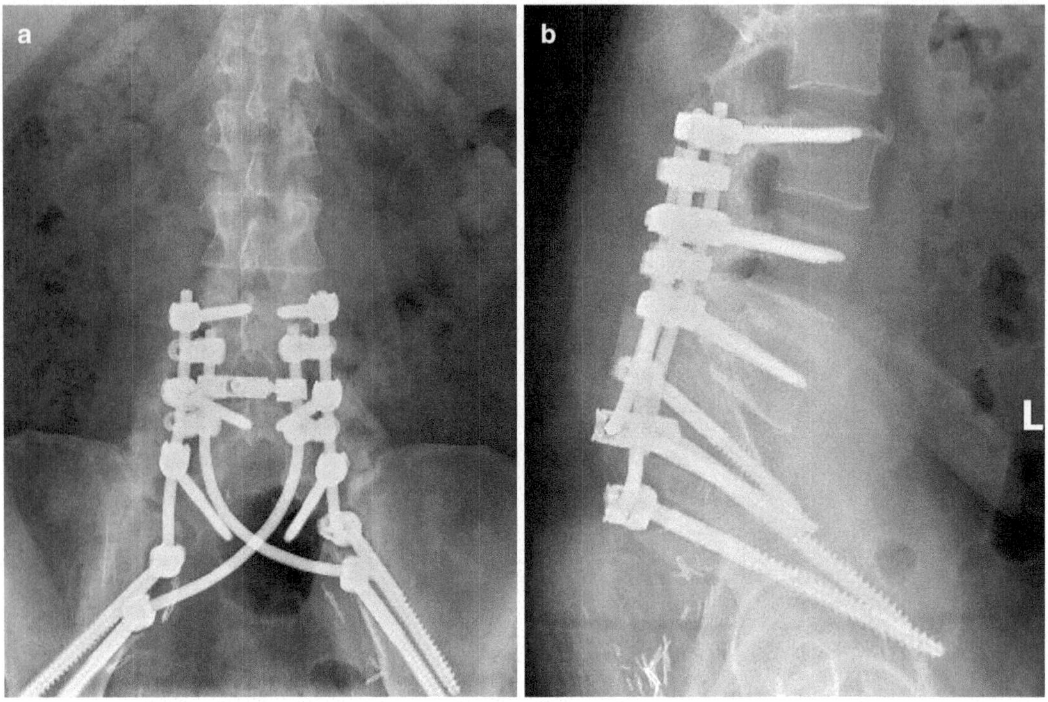

Fig. 10.7 (**a**) AP plain film X-ray of lumbo-pelvic reconstruction following total sacrectomy for chordoma. Patient ambulatory following surgery. (**b**) Lateral view of lumbo-pelvic reconstruction

a monopolar electrocautery knife. The sacrum should now be fully mobilized.

At this point, a penetrating towel clamp is used to secure the rostral aspect of the sacral specimen, which is then delivered posteriorly out of the pelvis (Fig. 10.6). It is critically important to avoid violation of the tumor capsule if at all feasible; furthermore, care must be taken to avoid injury to the rectum as it is dissected off the tumor capsule. At this point, the anococcygeal ligament is identified and divided permitting delivery of the specimen (Fig. 10.6).

Lumbo-Pelvic Reconstruction

As mentioned above, subtotal sacrectomy typically does not result in biomechanical instability; however, total sacrectomy may cause significant instability and often requires lumbo-pelvic reconstruction. Reconstruction begins with placement of pedicle screws at L3, L4, and L5 bilaterally, followed by bilateral iliac screws (Fig. 10.7). The iliac screws are connected to the pedicle screws on either side with a contoured rod. A trans-iliac rod may then be placed to further distribute weight evenly across the construct. A femoral shaft allograft is cut such that it spans the ilia transversely; the graft is then secured to the trans-iliac rod with titanium cables (Fig. 10.8). Subsequently, the areas to be fused are decorticated and the graft is packed from ilium to L3 along the facet joints and transverse processes to achieve arthrodesis.

Closure

If a myocutaneous rectus flap was harvested in the anterior portion of a two-staged procedure, it should now be visible through the sacral defect at which point it may be delivered posteriorly. Next, attention is turned to the rectum and pelvic contents; a piece of alloderm is sewn into the bony

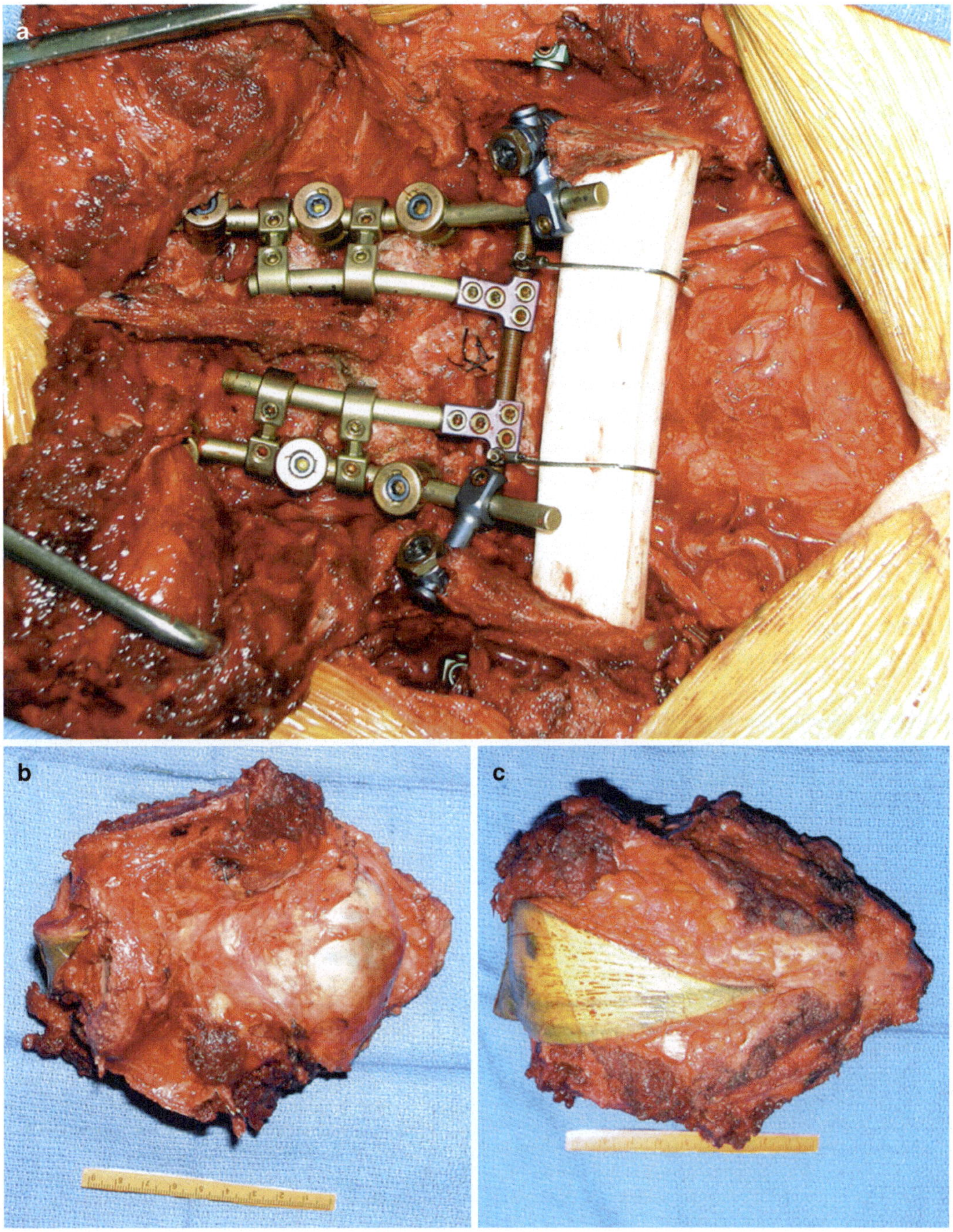

Fig. 10.8 (**a**) Lumbo-pelvic reconstruction following total sacrectomy with trans-iliac rod and femoral bone graft secured with titanium cables. (**b**) Specimen ventral aspect. (**c**) Specimen dorsal aspect with elliptical skin incision from biopsy tract incorporated

pelvis along the osteotomies to create a barrier to keep these elements ventral to the sacral defect. This decreases the risk of rectal herniation through the sacral defect and will keep the rectum sufficiently anterior if postoperative radiation is indicated.

Postoperative Care

Postoperative wound care is important to prevent wound breakdown/infection and improve outcomes following surgery. Patients should be on strict bed rest for 3–4 days in the immediate post-op period prior to mobilization; furthermore, it is key to minimize pressure on the wound, especially if a flap is used for closure. A pressure offloading bed such as a Clinitron may help minimize pressure over the wound.

Patients with bowel and bladder dysfunction following these surgeries must be appropriately managed with straight catheterization to minimize urinary tract infection and to keep the wound clean and dry. Likewise, bowel incontinence must be addressed with meticulous cleaning as well as a constipating diet and strict bowel regimen.

References

1. Menezes AH, Gantz BJ, Traynelis VC, McCulloch TM. Cranial base chordomas. Clin Neurosurg. 1997;44:491–509. Available from: http://www.ncbi.nlm.nih.gov/pubmed/10080023.
2. Cheng EY, Özerdemoglu RA, Transfeldt EE, Thompson RC. Lumbosacral chordoma: prognostic factors and treatment. Spine (Phila Pa 1976). 1999;24(16):1639–45.
3. Murphey MD, Andrews CL, Flemming DJ, Temple HT, Smith WS, Smirniotopoulos JG. From the archives of the AFIP. Primary tumors of the spine: radiologic pathologic correlation. RadioGraphics. 1996;16(5):1131–58. Available from: http://www.ncbi.nlm.nih.gov/pubmed/8888395.
4. McMaster ML, Goldstein AM, Bromley CM, Ishibe N, Chordoma PDM. Incidence and survival patterns in the United States, 1973-1995. Cancer Causes Control. 2001;12(1):1–11.
5. Higinbotham NL, Phillips RF, Farr HW, Hustu HO. Chordoma. Thirty-five-year study at memorial hospital. Cancer. 1967;20(11):1841–50.
6. Boriani S, Chevalley F, Weinstein JN, Biagini R, Campanacci L, De Iure F, et al. Chordoma of the spine above the sacrum. Treatment and outcome in 21 cases. Spine (Phila Pa 1976). 1996;21(13):1569–77.
7. Amendola BE, Amendola MA, Oliver E, McClatchey KD. Chordoma: role of radiation therapy. Radiology. 1986;158(3):839–43. Available from: http://www.ncbi.nlm.nih.gov/pubmed/3945761.
8. Chordoma MER. J Bone Joint Surg Am. 1981;63(3):501–5. Available from: http://www.ncbi.nlm.nih.gov/pubmed/7009618.
9. Hsu KY, Zucherman JF, Mortensen N, Johnston JO, Gartland J. Follow-up evaluation of resected lumbar vertebral chordoma over 11 years: a case report. Spine (Phila Pa 1976). 2000;25(19):2537–40. Available from: http://www.ncbi.nlm.nih.gov/pubmed/11013508.
10. Fourney DR, Gokaslan ZL. Current management of sacral chordoma. Neurosurg Focus. 2008;15(2)
11. Bergh P, Kindblom LG, Gunterberg B, Remotti F, Ryd W, Meis-Kindblom JM. Prognostic factors in chordoma of the sacrum and mobile spine: a study of 39 patients. Cancer. 2000;88(9):2122–34.
12. Boriani S, Bandiera S, Biagini R, Bacchini P, Boriani L, Cappuccio M, et al. Chordoma of the mobile spine: fifty years of experience. Spine. 2006;31(4):493–503.
13. York JE, Berk RH, Fuller GN, Rao JS, Abi-Said D, Wildrick DM, et al. Chondrosarcoma of the spine: 1954 to 1997. J Neurosurg. 1999;90(1 Suppl):73–8. Available from: http://www.ncbi.nlm.nih.gov/pubmed/10413129.
14. Boriani S, De Lure F, Bandiera S, Campanacci L, Biagini R, Di Fiore M, et al. Chondrosarcoma of the mobile spine: report on 22 cases. Spine (Phila Pa 1976). 2000;25(7):804–12.
15. Shives TC, McLeod RA, Unni KK, Schray MF. Chondrosarcoma of the spine. J Bone Joint Surg Am. 1989;71(8):1158–65. Available from: http://www.ncbi.nlm.nih.gov/pubmed/2777842.
16. Sheth DS, Yasko AW, Johnson ME, Ayala AG, Murray JA, Romsdahl MM. Chondrosarcoma of the pelvis: prognostic factors for 67 patients treated with definitive surgery. Cancer. 1996;78(4):745–50.
17. Rao G, Suki D, Chakrabarti I, Feiz-Erfan I, Mody MG, McCutcheon IE, et al. Surgical management of primary and metastatic sarcoma of the mobile spine. J Neurosurg Spine. 2008;9(2):120–8.
18. Fitzwilliams DCL. Hindquarter amputation for sarcoma. Proc Royal Soc Med. 2016;31(6):548–50.
19. Kellogg S. Hemipelvectomy. Ann Surg. 1932;95(2):167–73.
20. Enneking WF, Dunham WK. Resection and reconstruction for primary neoplasms involving the innominate bone. J Bone Joint Surg. 1978;60(6):731–46.
21. Puri A, Pruthi M, Gulia A. Outcomes after limb sparing resection in primary malignant pelvic tumors. Eur J Surg Oncol (EJSO). 2014;40(1):27–33.
22. Ozaki T, Flege S, Liljenqvist U, Hillmann A, Delling G, Salzer-Kuntschik M, et al. Osteosarcoma of the

spine: experience of the cooperative osteosarcoma study group. Cancer. 2002;94(4):1069–77.
23. Llauger J, Palmer J, Amores S, Bague S, Camins A. Primary tumors of the sacrum. Am J Roentgenol. 2000;174(2):417–24. Available from: http://www.ajronline.org/doi/10.2214/ajr.174.2.1740417.
24. Cade S. Osteogenic sarcoma; a study based on 133 patients. J R Coll Surg Edinb. 1955;1(2):79–111. Available from: http://www.ncbi.nlm.nih.gov/pubmed/13307660.
25. Savage SA, Mirabello L. Using epidemiology and genomics to understand osteosarcoma etiology. Sarcoma. 2011;2011:548151.
26. Seton M, Hansen MF. Osteosarcoma in Paget's disease of bone. In: Advances in Pathobiology and Management of Paget's Disease of Bone; 2016.
27. Fischgrund JS, American Academy of Orthopaedic Surgeons. OKU 9: orthopaedic knowledge update. American Academy of Orthopaedic Surgeons; 2008. 840 p.
28. Huang TL, Cohen NJ, Sahgal S, Tseng CH. Osteosarcoma complicating Paget??S disease of the spine with neurologic complications. Clin Orthop Relat Res. 1979;(141):260–5.
29. Sofka CM, Ciavarra G, Saboeiro G, Ghelman B. Paget's disease of the spine and secondary osteosarcoma. HSS J. 2006;2(2):188–90. Available from: http://www.ncbi.nlm.nih.gov/pubmed/18751835.
30. Mukherjee D, Chaichana KL, Parker SL, Gokaslan ZL, McGirt MJ. Association of surgical resection and survival in patients with malignant primary osseous spinal neoplasms from the surveillance, epidemiology, and end results (SEER) database. Eur Spine J. 2013;22(6):1375–82. Available from: http://www.ncbi.nlm.nih.gov/pubmed/23263168.
31. Shankar GM, Clarke MJ, Ailon T, Rhines LD, Patel SR, Sahgal A, et al. The role of revision surgery and adjuvant therapy following subtotal resection of osteosarcoma of the spine: a systematic review with meta-analysis. J Neurosurg Spine. 2017;27(1):97–104.
32. Anninga JK, Gelderblom H, Fiocco M, Kroep JR, Taminiau AHM, Hogendoorn PCW, et al. Chemotherapeutic adjuvant treatment for osteosarcoma: where do we stand? Eur J Cancer. 2011;47(16):2431–45.
33. Capanna R, Ayala A, Bertoni F, Picci P, Calderoni P, Gherlinzoni F, et al. Sacral osteoid osteoma and osteoblastoma: a report of 13 cases. Arch Orthop Trauma Surg. 1986;105(4):205–10. Available from: http://link.springer.com/10.1007/BF00435481.
34. Richard Winn H. Youmans & Winn Neurological Surgery. 2017.
35. Ruggieri P, Huch K, Mavrogenis AF, Merlino B, Angelini A. Osteoblastoma of the sacrum. Spine (Phila Pa 1976). 2014;39(2):E97–103. Available from: http://www.ncbi.nlm.nih.gov/pubmed/24108284.
36. Rosenthal DI, Hornicek FJ, Torriani M, Gebhardt MC, Mankin HJ. Osteoid osteoma: percutaneous treatment with radiofrequency energy. Radiology. 2003;229(1):171–5.
37. Cribb GL, Goude WH, Cool P, Tins B, Cassar-Pullicino VN, Mangham DC. Percutaneous radiofrequency thermocoagulation of osteoid osteomas: factors affecting therapeutic outcome. Skeletal Radiol. 2005;34(11):702–6.
38. Eckardt JJ, Grogan TJ. Giant cell tumor of bone. Clin Orthop Relat Res. 1986;(204):45–58. Available from: http://www.ncbi.nlm.nih.gov/pubmed/3514036.
39. Brien EW, Mirra JM, Kessler S, Suen M, Ho JKS, Yang WT. Benign giant cell tumor of bone with osteosarcomatous transformation ("dedifferentiated" primary malignant GCT): report of two cases. Skelet Radiol. 1997;26(4):246–55.
40. Nojima T, Takeda N, Matsuno T, Inoue K, Nagashima K. Case report 869. Benign metastasizing giant cell tumor of bone. Skelet Radiol. 1994;23(7):583–5.
41. Thomas D, Henshaw R, Skubitz K, Chawla S, Staddon A, Blay J-Y, Roudier M, Smith J, Ye Z, Sohn W, Dansey R, Jun S. Denosumab in patients with giant-cell tumour of bone: an open-label, phase 2 study. Lancet Oncol. 2010;11(3):275–80.
42. Yang Y, Li Y, Liu W, Xu H, Niu X. A nonrandomized controlled study of sacral giant cell tumors with preoperative treatment of denosumab. Medicine. 2018;97(46):e13139.
43. Sambri A, Medellin MR, Errani C, Campanacci L, Fujiwara T, Donati D, Parry M, Grimer R. Denosumab in giant cell tumour of bone in the pelvis and sacrum: long-term therapy or bone resection? J Orthop Sci. 2020;25(3):513–9.
44. Hosalkar HS, Jones KJ, King JJ, Lackman RD. Serial arterial embolization for large sacral giant-cell tumors: mid- to long-term results. Spine (Phila Pa 1976). 2007;32(10):1107–15.
45. Leggon RE, Zlotecki R, Reith J, Scarborough MT. Giant cell tumor of the pelvis and sacrum. Clin Orthop Relat Res. 2004;423(423):196–207. Available from: http://www.ncbi.nlm.nih.gov/pubmed/15232449.
46. Chakravarti A, Spiro IJ, Hug EB, Mankin HJ, Efird JT, Suit HD. Megavoltage radiation therapy for axial and inoperable Giant-cell tumor of bone. J Bone Jt Surg. 1999;81(11):1566–73.
47. Ruka W, Rutkowski P, Morysiński T, Nowecki Z, Zdzienicki M, Makula D, Ptaszyński K, Bylina E, Grzesiakowska U. The megavoltage radiation therapy in treatment of patients with advanced or difficult giant cell tumors of bone. Int J Radiat Oncol Biol Phys. 2010;78(2):494–8.
48. Turcotte RE, Sim FH, Unni KK. Giant cell tumor of the sacrum. Clin Orthop Relat Res. 1993;(291):215–21. Available from: http://www.ncbi.nlm.nih.gov/pubmed/8504603.
49. Schropp KP, Lobe TE, Rao B, Mutabagani K, Kay GA, Gilchrist BF, et al. Sacrococcygeal teratoma: the experience of four decades. J Pediatr Surg. 1992;27(8):1075–8.
50. De Backer A, Madern GC, Hakvoort-Cammel FGAJ, Haentjens P, Oosterhuis JW, Hazebroek FWJ. Study of the factors associated with recurrence in chil-

dren with sacrococcygeal teratoma. J Pediatr Surg. 2006;41(1):173–81.
51. Teich S, Caniano DA. Reoperative pediatric surgery. 2008.
52. Donnellan WA, Swenson O. Benign and malignant sacrococcygeal teratomas. Surgery. 1968;64(4):834–46. Available from: http://www.ncbi.nlm.nih.gov/pubmed/5683810.
53. Derikx JPM, De Backer A, Van De Schoot L, Aronson DC, De Langen ZJ, Van Den Hoonaard TL, et al. Factors associated with recurrence and metastasis in sacrococcygeal teratoma. Br J Surg. 2006;93(12):1543–8.
54. Dickman CA, Fehlings MG, Gokaslan ZL, editors. Spinal cord and spinal column tumors: principles and practice. Stuttgart: Georg Thieme Verlag; 2006. Available from: http://www.thieme-connect.de/products/ebooks/book/10.1055/b-002-52051.
55. Wu JT, Book L, Sudar K. Serum alpha fetoprotein (AFP) levels in normal infants. Pediatr Res. 1981;15(1):50–2.
56. Calaminus G, Vesterling-Hörner D, Bökkerink J, Gadner H, Günther G, Haas H, et al. Die prognostische Bedeutung des Serum α 1 -Fetoproteins (AFP) bei Kindern und Jugendlichen mit malignen extrakranialen nichttestikulären Keimzelltumoren. Klin Pädiatrie. 1991;203(04):246–50. Available from: http://www.ncbi.nlm.nih.gov/pubmed/1719268.
57. Rescorla FJ, Sawin RS, Coran AG, Dillon PW, Azizkhan RG. Long-term outcome for infants and children with sacrococcygeal teratoma: a report from the childrens cancer group. J Pediatr Surg. 1998;33(2):171–6.
58. Rescorla F, Billmire D, Stolar C, Vinocur C, Colombani P, Cullen J, et al. The effect of cisplatin dose and surgical resection in children with malignant germ cell tumors at the sacrococcygeal region: a pediatric intergroup trial (POG 9049/CCG 8882). J Pediatr Surg. 2001;36(1):12–7.
59. Göbel U, Schneider DT, Calaminus G, Jürgens H, Spaar HJ, Sternschulte W, et al. Multimodal treatment of malignant Sacrococcygeal germ cell tumors: a prospective analysis of 66 patients of the German cooperative protocols MAKEI 83/86 and 89. J Clin Oncol. 2001;19(7):1943–50. Available from: http://www.ncbi.nlm.nih.gov/pubmed/11283126.
60. Gonzalez-Crussi F, Winkler RF, Mirkin DL. Sacrococcygeal teratomas in infants and children. Relationship of histology and prognosis in 40 cases. Arch Pathol Lab Med. 1978;102(8):420–5.
61. Ein SH, Adeyemi SD, Mancer K. Benign sacrococcygeal teratomas in infants and children. A 25 year review. Ann Surg. 1980;191(3):382–4.
62. Engelskirchen R, Holschneider A, Rhein R, Hecker W, Höpner F. Steißbeinteratome im Kindesalter. Eur J Pediatr Surg. 1987;42(06):358–61. Available from: http://www.ncbi.nlm.nih.gov/pubmed/3439358.
63. Havránek P, Rubenson A, Güth D, Frenckner B, Olsen L, Åke Kornfält S, et al. Sacrococcygeal teratoma in Sweden: a 10-year national retrospective study. J Pediatr Surg. 1992;27(11):1447–50.
64. Bilik R, Shandling B, Pope M, Thorner P, Weitzman S, Ein SH. Malignant benign neonatal sacrococcygeal teratoma. J Pediatr Surg. 1993;28(9):1158–60. Available from: http://www.ncbi.nlm.nih.gov/pubmed/7508500.
65. Schmidt B, Haberlik A, Uray E, Ratschek M, Lackner H, Höllwarth ME. Sacrococcygeal teratoma: clinical course and prognosis with a special view to long-term functional results. Pediatr Surg Int. 1999;15(8):573–6.
66. Wakhlu A, Misra S, Tandon RK, Wakhlu AK. Sacrococcygeal teratoma. Pediatr Surg Int. 2002;18(5–6):384–7. Available from: http://www.ncbi.nlm.nih.gov/pubmed/12415361.
67. Perrelli L, D'Urzo C, Manzoni C, Pintus C, De Santis M, Masini L, et al. Sacrococcygeal teratoma. Outcome and management. An analysis of 17 cases. J Perinat Med. 2002;30(2):179–84.
68. Huddart SN, Mann JR, Robinson K, Raafat F, Imeson J, Gornall P, et al. Sacrococcygeal teratomas: the UK Children's Cancer Study Group's experience. I. Neonatal. Pediatr Surg Int. 2003;19(1–2):47–51. Available from: http://www.ncbi.nlm.nih.gov/pubmed/12721723.
69. Schneider DT, Wessalowski R, Calaminus G, Pape H, Bamberg M, Engert J, et al. Treatment of recurrent malignant Sacrococcygeal germ cell tumors: analysis of 22 patients registered in the German protocols MAKEI 83/86, 89, and 96. J Clin Oncol. 2001;19(7):1951–60. Available from: http://www.ncbi.nlm.nih.gov/pubmed/11283127.
70. Raque GH, Vitaz TW, Shields CB. Treatment of neoplastic diseases of the sacrum. J Surg Oncol. 2001;
71. Wuisman P, Lieshout O, Sugihara S, van Dijk M. Total sacretomy and reconstruction: Oncologic and functional outcome. Clin Orthop Relat Res. 2000;381:192–203.
72. Diel J, Ortiz O, Losada RA, Price DB, Hayt MW, Katz DS. The sacrum: pathologic spectrum, multimodality imaging, and subspecialty approach. RadioGraphics. 2001;21(1):83–104.
73. Disler DG, Miklic D. Imaging findings in tumors of the sacrum. Am J Roentgenol. 1999;173:1699.
74. Kollender Y, Meller I, Bickels J, Flusser G, Issakov J, Merimsky O, et al. Role of adjuvant cryosurgery in intralesional treatment of sacral tumors. Cancer. 2003;97(11):2830–8.
75. Cummings BJ, Ian Hodson D, Bush RS. Chordoma: the results of megavoltage radiation therapy. Int J Radiat Oncol Biol Phys. 1983;9(5):633–42.
76. Fornasier VL, Horne JG. Metastases to the vertebral column. Cancer. 1975;36(2):590–4.
77. Sundaresan N, Digiacinto GV, Hughes JEO, Cafferty M, Vallejo A. Treatment of neoplastic spinal cord compression: results of a prospective study. Neurosurgery. 1991;29(5):645–50.
78. Bradley Jacobs W, Perrin RG. Evaluation and treatment of spinal metastases: an overview. Neurosurg Focus. 2001;11(6):1–11.
79. Ozdemir MH, Gürkan I, Yildiz Y, Yilmaz C, Saglik Y. Surgical treatment of malignant tumours of

the sacrum. Eur J Surg Oncol. 1999;25(1):44–9. Available from: http://www.ncbi.nlm.nih.gov/pubmed/10188854.
80. Nader R, Rhines LD, Mendel E. Metastatic sacral tumors. Neurosurg Clin N Am. 2004;15(4):453–7. Available from: http://www.ncbi.nlm.nih.gov/pubmed/15450880.
81. Maranzano E, Trippa F, Chirico L, Basagni ML, Rossi R. Management of metastatic spinal cord compression. Tumori. 2019;89(5):469–75. Available from: http://www.ncbi.nlm.nih.gov/pubmed/14870766.
82. Loblaw DA, Laperriere NJ. Emergency treatment of malignant extradural spinal cord compression: an evidence-based guideline. J Clin Oncol. 1998;16(4):1613–24.
83. Todd LT, Yaszemski MJ, Currier BL, Fuchs B, Kim CW, Sim FH. Bowel and bladder function after major sacral resection. Clin Orthop Relat Res. 2002;397:36–9.
84. Guo Y, Palmer JL, Shen L, Kaur G, Willey J, Zhang T, et al. Bowel and bladder continence, wound healing, and functional outcomes in patients who underwent sacrectomy. J Neurosurg Spine. 2005;3(2):106–10.
85. Rose PS, Yaszemski MJ, Sim FH. A biomechanical approach to advances in sacropelvic reconstruction. Hamdan Med J. 2018;11(4):193.
86. Egund N, Olsson TH, Schmid H, Selvik G. Movements in the sacroiliac joints demonstrated with roentgen stereophotogrammetry. Acta Radiol Diagn. 2016;19(5):833–46.
87. Sturesson B, Selvik G, Udén A. Movements of the sacroiliac joints. Spine. 1989;14(2):162–5.
88. Pel JJM, Spoor CW, Pool-Goudzwaard AL, Hoek van Dijke GA, Snijders CJ. Biomechanical analysis of reducing sacroiliac joint shear load by optimization of pelvic muscle and ligament forces. Ann Biomed Eng. 2008;36(3):415–24.
89. Kiapour A, Joukar A, Elgafy H, Erbulut DU, Agarwal AK, Goel VK. Biomechanics of the sacroiliac joint: anatomy, function, biomechanics, sexual dimorphism, and causes of pain. Int J Spine Surg. 2020;14(s1):S3–S13.
90. Gunterberg B, Romanus B, Stener B. Pelvic strength after major amputation of the sacrum. Acta Orthop Scand. 2009;47(6):635–42.
91. Stener B, Gunterberg B. High amputation of the sacrum for extirpation of tumors. Spine. 1978;3(4):351–66.
92. Fourney DR, Rhines LD, Hentschel SJ, Skibber JM, Wolinsky J-P, Weber KL, Suki D, Gallia GL, Garonzik I, Gokaslan ZL. En bloc resection of primary sacral tumors: classification of surgical approaches and outcome. J Neurosurg Spine. 2005;3(2):111–22.
93. Michel A. Total sacrectomy and lower spine resection for giant cell tumor: one case report. Chir Organi Mov. 1990;75:117–8.
94. Simpson AH, Porter A, Davis A, Griffin A, McLeod RS, Bell RS. Cephalad sacral resection with a combined extended ilioinguinal and posterior approach. J Bone Joint Surg. 1995;77(3):405–11.
95. McLoughlin GS, Sciubba DM, Suk I, Witham T, Bydon A, Gokaslan ZL, Wolinsky J-P. En bloc total sacrectomy performed in a single stage through a posterior approach. Oper Neurosurg. 2008;63(suppl_1):ONS115–20.
96. Dickey ID, Hugate RR, Fuchs B, Yaszemski MJ, Sim FH. Reconstruction after total sacrectomy. Clin Orthop Relat Res. 2005;438:42–50.
97. Zileli M, Hoscoskun C, Brastianos P, Sabah D. Surgical treatment of primary sacral tumors: complications associated with sacrectomy. Neurosurg Focus. 2003;15(5):1–8.
98. Ohata N, Ozaki T, Kunisada T, Morimoto Y, Tanaka M, Inoue H. Extended total sacrectomy and reconstruction for sacral tumor. Spine. 2004;29(6):E123–6.
99. Wuisman P, Lieshout O, van Dijk M, van Diest P. Reconstruction after total en bloc sacrectomy for osteosarcoma using a custom-made prosthesis. Spine. 2001;26(4):431–9.
100. Tomita K, Tsuchiya H. Total sacrectomy and reconstruction for huge sacral tumors. Spine. 1990;15(11):1223–7.
101. Ruggieri P, Angelini A, Ussia G, Montalti M, Mercuri M. Surgical margins and local control in resection of sacral chordomas. Clin Orthop Relat Res. 2010;468(11):2939–47.
102. Kiatisevi P, Piyaskulkaew C, Kunakornsawat S, Sukunthanak B. What are the functional outcomes after total sacrectomy without spinopelvic reconstruction? Clin Orthop Relat Res. 2017;475(3):643–55.
103. Bederman SS, Shah KN, Hassan JM, Hoang BH, Kiester PD, Bhatia NN. Surgical techniques for spinopelvic reconstruction following total sacrectomy: a systematic review. Eur Spine J. 2014;23(2):305–19.
104. Guo W, Tang X, Zang J, Ji T. One-stage total en bloc sacrectomy. Spine. 2013;38(10):E626–31.
105. Arkader A, Yang CH, Tolo VT. High long-term local control with sacrectomy for primary high-grade bone sarcoma in children. Clin Orthop Relat Res. 2012;470(5):1491–7.
106. Asavamongkolkul A, Waikakul S. Wide resection of sacral chordoma via a posterior approach. Int Orthop. 2012;36(3):607–12.
107. Clarke MJ, Dasenbrock H, Bydon A, Sciubba DM, McGirt MJ, Hsieh PC, Yassari R, Gokaslan ZL, Wolinsky J-P. Posterior-only approach for en bloc sacrectomy. Neurosurgery. 2012;71(2):357–64.
108. Hsieh PC, Risheng X, Sciubba DM, McGirt MJ, Nelson C, Witham TF, Wolinksy J-P, Gokaslan ZL. Long-term clinical outcomes following en bloc resections for sacral chordomas and chondrosarcomas. Spine. 2009;34(20):2233–9.
109. Hugate RR, Dickey ID, Phimolsarnti R, Yaszemski MJ, Sim FH. Mechanical effects of partial sacrectomy. Clin Orthop Relat Res. 2006;450:82–8.
110. Yu B, Zheng Z, Zhuang X, Chen H, Xie D, Luk KDK, Lu WW. Biomechanical effects of transverse partial sacrectomy on the sacroiliac joints. Spine. 2009;34(13):1370–5.

111. Wuisman P, Lieshout O, Sugihara S, van Dijk M. Total sacretomy and reconstruction: oncologic and functional outcome. Clin Orthop Relat Res. 2000;381:192.
112. Gokaslan ZL, Fourney DR. 44 Surgical approaches for the resection of sacral tumors. In: Dickman CA, Fehlings MG, Gokaslan ZL, editors. Spinal cord and spinal column tumors: principles and practice. Stuttgart: Georg Thieme Verlag; 2006. https://doi.org/10.1055/b-002-52051.
113. Arnautović KI, Al-Mefty O. Surgical seeding of chordomas. J Neurosurg. 2009;95:798.
114. Kirshenbaum AH, Yang WC. Cervical chordoma with intradural invasion. A case report. Bull Hosp Jt Dis Orthop Inst. 1983;43(1):38–48. Available from: http://www.ncbi.nlm.nih.gov/pubmed/6309305.
115. McLoughlin GS, Sciubba DM, Suk I, Witham T, Bydon A, Gokaslan ZL, et al. En bloc total sacrectomy performed in a single stage through a posterior approach. Neurosurgery. 2008;63(1 Suppl 1):ONS115–20.
116. Clarke MJ, Dasenbrock H, Bydon A, Sciubba DM, McGirt MJ, Hsieh PC, et al. Posterior-only approach for en bloc sacrectomy: clinical outcomes in 36 consecutive patients. Neurosurgery. 2012;71(2):357–64.

Special Anatomical Zone: Craniocervical Junction Tumors

11

Mena G. Kerolus and John E. O'Toole

Abbreviations

ABC	Aneurysmal bone cyst
CSF	Cerebrospinal fluid
CT	Computed tomography
CVJ	Craniovertebral junction
DSA	Digital subtraction angiography
EBRT	External beam radiation therapy
EG	Eosinophilic granuloma
MEP	Motor evoked potential
MM	Multiple myeloma
MRA	Magnetic resonance angiogram
MRI	Magnetic resonance imaging
SINS	Spinal Instability Neoplastic Score
SRS	Stereotactic radiosurgery
SSEP	Somatosensory evoked potentials

Introduction

The craniovertebral junction (CVJ) encompasses the lower clivus, foramen magnum, the atlas (C1), the axis (C2), and the region between the occipital condyles and the atlantoaxial spine [1]. The CVJ contains several critical neurologic structures, major vasculature of the head and neck and an intricate network of ligamentous and osseous articulations. Treatment goals are dependent on the patient's clinical status, radiographic findings and ultimately histologic diagnosis. Tumors of the CVJ include pathology originating from bone (e.g., multiple myeloma), nervous system (e.g., schwannoma), nervous system associated tissue (e.g., meningioma), and soft tissues (e.g., hemangiomas).

Given the complexity of the region, surgery of the CVJ is challenging. A thorough understanding of regional anatomy, goals of surgery, and different surgical techniques are necessary to provide the best outcomes. In this chapter, we discuss the epidemiology, clinical evaluation, workup, and surgical options for primary and metastatic tumors of the CVJ.

Incidence

Craniovertebral junction (CVJ) tumors make up approximately 0.5% of all spinal malignancies, and it is the least affected region of the axial skeleton [2, 3]. The most common metastatic tumors of the CVJ originate from either the breast, lung or prostate during the sixth decade of life [1, 4]. The most common primary spinal cord tumor of the CVJ includes meningioma, myeloma, and chordoma. Of these, meningiomas are the most common and account for nearly 75% of intradural extramedullary tumors in this region.

M. G. Kerolus (✉) · J. E. O'Toole
Department of Neurosurgery, Rush University Medical Center, Chicago, IL, USA
e-mail: John_OToole@rush.edu

K. Singh, M. Colman (eds.), *Surgical Spinal Oncology*,
https://doi.org/10.1007/978-3-030-50722-0_11

In adults, the most common benign osseous tumors of the CVJ are aneurysmal bone cysts, giant cell tumors, osteoblastomas, eosinophilic granulomas, and solitary plasmacytomas. The most common malignant neoplasms, in decreasing frequency, are chordomas, myelomas, lymphomas, chondrosarcomas, osteosarcomas, and Ewing sarcomas. In children, the most common primary benign tumor of the CVJ are osteoid osteomas, osteoblastomas, and aneurysmal bone cysts. The most common malignant tumors in children are chordomas and Ewing sarcoma.

Diagnosis

An evaluation of the patient's clinical presentation, physical examination, laboratory workup, radiographic findings, and tissue histology will be needed in order to successfully create a treatment plan for patients with CVJ neoplasms.

Presentation

In patients with tumor involvement of the CVJ, presenting symptoms are variable and often ill-defined, mimicking symptoms commonly seen in patients with cervical degenerative disease. The most common symptom is upper cervical neck pain [5, 6]. Specifically, patient's present with significant rotational neck pain, rather than pain on flexion extension, given the large biomechanical rotational component of the atlantoaxial joint [7]. Various forms of neuralgia may occur including occipital or cervicobrachial neuralgia, retro auricular pain, cervical radiculopathy, localized pain, or headache. Local osseous destruction progresses to deformity and instability which is a major cause of mechanical pain. In rare cases of insidious growth, CVJ tumors can cause lower cranial nerve palsies, especially CN XI. Patients may develop progressive symptoms of dysphagia, dysarthria, and torticollis secondary to brainstem compression. These symptoms can be exacerbated with head movement or local pressure. In the late-stage disease, long tract signs, bladder or rectal dysfunction, spasticity, cerebellar ataxia, Brown–Sequard syndrome, and other cross-sectional neurologic syndromes may occur.

Laboratory Workup

Laboratory evaluation can help provide diagnostic information of the underlying malignancy. Hematologic abnormalities such as an elevated white blood cell count or low hemoglobin may indicate tumor involvement of the bone marrow. Serum or urine electrophoresis should be pursued if there is a concern for plasmacytoma or multiple myeloma.

Imaging

Various imaging modalities including static, dynamic, and vascular imaging are crucial for evaluation of tumor involvement of the CVJ. Static radiographs can help identify lytic destruction, pathologic fractures, and evaluate overall occipitocervical alignment. Dynamic flexion and extension radiographs should be pursued to determine upper cervical instability and the extent of subluxation with movement.

Magnetic resonance imaging (MRI) is considered the gold standard for the evaluation of spinal cord tumors. Especially in the region of the CVJ, an MRI is used to evaluate tumor compartment (extradural vs intradural), visualize the osseous and soft tissue boundaries of the tumor, and detail the neural and vascular anatomy in the vicinity of the tumor. Both noncontrast and contrast-enhanced sequences can determine potential surgical planes between pathologic and normal tissue. When treating a tumor of the CVJ, the vertebral arteries, venous vasculature, and lower cranial nerves should be identified. The specific anatomical details found on MRI strongly influence the surgical approach employed. A magnetic resonance angiogram (MRA) may be used for identification of the dominant vertebral artery and vascularity of the tumor.

Computed tomography (CT) or even CT myelogram is used to determine the extent of osseous tumor involvement and preoperative surgical planning. The width of the midline keel of the occipital bone can be measured on a preoperative CT to determine adequacy for occipital fixation. Additionally, a large transverse foramina of the axis may raise suspicion for a dominant or anomalous vertebral artery which may require an alternative C2 fixation option (e.g., C2 laminar screw). A CT scan is also used to evaluate the extent of lytic osseous involvement of the CVJ and subaxial cervical spine, which may influence the position of additional surgical fixation. Osseous changes on CT scan, such as hyperostosis at the dural site of origin or bone scalloping of the vertebral bodies or neural foramina, can help differentiate neoplasms such as a meningioma or schwannoma. CT myelogram is helpful to evaluate patients with prior instrumentation and the extent of brainstem or spinal cord compression secondary to tumor involvement when an MRI cannot be obtained. CT Angiogram might also be considered prior to instrumentation in patients with CVJ neoplasms as there is variability in the anatomy of the vertebral artery. Yamazaki et al. evaluated 100 consecutive patients that underwent CVJ instrumentation and found that 10% of patients had extraosseous anomalies of the vertebral artery (e.g., fenestrated vertebral artery or persistent first intersegmental artery) and 30% of patients had intraosseous vertebral artery anomalies [8].

Formal digital subtraction angiography (DSA) can detail tumor vascularity and provide the opportunity for preoperative embolization in tumors that are highly vascular (e.g., aneurysmal bone cyst or certain hypervascular metastatic tumors). If surgical ligation of the vertebral artery is anticipated, a balloon occlusion test can be performed.

Tissue Diagnosis

Primary osseous tumors of the cervical spine can often be confused with inflammatory, infectious or degenerative cervical spine disease, making histologic diagnosis vital for appropriate treatment [9]. Several metastatic and hematologic malignancies are highly sensitive to chemotherapy and radiation making tissue diagnosis imperative prior to a large surgical resection. Fluoroscopy or CT-guided needle biopsy is often used to obtain pathology. However, needle biopsy yields a 25% false-negative rate. Additionally, given the anatomic complexity of the CVJ, a needle biopsy may not be attainable. In these cases, an open biopsy should be considered. Significant osseous during should, if possible, be avoided as this may further destabilize the segment. Transoral biopsy may be necessary for purely ventral tumors [10].

Surgical and Anatomic Considerations

Surgical goals for metastatic and primary oncologic disease of the CVJ differ. Surgical intervention is largely reserved for patients with neurologic compromise, mechanical instability, intractable neck pain, and those with a primary tumor diagnosis. Surgery requires separation of the tumor from the vasculature and normal spinal cord followed by removal of the tumor. This may require multiple surgical approaches. Removal of osseous and structural components requires complex reconstruction techniques to stabilize the region. Surgical flexibility and adaptability between different approaches are crucial for success.

The anatomical complexity of the CVJ cannot be understated. Multiple critical structures reside in the vicinity of the CVJ, including major vasculature of the head and neck such as the carotid and vertebral arteries, cranial nerves, the brainstem, and spinal cord. Given the generous subarachnoid spacc at the CVJ, tumors can grow undetected for extended periods of time before neurological deficits occur, compounding the surgical difficulty of resection [6].

The foramen magnum is an oval ring formed by the occipital bone. The lowest portion of the clivus forms the anterior ring of the foramen magnum. The occipital condyles lie in the anterolateral portion of the foramen magnum. Drilling a portion of the posterior condyle and jugular tubercle during a far lateral approach can expose the lower lateral and ventral portion of the foramen magnum [11]. If the occipital condyle needs to be resected, the entire vertebral artery from the foramen transversarium to its dural entry needs to be dissected, which will entail drilling the foramen at C1. Extent of condylar dissection (50–70%) can lead to various degrees of CVJ instability resulting in pain, torticollis, and neurologic deficits. In the setting of disabling pain, patients may benefit from occipitocervical fusion [11, 12]. Directly lateral to the occipital condyle is the carotid canal and lateral to this is the jugular foramen. The stylomastoid foramen lies lateral to the jugular foramen. The facial nerve exits behind the posterior belly of the digastric muscle at its attachment to the digastric notch.

The CVJ protects multiple critical structures while also providing extensive motion of the head and neck. The ligaments of the CVJ play a vital role of maintaining surgical stability. The two main joints of the CVJ are the atlantooccipital joint and the atlantoaxial joint. The atlantooccipital joint mainly provides flexion and extension while the atlantoaxial joint is the largest contributor to axial rotation. Four layers of ligamentous stabilizers provide stability. The transverse ligament is the strongest and the major stabilizing ligament of the CVJ by retaining the odontoid against the anterior arch of C-1. The alar ligament is also a major stabilizing ligament of the CVJ and attaches the axis to the base of the skull. It limits axial rotation and lateral bending on the contralateral side. The apical ligament attaches the tip of the dens to the basion. The tectorial membrane is a three-layered membrane, posterior to the cruciform ligament that spans the foramen magnum and fuses into the posterior longitudinal ligament. The atlantooccipital membranes are thickest posteriorly and laterally and help stabilize the atlanto-ocipital joint [13–16]. Given the extensive ligamentous complex, it is often difficult for the tumor to extend into the foramen magnum.

The hypoglossal nerve travels in an anteromedial trajectory as it exits the intracranial compartment via the hypoglossal canal. The nerve then passes ventral to the C1 arch and dorsal to the digastric muscle before entering the tongue. The hypoglossal nerve is rarely involved in metastatic or primary tumors except for those originating from the lower clivus extending caudally into the spine. The nerve is frequently injured with high cervical anterior approaches. Patients can usually compensate for unilateral injury; however, bilateral injury can lead to dysphagia and even potentially life-threatening aspiration.

Major arterial and venous vasculature traverse the CVJ. Each vertebral artery arises from the subclavian artery, enters the transverse foramen of C6 and ascends the transverse foramina. The vertebral artery is positioned superolaterally at the transverse foramen of C2 and then enters laterally through the transverse foramina of C1. During the far lateral approach, the vertebral artery is found in the center of the suboccipital triangle, which is made up of the rectus capitis posterior major, the superior and inferior oblique muscles. The artery then passes on the posterior border of the lateral mass of C1and below the inferior border of the posterior atlantooccipital membrane before piercing the dura. The lateral mass of C1 and C2 are palpated in the suboccipital triangle which is approximately 1 cm below the tip of the mastoid process. Careful appreciation of vertebral artery anatomy is crucial to prevent a potentially devastating injury. Additionally, vertebral artery dominance can often be evaluated on preoperative imaging. A balloon occlusion test is used to determine if a vertebral artery can be safely sacrificed. Although there is no large single venous sinus of the CVJ, bleeding from the venous plexus in the region can be profound. Venous plexi at the region of the CVJ includes the suboccipital cavernous sinus, vertebral venous plexus, and the vertebral artery venous plexus [17].

Cervical nerve roots requiring sacrifice must be ligated proximal to the dorsal root ganglion to avoid neuroma formation and symptoms of neuralgia. The C2 nerve root is commonly sacrificed which may lead to occipital hypesthesia. C3 ligation in isolation is generally well tolerated but C3 and C4 injury can lead to diaphragmatic weakness, especially if bilateral sacrifice of the nerves occurs.

Surgical Approaches

Surgical approach to address CVJ pathology is based on multiple factors including: tumor location and extent of skull base involvement, tumor histology, tumor consistency, relationship of the tumor to the dural and neurovascular structures, the goal of the operation (biopsy, palliative decompression or complete resection), patient age, and CVJ stability. Complete resection may require multiple approaches. The three general surgical approaches are the dorsal/dosolateral approach, ventral/transoral approach, and the lateral/extreme lateral/transcondylar approach. A few case examples are described below.

Dorsal/Dorsolateral Approach

The approach most familiar to spine surgeons is the dorsal midline approach which is best used to address dorsal midline spinal tumors [6]. Ventral and lateral spine pathologies treated with a dorsal approach can lead to excessive spinal cord manipulation and neurologic injury. Extradural biopsies of the ventrolateral components of the CVJ could be considered using this approach in order to establish a diagnosis. A common variant is the dorsolateral approach, which allows for resection of tumor involving the ipsilateral facet, vertebral artery, and tumor involving the vicinity of the contralateral lamina. Both approaches provide the opportunity for simultaneous instrumentation and fusion.

Dorsolateral Approach: Case Example

A 55-year-old female presents with a one-year history of left upper extremity paresthesia and progressive right trunk and right lower extremity paresthesia. On physical examination, she has 5/5 motor strength in her extremities and 3+ reflexes in the right upper and lower extremities.

MRI with and without contrast of the cervical spine demonstrates severe spinal cord compression and ventrolateral displacement of the spinal cord due to a right dorsolateral intradural extramedullary heterogeneously enhancing neoplasm consistent with a meningioma. The neoplasm lies adjacent to the proximal intradural portion of the right vertebral artery (Fig. 11.1).

Due to her progressive myelopathy and imaging findings, she undergoes an occiput to C2 posterior laminectomy for resection of intradural-extramedullary neoplasm.

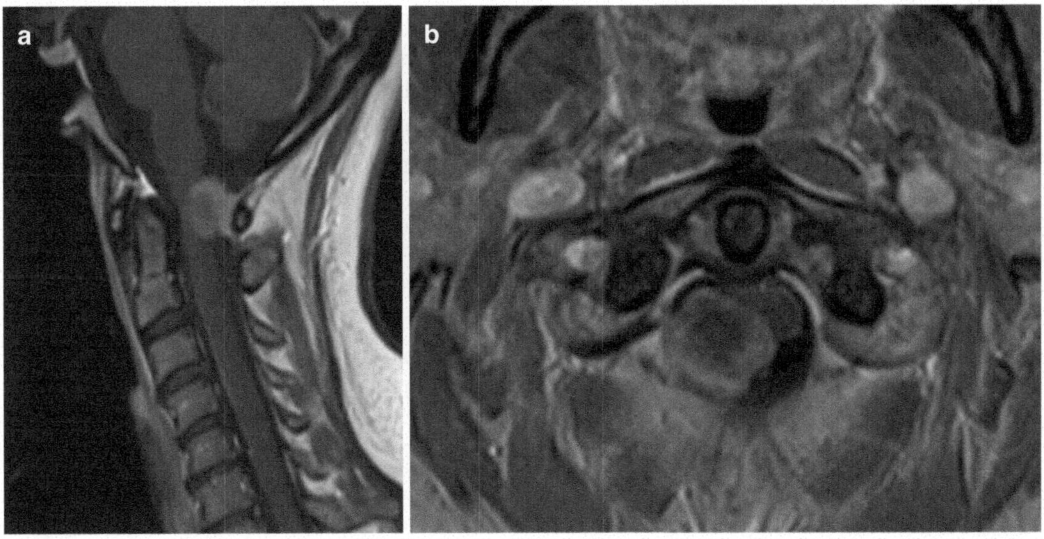

Fig. 11.1 (**a**) Postcontrast T1-weighted sagittal and (**b**) axial magnetic resonance imaging (MRI) demonstrates tumor and brainstem compression in the right dorsolateral spinal canal with severe compression of the spinal cord due to an intradural-extramedullary meningioma

Dorsolateral Approach: Surgical Technique

The procedure is performed with the patient under general anesthesia. Postpositioning somatosensory-evoked potentials (SSEP) and motor-evoked potentials (MEP) are monitored duration of surgery. The patient is placed in Gardner–Wells tongs or Mayfield head holder and the patient placed prone on the radiolucent Jackson table. The posterior neck is marked, prepped, and draped in a sterile fashion. A midline incision is made sharply from the base of the occiput to C2. The subcutaneous tissue is divided in the midline over the base of the occiput, C1 arch, and top of the C2 spinous process and lamina. Self-retaining retractors are used to maintain exposure. The lateral portions of the C1 arch are identified and cut using a high-speed drill. Angled curettes are used to remove the floating C1 arch. The bottom of the occiput and top of the C2 lamina are drilled to increase the dural exposure. An intraoperative ultrasound is brought into the field to visualize the intradural tumor and ensure that surgical exposure is adequate.

A midline durotomy is made and the dural edges are tented using 4-0 Nurolon suture. The arachnoid is sharply dissected off the tumor, noting that the spinal cord is displaced to the left anterolateral aspect of the thecal sac. The intradural vertebral artery is identified and carefully dissected free of the tumor. The tumor is circumferentially dissected, separated from its dural base, freed from the spinal cord, and removed as a single specimen if possible. If the tumor cannot be dissected free of the spinal cord without undue manipulation of the spinal cord, it should be internally debulked with an ultrasonic aspirator first. The dural base of the tumor is cauterized with low power bipolar cautery in an attempt to reduce the risk of recurrence. The dura is then closed with running suture and a fibrin dural sealant is placed. The fascia and soft tissues are closed in serial layers in a standard manner.

Ventral/Transoral Approach

The ventral/transoral approach is best used for ventral midline extradural tumors. The transoral approach provides access to the ventral clivus, atlas, and axis about 2 cm from midline. Lateral dissection is limited secondary to the vertebral artery, eustachian tube, and hypoglossal nerve. Other challenges include dural closure. Infectious risks occur because of the contaminated oropharynx. This approach is often combined with a second-stage posterior instrumentation and fusion.

Transoral Approach: Case Example

The patient is a 35-year-old male with new onset severe neck pain. A CT and MRI of cervical spine demonstrates a pathological fracture of C2 with an intrinsic erosive neoplasm with epidural and paraspinal involvement (Fig. 11.2). A CT-guided biopsy reveals a chordoma. Given tissue diagnosis, surgical resection is indicated.

Transoral Approach: Surgical Technique

The patient is placed under general anesthesia and remains in the supine position. The head is positioned in a 3-point Mayfield head fixation device in a gentle extension. A prophylactic tracheostomy is performed for airway protection and to allow for adequate transoral exposure. The pharynx, face, and neck are prepped. A retractor is placed so that the midportion of C3 is visible caudally. In order to obtain exposure of the clivus, the palate is split and a mucoperiosteal flap is elevated. Monopolar cautery is used to divide the pharynx from the level of the eustachian tubes to the mid portion of the C3 vertebral body. The submucosa and constrictors are divided. The pharyngeal flaps are elevated and retracted laterally. For cases requiring more extensive exposure, mandibular splitting may be necessary.

Self-retaining retractors are placed in the oropharynx and the microscope is brought into the operating field. Using a subperiosteal dissection, the longus colli muscles are dissected off the arch of C1, the tip of the clivus, the body C2, and the disc of C3. The prespinal tumor over C2 is visualized. Image-guided navigation can be helpful in some of these cases. The lateral border of the anterior arch of C1 is identified and removed using a high-speed drill and pituitary rongeurs. The dens is then dissected carefully and using an osteo-

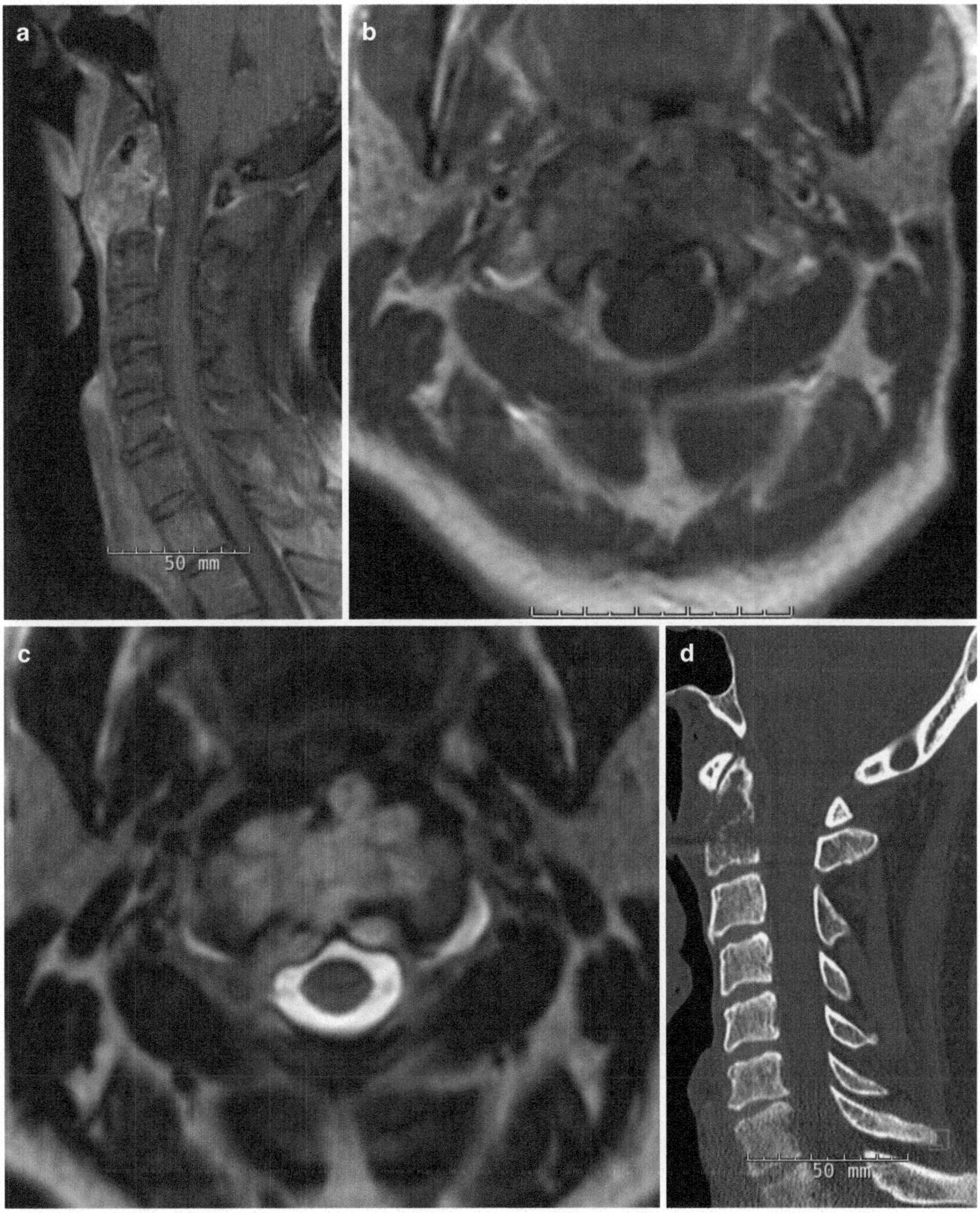

Fig. 11.2 C2 Chordoma (**a**) Postcontrast T1-weighted sagittal (**b**) axial MRI demonstrating a heterogeneously enhancing lytic lesion of the dens with epidural and prevertebral paraspinal soft tissue tumor involvement. (**c**) T2-weighted axial MRI demonstrating the lobulated, hyperintense appearance of the tumor. (**d**) Noncontrast computed tomography (CT) sagittal and (**e**) axial lytic lesion involving the C2 dens and vertebral body. (**f**) Plain lateral radiographs of the anterior and posterior instrumentation

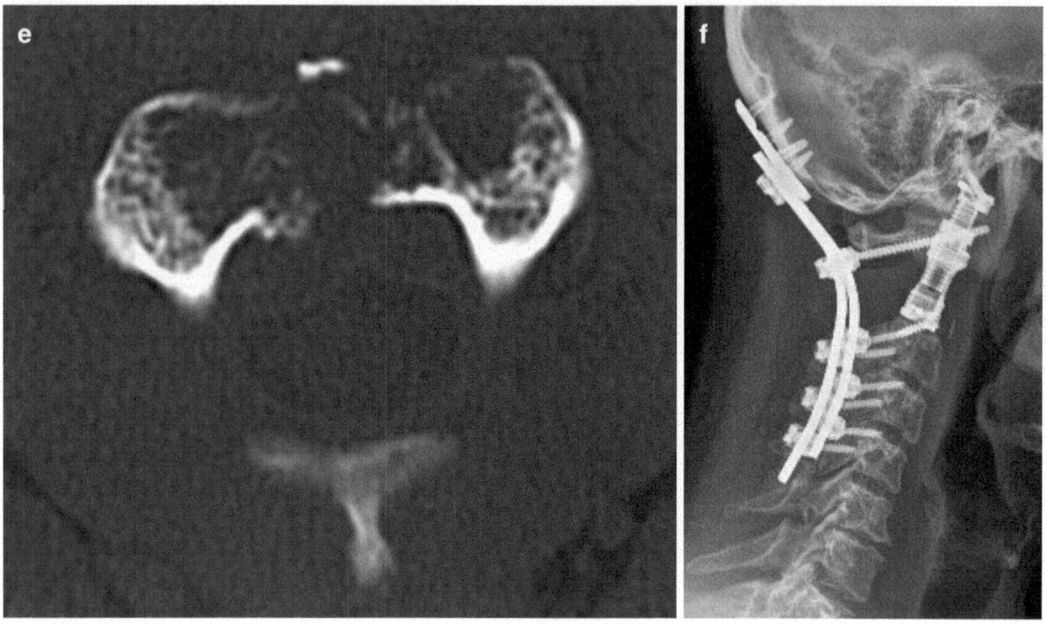

Fig. 11.2 (continued)

tome, two osteotomies are made at the base of the dens and the ligamentous attachments, allowing the dens to be removed in a single piece. The prespinal soft tissue tumor is debulked and carefully dissected off the longus colli. Osteotomies are made on the lateral aspect of the C2 vertebral body just medial to the pedicle and removed in a piecemeal fashion to the posterior longitudinal ligament. The pedicles are then resected. The transverse atlantal ligament is also divided and resected using Kerrison rongeurs. The posterior longitudinal ligament and ventral tumor behind the C2 vertebral body is removed clearing the ventral epidural space between the C3 endplate and tip of the clivus. The C3 endplate and the tip of the clivus are prepared for arthrodesis. Under direct fluoroscopy, an interbody biomechanical device is placed and integrated screws inserted into the clivus and C3 body. Final fluoroscopic images are obtained revealing appropriate placement. The oropharynx is closed with interrupted Vicryl. A Dobhoff is placed under direct vision and a cervical collar is placed prior to repositioning. The patient is then carefully placed in the prone position in a Mayfield head holder and the neck repositioned under fluoroscopy.

As is often needed with transoral resection, posterior stabilization is performed during the completion of the C2 spondylectomy. The posterior neck is prepped and draped in a sterile fashion. A midline incision is made sharply from the inion to the C6 spinous process. The subcutaneous tissue is divided using monopolar cautery from the occiput over the edge of the lateral masses from C1 through C5. The C2 nerve roots are dissected bilaterally and ligated, using bipolar cautery and tenotomy scissors making sure that the nerve roots are cut proximal to the dorsal root ganglia. An occipital plate is fixed to the occipital keel and screws placed in the lateral masses of C1 and C3–5.

The remaining spondylectomy is then performed by removing all the posterior elements including lamina, lateral masses/facets, and spinous process of C2 using osteotomes and the high-speed drill to create appropriate osteotomy cuts. The pedicle–pars complex and superior articular process of C2 are removed from both sides by dissecting out the posterolateral aspect of the transverse process and removing the posterior wall. The pedicle is divided using the high-speed drill. The pars, inferior and superior articular processes, and pedicle are removed separately on both sides. At this point, the entire C2 spondylectomy is complete resulting in a gross total resection. The C3 nerve roots and vertebral arteries are carefully dissected out and protected during this entire procedure. Appropriately sized rods are measured, cut, and contoured to fit the occipital plate and screw heads. Posterolateral arthrodesis is performed with morselized allograft over the occiput, C1 arch, and from C3 to C5 posterolateral regions. The wound is closed in layers in a standard manner.

Lateral/Far Lateral Approach

The lateral/far lateral/extreme lateral or transcondylar approach is used for intra- and extradural tumors (e.g., meningiomas and neurofibromas) of the lower clivus and upper cervical spine ventral to the foramen magnum. These cases often have concomitant rotatory or axial pathology. This approach provides direct access to the anterior rim of the foramen magnum without brainstem or cerebellar retraction. The lateral approach involves risk of facial nerve injury and requires dissection of the submandibular gland. The accessory nerve is identified and protected. The vertebral artery is also often identified on the superior surface of the sulcus arteriosus and reflected superiorly during C1 laminectomy. Posterior stabilization is considered if a large portion of the occipital condyle is resected (discussed further in surgical considerations).

Far Lateral Approach: Case Example

A 62-year-old male presents with a 5-month history of right upper extremity paresthesia involving his hand that progressed to his left hand resulting in loss of hand dexterity. On examination, he was noted to have 3+ reflexes of his right brachioradialis.

CT and MRI of the cervical spine demonstrates a left-sided intradural extramedullary tumor at the level of C1–3 with extradural involvement of the left C1–3 foramina. There is also extension of the tumor involving the V3–V4 junction. The tumor is partially calcified with a significant compression of the upper cervical spinal cord (Fig. 11.3).

Given his progressive symptoms of myelopathy and imaging findings, the patient undergoes a left-sided far lateral approach for C1–3 laminectomies with resection of both the intradural extramedullary and extradural tumor.

Far Lateral Approach: Surgical Technique

Under general anesthesia, the patient is placed in the lateral decubitus or three-quarter prone position in a Mayfield head holder. The head is placed in the lateral position, slightly rotated to the right and in flexion to expose the posterior neck and left suboccipital region. Postpositioning SSEPs and MEPs are obtained to confirm appropriate baseline neuromonitoring.

An inverted hockey stick incision is marked from the base of the mastoid to the inferior nuchal line just below the inion and then along the midline to the C4 spinous process. Using a monopolar cautery, the spinous process of C2, posterior arch of C1, and occiput are identified and a myocutaneous flap is created. The occiput, the left C1 arch, the left side of the C2–3 spinous processes, lamina and lateral masses are identified. The vertebral artery is then identified and carefully dissected off the sulcus arteriosus on the superolateral portion of the C1 posterior arch to protect it. An ultrasonic scalpel is used to perform a C1, C2, and superior portion of C3 laminectomies. The epidural plexus is controlled using a combination of hemostatic agents and bipolar cautery. The C2 nerve root in this case was enlarged as there was a tumor extending extradurally through the nerve root sleeve.

An intraoperative ultrasound is used to assess adequate bony exposure prior to addressing the intradural pathology. Under the microscope, the dura is opened sharply in a curvilinear fashion with the base of the dura retracted laterally (Fig. 11.4). The arachnoid is opened sharply and the tumor is immediately identified on the ventral aspect of the spinal canal. The accessory nerve is identified using intraoperative evoked EMG nerve stimulation and is subsequently dissected free and protected. The dorsal intradural C2 nerve rootlets are ligated. The dentate ligament is sectioned. The rostral and caudal poles of the tumor are identified. The dentate ligament is elevated using a 6-0 prolene suture to protect the spinal cord during resection. The tumor is easily identified, cauterized, and debulked using an ultrasonic aspirator. Using microdissection techniques, the tumor is sharply resected from the spinal cord. Dural feeding vessels and the lateral surface of the dura is cauterized to prevent recurrence. The intradural component of the tumor is completely resected.

The extradural extent of the tumor is then addressed. The C2 nerve root is dissected circumferentially and ligated at the normal-appearing root distal to the tumor. The extradural portion of the tumor is sectioned at the nerve root sleeve and

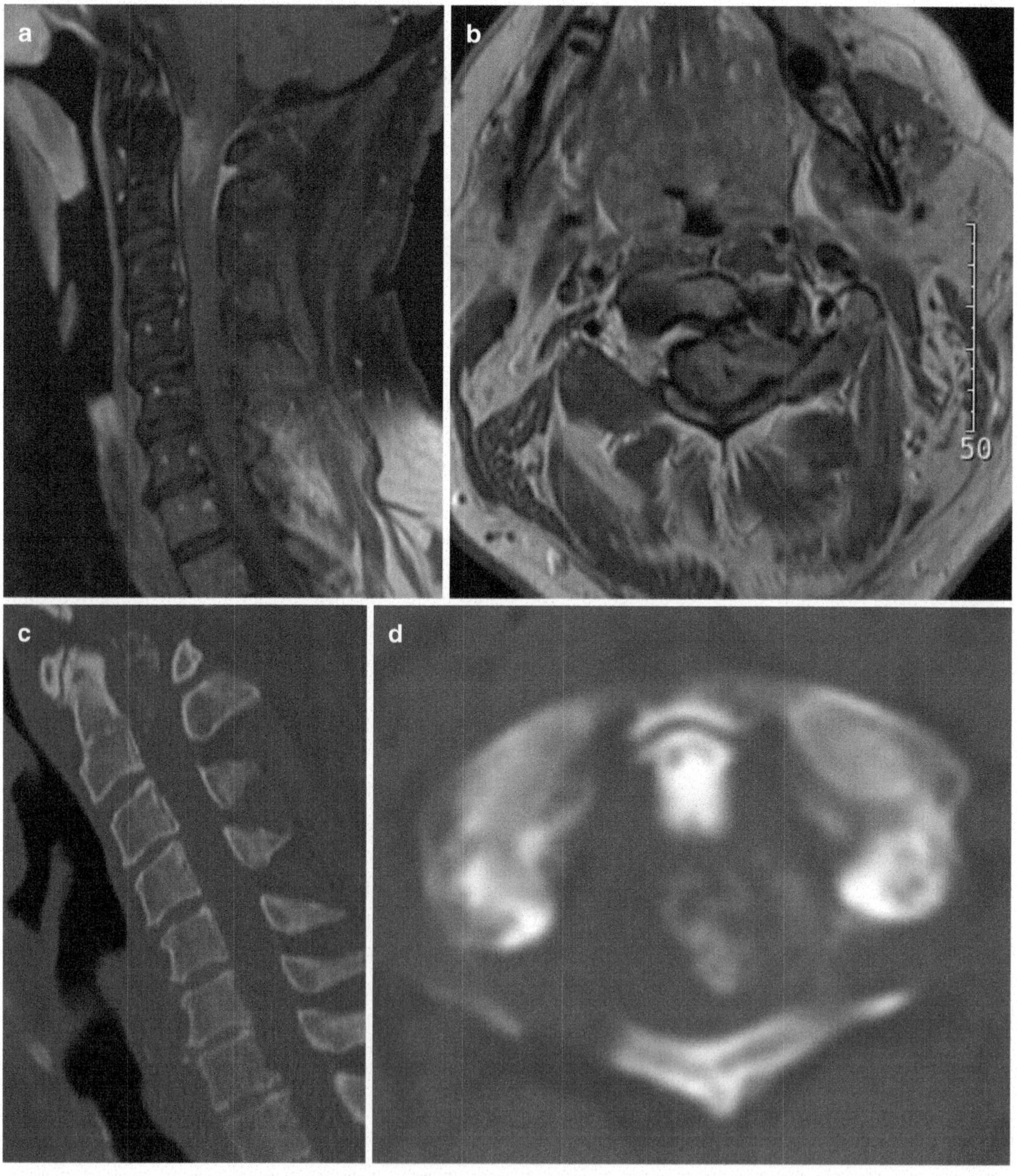

Fig. 11.3 (**a**) Noncontrast sagittal (**b**) axial cervical spine demonstrating a partially calcified osseous centered behind the axis and eccentric to the left of the spinal canal. Postcontrast T1-weighted (**c**) sagittal (**d**) axial (**e**) MRI angiography demonstrating a homogeneously enhancing extradural and intradural meningioma eccentric to the left. Note tumor involvement adjacent to the left vertebral artery

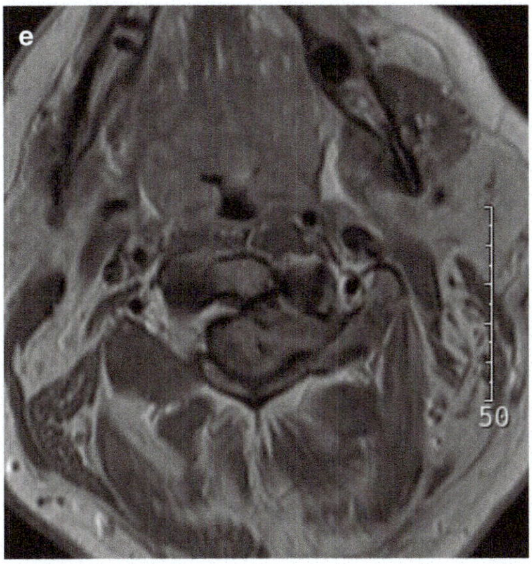

Fig. 11.3 (continued)

gross total resection is accomplished. After hemostasis is achieved, the dura is closed with a running suture and the dural patch graft for a watertight closure. A dural sealant is used over the dural closure. The myocutaneous flap is closed in serial layers.

Tumor Classification

Metastatic CVJ Pathology

In patients with metastatic disease of the CVJ, patients are more likely to present with neck pain and findings of instability rather than symptoms of cord compression or myelopathy [10]. Surgical treatment is often palliative with a predilection to the anterior spinal elements (e.g., clivus or odontoid). Surgery should be reserved for patients with

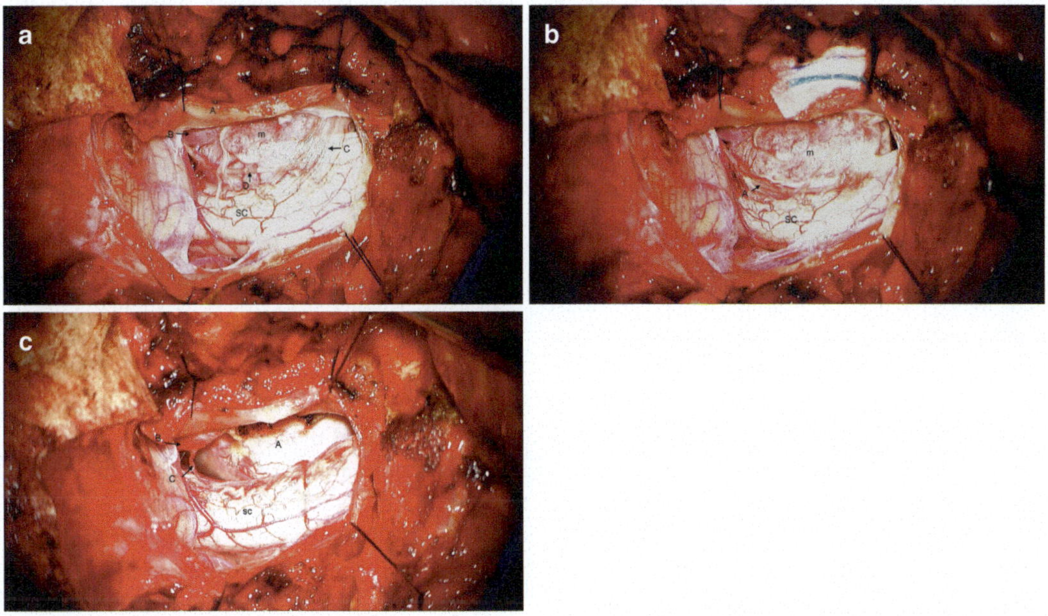

Fig. 11.4 Intraoperative photograph of a right transcondylar approach to an intradural foramen magnum meningioma. Note posterior displacement of the spinal cord. (**a**) The dura (a) is reflected open to visualize the spinal cord (sc), foramen magnum meningioma (m), intradural vertebral artery (b) C2 nerve roots (c), and accessory nerve (d). (**b**) Intradural exposure after ligation of the C2 nerve roots. The accessory nerve (a) is reflected posteriorly. (**c**) Post-tumor resection. Note that the spinal cord (sc) has been decompressed falling into the surgical cavity (a). Additionally, note the posterior spinal artery (b) a branch of the vertebral artery (c). These need to be spared to avoid serious neurologic consequence

more than 3 months of expected survival with the goals of preserving neurologic function, addressing instability and progressive deformity, treating incapacitating pain, and for long-term local tumor control. Given the large cerebrospinal fluid (CSF) space of the CVJ, patients with metastatic disease of the CVJ are more likely to present with symptoms of mechanical neck pain secondary to subluxation rather than direct extension of the tumor against the spinal cord. In cases of instability, reduction and stabilization with posterior instrumentation has been shown to provide durable pain relief with neurologic preservation [5, 7]. A decompression (e.g., laminectomy or partial facetectomy) and reconstitution of the thecal sac may also be needed [5]. Adjuvant radiotherapy and systemic chemotherapy are most frequently a component of the treatment algorithm.

Primary CVJ Pathology

Surgical resection is the first line treatment for most primary tumors of the CVJ (hematologic malignancies being a notable exception). En bloc resection can provide prolonged disease-free survival. However, such resection is often not feasible given the anatomic complexity of the CVJ and the typically infiltrating nature of these tumors around critical structures. In patients with primary tumors, maximal excision is done followed by instrumentation if needed [5]. Adjuvant radiotherapy often requires stereotactic ablative doses or alternate particle therapy (e.g., proton or carbon). A brief summary of a few common primary tumors of the CVJ are described below. Readers are directed to Chaps. 6 and 7 for a complete discussion of the presentation and management of benign and malignant spine tumors, respectively. Below, we discuss the specific considerations for these presenting in the complex anatomic environment of the CVJ.

Malignant Tumors

Multiple myeloma (MM) is the most common primary malignant tumor of the spine, especially in the upper cervical spine and skull [18]. MM arises from an abnormal proliferation of plasma cells. Patients most often present with mechanical axial neck pain secondary to osseous involvement or instability rather than cord compression or acute neurologic deficits. CT imaging can demonstrate punched out lesions, osteopenia, and fractures. An MRI may be useful to evaluate epidural extension into the spinal canal. Surgical intervention is reserved for patients with clinical instability or neurological compressive syndromes. Systemic treatment includes chemotherapy and radiation along with bisphosphonates. Median survival is variable but ranges from 2 years to more than 10 years [18].

Chordoma is the second most common primary tumor of the spine and is commonly diagnosed in the fifth and sixth decades of life. Chordomas are malignant tumors arising from remnants of the primitive notochord [19]. Although most common in the sacrum, about 30% will arise in the skull base (e.g., clivus) and about 15% will arise in the C1–2 region of the cervical spine. When involving the CVJ, chordomas frequently cause neck pain, cranial nerve deficits, myelopathy, or a symptomatic retropharyngeal mass. These lesions are slow growing and hence at the time of diagnosis, are often extensive. En bloc resection is the main treatment option as these tumors are radioresistant. More than 50% of patients have destruction of the occipital condyle and atlantal masses at time of diagnosis [20]. En bloc resection is the main treatment option as these tumors are radioresistant [21]. Adjuvant proton beam therapy is often employed following surgery and newer treatment regimens may include neo-adjuvant radiotherapy [22]. Recent prospective trials have included patients undergoing proton beam therapy as definitive-intent therapy in nonsurgical patients with local control. In these cases, stabilization may be the only indication for surgery [23]. Death is most likely to occur from a recurrent tumor rather than metastasis.

Osteosarcoma most commonly occurs in the second to third decade of life. These tumors are locally aggressive tumors that typically affect the appendicular skeleton. Only 3–5% of osteosarcomas affect the axial skeleton with no particular region of preference. They are locally aggressive tumors. When involving the CVJ, patients commonly present with focal pain and less likely neurologic symptoms. CT will demonstrate lytic patterns. PET scan demonstrates increased uptake due to bone turnover. Aggressive en bloc surgical resection followed by chemotherapy is needed for a potential cure as these tumors are generally radioresistant. Survival is around 2 years depending upon the extent of the disease [24].

Benign Tumors

Readers are directed to Chap. 6 for a complete discussion of the presentation and management of benign spine tumors. Below we will discuss the specific considerations for these presenting in the complex anatomic environment of the CVJ.

Aneurysmal bone cysts (ABCs) are benign vascular expansile tumors that most commonly occur in the second to third decade of life with a predilection for females. ABCs comprise about 15% of primary spine tumors with approximately 30% occurring in the cervical spine and 16% in the atlantoaxial spine. ABCs have a predilection for the posterior elements [25]. Although benign, these tumors can grow rapidly and cause bone destruction. CT findings may include a thin cortical shell with a highly vascular honeycomb central cavity. Radiographic findings of ABC involving the CVJ include the posterior atlas cyst, odontoid fracture, and vertebral body collapse. MRI may identify fluid–fluid levels which is characteristic for an ABC. Nonsurgical treatment options include percutaneous doxycycline, bisphosphonates, and radiotherapy although these case series' and results are limited [26]. Definitive surgical resection can be curative and residual tumor has a high recurrence rate. Preoperative embolization may be helpful as these tumors are hypervascular [20].

Eosinophilic granulomas (EG) is most commonly diagnosed in the first decade of life, rarely involving the spine. X-ray or CT images demonstrate vertebrae plana or lytic vertebra destruction with vertebral body collapse. MRI will often be isointense on T1 and hyperintense on T2. Patients commonly present with pain and most patients may present with neurologic deficit. In cases of atypical lytic lesions, CT-guided biopsy may need to be considered to differentiate between plasmacytoma, osteochondritis, and Ewing's sarcoma. Systemic forms of EG include Letterer-Siwe and Hand-Schuller-Christian disease which require aggressive treatment. Adjunct treatment strategies are unclear but low dose radiation and chemotherapy may be effective [27].

Osteoid osteomas are benign expansile lytic lesions with sclerotic margins. They are of osteogenic origin and localize to the cervical and lumbar spine. Percutaneous thermal ablation is a potential treatment option. Osteoblastomas are larger and generally more aggressive than osteoid osteomas with a potential for malignant transformation if not adequately resected. Osteoblastoma occurs in adolescents and young adults with a predilection for the posterior spinal elements, including the lamina and pedicle. The lesion is typically osteolytic with soft tissue expansion often involving the spinal canal. When in the cervical spine, patients most commonly present with unusual neck pain, painful torticollis, and reduced range of motion. Primary treatment is complete resection with favorable outcomes. Aspirin may help with long-term bone healing in patients with osteoid osteoma [25]. Osteochondromas arise as an epiphyseal herniation of displaced cartilage forming a cartilaginous cap. Although this benign lesion most commonly involves the appendicular skeleton, up to 4% of cases involve the spine. Spinal osteochondromas most commonly occur at transitional levels with reports of up to 43% in the atlantoaxial region [25].

Foramen magnum meningiomas account for up to 3% of all meningiomas and are most commonly diagnosed in the fifth decade of life. On CT, meningiomas often can demonstrate findings of hyperostosis, diffuse dural thickening, enlargement of meningeal channels, and calcification. Meningiomas are often isointense on MRI, but enhance avidly on postcontrast gadolinium studies. Controversies exist regarding optimal surgical position and approach but the goal of surgery is complete resection during the initial operation. These tumors often involve the vasculature (e.g., extradural or intradural vertebral artery) and multiple cranial nerves, especially IX–XII. Postoperative radiation is rarely used given the proximity to important neurological structures except in higher grade meningioma (e.g., atypical or anaplastic) [20, 28].

Instrumentation and Fusion

With the evolution of spinal instrumentation, aggressive resection and stabilization has become a feasible and durable option for patients with oncologic CVJ pathology. The opportunity for extensive resection while maintaining neurologic stability has been successful with and without adjunctive chemotherapy and radiotherapy [5, 7, 13, 16, 17].

Instability in this region can be due to tumor destruction or as a result of bone removal for tumor resection. Assessing instability of the CVJ is determined by a combination of clinical status and radiographic findings which includes degree of subluxation, angulation (>11 degrees), and displacement (>5 mm). Appreciation of the biomechanical properties of the CVJ also aids in the surgical decision making. Several case series have demonstrated either improvement or maintenance of neurologic function and improvement in neck pain in patients undergoing stabilization for instability secondary to neoplasms of the CVJ [5, 7, 14, 29–31].

In the past, fusion techniques of the CVJ initially involved contoured loop instrumentation and braided titanium cables [14, 29]. With the development of more recent spinal instrumentation, there are fewer complications, longer maintenance of alignment, and higher fusion rates with occipital plate and screw constructs. Biomechanical studies have showed increased stiffness with the screw-occipital plate techniques when compared to prior wiring techniques [32–34]. Additionally, with newer modifications of instrumentation, such as the multiaxial screw, the articulating saddle of the screw head, and lateral offset connectors, have provided a greater degree of screw head angulation and easier rod placement.

Occipital screw and plate fixation is one of the stiffest biomechanical instrumentation options of the entire spine. Optimizing screw placement is crucial to enhancing stiffness and potential fusion. Occipital screws should be placed in the thickest part of the occipital keel, inferior to the superior nuchal line and as close to the midline as possible. Anatomical studies have determined that the occipital screw length should be 8–12 mm in length, given the thickness of the occipital midline keel is approximately 8 mm and the buttress plate 3–5 mm in thickness. Screws should be placed in a bicortical fashion as the pullout strength is 50% more than that of the unicortical purchase [35]. If screws are placed lateral to the midline keel, the drill may pierce the bone at a shorter length. Laterally placed screws may reduce screw load with lateral bending and increase the moment arm, hence decreasing fusion rate [36–38].

C1 lateral mass and C2 instrumentation may not always be feasible given rod placement and osseous lytic destruction by the tumor. Additional fixation options include the pars or pedicle screws at C2, lateral mass screws in the subaxial spine and pedicle screws in the thoracic spine. Ideally, the shortest construct is desired but there should be at least four points of fixation below the resected level. In patients with poor bone quality, osteoporosis, or multiple areas of subaxial disease, longer constructs may be needed to maintain stability and aid in fusion [5].

With occipital plate and screw constructs, fusion rates have been reported in small patient series to range from 89% to 100%. Structural autograft (e.g., rib) or allograft is often used to aid in fusion [17]. Zou et al. reported 100% fusion rate at 6 months in 24 patients with oncologic disease of the CVJ requiring instrumentation [21]. In a single cohort of 120 patients with a mean follow-up of 35 months, Martinez et al. reported 89% fusion rate in 107 patients undergoing OC fusion, in which 10 patients were lost to follow-up [34]. Improvement in VAS neck pain scores, stability, and improved neurologic function have been reported after stabilization in patients with neoplasms involving the CVJ [5, 31, 33].

Surgical Complications, Management, and Avoidance

The development of improved surgical techniques and modified approaches have significantly decreased the overall morbidity and mortality of tumor surgery involving the CVJ. However, given the anatomic complexity of the CVJ, careful evaluation of the neurovascular anatomy on preoperative imaging is vital to help prevent a potential catastrophic injury.

Iatrogenic vertebral artery injury ranges from 0.5% to 4.1% in patients undergoing both anterior and posterior cervical approaches, respectively [10, 39]. In patients undergoing anterior cervical surgery, 14% of iatrogenic vertebral artery injuries occur in the setting of cervical spinal tumors [39]. Congenital anomalies on preoperative CT or MRI may raise suspicion of an abnormal vertebral artery anatomy and the need to pursue further vascular imaging (i.e., CTA, MRA, or DSA). During anterior approaches to the cervical spine, lateral dissection is a major contributor to vertebral artery injury. During lateral or posterior approaches to the cervical spine, screw placement during instrumentation is vital to avoid vertebral artery injury. Transarticular screw fixation carries the highest risk of iatrogenic vertebral artery injury [10]. If brisk arterial bleeding is identified during an anterior or posterior cervical approach, temporary clips may be applied and primary repair attempted. Surgical ligation or tamponade with pressure or screw placement may be used on a more urgent basis but has a high rate of pseudoaneurysm [39]. It may be prudent to perform a preoperative angiogram and balloon occlusion test prior to surgery if there is high suspicion of potential vertebral artery involvement.

Often a significant amount of venous bleeding can occur during posterior dissection of the CVJ. This is especially true in the setting of venous hypertension which is exacerbated by patient positioning (i.e., prone position with neck flexion). Venous bleeding can be controlled with thrombin-soaked gel foam and packing. Aggressive cauterization during exposure can help avoid iatrogenic vertebral artery injury.

Tumors of the CVJ often involve the basilar and /or vertebral artery and its branches. Vascular spasm often occurs in a delayed fashion after prolonged operations with significant neurovascular manipulation. Although gross total tumor resection is often a major goal of the operation, it is often necessary to leave the residual tumor on a diseased vessel wall, rather than induce a neurologic or vascular injury. In the setting of vascular spasm, elevating the mean arterial pressure and administration of calcium channel blockers are initial treatment options. Endovascular angioplasty may be an option in advanced cases. (Alotaibi)

CSF dynamics may change after intradural tumor resection of the CVJ. Postoperative sequelae include pseudomeningocele formation, CSF leak, and hydrocephalus. CSF leak and pseudomeningocele may be due to inadequate dural closure or underlying hydrocephalus. Obstructive hydrocephalus is most likely due to an acute etiology (i.e., subarachnoid hemorrhage in the cisterns/foramen magnum) whereas communicating hydrocephalus may present in a delayed fashion. The risks of postoperative CSF leak are decreased with a watertight dural closure, replacement of the bone flap, the use of dural sealant, and fat graft. If adequate dural closure is unable to be performed, immediate lumbar drain should be considered. If persistent CSF leaking occurs despite lumbar drain placement, surgical exploration is often required. The need for permanent CSF drainage may be needed depending on evidence of reaccumulating CSF or persistent leaking. Meningitis is often a complication of CSF leak which is increased with a transoral approach. A well vascularized reconstruction may be necessary to aid with wound closure. Antibiotic coverage should be considered.

Additional Considerations

Radiation treatment strategies have also evolved in the treatment of CVJ pathology. External beam radiation therapy (EBRT) has been used for the treatment of metastatic disease of the

CVJ. In a cohort of 25 patients with radiosensitive tumors of the CVJ, median survival rate in patients undergoing surgery plus radiotherapy was 16 months vs. 5 months with EBRT alone. This finding was attributed to selection bias as patients who had widely metastatic disease or were too sick to undergo surgery were more likely to undergo radiation alone [7]. Stereotactic radiosurgery (SRS) provides high energy radiation to isolated lesions in the spine. It has been shown that SRS may improve local tumor control with lower complication rates in patients with metastatic spinal disease compared to EBRT [40]. Tuchman et al. reported on a series of nine patients with metastatic disease to CVJ undergoing SRS with a median survival of 4 months and none of these patients required subsequent surgery [41]. In one of the largest published series to date of patients undergoing SRS for neoplasms of the CVJ, Azad et al. retrospectively reviewed 25 patients with metastatic spine disease to the CVJ. All patients were stable based on the Spinal Instability Neoplastic Score (SINS) and thus did not require stabilization prior to surgery. All 25 patients received SRS and only two patients required surgical intervention post-SRS to stabilize the spine. They concluded that SRS can provide palliative pain relief with little morbidity in patients without cervical instability [42].

Conclusion

Neoplasms of the CVJ require prompt diagnosis and careful implementation of a treatment strategy. Treatment is driven by histologic diagnosis, tumor location, and involvement of local anatomy, neurologic status, and pain. Identifying appropriate surgical goals and determining the appropriate surgical approach remains the foundation of successful treatment. Modern surgical techniques and spinal instrumentation as well as advanced radiotherapy options have all enhanced our ability to achieve higher rates of tumor control/cure, satisfactory clinical outcomes, and the successful rates of fusion in this highly complex anatomic location.

References

1. Moulding HD, Bilsky MH. Metastases to the craniovertebral junction. Neurosurgery. 2010;66:113–8.
2. Sherk HH. Lesions of the atlas and axis. Clin Orthop. 1975:33–41.
3. Jeszenszky DJ, Haschtmann D, Pröbstl O, Kleinstück FS, Heyde CE, Fekete TF. Tumors and metastases of the upper cervical spine (C0-2). A special challenge. Orthopade. 2013;42:746–54.
4. Bambakidis NC, Dickman CA, Spetzler R, Sonntag VKH, editors. Primary osseous and metastatic neoplasms of the craniovertebral junction. Surg Craniovertebr Junction. 2013; https://doi.org/10.1055/b-0034-84441.
5. Zuckerman SL, Kreines F, Powers A, Iorgulescu JB, Elder JB, Bilsky MH, Laufer I. Stabilization of tumor-associated craniovertebral junction instability: indications, operative variables, and outcomes. Neurosurgery. 2017;81:251–8.
6. Fehlings MG, David KS, Vialle L, Vialle E, Setzer M, Vrionis FD. Decision making in the surgical treatment of cervical spine metastases. Spine. 2009;34:S108–17.
7. Bilsky MH, Shannon FJ, Sheppard S, Prabhu V, Boland PJ. Diagnosis and management of a metastatic tumor in the atlantoaxial spine. Spine. 2002;27:1062–9.
8. Yamazaki M, Okawa A, Furuya T, Sakuma T, Takahashi H, Kato K, Fujiyoshi T, Mannoji C, Takahashi K, Koda M. Anomalous vertebral arteries in the extra- and intraosseous regions of the craniovertebral junction visualized by 3-dimensional computed tomographic angiography: analysis of 100 consecutive surgical cases and review of the literature. Spine. 2012;37:E1389–97.
9. George B, Archilli M, Cornelius JF. Bone tumors at the cranio-cervical junction. Surgical management and results from a series of 41 cases. Acta Neurochir (Wien). 2006;148:741–9; discussion 749
10. O'Sullivan MD, Lyons F, Morris S, Synnott K, Munigangaiah S, Devitt A. Metastasis affecting craniocervical junction: current concepts and an update on surgical management. Global Spine J. 2018;8:866–71.
11. Shiban E, Török E, Wostrack M, Meyer B, Lehmberg J. The far-lateral approach: destruction of the condyle does not necessarily result in clinically evident craniovertebral junction instability. J Neurosurg. 2016;125:196–201.
12. Bejjani GK, Sekhar LN, Riedel CJ. Occipitocervical fusion following the extreme lateral transcondylar approach. Surg Neurol. 2000;54:109–15; discussion 115–116
13. Harris MB, Duval MJ, Davis JA, Bernini PM. Anatomical and roentgenographic features of atlantooccipital instability. J Spinal Disord. 1993;6:5–10.
14. Shin H, Barrenechea IJ, Lesser J, Sen C, Perin NI. Occipitocervical fusion after resection of cra-

niovertebral junction tumors. J Neurosurg Spine. 2006;4:137–44.
15. Panjabi M, Dvorak J, Crisco J, Oda T, Hilibrand A, Grob D. Flexion, extension, and lateral bending of the upper cervical spine in response to alar ligament transections. J Spinal Disord. 1991;4:157–67.
16. Tubbs RS, Hallock JD, Radcliff V, Naftel RP, Mortazavi M, Shoja MM, Loukas M, Cohen-Gadol AA. Ligaments of the craniocervical junction. J Neurosurg Spine. 2011;14:697–709.
17. Wang Z, Wang X, Wu H, Chen Z, Yuan Q, Jian F. C2 dumbbell-shaped peripheral nerve sheath tumors: surgical management and relationship with venous structures. Clin Neurol Neurosurg. 2016;151:96–101.
18. Ahmadi SA, Slotty PJ, Munoz-Bendix C, Steiger H-J, Cornelius JF. Early surgical occipitocervical stabilization for plasma cell neoplasms at the craniocervical junction: systematic review and proposal of a treatment algorithm. Spine J Off J North Am Spine Soc. 2016;16:91–104.
19. Chambers KJ, Lin DT, Meier J, Remenschneider A, Herr M, Gray ST. Incidence and survival patterns of cranial chordoma in the United States. The Laryngoscope. 2014;124:1097–102.
20. Menezes AH. Craniovertebral junction neoplasms in the pediatric population. Childs Nerv Syst ChNS Off J Int Soc Pediatr Neurosurg. 2008;24:1173–86.
21. Molina CA, Ames CP, Chou D, Rhines LD, Hsieh PC, Zadnik PL, Wolinsky J-P, Gokaslan ZL, Sciubba DM. Outcomes following attempted en bloc resection of cervical chordomas in the C-1 and C-2 region versus the subaxial region: a multiinstitutional experience. J Neurosurg Spine. 2014;21:348–56.
22. Barrenechea IJ, Perin NI, Triana A, Lesser J, Costantino P, Sen C. Surgical management of chordomas of the cervical spine. J Neurosurg Spine. 2007;6:398–406.
23. Konieczkowski DJ, DeLaney TF, Yamada YJ. Radiation strategies for spine chordoma: proton beam, carbon ions, and stereotactic body radiation therapy. Neurosurg Clin N Am. 2020;31:263–88.
24. Feng D, Yang X, Liu T, et al. Osteosarcoma of the spine: surgical treatment and outcomes. World J Surg Oncol. 2013;11:89.
25. Menezes AH, Ahmed R. Primary atlantoaxial bone tumors in children: management strategies and long-term follow-up: clinical article. J Neurosurg Pediatr. 2014;13:260–72.
26. Parker J, Soltani S, Boissiere L, Obeid I, Gille O, Kieser DC. Spinal aneurysmal bone cysts (ABCs): optimal management. Orthop Res Rev. 2019;11:159–66.
27. Prasad GL, Divya S. Eosinophilic granuloma of the cervical spine in adults: a review. World Neurosurg. 2019; https://doi.org/10.1016/j.wneu.2019.01.230.
28. Wu Z, Hao S, Zhang J, Zhang L, Jia G, Tang J, Xiao X, Wang L, Wang Z. Foramen magnum meningiomas: experiences in 114 patients at a single institute over 15 years. Surg Neurol. 2009;72:376–82; discussion 382
29. Piper JG, Menezes AH. Management strategies for tumors of the axis vertebra. J Neurosurg. 1996;84:543–51.
30. Sanpakit S, Mansfield TL, Liebsch J. Role of onlay grafting with minimal internal fixation for occipitocervical fusion in oncologic patients. J Spinal Disord. 2000;13:382–90.
31. Zou J, Yuan C, Zhu R, Zhang Z, Jiang W, Yang H. Effect of occipitocervical fusion with screw-rod system for upper cervical spine tumor. BMC Surg. 2014;14:30.
32. Hurlbert RJ, Crawford NR, Choi WG, Dickman CA. A biomechanical evaluation of occipitocervical instrumentation: screw compared with wire fixation. J Neurosurg. 1999;90:84–90.
33. Deutsch H, Haid RW, Rodts GE, Mummaneni PV. Occipitocervical fixation: long-term results. Spine. 2005;30:530–5.
34. Martinez-Del-Campo E, Turner JD, Kalb S, Rangel-Castilla L, Perez-Orribo L, Soriano-Baron H, Theodore N. Occipitocervical fixation: a single surgeon's experience with 120 patients. Neurosurgery. 2016;79:549–60.
35. Haher TR, Yeung AW, Caruso SA, Merola AA, Shin T, Zipnick RI, Gorup JM, Bono C. Occipital screw pullout strength. A biomechanical investigation of occipital morphology. Spine. 1999;24:5–9.
36. Logroscino CA, Genitiempo M, Casula S. Relevance of the cranioaxial angle in the occipitocervical stabilization using an original construct: a retrospective study on 50 patients. Eur Spine J Off Publ Eur Spine Soc Eur Spinal Deform Soc Eur Sect Cerv Spine Res Soc. 2009;18(Suppl 1):7–12.
37. Heywood AW, Learmonth ID, Thomas M. Internal fixation for occipito-cervical fusion. J Bone Joint Surg Br. 1988;70:708–11.
38. Frush TJ, Fisher TJ, Ensminger SC, Truumees E, Demetropoulos CK. Biomechanical evaluation of parasagittal occipital plating: screw load sharing analysis. Spine. 2009;34:877–84.
39. Guan Q, Chen L, Long Y, Xiang Z. Iatrogenic vertebral artery injury during anterior cervical spine surgery: a systematic review. World Neurosurg. 2017;106:715–22.
40. Hall WA, Stapleford LJ, Hadjipanayis CG, Curran WJ, Crocker I, Shu H-KG. Stereotactic body radiosurgery for spinal metastatic disease: an evidence-based review. Int J Surg Oncol. 2011; 2011:979214.
41. Tuchman A, Yu C, Chang EL, Kim PE, Rusch MC, Apuzzo MLJ. Radiosurgery for metastatic disease at the craniocervical junction. World Neurosurg. 2014;82:1331–6.
42. Azad TD, Esparza R, Chaudhary N, Chang SD. Stereotactic radiosurgery for metastasis to the craniovertebral junction preserves spine stability and offers symptomatic relief. J Neurosurg Spine. 2016;24:241–7.

Part III

Metastatic Spinal Disease

Joe Schwab

Prognosis and Decision-Making in Spinal Metastases

12

Andrew J. Schoenfeld and Marco L. Ferrone

Introduction

Spinal metastatic disease has increased in frequency over the last two decades, in concert with improved treatment modalities and enhanced patient survival, overall [1–3]. The annual incidence of new cases of spinal metastases is now estimated at 20,000 and there are approximately over five million patients living with this spinal disorder at present in the United States [1–3]. Following the diagnosis of spinal metastatic disease, patients, their families, and clinicians are confronted with numerous challenges including formulating a treatment plan, making decisions regarding surgery, and coordinating expeditious care delivery [1–5]. These factors are frequently compounded by the enormous emotional weight and clouded judgment that can follow in the wake of a new diagnosis of spinal metastases, not to mention clinical deterioration and consequent impact on independent function and quality of life [1, 5].

Within 1 year of a diagnosis, nearly half of all patients with spinal metastases may have died and the post-treatment complication rate following surgery is generally reported in the range of 20–40% [6, 11]. Unfortunately, recent estimates reveal that morbidity following nonoperative care is often not significantly different from that of surgery, although the complication profile is altered [5]. In the setting of a new diagnosis of spinal metastases, patients and their clinicians have a shared goal of initiating the most appropriate and efficient treatment regimen capable of maximizing quality of life, mitigating disease progression, and minimizing the potential for post-treatment morbidity and clinical deterioration. Depending on a variety of factors, including the primary cancer diagnosis, extent of metastatic spread, medical comorbidities, nutritional status, and functional capacity, the outlook for patients with spinal metastases can be dramatically different, as can the selected treatment modalities used to support their care [1, 5]. Approaches to management have changed fairly rapidly in the last two decades commensurate with advances in oncology, medical management, operative techniques and understanding regarding the impact of spine surgical intervention on ambulatory function and longevity [1, 3]. Since the publication of the randomized trial of Patchell et al. in 2005 [12], spine surgical intervention has been increasingly accepted as a viable treatment option for patients with metastatic disease, especially in the event of pathologic fracture or epidural compression [1, 3]. Emerging literature has also identified that patients with certain types of primary cancer and independent functional ability at the time of

A. J. Schoenfeld (✉) · M. L. Ferrone
Department of Orthopaedic Surgery, Brigham and Women's Hospital, Harvard Medical School, Boston, MA, USA
e-mail: ajschoen@neomed.edu; mferrone@bwh.harvard.edu

K. Singh, M. Colman (eds.), *Surgical Spinal Oncology*,
https://doi.org/10.1007/978-3-030-50722-0_12

presentation may benefit more from operative intervention than nonsurgical care [5, 13].

The challenge confronting clinicians at the time of patient presentation is to meaningfully convey anticipated longevity and the risks and benefits of various treatment approaches to individuals and their families such that an informed decision regarding initial treatment strategy can be made. Patients who stand to tolerate surgery the best might also benefit from nonoperative care without the attendant risks of surgery [1, 5]. At the same time, if initial nonsurgical care fails and operative treatment is performed at a later date, outcomes including survival and the risks of post-treatment morbidity may be compromised [1, 13]. The most efficient means of conveying estimates and anticipated outcomes to patients and families is through prognostic models or scoring systems which have gained increased popularity in the last 5–10 years [14–20]. These tools are not always appropriate for specific individuals; however, many of the scoring systems available have not been independently validated [1, 14]. Some were not even developed for the specific purpose of prognosticating outcomes in all clinical contexts, and real-time clinical determinations may be specious as a result. The goal of this chapter is to present important considerations for discussing prognosis and making recommendations regarding treatment for patients with spinal metastases, including the appropriate selection and application of existing prognostic measures and scoring systems.

General Considerations

The ideal prognostic tool is easy to use and understand for clinicians at all levels of training/experience, patients, and family members [1, 14]. In addition, the tool should be generally applicable to all patients with spinal metastatic disease, inform clinical care and/or anticipated outcomes, and be independently validated in the population in which it is being applied. Unfortunately, very few (if any) of the current systems available truly meet these criteria in full [1, 14, 21].

Most were developed in curated populations (single practice, only operative cases, specific primary tumor types, etc.) and few have undergone rigorous external validation. For example, the Spinal Instability Neoplastic Score (SINS) was developed for the purposes of forecasting instability in the setting of spinal metastases, not survival or other outcomes following treatment [14]. As such, clinicians should review the parameters of the specific scoring systems, the populations used in their development, and the means by which they were created, before applying them in direct patient care [1]. The clinical and sociodemographic characteristics of the patient in whom the prognostic tool is being applied should generally appear similar to the individuals in which the score was developed (as reported in the literature). While numerous scoring systems and predictive tools abound [14, 21], including emerging 'plug and play' machine learning platforms [17, 18], this chapter focuses on the most widely investigated utilities: the Tokuhashi Score, the Tomita Scale, the Spine Oncology Research Group (SORG) nomogram, and the New England Spinal Metastasis Score (NESMS), which incorporates the modified Bauer system.

The Tokuhashi Score

This utility was among the first spinal metastatic scoring systems developed and is probably the most widely studied as a result [14, 22]. First published in 1990, the score was revised in 2005 and takes into account general function as measured by performance status, primary tumor, extent of metastatic spread, and neurologic involvement. The score ranges from 0 to 15, with higher scores being more favorable (Table 12.1). There are appendant estimates of survival that are primarily intended to inform whether surgery could/should be offered. The score was not developed or advertised as a means to inform other aspects of patient care. It has also not been independently validated using rigorous methodologic techniques [14].

Table 12.1 The Tokuhashi scoring system

Characteristics	Points
Performance status	
Poor: 10–40%	0
Moderate: 50–70%	1
Good: 80–100%	2
Extraspinal metastases	
3 or more	0
1–2	1
0	2
Number of vertebral metastases	
3 or more	0
2	1
1	2
Metastases to other organs	
Not resectable	0
Resectable	1
Absent	2
Neurologic function	
Frankel A or B	0
Frankel C or D	1
Frankel E	2
Primary cancer	
Lung, osteosarcoma, gastric, bladder, pancreas	0
Liver, gallbladder, unknown	1
Other	3
Renal, uterine	4
Thyroid, breast, prostate, carcinoid	5
Total score	*Predicted survival*
0–8	Less than 6 months
9–11	Greater than 6 months
12–15	Greater than 1 year

Perhaps due to its longevity, the score has gained wide recognition and general acceptance in the literature [14]. It can serve as a useful stepwise construct for processing the factors necessary to determine a treatment regimen for patients with spinal metastases. The scoring system is cumbersome, however, and may be difficult to apply and understand, especially for nonsurgeons and patients. Metastatic disease in other organs is graded as absent, resectable, or unresectable, and information such as treatment approach for nonspinal metastases could be difficult to accurately determine at the time of presentation, or when the score is being calculated. The point derivations may also not be accurately weighted.

The score has not always performed well in confirmatory research, with a reported accuracy widely ranging from 39% to 88% [14]. Importantly, the higher estimates are derived from Tokuhashi's own group and may reflect concerns for expertise bias or other confounding due to intimate familiarity with the scheme's application. Moreover, some have raised the possibility that the Tokuhashi score is not useful in prognosticating outcomes in patients with lung cancer or myeloma [14, 23–25]. In a systematic review, Cassidy et al. maintained that the tool is more useful for patients anticipated to survive for a period of 1-year or longer based on their clinical presentation, as opposed to individuals with shorter anticipated longevity [14]. In a comparative study published by Ahmed et al. using patient data collected from Johns Hopkins University, the revised Tokuhasi score was determined to be inferior to the original scheme and did not have sufficient accuracy regarding predicting survival at 30-days, 90-days, and 1-year following surgery [19]. Similarly, in recent work conducted among 1400+ patients collected from different centers, the Tokuhashi score failed to achieve the performance threshold deemed necessary by the authors to be designated a good predictive tool [20].

The Tomita Scale

The Tomita Scale was published in 2001 and is among the mostly widely utilized scoring systems for spinal metastatic disease at present [26]. This stems from the fact that several studies have supported its use in the past, the system incorporates fewer variables, and is easier to apply as compared to the more cumbersome Tokuhashi system [14]. The Tomita Scale develops a score based on the growth rate of the primary tumor (classified as slow, moderate, or rapid), the number of visceral metastases, and the number of bone metastases (Table 12.2). The scale ranges from 2 to 10 with a relative weight applied for each variable and higher scores indicative of a worse prognosis. Appendant survival estimates also exist for vari-

Table 12.2 The Tomita scoring system

Characteristics	Points
Primary tumor	
Slow growth	1
Moderate growth	2
Rapid growth	3
Bone metastases	
Solitary	1
Multiple	2
Visceral metastases	
Treatable	2
Not treatable	4
Total score	*Predicted survival*
2–3	Greater than 2 years
4–5	1–2 years
6–8	6–12 months
9–10	<3 months

ous derivations of the score, ranging from <3 months for those with 8–10 points to >2 years for individuals with a score of <4.

The Tomita system is advantaged by reliance on easily accessible data, fewer data points, and easier comprehension among nonsurgeons and nonclinicians. The scheme does not take into account symptoms at presentation or the patient's functional capacity. It also does not account for the integrity of the spinal column or the epidural space. The anticipated growth rate of certain tumor subtypes may also not be readily apparent or prone to misclassification, especially in the context of end-stage disease such as metastatic spread.

The most damaging critique of the score, however, is that it was designed in the setting of a retrospective review of 67 patients treated in a single practice [26]. The methodology employed in the development of the original score was such that findings may be parochial to the clinical context in which the data were developed and other determinations could be spurious [1, 14]. As a result, and perhaps not surprisingly, the score has been reported to have suboptimal reliability. Similar to the Tokuhashi system, some authors have cautioned that the system does not predict well for certain types of primary cancer [24, 25] and in head-to-head comparison, the Tokuhashi score has generally outperformed the Tomita Scale [14, 19]. Choi et al. reported that the Tomita Scale performed comparably to the Tokuhsahi in their prospective international study of 1469 patients, but cautioned that neither met the criteria for a good predictive tool [20]. In the work of Ahmed et al., however, the Tomita system was among the worst performers overall, as well as in the specific subcategories of breast, lung, prostate, renal cell, and all nonhematologic malignancies [19]. Conversely, in the study of Choi and colleagues, the Tomita system was one of the better performing scoring systems [20].

Spine Oncology Research Group (SORG) System

In 2016, the Spine Oncology Research Group (SORG) published a utility based on machine learning platforms, which has subsequently undergone fairly intense investigation and revision [11, 17, 18]. In general, the SORG scheme and its derivatives (including the nomogram) account for a variety of patient-specific factors including age, performance status, primary cancer, number of spinal, and other nonosseous metastases, prior systemic therapy, white blood cell, and hemoglobin counts (Table 12.3) [11, 17–19]. Most notably, the system does not address symptoms at presentation or physical function. It is also unclear at what time-point the measured laboratory values should be applied. Presumably, these would be at presentation or when the score is calculated. But such laboratory values can vary substantially, even within the

Table 12.3 The Spine Oncology Research Group (SORG) system

Characteristics	Points
Age 65 or older	1
Performance status of 3–4	2
Primary tumor is other than breast, renal, lymphoma or myeloma, prostate or thyroid	2
More than one spinal metastasis	1
Lung or liver metastases	1
Brain metastases	2
Modified Bauer score ≥3	2
Prior systemic therapy	2
Hemoglobin level ≤10 g/dL	1
White blood cell count ≥11	1

span of a few days and it is unclear if alterations (or corrections) in these data should influence the score or otherwise alter its prognostic capacity.

The SORG system includes several variables, but in general, these are readily understood by clinicians, nonsurgeons, patients, and family members alike. The automated SORG calculator also makes determining the score more user-friendly and its application may be scalable to most centers that treat patients with spinal metastatic disease. It should be noted that the SORG nomogram is a specific tool which was developed using machine-learning models, but the instrument and the machine learning models themselves are not equivalent.

In the work of Ahmed et al., conducted among 176 patients treated at a single center, the SORG nomogram was reported to be the most accurate at predicting mortality at 30-days and 3-months following surgery, but was outperformed at 1-year by the original Tokuhashi Score [19]. In subset analysis, the SORG nomogram appeared to perform more favorably in the context of patients with lung cancer and hematologic malignancies [19]. Outside of prognosticating survival, the ability of the SORG system to directly inform patient care has not been well characterized [1].

The New England Spinal Metastasis Score (NESMS)

At the same time as the SORG was being developed, a consortium of four academic medical centers in New England collaborated to develop the New England Spinal Metastasis Score (NESMS) [6–8]. This system was specifically intended to be user friendly, easily understood by providers and patients, and clinically applicable to the prognostication of outcomes in patients treated operatively and nonoperatively [7]. The NESMS relies on the modified Bauer Score as a base to characterize the primary tumor characteristics and extent of the tumor burden. The modified Bauer Score alone is one of the more widely used systems for grading metastatic disease but has been criticized for poor performance in populations with spinal metastases and insufficient detail specific to directing patient care [14]. The NESMS attempted to correct some of these issues by including assessments for ambulatory function (intended to account for serious neurologic issues in conjunction with functional ability) and serum albumin (as a proxy of nutritional status and capacity to tolerate treatment, including surgery) [7, 8]. Individual performance for each measure was used to develop a final weighted point system that ranged from 0 to 4 with higher scores indicative of more favorable patient states (Table 12.4). The modified Bauer Score was dichotomized as high or low, with 2 points designated for scores ≥3. Independent ambulatory function and serum albumin at presentation ≥3.5 g/dL were also eligible for one point each. The score, however, is capped at 3, such that patients with a high modified Bauer Score and either one of the other positive general health attributes are considered the same as patients having all three positive characteristics [7, 8].

The NESMS was originally developed using 1-year survival as the outcome of interest [8]. In subsequent analysis using data from the National Surgical Quality Improvement Program (NSQIP), the score was found to adequately predict 30-day mortality, major systemic complications, and failure to rescue (a measure of the likelihood of mortality following development of a sentinel complication event) [7]. As compared to patients with the worst score of 0, those with a NESMS of 1 were found to have a 64% reduction in the likeli-

Table 12.4 The New England Spinal Metastasis score

Characteristics	Points
Modified Bauer score	
No visceral metastases (1 point)	–
Primary tumor is not lung cancer (1 point)	–
Primary tumor is breast, renal, lymphoma or myeloma (1 point)	–
Single skeletal metasasis (1 point)	–
Modified Bauer score ≤2	0
Modified Bauer score ≥3	2
Ambulatory function	
Dependent ambulatory/nonambulatory	0
Independent ambulatory	1
Serum albumin	
<3.5 g/dL	0
<3.5 g/dL	1

hood of mortality, 70% reduction in odds of complications, and 58% reduction in the likelihood of failure to rescue. Individuals with a score of 2 demonstrated an 81% reduction in mortality, 70% declination in complications, and similar reduction in the chance of failure to rescue. With the highest score of 3, patients were found to have an 89% decrease in the likelihood of mortality, 88% reduction in the odds of failure to rescue, and 74% decrease in the likelihood of complications [7].

The NESMS was independently validated and found to adequately predict outcomes in a cohort of patients receiving surgery at Johns Hopkins [10]. Most importantly, the scoring system was also found to perform successfully in patients treated nonoperatively for spinal metastatic disease [9]. At the present time, prospective observational work is being completed with the intent of validating the NESMS score and comparing its performance to other commonly employed prognostic tools [1].

The advantages of the NESMS include its independent external validation, reliance on a limited number of variables that are easy to obtain and comprehend, ability to inform care and expectations beyond that of survival, and applicability to patients receiving operative and nonoperative treatment. A key limitation consists of the fact that head-to-head comparisons of the NESMS with other scoring systems are not yet available in the literature. The NESMS is also unable to inform surgical approach or the ideal procedure if surgery is selected.

Recent work has delineated the importance of baseline laboratory values at presentation beyond albumin, such as measures of inflammation (e.g., platelet-lymphocyte ratio), serum creatinine, and serum glucose as mediators of outcome [4, 27]. Once the true value of these laboratory factors in forecasting outcomes is defined to a greater extent, their incorporation into existing scoring systems such as the NESMS may become necessary.

Case Example

To demonstrate a comparison between the various scoring utilities and how these may, or may not, prove useful in direct application to patient care; consider the case of a 72-year-old female who presented with prior history of lung and breast cancer, both in remission for several years. She presented with relatively new onset back and lower extremity pain, including radiation in an L2–3 distribution in the right leg. Magnetic resonance imaging of the spine (Fig. 12.1) revealed

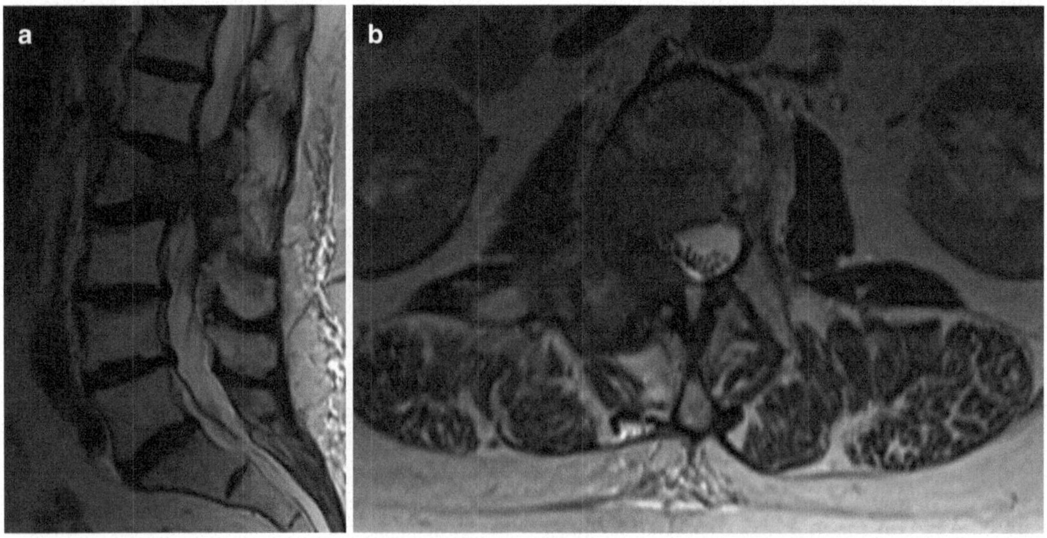

Fig. 12.1 Sagittal reconstruction (**a**) and axial (**b**) sections at the level of the L2 vertebra from a magnetic resonance imaging study of a 72-year-old female with back and lower extremity symptoms, including radiation in an L2–3 distribution in the right leg. Magnetic resonance imaging revealed metastatic involvement of the L2 vertebral body, pedicle, and right-sided posterior elements with some epidural extension and compression of the lateral recess (**b**)

metastatic involvement of the L2 vertebral body, pedicle, and right-sided posterior elements with some epidural extension and compression of the lateral recess. Biopsy confirmed metastatic squamous cell carcinoma of the lung. Gastrohepatic and portocaval involvement were also detected during staging studies performed subsequently. The patient was independently ambulatory at the time of presentation with an albumin of 4.0 g/dL, a white blood cell count of 9.34, and a hemoglobin of 11.9.

Given these parameters, she would receive a Tokuhashi score of 5, a Tomita score of 6, a SORG score of 6, and a NESMS score of 2. Based on the Tokuhashi score, the patients estimated survival would be anticipated at <6 months, but would stand at 1–2 years per the Tomita grade. Taking into account the SORG and Tomita scores, she would be considered a reasonable surgical candidate, but less so based on the Tokuhashi determination. Using the NESMS score, she would perhaps be considered a reasonable candidate for surgery with a 54% estimated survival at one-year. Near-term prognostications based on the NESMS score would include 7% chance of 30-day mortality, 9% major complications, and 17% chance of readmission following surgery.

After considering operative and nonoperative treatment, the patient decided to proceed with spinal radiation in combination with carboplatin, taxol, and pembrolizumab. Following radiation, the patient's lower extremity symptoms and back pain resolved and she did not develop instability, pathologic fracture, or require later spine surgery. One year after diagnosis, the patient remains on pembrolizumab with low levels of back pain and she ambulates without assistive device.

In this particular example, the Tokuhashi score underestimated the patient's prospects for survival, while more reasonable determinations were generated by using the Tomita and SORG systems. Only the NESMS tool was able to present estimates to the patient of anticipated outcomes beyond survival in the near-term, with additional predictions regarding the prospect of mortality out to 1 year.

Applying Prognostic Tools in the Clinical Context

At this time, there are several prognostic utilities and scoring systems intended to facilitate treatment for patients with spinal disease, including many that have not been discussed in this chapter [14]. As the above case illustrates, beyond providing a structured rubric around which to discuss important factors for decision-making, the different scoring schemes may not be congruent and estimates can certainly be incorrect [1, 14, 19–21]. Disagreements in reliability may stem from differences between the populations from which the scores were developed and the context in which they are being applied, advancements in oncology, radiation, and surgical care in the present day, clinical realities at the time a scoring system was developed, and other (unmeasured) factors that may be important to prognosis and are not encapsulated in the scoring system employed [1, 14, 20].

Furthermore, putative validation studies may not be true efforts that independently verify the integrity of a scoring system, particularly if they are not well designed and subject to rigorous methodologic considerations [1]. At best, retrospective case series without adequate adjustment for selection, indication, and information (not to mention expertise) bias can at best support the use of a scoring rubric in the clinical context in which the study was performed. At worst, such investigations are nothing more than an assessment of how well the authors are able to align their scoring regimen and clinical practice with those who developed the prognostic tool in the first place.

Cassidy et al. have suggested that the rapid advances in clinical medicine at present render any prognostic score potentially outdated by the time it would appear in print [14]. Similarly, Choi and colleagues cautioned that scoring systems developed before 2010 should be considered of limited reliability and they encouraged revising prognostic tools in real-time or with current data [20]. As such in depth re-examination of the classic predictive scores has not appeared in print, it is up to the individual provider to examine and determine which systems perform best in their hands and within the populations they serve [1].

The important factors to recognize are that at present the scoring utilities should not be viewed as oracles or tools that predict any patient's course of care with high reliability. Instead, they are, when most appropriately applied, a scheme for evaluating and presenting estimations in a more systematic fashion which can help patients and providers think about important parameters for care, treatment planning, and anticipated outcomes in an accessible way. It is up to the provider to select the scoring tool that they feel works best for them and their patients and which seems to reasonably prognosticate outcomes in their specific practice. If real time, adaptable estimates are favored, using a machine learning algorithm such as the SORG nomogram could be appropriate. If the preference is for a single tool that would be applicable to patients irrespective of operative or nonoperative treatment, then the NESMS may be a more reasonable choice as of this writing.

Funding and Disclosure Dr. Schoenfeld is supported by the National Institutes of Health (NIH-NIAMS) grant (K23-AR071464). The views expressed in this chapter are those of the authors and do not necessarily reflect the position or policy of the NIH or the Federal government.

References

1. Schoenfeld AJ, Ferrone ML. The next generation in surgical research for patients with spinal metastases. Spine J. 2018;18(10):1956–8.
2. Cole JS, Patchell RA. Metastatic epidural spinal cord compression. Lancet Neurol. 2008;7:459–66.
3. Rose PS, Buchowski JM. Metastatic disease in the thoracic and lumbar spine: evaluation and management. J Am Acad Orthop Surg. 2011;19:37–48.
4. Schoenfeld AJ, Ferrone ML, Passias PG, Blucher JA, Barton LB, Shin JH, Harris MB, Schwab JH. Laboratory markers as useful prognostic indicators for survival in patients with spinal metastases. Spine J. 2019; e-pub ahead of print.
5. Schoenfeld AJ, Losina E, Ferrone ML, Schwab JH, Chi JH, Blucher JA, Silva GS, Chen AT, Harris MB, Kang JD, Katz JN. Ambulatory status after surgical and non-surgical treatment for spinal metastasis. Cancer. 2019; e-pub ahead of print.
6. Schoenfeld AJ, Leonard DA, Saadat E, Bono CM, Harris MB, Ferrone ML. Predictors of 30- and 90-day survival following surgical intervention for spinal metastases: a prognostic study conducted at four academic centers. Spine. 2015. (Accepted for publication 9/25/2015).
7. Schoenfeld AJ, Le HV, Marjoua Y, Leonard DA, Belmont PJ Jr, Bono CM, Harris MB. Assessing the utility of a clinical prediction score regarding 30-day morbidity and mortality following metastatic spine surgery: the New England Spinal Metastasis Score (NESMS). Spine J. 2015. (Accepted for publication 9/21/ 2015).
8. Ghori AK, Leonard DA, Schoenfeld AJ, Saadat E, Scott N, Ferrone ML, Pearson A, Harris MB. Modeling one-year survival after surgery on the metastatic spine. Spine J. 2015;15:2345–50.
9. Shi DD, Chen YH, Lam TC, Leonard D, Balboni TA, Schoenfeld A, Skamene S, Cagney DN, Chi JH, Cho CH, Harris M, Ferrone ML, Hertan LM. Assessing the utility of a prognostication model to predict 1-year mortality in patients undergoing radiation therapy for spinal metastases. Spine J. 2018;18:935–40.
10. Goodwin CR, Schoenfeld AJ, Abu-Bonsrah NA, Garzon-Muvdi T, Sankey EW, Harris MB, Sciubba DM. Reliability of a spinal metastasis prognostic score to model 1-year survival. Spine J. 2016;16(9):1102–8.
11. Karhade AV, Thio QCBS, Ogink PT, Bono CM, Ferrone ML, Oh KS, Saylor PJ, Schoenfeld AJ, Shin JH, Harris MB, Schwab JH. Predicting 90-Day and 1-year mortality in spinal metastatic disease: development and internal validation. Neurosurgery. 2019 Mar 14. pii: nyz070. https://doi.org/10.1093/neuros/nyz070. [Epub ahead of print].
12. Patchell RA, Tibbs PA, Regine WF, Payne R, Saris S, Kryscio RJ, Moiuddin M, Young B. Direct decompressive surgical resection in the treatment of spinal cord compression caused by metastatic cancer: a randomised trial. Lancet. 2005;366:643–8.
13. Lo WY, Yang SH. Metastatic spinal cord compression (MSCC) treated with palliative decompression: surgical timing and survival rate. PLoS One. 2017;12:e0190342.
14. Cassidy JT, Baker JF, Lenehan B. The role of prognostic scoring systems in assessing surgical candidacy for patients with vertebral metastasis: a narrative review. Global Spine J. 2018;8:638–51.
15. Nater A, Tetreault LA, Kopjar B, Arnold PM, Dekutoski MB, Finkelstein JA, Fisher CG, France JC, Gokaslan ZL, Rhines LD, Rose PS, Sahgal A, Schuster JM, Vaccaro AR, Fehlings MG. Predictive factors of survival in a surgical series of metastatic epidural spinal cord compression and complete external validation of 8 multivariate models of survival in a prospective North American multicenter study. Cancer. 2018;124(17):3536–50.
16. Choi D, Pavlou M, Omar R, Arts M, Balabaud L, Buchowski JM, Bunger C, Chung CK, Coppes MH, Depreitere B, Fehlings MG, Kawahara N, Lee

CS, Leung Y, Martin-Benlloch JA, Massicotte EM, Mazel C, Meyer B, Oner FC, Peul W, Quraishi N, Tokuhashi Y, Tomita K, Ulbricht C, Verlaan JJ, Wang M, Crockard HA. A novel risk calculator to predict outcome after surgery for symptomatic spinal metastases; use of a large prospective patient database to personalise surgical management. Eur J Cancer. 2019;107:28–36.

17. Paulino Pereira NR, Janssen SJ, van Dijk E, Harris MB, Hornicek FJ, Ferrone ML, Schwab JH. Development of a prognostic survival algorithm for patients with metastatic spine disease. J Bone Joint Surg Am. 2016;98:1767–76.
18. Paulino Pereira NR, Mclaughlin L, Janssen SJ, van Dijk CN, Bramer JAM, Laufer I, Bilsky MH, Schwab JH. The SORG nomogram accurately predicts 3- and 12-months survival for operable spine metastatic disease: external validation. J Surg Oncol. 2017;115(8):1019–27.
19. Ahmed AK, Goodwin CR, Heravi A, Kim R, Abu-Bonsrah N, Sankey E, Kerekes D, De la Garza RR, Schwab J, Sciubba DM. Predicting survival for metastatic spine disease: a comparison of nine scoring systems. Spine J. 2018;18:1804–14.
20. Choi D, Ricciardi F, Arts M, et al. Prediction accuracy of common prognostic scoring systems for metastatic spine disease: results of a prospective international multicentre study of 1469 patients. Spine. 2018;43:1678–84.
21. Bollen L, Wibmer C, Van der Linden YM, Pondaag W, Fiocco M, Peul WC, Marijnen CA, Nelissen RG, Leithner A, Dijkstra SP. Predictive value of six prognostic scoring systems for spinal bone metastases: an analysis based on 1379 patients. Spine. 2016;45:E155–62.
22. Tokuhashi Y, Matsuzaki H, Toriyama S, Kawano H, Ohsaka S. Scoring system for the preoperative evaluation of metastatic spine tumor prognosis. Spine. 1990;15:1110–3.
23. Oliveira MF, Barros Bde A, Rotta JM, Botelho RV. Tokuhashi scoring system has limited applicability in the majority of patients with spinal cord compression secondary to vertebral metastasis. Arq Neuropsiquiatr. 2013;71:798–801.
24. Tan JH, Tan KA, Zaw AS, et al. Evaluation of scoring systems and prognostic factors in patients with spinal metastases from lung cancer. Spine. 2016;41:638–44.
25. Amelot A, Cristini J, Saluad C, et al. Overall survival in spine myeloma metastases: difficulties in predicting with prognostic scores. Spine. 2017;42:400–6.
26. Tomita K, Kawahara N, Kobayashi T, Yoshida A, Murakami H, Akamaru T. Surgical strategy for spinal metastases. Spine. 2001;26:298–306.
27. Thio QCBS, Goudriaan WA, Janssen SJ, Paulino Pereira NR, Sciubba DM, Rosovksy RP, Schwab JH. Prognostic role of neutrophil-to-lymphocyte ratio and platelet-to-lymphocyte ratio in patients with bone metastases. Br J Cancer. 2018;119:737–43.

Economic Value in Spinal Tumor Surgery

13

Aditya Mazmudar and Alpesh A. Patel

Introduction

Spinal tumors are uncommon diagnoses that are associated with high morbidity, mortality, and a cost burden which reflects not only surgical care but also many other cost centers such as medical, radiation, and rehabilitation treatments [1]. As health expenditures continue to rise as a percentage of gross domestic product in the United States, there is a strong focus on value-based healthcare as a potential solution for curbing direct and indirect healthcare costs. The passage of the Patient Protection and Affordable Care Act in 2010 enacted meaningful healthcare policy changes, particularly through payment reform and reportable metrics that continue to impact the practice and economics of spine surgery today. The field of spine surgery, including spine oncology, may be a unique target of future efforts to encourage appropriate patient selection, promote more efficient resource allocation, and decrease sizable end-of-life care costs.

The surgical treatment of primary and metastatic spinal tumors has been utilized to provide improvements in patient symptoms, healthcare-related quality of life, and survival. The decision to proceed with surgical management of spinal oncologic conditions depends upon myriad factors. Tumor grading, staging, and location, presence of spinal instability, neurologic status, success of antecedent treatments, and other host factors all affect surgical decision-making [2, 3]. Accordingly, the goals of surgical treatment vary significantly and may include palliative pain control, neural decompression, spinal stability, local tumor control, and patient function [2, 3].

Over the last two decades, there have been significant improvements in surgical and medical technologies including magnetic resonance imaging, minimally invasive spine surgery, intraoperative neuromonitoring, and others. These enable better surgical care and improved patient outcomes for increasingly complex and diverse patient populations [4]. Although these interventions may improve quality and outcomes, they frequently are associated with an elevated cost. Thus, in the transition to a value-based healthcare system, the focus on surgical innovation and postsurgical patient outcomes must be coupled with a closer look at the economic impact of these surgical interventions. Accordingly, the future practice of oncologic spine surgery may need to clear a higher economic value threshold than its current form.

Nevertheless, spinal tumors provide an interesting forum for value discussion, since issues of survivorship, patient preference, and quality of life are paramount. For example, one must ask not only about the economic impact of treating

A. Mazmudar (✉) · A. A. Patel
Department of Orthopaedic Surgery, Feinberg School of Medicine, Northwestern University, Chicago, IL, USA

K. Singh, M. Colman (eds.), *Surgical Spinal Oncology*,
https://doi.org/10.1007/978-3-030-50722-0_13

spine tumors with surgical technology, but also about the economic impact of nonoperative and palliative care.

This chapter examines recent trends, defines the measurement of economic value, and elucidates economic value within the context of specific spinal tumor interventions. The case studies at the end of the chapter help apply the concepts of quality and cost in spine surgery which guide discussions of economic value.

Important Trends and Considerations in Spinal Tumor Interventions

There are several important trends in oncologic spine surgery that are relevant to discussions of economic value. Most importantly, the incidence of metastatic spinal tumors is increasing with aging populations and longer life expectancies [5, 6]. This increased incidence coupled with improving interventions will increase the prevalence of patients living with oncologic spine conditions [5, 6]. As surgical resection remains an important strategy in many of the treatment algorithms for primary and metastatic spinal tumors, this demographic trend will continue to drive increased utilization of surgical and ancillary services in the near future. As the utilization of these services increases more drastically relative to the utilization of other healthcare services, the field may attract the attention of policy-makers and the Center for Medicare and Medicaid Services.

In addition, the growth and availability of new technologies such as advanced imaging, 3-dimensional printing of implants and surgical guides, computer navigation, robotics, novel minimally invasive surgical techniques, intraoperative neurophysiological monitoring, and advanced radiotherapy modalities, to name a few, may result in improved surgical outcomes [4]. However, it is important to recognize the learning and cost curves associated with new technologies. For example, stereotactic radiosurgery, while promising as a technology, given its lower radiotoxicity profiles compared to conventional radiation, is also clearly more costly [7]. New technologies may drive significantly higher costs for marginal benefit, especially at their introduction. In the spine oncologic patient population, it can be particularly difficult to study these technologies due to low cohort size, ethical considerations, and significant loss to follow-up.

Defining and Measuring Economic Value

Definitions of economic value vary marginally depending upon different healthcare stakeholders (providers, payers, device companies, and others). The principal definition of economic value in healthcare is quality relative to cost of the intervention [8, 9]. Quality, the numerator of the economic value equation, is not defined by any single measure but rather the combination of multiple types of outcome measures. Even through the combination of measures, quality of care has been difficult to define in a reproducible manner. Cost, the denominator of the economic value equation, is defined as the total aggregate cost of an intervention and is equally challenging to measure. The complexities and heterogeneity of payer–provider dynamics make it difficult to define all of the direct and indirect costs associated with an intervention. Economic value of care is maximized when high quality of care is accompanied by low cost of care, and benefits are sustained over time. Therefore, the potentially low durability of outcomes and high recurring costs of adjuvant treatments are particularly relevant factors in discussions of value in spine oncologic surgery.

Economic value is studied primarily through cost-effectiveness analyses and cost-utility analyses (CEA and CUA, respectively) in the scientific literature. The threshold for cost-effectiveness is not exactly defined, but tends to be quoted as less than \$100,000 dollars (cost/quality-adjusted life year gained) [10]. These types of studies and publications have increased over the last decade, especially in the spine literature. Given the inherent difficulties of measuring outcomes and costs, vastly different methodologies are employed, leading to a significant amount of heterogeneity in cost-effectiveness analyses published to date.

Consistent methodology, meticulous accounting, and transparency of costs included are critical to the quality of CEAs. The US Panel on Cost-Effectiveness in Health and Medicine has set forth recommendations to guide CEA design, including definitions of cost depending on healthcare sector or societal perspective, discounting of cost to account for the time value of money, and methodology for sensitivity analyses [11]. Additionally, the Second Panel on Cost-Effectiveness in Health and Medicine recently noted that condition-specific health measures may be more sensitive measures of outcomes compared to the general health measures traditionally used to calculate the ubiquitous quality-adjusted life years (QALYs) [12].

Measuring Quality

The Institute of Medicine (IOM) defines healthcare quality as "the degree to which healthcare services for individuals and populations increase the likelihood of desired health outcomes and are consistent with current professional knowledge" [13]. Quality can be measured in a variety of ways, including process measures, such as length of hospital stay and readmission rates, and outcome measures, such as postsurgical complications, physical functioning, and mortality. The increased focus on quality reporting, particularly over the last decade, has led to the development of numerous generic and condition-specific patient-reported outcome measures (PROs) to better describe healthcare quality. Patient-reported outcomes (PROs), including EuroQoL (EQ)-5D, Short Form (SF)-12/36, Patient-Reported Outcomes Measurement Information (PROMIS), and National Institutes of Health Toolbox, Visual Analog Scale (VAS), Neck Disability Index (NDI), Oswestry Disability Index (ODI), and others, have been extensively studied in the spine literature to serve as proxies for healthcare-related quality of life. Similarly, numerous scales have been studied in the cancer literature for this purpose (e.g., ECOG Performance Status, Symptom Distress Scale, and EORTC QLQ-C30).

Together, these single metrics better elucidate quality of care provided to patients but are difficult to compare across disease states and among patient cohorts. Therefore, the quality-adjusted life year (QALY) has been primarily used in cost-effectiveness literature to communicate the relative impact of different interventions across various disease and health states [14]. QALY is calculated as the utility of an intervention times the duration of benefit. The relative QALYs' gained can distinguish two interventions. The utility of an intervention is derived from existing general measures such as EuroQoL (EQ)-5D and Short Form (SF)-12/36 via conversion calculators and algorithms. Historically, utility scores have primarily been derived from general health outcome measures, but there is increasing research supporting development of conversion models for specific disease measures, such as ODI [15].

While QALYs have useful characteristics, particularly in the communication of healthcare-related quality of life, and are extensively used in cost-effectiveness and cost-utility literature, it is important to recognize their limitations, specifically in the setting of oncologic spine surgery [16]. QALYs assume homogenous utility for a given health state and identical provider skill. Individual patients vary in the evaluation of their health state and, therefore, the benefit gained from an intervention. In addition, provider skill is not homogenous and affects the QALYs gained from each individual intervention. For example, in disease states with low prevalence and incidence, variations in provider skill and perception of utility become more relevant, and the average QALY gain becomes less reliable. As such, in the evaluation of any particular quality measure, the difference between statistical and clinical significance must be considered.

Measuring Costs

Determining the total all-in cost of spinal oncologic interventions is a challenging task. The interdisciplinary approach of oncologic surgery, specifically, involves many different inpatient cost centers and significant rehabilitation costs. While intended to study surgical versus nonoperative management for degenerative spinal disorders, the multicenter Spine Patient Outcomes

Research Trial (SPORT) trial identified components of cost, including a breakdown of direct and indirect costs [17, 18].

The direct costs of spine-related care include the associated healthcare visit costs, diagnostic testing costs, medication costs, surgical costs, provider costs, and facility costs, among others. Direct costs vary based on patient, demographic, and hospital factors. After analyzing spinal cord tumor surgery from 2003 to 2010 in the Nationwide Inpatient Sample (NIS), an all-payer database, Sharma et al. found that direct cost of hospitalization after tumor resection varied significantly based on age, postoperative complication, high comorbidity index, admission day and status, as well as hospital size, volume, and region [19].

Indirect costs are loosely tied to the concept of opportunity cost and are primarily determined by estimating the costs associated with productivity loss. Indirect costs include days of missed work, days worked with restrictions, transportation costs, and caregiver costs. Indirect costs are often difficult to calculate and vary significantly based on compensation level. For example, potential change in type of work or profession or potential loss of higher salaried work is challenging to take into consideration.

Understanding the data source for direct and indirect costs is imperative. In most studies, direct costs tend to be determined based on average national costs, typically from Medicare data [20]. While these costs are typically extrapolated to a privately insured study population, it is important to recognize that heterogeneity does exist based on insurance status and type. In addition, hospital charge data may not be consistent and reflective of true direct cost [20, 21].

Cost-effectiveness studies must clearly state whether the study is conducted from a societal or a healthcare sector perspective in their methodology [11]. The perspective impacts the type of costs included in the study. Typically, many indirect costs such as time costs for patients and caregivers, transportation costs, and non-healthcare sector costs are only included in the societal perspective. The time horizon of the study, costing year, and discount rate applied to included costs are other methodological considerations that impact interpretation as well [11]. While it is important to recognize that limitations exist with every study or analysis, transparency about methodology is the most crucial element needed for comparability and external validity.

Economic Value of Selected Spinal Tumor Interventions

In this section, economic value principles are applied to two selected topics: metastatic epidural spinal cord compression (MESCC) and intradural extramedullary (IDEM) spinal tumors. An economic value assessment is performed using currently available scientific literature.

Metastatic Epidural Spinal Cord Compression

Up to 10% of oncologic patients develop symptomatic metastatic epidural spinal cord compression (MESCC). MESCC is among the most common conditions evaluated by oncologic spine surgeons, and surgical treatment modalities have expanded significantly with the advent of new surgical technologies [22]. As a result, the cost effectiveness of surgical intervention with radiotherapy versus radiotherapy alone has been of significant interest [22].

In 2005, Patchell et al. performed a randomized, multi-institutional, and nonblinded trial with 101 patients to assess the role and efficacy of direct decompressive surgery in MESCC [23]. The trial was stopped prematurely after interim analysis because the direct decompressive surgery plus postoperative radiotherapy treatment arm had longer survival, significantly higher odds of being able to walk after treatment, retained the ability to walk for longer periods, and required less corticosteroids and opioid analgesics compared to the radiotherapy alone treatment arm [23]. Since the trial, other studies have shown similar results with regard to ambulation, pain control, and survival [22–25].

Furthermore, two high-quality cost-effectiveness and cost-utility analyses have been published. Thomas et al. examined the cost effectiveness of direct decompressive surgery plus radiotherapy versus radiotherapy alone from a societal perspective [24]. Clinical outcomes data from Patchell et al. were utilized to determine the incremental cost-effectiveness ratio (ICER). Direct and indirect costs of acute and postoperative care were estimated from existing literature. Of note, the study was published in Canadian dollars (CDN$) and discounting was not applied given the short time horizon. The study found that the surgical intervention plus radiotherapy arm ambulated an additional 220 days and survived an additional 156 days. In 2003 US dollars, this yielded a $48 cost per additional day of ambulation and $24,750 cost per QALY gained [24]. A CUA published by Furlan et al. based on the trial data from Patchell et al. found an ICER of $250,310 per QALY gained [25]. Furlan et al. concluded that the surgery plus radiotherapy treatment approach for patients with MSCC was likely to result in both improved patient outcomes and increased total healthcare expenditures. Future studies with prospectively collected cost data will be important to further evaluate the cost effectiveness of the additive value of surgery in patients with MESCC.

The conclusions reached about cost-effectiveness after this evaluation depend upon perspective and budgetary constraints. According to data from patients with advanced prostate cancer, MESCC treated with direct spinal decompression and concurrent bone surgery is the most expensive skeletal-related event, costing almost $83,000 [26]. In addition, inpatient costs accounted for nearly two-thirds of the total cost of care for skeletal-related events [26]. Therefore, with expensive interventions, quality and cost considerations are heavily impacted by stringency of indications for surgical intervention. Further research into appropriate patient selection and risk stratification may facilitate increased economic value of surgical intervention for MESCC [27].

Intradural Extramedullary (IDEM) Spinal Tumors

Intradural extramedullary spinal tumors, particularly meningiomas and nerve sheath tumors, are among the most commonly encountered primary tumors of the spine [28]. Surgical resection is the major treatment modality for these lesions. Recently, minimally invasive surgery (MIS) techniques have been applied for the treatment of IDEM tumors and have been accompanied by a developing research interest in comparing outcomes between minimally invasive and open techniques.

Studies have shown high patient satisfaction and significant improvements in disability, pain, general physical and mental health, and quality of life following open IDEM tumor resection [28, 29]. Wong et al. found that, relative to the open technique, the MIS approach is associated with lower average hospital stay and perioperative blood loss [28]. There were no significant differences in the rates of complications and reoperation between the two cohorts. Of note, a gross-total resection was achieved in 92.6% of MIS cases and 94.4% of open cases with a p-value of 0.81. There appears to be a trend toward equivalence between MIS and open techniques for IDEM tumor resection in the appropriately selected patients. The power of post-IDEM surgical outcomes studies is often limited because of the small sample size of the relevant study population.

Chotai et al. analyzed healthcare resource utilization during the postoperative period following open resection of IDEM spine tumors [1]. In a breakdown of direct costs (healthcare visit cost, diagnostic cost, medication cost, surgeon professional fee, and hospital cost) and indirect costs (patient income loss, family income loss, and caregiver cost), the study found mean direct costs of $23,717 ± $7412 and mean indirect costs of $5544 ± $4336, resulting in mean total 1-year costs of $29,177 ± $9314 [1]. Direct costs were calculated based on Medicare payments, and indirect costs were calculated based on self-reported gross-of-tax wage rate. Furthermore, a perioperative hospital charge analysis by Fontes et al. found that hospital charges and postoperative charges were significantly different between open and MIS techniques for resection of IDEM tumors [21]. Hospital costs ($21,307 open, $15,015 MIS, $p < 0.01$), postoperative costs ($75,383 open, $56,006 MIS, $p < 0.01$), and total charges ($100,779 open, $76,100 MIS, $p < 0.01$) were significantly lower in the MIS group [21]. The approximately 30% decrease in hospital costs for the MIS cohort was primarily attributed to decreased complication rate as well as reduced postoperative intensive care unit and hospital stays. This analysis focused on charge data rather than actual reimbursement data and, therefore, may overestimate the MIS versus open cost savings it reports.

While the outcomes and cost literature for IDEM open versus MIS surgical technique is not as developed as that of MESCC, the economic value framework may still be applied. In the appropriately selected patient, MIS technique for IDEM tumor resection may be a cost-effective option, demonstrating a trend toward outcomes equivalence and increased cost savings. The potential for selection and author bias are additional confounders in this area, and studies should be read critically.

Conclusion and Future Directions

The economic value framework of assessing outcomes relative to costs over time is a useful tool for studying and interpreting the benefits of oncologic spine interventions. When comparing the cost-effectiveness of new interventions and technologies or analyzing current strategies being utilized to increase value, it is important to critically examine the methodology used to benchmark associated outcomes and costs.

Quality of care for cost-effectiveness studies has been difficult to define due to the certain limitations of QALYs in oncologic patients and lack of generalizability of oncologic interventions relative to more homogenous, elective procedures. Additionally, cost accounting of oncologic spine-related care is complex due to the number of direct cost centers typically involved in patient care and variability of perspectives involved. Therefore, interpreting economic value in spine oncologic surgery must be done in a thoughtful manner. Further research must be conducted on stage-based cost-effectiveness of surgical interventions, as well as neoadjuvant or adjuvant treatments, as outcomes and costs significantly vary based on these factors [29]. Thus, as the impact of value-based care continues to grow in this field and in the United States healthcare system as a whole, the ability to critically analyze economic value will become a useful skill.

References

1. Chotai S, et al. Healthcare resource utilization and patient-reported outcomes following elective surgery for intradural extramedullary spinal tumors. Neurosurgery. 2017;81(4):613–9.
2. Bell GR. Surgical treatment of spinal tumors. Clin Orthop Relat Res. 1997;335:54–63.
3. Sciubba DM, et al. Diagnosis and management of metastatic spine disease: a review. J Neurosurg Spine. 2010;13(1):94–108.
4. Jallo GI, Kothbauer KF, Epstein FJ. Intrinsic spinal cord tumor resection. Neurosurgery. 2001;49(5):1124–8.
5. Schellinger KA, et al. Descriptive epidemiology of primary spinal cord tumors. J Neuro-Oncol. 2008;87(2):173–9.
6. Duong LM, et al. Descriptive epidemiology of malignant and nonmalignant primary spinal cord, spinal meninges, and cauda equina tumors, United States, 2004–2007. Cancer. 2012;118(17):4220–7.
7. Haley ML, Gerszten PC, Heron DE, Chang YF, Atteberry DS, Burton SA. Efficacy and cost-effectiveness analysis of external beam and stereotactic body radiation therapy in the treatment of spine metastases: a matched-pair analysis. J Neurosurg Spine. 2011;14(4):537–42.
8. Porter ME. What is value in health care? N Engl J Med. 2010;363(26):2477–81.
9. Porter ME. A strategy for health care reform—toward a value-based system. N Engl J Med. 2009;361(2):109–12.
10. Neumann PJ, Cohen JT, Weinstein MC. Updating cost-effectiveness—the curious resilience of the $50,000-per-QALY threshold. N Engl J Med. 2014;371(9):796–7.
11. Weinstein MC, et al. Recommendations of the panel on cost-effectiveness in health and medicine. JAMA. 1996;276(15):1253–8.

12. Carias C, et al. Recommendations of the second panel on cost effectiveness in health and medicine: a reference, not a rule book. Am J Prev Med. 2018;54(4):600–2.
13. McGlynn EA. Six challenges in measuring the quality of health care. Health Aff. 1997;16(3):7–21.
14. Detsky AS, Laupacis A. Relevance of cost-effectiveness analysis to clinicians and policy makers. JAMA. 2007;298(2):221–4.
15. Patel SA, Rihn JA. Understanding value in spine surgery: part I—Understanding quality. Contemp Spine Surg. 2014;15(4):1–5.
16. Garau M, et al. Using QALYs in cancer. PharmacoEconomics. 2011;29(8):673–85.
17. Birkmeyer NJO, et al. Design of the spine patient outcomes research trial (SPORT). Spine. 2002;27(12):1361.
18. Weinstein JN, et al. The SPORT value compass: do the extra costs of undergoing spine surgery produce better health benefits? Med Care. 2014;52(12):1055.
19. Sharma M, et al. Discharge dispositions, complications, and costs of hospitalization in spinal cord tumor surgery: analysis of data from the United States Nationwide Inpatient Sample, 2003–2010. J Neurosurg Spine. 2014;20(2):125–41.
20. Patel SA, Rihn JA. Understanding value in spine surgery: part I—Understanding costs. Contemp Spine Surg. 2014;15(4):1–5.
21. Fontes RBV, Wewel JT, O'Toole JE. Perioperative cost analysis of minimally invasive vs open resection of intradural extramedullary spinal cord tumors. Neurosurgery. 2015;78(4):531–9.
22. Fehlings MG, Nater A, Holmer H. Cost-effectiveness of surgery in the management of metastatic epidural spinal cord compression: a systematic review. Spine. 2014;39(22S):S99–S105.
23. Patchell RA, et al. Direct decompressive surgical resection in the treatment of spinal cord compression caused by metastatic cancer: a randomised trial. Lancet. 2005;366(9486):643–8.
24. Thomas KC, et al. Cost-effectiveness of surgery plus radiotherapy versus radiotherapy alone for metastatic epidural spinal cord compression. Int J Radiat Oncol Biol Phys. 2006;66(4):1212–8.
25. Furlan JC, et al. The combined use of surgery and radiotherapy to treat patients with epidural cord compression due to metastatic disease: a cost-utility analysis. Neuro-Oncology. 2012;14(5):631–40.
26. Jayasekera J, et al. The economic burden of skeletal-related events among elderly men with metastatic prostate cancer. PharmacoEconomics. 2014;32(2):173–91.
27. Lau D, et al. Costs and readmission rates for the resection of primary and metastatic spinal tumors: a comparative analysis of 181 patients. J Neurosurg Spine. 2016;25(3):366–78.
28. Wong AP, et al. Comparison of open and minimally invasive surgery for intradural-extramedullary spine tumors. Neurosurg Focus. 2015;39(2):E11.
29. Choi D, et al. Review of metastatic spine tumour classification and indications for surgery: the consensus statement of the Global Spine Tumour Study Group. Eur Spine J. 2010;19(2):215–22.

State of the Art for Metastatic Histologies

14

Varan Haghshenas, Arash J. Sayari, Ahmed N. Shehabeldin, and Rex A. W. Marco

Introduction

The spine remains one of the most frequent sites for metastases, and treatment algorithms for patients with metastatic spine disease are constantly evolving. Cancers once thought incurable are now contained with modern treatments. Treatment plans need to be consistently tailored to a patient's individual characteristics, and surgical, radiation, or systemic therapies must be combined in a coordinated way. Therefore, a multidisciplinary approach is a key step in formulating an appropriate plan for each individual patient.

For example, tumors that were historically relatively radioresistant (renal cell carcinoma, lung carcinoma, and most soft-tissue sarcomas) are now being treated with stereotactic radiation therapy, which delivers high doses of radiation to the tumor without exposing the spinal cord to unsafe levels of radiation. Furthermore, the combination of stereotactic radiation therapy and targeted chemotherapy or immune therapy probably potentiates the effectiveness of these modalities and provides improved local control for patients with metastatic spinal disease. The ever-changing treatment options have placed patient-centered multidisciplinary approaches at the forefront of treatment algorithms.

While prognostic factors vary depending on specific factors unique to each spinal metastasis, general parameters have been closely investigated to develop scoring systems that predict outcomes. The state of the art for these scoring systems is discussed in detail in Chap. 11. In addition to patient prognosis, myriad other factors must be considered. Like the popular NOMS framework, another up-to-date and fluid patient-centered approach used by the authors is the MOSS treatment algorithm [1, 2]. MOSS (Medical/Mental, Oncologic, Stenosis, Stability) is a multidisciplinary approach that prioritizes the patient's medical and mental condition to ensure that the patient is well enough to undergo appropriate treatment with chemotherapy, hormonal therapy, immunotherapy, radiation therapy, or surgery. Patients with metastatic spinal cord compression who are very ill would not be appropriately treated with surgery, whereas a healthy patient with high-grade spinal cord compression from a relatively radioresistant tumor may be optimally treated with surgery. The second priority in the MOSS system is the oncologic diagnosis.

V. Haghshenas (✉) · R. A. W. Marco
Department of Orthopedic Surgery, Houston Methodist Hospital, Houston, TX, USA
e-mail: Vhaghshenas@houstonmethodist.org

A. J. Sayari
Department of Orthopaedic Surgery, Rush University Medical Center, Chicago, IL, USA

A. N. Shehabeldin
Department of Anatomic and Clinical Pathology, Houston Methodist Hospital, Houston, TX, USA
e-mail: Anshehabeldin@houstonmethodist.org

K. Singh, M. Colman (eds.), *Surgical Spinal Oncology*,
https://doi.org/10.1007/978-3-030-50722-0_14

The new chemotherapeutic agents and radiation therapy modalities have dramatically improved nonoperative treatment of most patients presenting with metastatic spinal cord compression. It is, thus, imperative that the multidisciplinary team of oncologists, radiation therapists, internists, and surgeons identify the type of cancer present in the spine and determine whether this patient is likely to respond to the newer nonoperative treatment modalities. Identifying the type of cancer, obtaining staging studies, and determining the probable response to new antitumor agents and stereotactic radiation therapy also help determine the patient's prognosis, which, in turn, helps determine the treatment plan. The revised Tokuhashi score is helpful for estimating prognosis and guiding treatment and is favored by the authors [3, 4]. The third and fourth priorities in the MOSS system evaluate the degree of stenosis and the stability of the spine. Modern chemotherapy and radiation therapy have allowed most ambulatory patients with high-grade spinal cord compression from sensitive tumor histologies to be treated without surgery. On the other hand, most otherwise healthy, nonambulatory patients with high-grade spinal cord compression associated with a relatively radioresistant tumor are probably best treated with surgery. A multidisciplinary discussion with the patient will help guide them through the treatment options. Spinal instability is difficult to treat without surgical intervention. Some authors use the SINS score to help decide whether a consultation with a spine surgeon is warranted [5]. Our preference is to use the White-Panjabi definition of physiologic instability [6]. White-Panjabi defined physiologic instability as progressive neurological dysfunction, progressive deformity, or uncontrolled pain after appropriate medical treatment under normal physiologic loads. Patients with a physiologic instability may benefit from surgery if they are medically well, have a life expectancy of greater than 3 months, and have a relatively radioresistant tumor.

In summary, patient-centered factors must be married to a thorough understanding of tumor tissue at a microscopic level when seeking to control tumor metastases. This chapter highlights advancements in histologic understanding and its application to diagnosis and management of metastatic disease for the most common metastatic histologies.

Breast Cancer

Evaluation first begins with assessment of tumor biology. Breast cancer biomarkers include estrogen receptor (ER), progesterone receptor (PR), and HER2 overexpression. Tumors with high expression of ER form a continuum ranging from well-differentiated carcinoma with low proliferation indices to poorly differentiated carcinomas with high proliferation indices. Tumors with overexpression of HER2 are typically high grade with high proliferation rate. However, HER2 overexpression opens the door for treatment with targeted monoclonal antibody therapy. ER, PR, and HER2-negative tumors, that is, triple-negative breast cancers, are a distinctly different group, with marked genomic instability, high proliferative rate, and generally poor prognosis. Testing the tumor biomarkers is particularly important for triple-negative cancers since conversion to receptor positivity during the metastatic process could dramatically change therapy and prognosis. In cases where the source of the metastatic tumor is obscure or when the morphology of the tumor is not typical, immunohistochemical stains that point to a breast primary, including GATA3, gross cystic disease fluid protein 15 (GCDFP15), and mammaglobin, can be used [7, 8].

In general, hormonal therapy is favored for hormone receptor-positive cancers; however, addition of chemotherapy in rapidly progressive disease may confer more favorable responses. Targeted cancer therapies target specific characteristics on cancer cells and may have less systemic side effects. Immune-targeted therapy with monoclonal antibodies is named with the suffix "-mab" (monoclonal antibody). Trastuzumab (herceptin) is a monoclonal antibody that targets HER2 overexpressing cancer cells causing growth arrest and reduced cell proliferation. Other targeted therapies inhibit CDK4/6 [palbociclib (Ibrance), ribociclib (Kisqali), and abemaciclib (Verzenio)], HER2 [lapatinib (Tykerb)], HER [neratinib (Nerlynx)], and PI3K [alpelisib (Piqray)]. CDK4/6 inhibitors are named with the suffix "-ciclib," while tyrosine kinase inhibitors are named with the suffix "-tinib." mTOR inhibitors like everolimus (Afinitor) inhibit the mammalian target of rapamycin (mTOR). Everolimus is used against hormone receptor-positive breast cancers that no longer respond to Arimidex or Femara.

For patients with metastatic HER2-negative breast cancer who have a germ line *BRCA* mutation, two trials have demonstrated the single-agent activity of the oral inhibitors of polyadenosine diphosphate-ribose polymerase (PARP) *olaparib* and *talazoparib* [9, 10]. In both trials, the PARP inhibitor was superior to chemotherapy for progression-free survival (PFS), the primary endpoint, as well as for response and toxicity. PARP inhibitors are named with the suffix -parib.

Addition of denosumab or osteoclast inhibitors has shown to decrease the rate of skeletal-related events in patients with bony metastases [11, 12].

Recurrence and Survival Rates

Breast carcinoma remains one of the most common cancer diagnoses, accounting for 15% of cancer deaths among women [13]. Breast cancer includes more than 4 distinct molecular subtypes and 20 histological subtypes, which have been demonstrated to vary in their diagnostic intricacies, management options, and survival rates [14]. Furthermore, the presence or absence of progesterone or estrogen receptors (PR, ER) and unique proteins such as HER2 play a role in response to treatment. In general, the incidence, mortality, and survival vary throughout the world, and breast cancer is more commonly diagnosed in Western countries, though imparts lower survival rates in less-developed countries. Fortunately, survival rates in North America remain above 90% at 5 years for early-stage disease, and modern clinical practices including routine mammography have led to a 36% reduction in death rates over 23 years from 1989 to 2012 in the United States [15].

Metastatic breast cancer confers a worse prognosis, and up to two-thirds of bony metastases involve the spinal column. A meta-analysis in 2018 analyzed 15 studies of metastatic breast cancer, demonstrating a median survival rate in 2010 of 47 months, as high as 57 months in ER+, and 33 months in ER– patients, though lead-time bias likely plays a role in the improved statistics [16]. Survival rates starkly decline in metastatic disease to 15–26% at 5 years. Tumor grade, hormone receptor status, and HER2 status have all been demonstrated to influence survival, as those with "triple-negative" status of hormone and growth factor receptors have the worst over all and disease-free survival rates [17, 18]. ER/PR– and HER2+ had an overall 5-year survival rate of 78.8% and disease-free survival rate of 66% [19]. A smaller study of 311 patients demonstrated survival in bone-only metastases to average 55.5 months [20].

Briasoulis et al. evaluated 2514 patients over a 20-year duration and analyzed 104 of them who had confirmed bony metastases. They were found to develop metastases at roughly 38 months following surgery for the primary tumor. Survival in this group was 72 months, and there was no improvement in survival based on tumor grade or anatomic distribution [21]. Metastases confined to bone have been suggested to be more indolent and more responsive to systemic therapies, and they may have better survival rates than patients with extraosseous metastases [22, 23]. Spinal cord compression may occur in roughly 7% of patients with skeletal metastases, and though this stems from a single study, the clinical implications can vary from pain to neurologic compromise requiring surgical intervention [21].

In general, both hormone receptor status and molecular heterogeneity influence recurrence rates following successful treatment of breast cancer, and studies have suggested that hormone-positive patients have lower recurrence rates at 5 years [18]. Alternative subtypes such as luminal A, luminal B, basal, HER2 enriched, and alternative molecular factors have also been shown to play a role in recurrence rates, though recent advancements in adjuvant therapies have further increased the recurrence-free interval [16, 24]. A large French cohort study of 4926 patients with breast cancer over an 18-year period found a recurrence rate of 18% at an average 7.2 years, with a 36% chance of death within 5 years in patients with two recurrences [25]. However, their study followed patients before and after the release of multiple prognosis-influencing breast cancer therapies such as trastuzumab, which likely influenced their findings. In another study with 15-year follow-up of patients with metastatic breast cancer, only 1.8% of patients were disease free after receiving chemotherapy alone, suggesting that more aggressive treatment to consolidate remission, especially in cases of oligometastatic disease, may be beneficial [26, 27].

Imaging and Diagnostic Characteristics

Surveillance and screening have allowed for improved management and earlier diagnosis of primary breast cancer, while MRI and mammography have demonstrated both pros and cons in this arena [28]. In the setting of diagnosing metastatic lesions, the choice of imaging modality can often follow an algorithmic approach. Pain is the presenting symptom in nearly 90% of patients, though descriptors will vary widely and may result in a delay in diagnosis for up to 2 months [29, 30]. Mid-thoracic back pain or nonmechanical back pain is less often related to degenerative spinal disease in such a clinical scenario and is more often involved in metastatic disease of the spine [31]. Neurologic compromise may be radicular or progressive and result in compression of the spinal cord or cauda equina, depending on the level, each having a unique neurologic presentation [32].

In the setting of a history of active or latent breast cancer with new-onset back pain, it is prudent to obtain full-spine radiographs with a thorough evaluation and high suspicion for spinal metastases. Metastatic breast cancer to bone often presents with osteolytic lesions, though blastic and mixed forms can be seen, along with pathologic fractures and impending canal compromise. Lytic lesions are usually seen when bone demineralization exceeds 30–50%, and scintigraphy is more sensitive in such scenarios [33]. CT and MRI are useful modalities for identifying the lesion. CT allows for a more precise identification of tumor extension and osseous anatomy. On the other hand, MRI has become the gold standard for evaluating metastatic spinal tumors (Fig. 14.1). Improved sensitivity, clearer identification of margins, and understanding of osseous, neurovascular, and soft-tissue anatomy allow for diagnostic and therapeutic applications (Figs. 14.2 and 14.3). Addition of gadolinium improves vascular understanding and better delineates metastatic breast lesions. Finally, PET utilizes glucose metabolism to identify tumor activity and tracer uptake, and when added to CT (PET-CT), it has a remarkable ability to provide diagnostic and therapeutic advantages. New biomarkers in PET imaging are also a valuable tool in evaluating the efficacy of endocrine therapies and in developing new endocrine drugs.

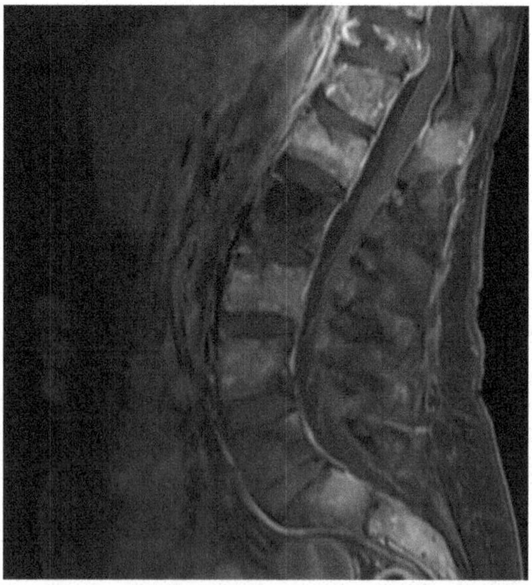

Fig. 14.1 Lumbar MRI of patient with diffusely metastatic breast ductal carcinoma demonstrating several pathologic fractures and cord compression at T11

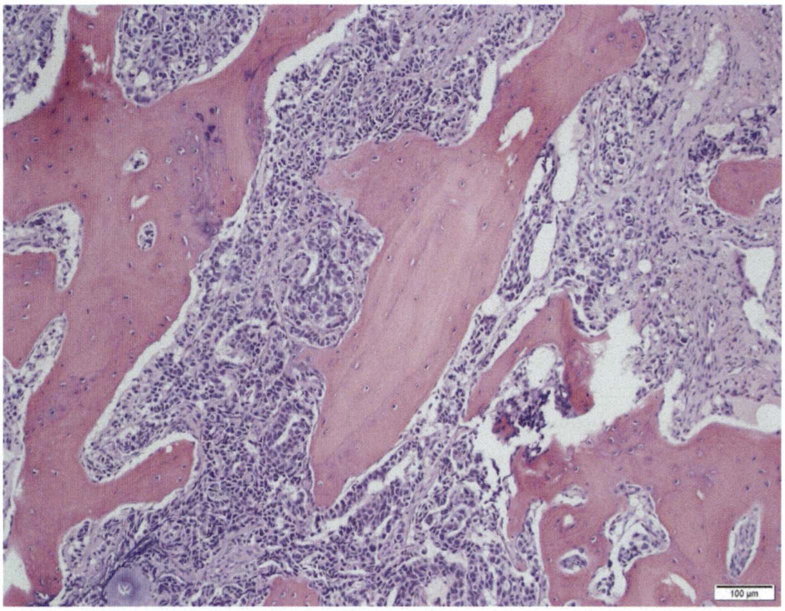

Fig. 14.2 Biopsy of T11 lesion shows bone with metastatic carcinoma infiltrating the marrow spaces [hematoxylin–eosin, original magnification ×100]

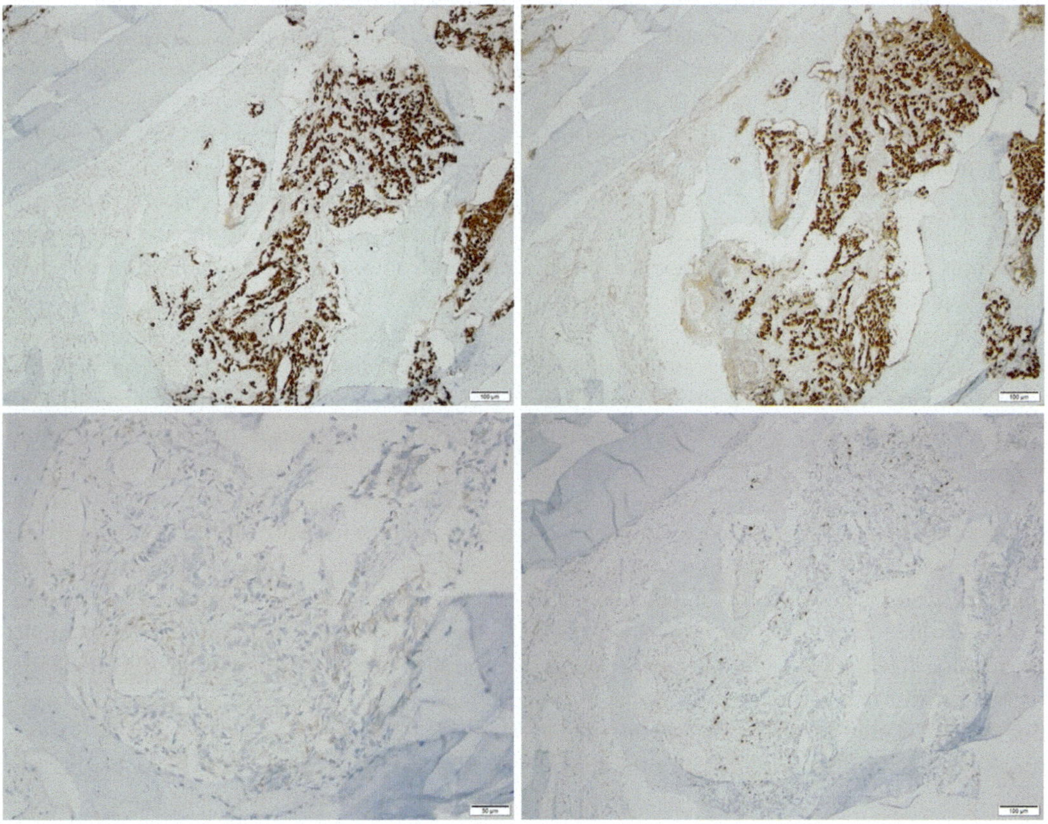

Fig. 14.3 Image 1 shows strong and diffuse nuclear positivity with GATA3, supporting of a breast primary of the metastatic carcinoma. Image 2 shows strong and diffuse nuclear positivity with ER. Image 3 shows weak focal nuclear positivity with PR, and Image 4 shows weak focal membranous positivity with HER2, both considered negative

Lung Cancer

Treatment for patients with metastatic non-small-cell lung cancer (NSCLC) has historically consisted of systemic cytotoxic chemotherapy. An improved understanding of the molecular pathways that drive malignancy in NSCLC led to the development of agents that target specific molecular pathways in malignant cells beginning in the early 2000s. The hope is that these agents will be able to preferentially kill malignant cells but will be relatively innocuous to normal cells. Mutations in the epidermal growth factor receptor (*EGFR*) or rearrangements of the anaplastic lymphoma kinase (*ALK*) gene or c-ROS oncogene 1 (*ROS1*) gene have led to a paradigm shift and the development of specific molecular treatments for patients.

Mutations in the *EGFR* tyrosine kinase are observed in approximately 15% of NSCLC adenocarcinomas in the United States and occur more frequently in nonsmokers and up to 62% of Asians [34, 35]. The presence of an *EGFR* mutation confers a more favorable prognosis and strongly predicts for sensitivity to EGFR tyrosine kinase inhibitors (TKIs) (erlotinib, gefitinib, afatinib, and osimertinib).

ALK gene rearrangement (*ALK*+ NSCLC) is present in about 4% of the population and strongly predicts for sensitivity to ALK TKIs (crizotinib, ceritinib, alectinib).

c-ROS oncogene 1 (ROS1) is a receptor tyrosine kinase that acts as a driver oncogene in 1–2% of NSCLC via a genetic translocation between *ROS1* and other genes, the most common of which is *CD74* [36–38]. Treatment with crizotinib is FDA approved and recommended for patients with the ROS1 translocation, including those who have received chemotherapy and those who are treatment naïve with median progression-free survival of 19.2 months. Case reports suggest that cabozantinib may be effective in ROS1-translocated cancers that have become resistant to crizotinib [39, 40]. *BRAF* mutations have been observed in 1–3% of NSCLCs and are usually associated with a history of smoking. These are generally treated with chemotherapy, and addition of TKIs, such as vemurafenib and dabrafenib, appears to be an effective strategy in the treatment of progressive disease [41–43].

Recurrence and Survival Rates

Unlike breast cancer, patients diagnosed with lung cancer are often part of an older cohort. In fact, 75% are older than 65 years at the time they are diagnosed with small-cell lung cancer (SCLC) or non-small-cell lung cancer. At the time of presentation, SCLC has already reached a metastatic state, and therefore, it confers a worse prognosis than NSCLC. The overall survival rate of lung cancer has only increased by roughly 13% from 34% in the late 1970s to 47% in the early 2010s [17]. This is, in part, due to the asymptomatic nature of the disease in the early stages. In fact, the 5-year survival rate was 57% in 2019 in patients with stage I lung cancer versus 4% for patients with stage IV, and it tends to be lower across the board for SCLC when compared to NSCLC.

Specific to spinal metastases, molecule-targeting therapies, such as gefitinib, and bone-modifying agents, such as zoledronate and denosumab, have improved the overall survival rate since 2006, and studies have since challenged the Tokuhashi score of predicting survival rates of metastatic lung cancer [44]. However, despite these modern advances, the median survival following diagnosis of spinal metastases in the setting of lung cancer has been suggested to be only around 1 year [45].

Local recurrence rates following NSCLC resection range from 30% to 55%. A majority are distant metastases, and 80% of them occur within 2 years [46, 47]. A separate study of 106 patients following lobectomy for NSCLC demonstrated a recurrence rate of 43% at a mean of 57.9 months [48]. Recognition of different histological subtypes has allowed for assessment of various markers that have been used to better predict and identify recurrence of distal metastases, including Ki-67, MACC, and TS [49, 50]. Similarly, as with localized disease, EGFR mutations are used in dictating treatment such as gefitinib after recurrent or metastatic disease. Lastly, time from treatment of primary disease to distant recurrence has been demonstrated to play a role in postrecurrent survival rates [51].

Imaging and Diagnostic Characteristics

At the time of diagnosis, 20–30% of patients with lung cancer already have skeletal metastases, most commonly to the bone. Via lymphatic or hematogenous spread, the thoracic spine is the most common site of such metastases. Though a majority of patients will present with back pain, metastatic spinal cord compression is a frequently presenting sign necessitating further evaluation. In addition, elevated serum calcium or alkaline phosphatase levels as a result of osteolysis should also prompt such evaluation. After scrutinization of osteolysis in plain radiographs, CT and MRI are viable options for evaluation of the spinal elements, though CT myelography should be implemented in patients who cannot undergo MRI and lends a useful adjunct of allowing for pathologic evaluation of cerebrospinal fluid. SPECT, PET, and PET-CT are alternative options that can be employed using a multidisciplinary approach alongside nuclear medicine and radiation oncology teams. Low-dose CT has gained significant popularity in screening for lung cancer, though with much debate. It offers a higher sensitivity in diagnosing higher risk patients, and multiple studies have been recently published evaluating the usefulness of this modality [52].

Histological analysis of lung tumor tissue should allow for identification of tumor type (Fig. 14.4). The most common tumor types are adenocarcinoma, squamous cell carcinoma, small-cell carcinoma, and large-cell carcinoma [53]. Tissue can be analyzed for epidermal growth factor receptor (EGFR) mutations as it can have prognostic implications, provide treatment targets, and predict metastatic sites [54]. ALK and ROS1 gene translocations are found infrequently, often in male nonsmokers [55, 56]. Similarly, immunologic testing via antibodies has assisted in diagnosing lung cancer. Antibodies to p53 can aid in diagnosis in roughly 12% of cases, though adding six others, including Hu-D, SOX-2, MAGE-A4, CAGE, GBU4-5, and NY-ESO-1, can increase the sensitivity and specificity to 47% and 90%, respectively [57, 58]. Such mutations present targets for future therapies.

Prostate Cancer

Androgen deprivation therapy (ADT) is a component of the initial approach for patients with metastatic disease. Combining ADT with either abiraterone or docetaxel increases overall survival compared with ADT alone in patients with high risk and/or de novo presentation with metastases [59–62]. Progression of disease after surgical or medical orchiectomy is deemed castration-resistant prostate cancer (CRPC). In these patients, ADT should be continued, but gonadotropin-releasing hormone (GnRH) agonists should be stopped before initiating alternative therapy. Alternate therapies for these patients include cellular immunotherapy with sipuleucel-T, taxane chemotherapy, and bone-targeting radioisotope radium-223. Sipuleucel-T has shown to improve overall survival but has not significantly increased progression-free survival or affected serum prostate-specific antigen (PSA) [63].

In patients with disease limited to skeletal metastases, radium-223 was well tolerated and increased both overall survival and time to first symptomatic skeletal-related event (external beam radiation therapy to relieve skeletal symptoms, new symptomatic pathologic fracture, occurrence of spinal cord compression, or tumor-related orthopedic surgical intervention) [64].

Recurrence and Survival Rates

Lead-time bias and overdiagnosis with the frequent measurement of prostate-specific antigen (PSA) during screening have increased the 5-year survival rate following prostate cancer diagnosis to 99% by 2014 [17]. Such an increase in surveillance has influenced treatment as well, as rates of radical prostatectomy have declined 16% between 2010 and 2015 [65]. Prostate cancer is

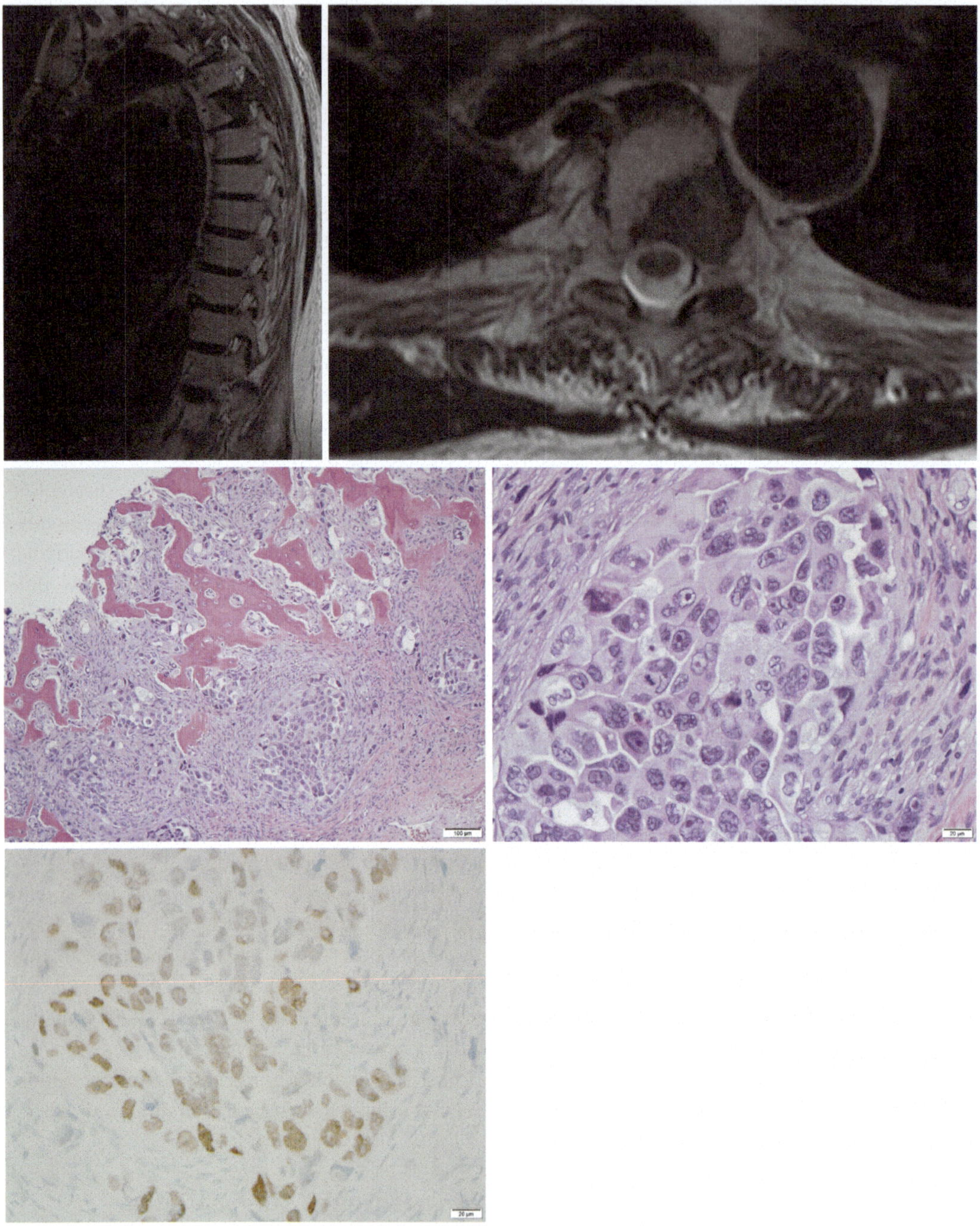

Fig. 14.4. Images 1 and 2 demonstrate pathologic vertebral body compression fracture of T2 with left epidural extension of tumor resulting in mild spinal canal stenosis. Image 3 is a low power micrograph of the lesion which shows trabecular bone involved by a poorly differentiated carcinoma with the tumor cells forming cohesive groups. This is better seen in image 4 at 400× magnification with markedly enlarged and irregular nuclei with prominent nucleoli. Image 5 shows TTF-1 immunohistochemical stain with nuclear staining of the tumor cells, consistent with lung adenocarcinoma as the primary tumor

frequently diagnosed while still in a local stage, though survival drops by nearly 70% to 30% when metastases are present. In cases of spinal metastases, concomitant visceral metastases and higher PSA at time of spinal metastases diagnosis confer worse survival rates, while bisphosphonate treatment and hormone status have less of an effect on survival [66, 67]. Classically, median survival has been quoted to be 53 months in cases of bony metastases and 12–30 months when visceral metastases are present [68].

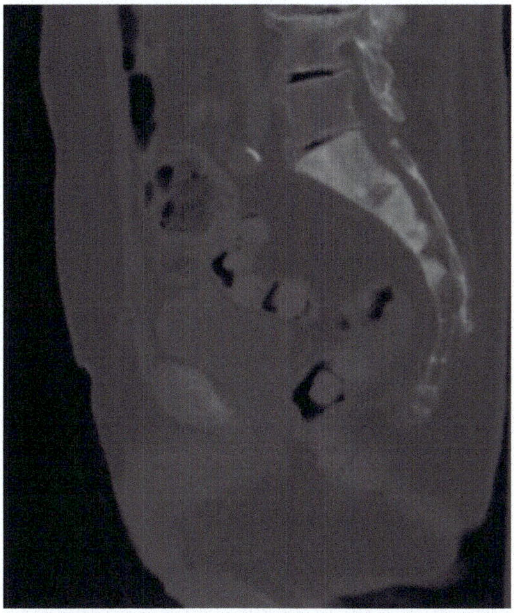

Fig. 14.5 CT of patient with metastatic prostate cancer to sacrum

Given the various levels of treatments in prostate cancer, recurrence rates can vary widely, though the general reported definition revolves around biochemical recurrence, with PSA levels >0.2 ng/mL. Recurrence rates generally improve with negative margins during radical prostatectomy and worsen with Gleason scores of 8–10, or worse preoperative stage [69, 70]. Various tools have been suggested as predictors of recurrence, but none has been validated [71, 72].

Imaging and Diagnostic Characteristics

Unlike renal, breast, and lung cancers, metastatic prostate cancer almost always clinically presents as an osteoblastic lesion (Fig. 14.5). As such, intraspinal blastic tumor encroachment can create particular challenges with regard to neural compression. Decompression of these zones often requires extensive tumor-laden bone resection, in contradistinction to other histologies which create soft-tissue epidural extension. Bony metastases from prostate cancer are likely related to the prostate venous plexus draining to the vertebral veins (Figs. 14.6 and 14.7). While back pain is nearly always a symptom in spinal metastases, motor impairment occurs in fewer than a fourth of these patients and bladder dysfunction in 3% [73]. Ultrasonographic techniques have been useful in detecting prostate lesions, though patients with hormone-resistant prostate cancer who

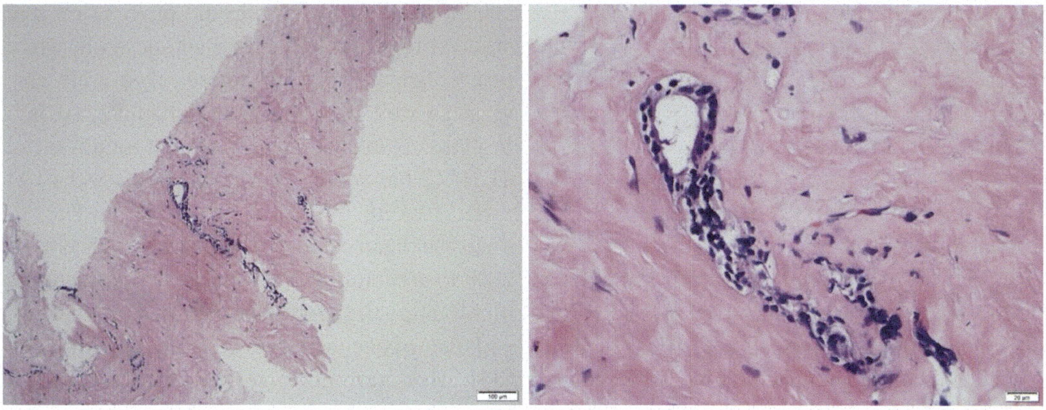

Fig. 14.6 Sections from a sacral mass demonstrate small cores of fibrous tissue which contain an adenocarcinoma [hematoxylin–eosin, original magnification ×100 (left), ×400 (right)]

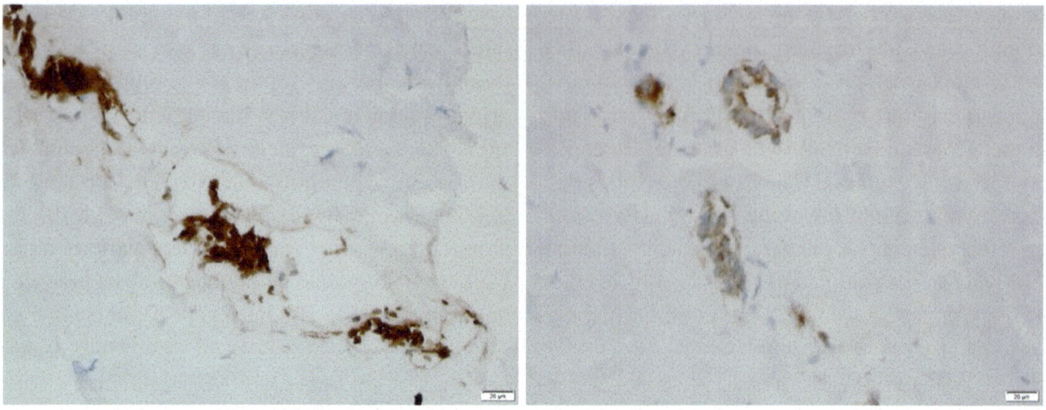

Fig. 14.7 Prostate-specific antigen (PSA) (left) and prostatic acid phosphatase (PAP) (right) immunohistochemical staining show positivity in tumor cells, confirming the diagnosis of metastatic prostatic adenocarcinoma [original magnification ×400]

report back pain should be thoroughly evaluated for spinal metastases and often require advanced imaging beyond plain radiographs and bone scans. Multiparametric ultrasound and MRI have demonstrated utility in evaluating primary as well as recurrent prostate cancer [74]. Specifically, diffusion-weighted series are helpful delineating tumor tissue, and T1-weighted images demonstrate hypointense signal when compared to adjacent muscle. Magnetic resonance spectroscopic imaging (MRSI) similarly is a useful tool emerging with utility in detecting recurrent prostate cancer. As a surface glycoprotein, prostate-specific membrane antigen has gained traction as a potential target for radiotracers and as a tool for identifying prostate cancer in cases where PSA levels are greater than 0.5 ng/mL, though traditional PET scans are useful when PSA levels increase to greater than 2 ng/mL [70].

Renal Cell Carcinoma

Recurrence and Survival Rates

One-third of those with renal cell carcinoma (RCC) will present with metastases (mRCC), 30% of which are to the spine, and are of the clear cell histologic subtype (CCRCC) [75, 76]. Only 50% of patients with bony metastases survive beyond 1 year, and survival continues to decline to 10% at 5 years, with a median survival rate of roughly 8 months [77]. In the last 20 years, there has been a shift in treating RCC with cytotoxic to more targeted molecular therapies, resulting in a more favorable trend in mRCC survival [78]. Despite this, survival rates are worse with multiple metastases, and axial metastases worsen survival rates compared to appendicular metastases [79]. First-line therapy for patients with advanced disease or unresectable metastases involves systemic immunotherapy following cytoreductive nephrectomy. In the era of interferon immunotherapy, patients who underwent nephrectomy prior to systemic therapy had a median survival rate of 17 months versus 7 months in those with therapy alone [80, 81]. Combination of immune checkpoint inhibitors and antiangiogenic therapies (pembrolizumab/axitinib and avelumab/axitinib) improved progression-free survival relative to single-agent sunitinib, while pembrolizumab/axitinib improved overall survival as well [82, 83]. Pembrolizumab/axitinib is an acceptable frontline treatment for advanced CCRCC, but comparison to existing standard of care is lacking.

In localized cases, recurrence rates vary from 20% to 40% following successful nephrectomy, highlighting the aggressive nature of this disease, and recurrence to bone is often disseminated [84]. However, other reviews have suggested that bone metastases occur in less than 2–8% of cases following nephrectomy [85–87]. Most recurrences are thought to occur within 2 years, though a recent study found that 26% of patients with primary RCC undergoing curative nephrectomy had a recurrence at more than 5 years [88].

Imaging and Diagnostic Characteristics

RCC lesions are most commonly extradural, eccentrically displacing the thecal sac with varying degrees of cord compression as measured by the Metastatic Epidural Spinal Cord Compression Scale [89]. Following hematogenous spread, mRCC is destructive to local bone, resulting in varying amounts of pain and mechanical instability; nerve root or spinal cord compression may be as common as 28% [90, 91].

Advanced mRCC can be seen radiographically, both as destroyed local bone as a "soap-bubble" appearance and as pedicular bone as a "winking owl" on AP radiographs. MRI and CT (Figs. 14.8 and 14.9) findings are not unique in mRCC, and trend similar to others, with hypointense T1-weighted signals and hyperintense diffusion-weighted signals. However, given the increased vascularity of RCC, gadolinium

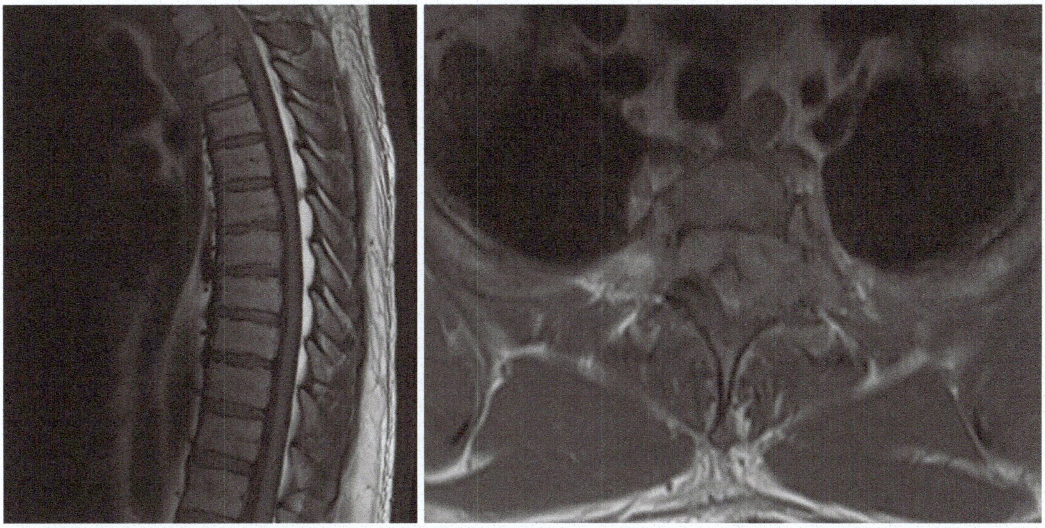

Fig. 14.8 Sagittal and axial T1 MRI demonstrate metastatic RCC pathologic compression fracture of the T2 vertebral body with dorsal bony retropulsion resulting in spinal stenosis and cord compression

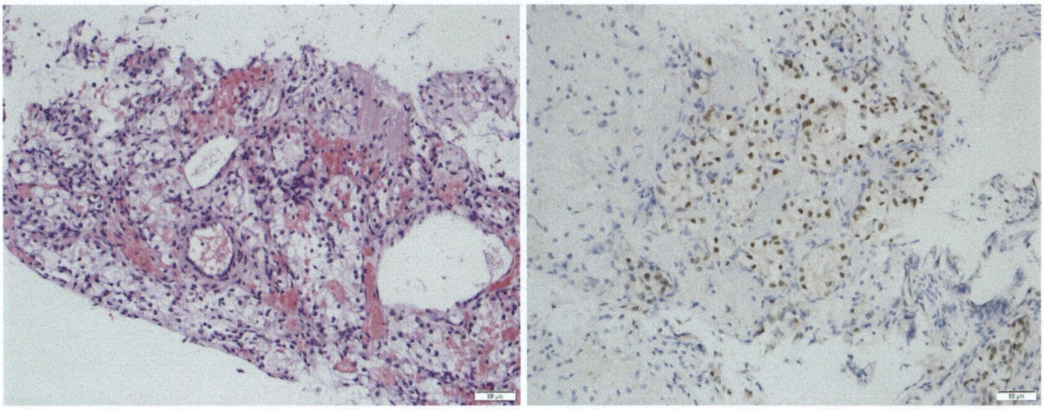

Fig. 14.9 Biopsy from vertebral mass of same patient shows large neoplastic cells with clear cytoplasm and delicate vasculature. Nuclear positivity with PAX8 immunohistochemical staining (a transcription factor expressed in the thyroid gland, upper urinary tract, and Müllerian organs) and the morphologic appearance on hematoxylin–eosin confirm the diagnosis of conventional clear cell renal cell carcinoma

contrast can starkly increase the signal of such lesions. Similarly, a topography of arterial vessels has diagnostic and therapeutic utility involving selective angiography and planned embolizations during treatment [92].

Lymphoma

Recurrence and Survival Rates

Lymphomas, made up of Hodgkin (HL) and non-Hodgkin types (NHL), are defined by blood cancers of the lymph nodes, and spinal lymphomas are late manifestations of disseminated disease. Furthermore, spinal metastases as the initial presentation of NHL uncommonly occur in less than 5% of patients [93]. Primary non-Hodgkin lymphoma of bone (PLB) is quite rare, accounting for 3% of primary bone malignancies [94]. Arising from the paraspinal soft tissues and then entering the epidural spaces, PLB causes direct neural compression, unlike other spinal metastases which reach the thecal sac through vertebral destruction. The 2-year survival rate after diagnosis of PLB is made has been suggested to be 36% [95, 96]. A separate retrospective evaluation of 30 patients with spinal lymphomas demonstrated a mean survival of 87.6 months, suggesting improvement in diagnosis and management [97]. Rarely, clinically indolent lymphomas, such as follicular lymphoma, small lymphocytic lymphoma, and marginal zone lymphoma, may present as PLB.

Immunocompromised state, increasing age, aggressive histological grade, neurologic involvement, and elevated CSF protein levels have been associated with a worse prognosis [98, 99].

Imaging and Diagnostic Characteristics

PLB and metastatic lymphoma to the spine generally present in an initial, insidious onset that may last up to a year before more rapid neural involvement, thereby often being confused with other diagnoses such as lumbar disc herniations or spondylitis [100, 101]. Plain radiographs are useful in the evaluation of suspected spinal lymphoma. Whereas metastatic lesions cause bony lesions such as local erosion, PLB rarely causes bony destruction. Rather, epidural sites are more common, noted as hypo- or iso-intense signal on contrast-enhanced MRIs (Fig. 14.10). Similarly, metastatic NHL can extend adjacent soft tissues

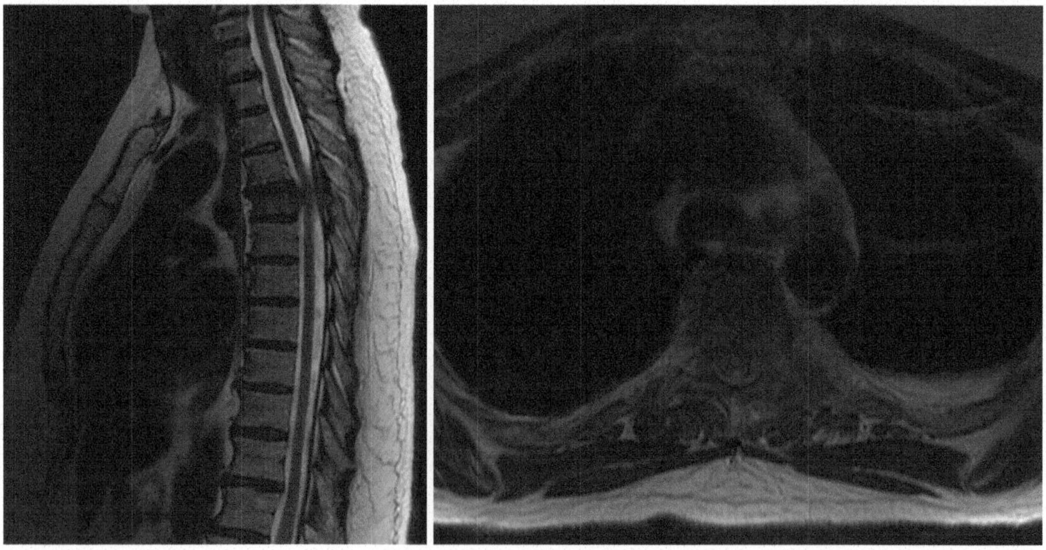

Fig. 14.10 MRI demonstrating T5 pathologic fracture with epidural extension and associated mild cord compression

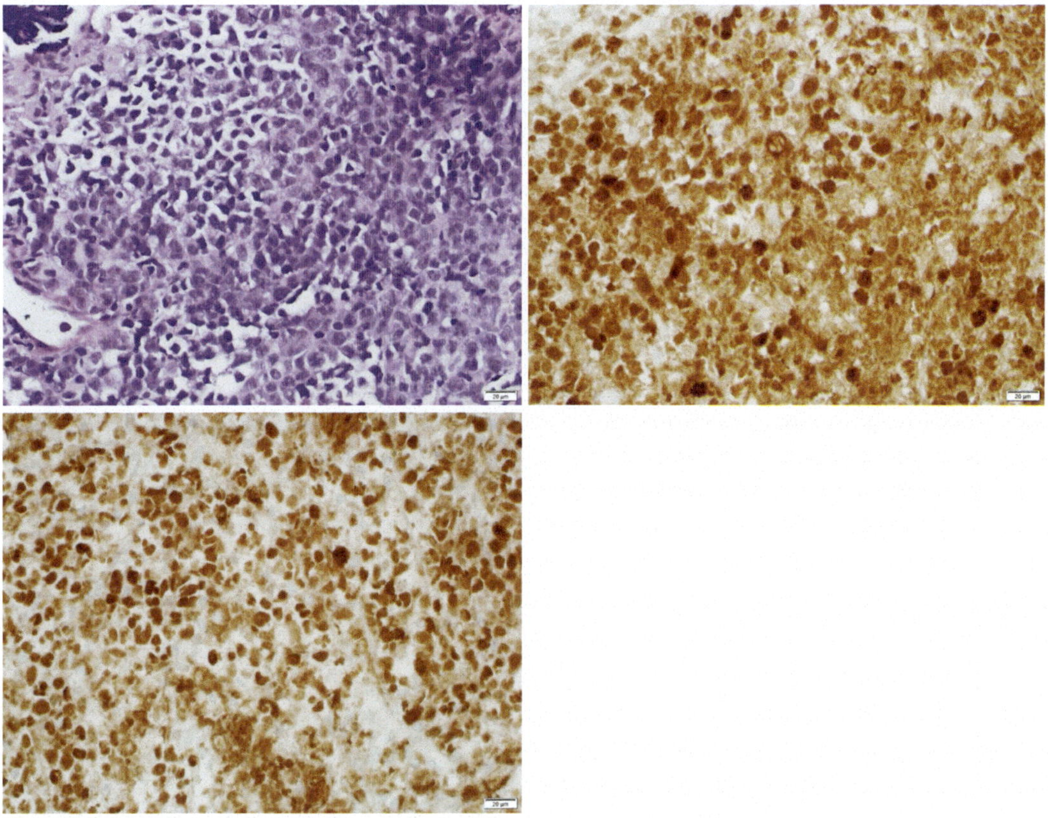

Fig. 14.11 Image 1 demonstrates T5 paraspinal mass biopsy showing diffuse infiltrate of large lymphocytes with oval to irregular nuclei and occasional prominent nucleoli. Image 2 is immunohistochemical stains for MUM1. Image 3 is BCL-6 staining which shows nuclear positivity in the neoplastic cells. The corresponding flow cytometry demonstrated B-cell lymphoma CD5 negative, CD10 negative, lambda light-chain restricted. The morphologic features, CD10 negativity, and MUM1 and BCL-6 positivity are consistent with a diffuse large B-cell lymphoma, nongerminal center type

and local bone, inducing thecal sac compression (Fig. 14.11). Unfortunately, cytologic CSF analysis and CT-guided needle biopsies rarely allow for diagnosis, whereas surgical pathology is a more useful means of achieving accurate diagnosis. Despite this, the low risk of needle biopsy suggests this as a useful tool in the diagnostic algorithm [102].

Myeloma

The first step in evaluating a new patient with MM is to verify the diagnosis since the premalignant stages of myeloma, namely monoclonal gammopathy of undetermined significance (MGUS) and smoldering multiple myeloma (SMM), may be easily misdiagnosed as MM. Evaluation with fluorescence in situ hybridization (FISH) for specific translocations is used for risk stratification and helps with prognosis.

Treatment of standard-risk MM depends on hematopoietic cell transplantation (HCT) eligibility and comorbidities. For most patients, initial treatment with bortezomib, lenalidomide, and dexamethasone (VRd) is recommended unless there are contraindications to lenalidomide (e.g., acute renal failure) in which case bortezomib can be used as a substitute [103].

Proteasome inhibitors such as carfilzomib have shown improved survival in relapsed disease. The use of carfilzomib in place of bortezomib in previously untreated MM has not shown to be beneficial [104]. The anti-CD38 monoclonal antibody daratumumab is another preferred agent for the treatment of relapsed multiple myeloma (MM). In recent trials, the use of daratumumab on newly diagnosed MM has shown deepened response and improved progression-free survival although further follow-up is still pending [105, 106].

Recurrence and Survival Rates

As the second most common hematologic malignancy after NHL, multiple myeloma (MM) is a neoplastic proliferation of plasma cells, and the spine is the most frequent site of metastasis, as 60% of patients are present with spinal metastases at the time of diagnosis [107]. Median survival ranges from months to more than 10 years, though translocations such as t(14;16)(q32;q23) or t(4;14)(p16.3;q32) are associated with a worse prognosis. Median survival rates of 24.5–36.1 months have been suggested with such translocations [108, 109]. Prognostic factors have been demonstrated to be based on involved light-chain ratio of ≥100, >60% bone marrow plasma cell burden, and more than one lytic lesion in the spine [110]. The surveillance, epidemiology, and end results (SEER) data have suggested 5-year survival rates of 49% through 2011, nearly a 25% improvement from 30 years earlier [111]. Similarly, evaluation of the Swedish registry demonstrated improvement in 5-year survival rates in all four periods examined, 41% at 5 years and 20% at 10 years [112]. Such results demonstrate how survival rates have improved with increased availability of autologous stem cell transplantation and agents, such as thalidomide, bortezomib, and lenalidomide.

Imaging and Diagnostic Characteristics

In cases of monoclonal gammopathy of unknown significance (MGUS), serum M protein levels are <3 g/DL with <10% monoclonal plasma cells found in the bone marrow. MGUS progresses to smoldering (asymptomatic) MM when these numbers increase, and MM is ultimately diagnosed with end-organ damage as determined by the "CRAB" criteria, which includes hypercalcemia, renal failure, anemia, and lytic bony lesions larger than 5 mm. Clinically, because MM is highlighted by progressive bony destruction, back pain is a leading symptom in patients with spinal metastases. Roughly 5% of patients with MM will have lesions causing spinal cord compression [113].

Radiographically, well-circumscribed lesions that are identified within the spine are more common than expansile lesions, which are more commonly found in other bony structures such as the ribs [114]. CT findings are similar to those on XR; however, low-dose whole-body CT may identify other lesions and delineate any cortical breach or extension into adjacent tissue as bony destruction may be missed until 30% of trabecular volume loss [115]. In fact, a recent systematic review comparing various imaging modalities suggested that low-dose CT, MRI, and PET-CT were superior to plain radiography in identifying MM bone lesions in all cases except the skull and ribs [116]. MRI should be obtained with contrast enhancement to identify discrete lesions that may be missed due to marrow infiltration. Such marrow changes can be highlighted by using fat-suppression sequences. MM lesions appear hypointense on T1-weighted images, owing to a fat content lower than the adjacent intervertebral disc. Increased water content and cellularity translates to hyperintensity as seen on fat-suppressed imaging series. MM can be confused with hemangiomas, which often contain fat, which is readily differentiated on weighted MRI series. Stäbler et al. classified five various appearances of vertebral marrow involvement: normal marrow, focal lesions, diffuse infiltration, combined (heterogeneous) focal and diffuse infiltration, and salt-and-pepper lesions [117].

PET-CT also allows for visualization of spine marrow infiltration, as MM is FDG-PET-CT positive in patients with such marrow involvement. However, PET-CT is less sensitive than MRI for diffuse marrow involvement; PET-CT is also negative in patients with MGUS or low disease burden [118]. Other radiotracers such as F-sodium fluoride have also been implemented in evaluation, though MRI remains the preferred imaging modality thus far. Introduction of PET-MRI is useful and highlights hybrid technology, and early investigations have been promising [119, 120].

The combination of WBCT with 18F-fluorodeoxyglucose (FDG) positron emission tomography (PET-CT) provides an alternative method of visualizing bone marrow infiltration while also allowing visualization of total body tumor burden. Metabolic activity of lesions of interest is calculated based on FDG uptake in cells with high glucose demand and compared with standardized uptake values. CT images are then combined with PET images to provide anatomic localization. Importantly, hypermetabolic bone lesions can be identified in the absence of underlying lytic lesions. Active MM is FDG-PET-CT positive in the marrow space, although FDG-PET-CT is less sensitive than MRI for evaluation of diffuse marrow infiltration (Fig. 14.12) [106]. FDG-PET-CT is negative in patients with MGUS and SMM with low disease burden [121]. Therapeutic response to treatment is characterized by a reduction or elimination of FDG accumulation in involved bone structures.

Multiple studies comparing whole-body (WB) MRI or SS with MRI of the spine and pelvis to FDG-PET-CT in patients with active MM have demonstrated that MRI is superior to CT for detection of skeletal lesions (Figs. 14.13 and 14.14). Results of studies comparing WBMRI to FDG-PET-CT, however, are mixed, and it is likely that the imaging modalities are of equal sensitivity, except for when evaluating the spine, where MRI is preferred. PET-MRI is a promising new hybrid technology, which in initial investigations appears to be at least as sensitive as PET-CT.

Sarcoma

Recurrence and Survival Rates

The spine is an infrequent site of primary osteosarcoma, making up less than 3% of cases, and conferring a poor prognosis. A study of 25 patients with spinal sarcomas treated over

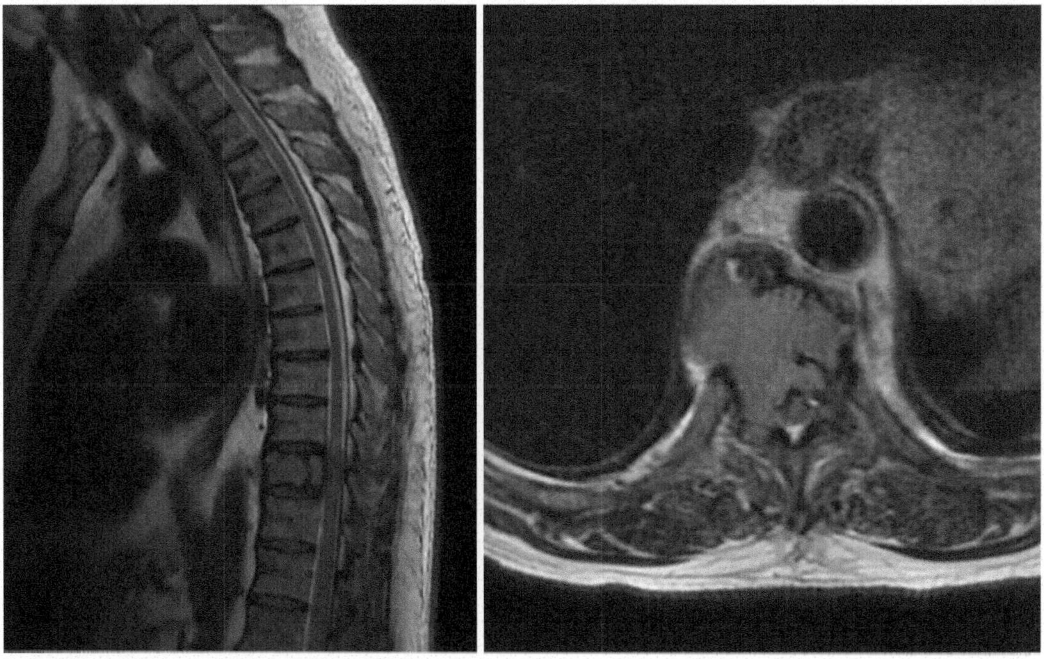

Fig. 14.12 MRI demonstrating T10 pathologic fracture with retropulsion and mild canal stenosis. Multiple myeloma often has normal bone marrow signal with diffuse involvement

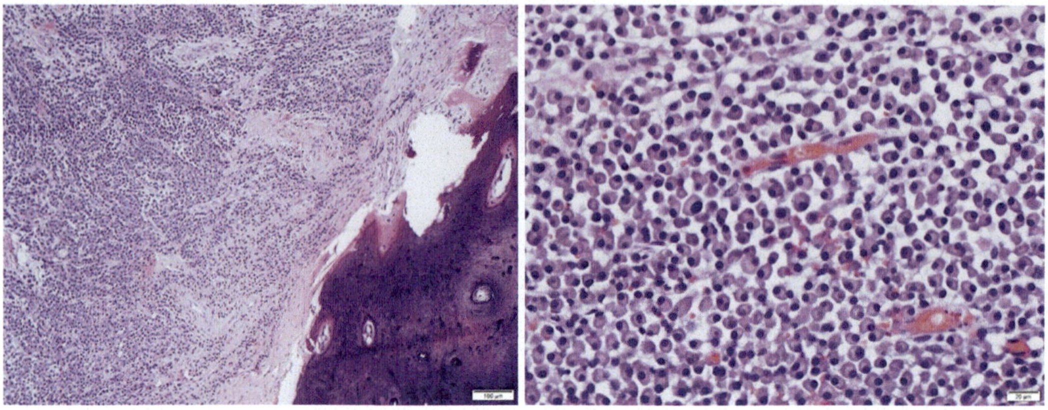

Fig. 14.13 Biopsy of a lesion shows a fragment of cancellous bone and sheets of plasma cells [hematoxylin–eosin, original magnification ×100 (left), ×400 (right)]

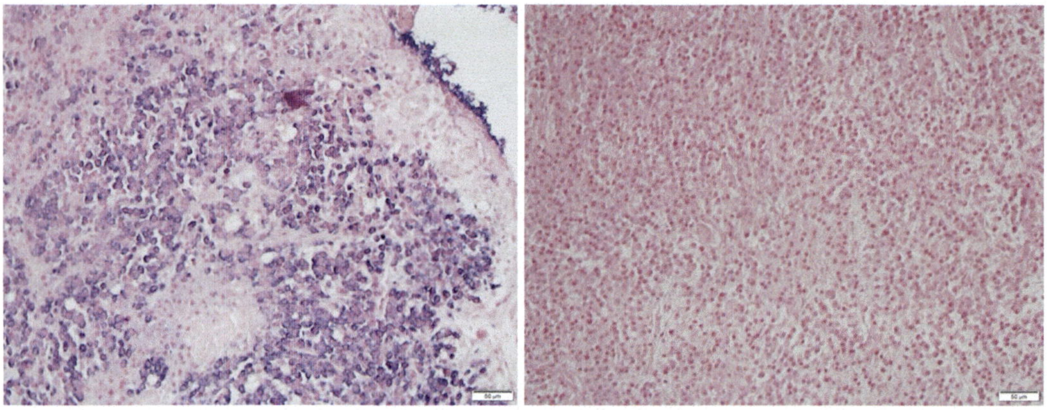

Fig. 14.14 Kappa light-chain in situ hybridization (left) and lambda light-chain in situ hybridization (right) show kappa light-chain restriction of the neoplastic plasma cells [original magnification ×200]

10 years demonstrated a median survival rate of 59.5 months in those with chondrosarcoma versus 16.8 months in those with osteosarcoma. Patients who underwent intralesional resection had a median survival of 17.8 months [122]. A separate study of 17 patients with osteosarcoma demonstrated a median survival of 38.1 months, which improved to 77.3 months in those who underwent en bloc resection. In their cohort, 35% developed a local recurrence [123].

Metastatic spinal sarcomas include chondrosarcoma, rhabdomyosarcoma, liposarcoma, leiomyosarcoma, and synovial cell sarcoma. In patients with CNS metastases, recurrence rates have been reported to range 0.2–6.9 years, with a median of 1.6 years [124], whereas other literature has demonstrated 42% 5-year survival in cases of metastatic Ewing sarcoma, highlighting the wide range of survival depending on sarcoma type [125]. A review of 80 patients with primary and metastatic spinal sarcoma found a median survival of 40.2 months in those with primary sarcoma versus 17.3 months in those with metastatic sarcomas to the spine [126]. The same analysis found that primary versus metastatic status had no influence on recurrence rates, nor did patient age. However, osteosarcoma and high tumor grade were associated with higher rates of local recurrence. Recurrence rates were also improved from 35% in metastatic spine sarcomas undergoing intralesional resection to 25% in those undergoing en bloc resection, with a median time to recurrence of 22.7 months.

Nearly half of patients with soft-tissue sarcomas (STS) develop metastatic disease, often within 3 years of diagnosis [127]. Diagnosis of metastatic STS to the spine confers a median survival rate of 5 months, ranging from 1 to 21 months [128]. Metastatic STS such as synovial sarcoma can metastasize within the spine, reported to metastasize from the lumbar to cervical spine with recurrence rates of 28–70% [129]. Unlike other soft-tissue sarcomas, myxoid liposarcomas have a propensity to metastasize to the axial skeleton and have an overall survival rate suggested to be 81% at 5 years and 72% at 10 years [130, 131].

Imaging and Diagnostic Characteristics

Spinal cord compression secondary to metastatic STS occurs in 3% of patients, most commonly in the lumbosacral spine [128]. More commonly, insidious onset back pain with or without radiculopathy is a presenting symptom. Metastatic sarcoma to the spine is often destructive to bone and adjacent tissues, increasing the need for multiple imaging modalities.

Plain radiographs are useful in identifying a majority of benign lesions and metastatic lesions with greater than 50% bony destruction [132]. Diagnoses of soft-tissue sarcomas have been found incidentally in several reports, often prompted by imaging obtained after a trauma [133]. The same study found MRI to be increasingly more sensitive in identifying such lesions, with a sensitivity of only 14% when using PET scan. Despite some patients having negative PET scans, positive MRI confirmed diagnosis. Overall, FDG-PET scans had a positive predictive value of 100% and negative predictive value of 85%, though they miss sarcoma spinal metastases that would be otherwise found on axial MRI imaging [131, 133]. In cases of metastatic STS to the spine, MRI can demonstrate paravertebral masses extending posteriorly, causing local destruction and involvement of the spinal canal and resulting in spinal cord compression. T1-weighted post-gadolinium-enhanced sequences demonstrate hyperintense lesions, as contrast enhancement can also assist in distinguishing between intradural and extradural tumors. Diffusion-weighted imaging has been further validated in the literature, and similar series are used in surveillance imaging (often paired with CT of the chest, abdomen, and pelvis) [134]. Given the heterogeneity of metastatic sarcomas to the spine, ultimately, histological analysis leads to an accurate diagnosis that will further guide treatment.

The Future

The management of spine metastases remains challenging, but the future is promising. With advancements in high-dose stereotactic radiation, targeted chemotherapy, and immunotherapy, tumors once thought incurable can now be better controlled. New tools such as 3D printing assist in preoperative planning of the complex and often distorted anatomy. Furthermore, advances in navigation and robotic surgery continue to give the surgeon additional tools to attack these complex cases.

Many further advances in the medical surgical treatment of cancer will continue to be made. However, some things remain the same such as keeping the patient at the center of the treatment algorithm. Each patient is unique with their own medical, mental, oncologic, osteoporotic, social, and emotional variables that should be taken into consideration with the use of a multidisciplinary approach. We believe that by using a patient-centered algorithm, such as MOSS, high-quality individualized care can be delivered with the use of the latest available treatment modalities.

Acknowledgments We would like to give a special thanks to the team that supported us, including Paul Holman, MD, Christoph B. Meyer, MD, Hosun Hwang, MD, Alberto Ayala, MD and Jonathan Y. Zhang, MD.

References

1. Laufer I, Rubin DG, Lis E, et al. The NOMS framework: approach to the treatment of spinal metastatic tumors. Oncologist. 2013;18(6):744–51. https://doi.org/10.1634/theoncologist.2012-0293.

2. Marco RAW, Brindise J, Dong D. MOSS: a patient-centered approach. In: Marco RAW, editor. Metastatic spine disease: a guide to diagnosis and management. Cham: Springer International Publishing; 2018. p. 1–20. https://doi.org/10.1007/978-3-319-76252-4_1.
3. Tokuhashi Y, Matsuzaki H, Oda H, Oshima M, Ryu J. A revised scoring system for preoperative evaluation of metastatic spine tumor prognosis. Spine (Phila Pa 1976). 2005;30(19):2186–91. https://doi.org/10.1097/01.brs.0000180401.06919.a5.
4. Tokuhashi Y, Matsuzaki H, Toriyama S, Kawano H, Ohsaka S. Scoring system for the preoperative evaluation of metastatic spine tumor prognosis. Spine (Phila Pa 1976). 1990;15(11):1110–3. https://doi.org/10.1097/00007632-199011010-00005.
5. Fisher CG, DiPaola CP, Ryken TC, et al. A novel classification system for spinal instability in neoplastic disease: an evidence-based approach and expert consensus from the Spine Oncology Study Group. Spine (Phila Pa 1976). 2010;35(22):E1221–9. https://doi.org/10.1097/BRS.0b013e3181e16ae2.
6. Panjabi MM. Clinical spinal instability and low back pain. J Electromyogr Kinesiol. 2003;13(4):371–9. https://doi.org/10.1016/s1050-6411(03)00044-0.
7. Shaoxian T, Baohua Y, Xiaoli X, et al. Characterisation of GATA3 expression in invasive breast cancer: differences in histological subtypes and immunohistochemically defined molecular subtypes. J Clin Pathol. 2017;70(11):926–34. https://doi.org/10.1136/jclinpath-2016-204137.
8. Zaha DC. Significance of immunohistochemistry in breast cancer. World J Clin Oncol. 2014;5(3):382–92. https://doi.org/10.5306/wjco.v5.i3.382.
9. Robson ME, Tung N, Conte P, et al. OlympiAD final overall survival and tolerability results: olaparib versus chemotherapy treatment of physician's choice in patients with a germline BRCA mutation and HER2-negative metastatic breast cancer. Ann Oncol Off J Eur Soc Med Oncol. 2019;30(4):558–66. https://doi.org/10.1093/annonc/mdz012.
10. Litton JK, Rugo HS, Ettl J, et al. Talazoparib in patients with advanced breast cancer and a germline BRCA mutation. N Engl J Med. 2018;379(8):753–63. https://doi.org/10.1056/NEJMoa1802905.
11. Van Poznak C, Somerfield MR, Barlow WE, et al. Role of bone-modifying agents in metastatic breast cancer: an American Society of Clinical Oncology-Cancer Care Ontario focused guideline update. J Clin Oncol. 2017;35(35):3978–86. https://doi.org/10.1200/JCO.2017.75.4614.
12. Coleman R, Body JJ, Aapro M, Hadji P, Herrstedt J, Group EGW. Bone health in cancer patients: ESMO clinical practice guidelines. Ann Oncol Off J Eur Soc Med Oncol. 2014;25(Suppl 3):iii124–37. https://doi.org/10.1093/annonc/mdu103.
13. Gennari A. The impact of new chemotherapeutic and hormone agents on survival in a population-based cohort of women with metastatic breast cancer. Breast Dis A Year B Q. 2008;19(2):180. https://doi.org/10.1016/S1043-321X(08)80124-5.
14. Cheang MCU, Martin M, Nielsen TO, et al. Defining breast cancer intrinsic subtypes by quantitative receptor expression. Oncologist. 2015;20(5):474–82. https://doi.org/10.1634/theoncologist.2014-0372.
15. DeSantis CE, Fedewa SA, Goding Sauer A, Kramer JL, Smith RA, Jemal A. Breast cancer statistics, 2015: convergence of incidence rates between black and white women. CA Cancer J Clin. 2016;66(1):31–42. https://doi.org/10.3322/caac.21320.
16. Caswell-Jin JL, Plevritis SK, Tian L, et al. Change in survival in metastatic breast cancer with treatment advances: meta-analysis and systematic review. JNCI cancer Spectr. 2018;2(4):pky062. https://doi.org/10.1093/jncics/pky062.
17. Miller KD, Nogueira L, Mariotto AB, et al. Cancer treatment and survivorship statistics, 2019. CA Cancer J Clin. 2019;69(5):363–85. https://doi.org/10.3322/caac.21565.
18. Lin J, Goldstein L, Nesbit A, Chen MY. Influence of hormone receptor status on spinal metastatic lesions in patients with breast cancer. World Neurosurg. 2016;85:42–8. https://doi.org/10.1016/j.wneu.2015.07.068.
19. Onitilo AA, Engel JM, Greenlee RT, Mukesh BN. Breast cancer subtypes based on ER/PR and Her2 expression: comparison of clinicopathologic features and survival. Clin Med Res. 2009;7(1–2):4–13. https://doi.org/10.3121/cmr.2009.825.
20. Ahn SG, Lee HM, Cho S-H, et al. Prognostic factors for patients with bone-only metastasis in breast cancer. Yonsei Med J. 2013;54(5):1168–77. https://doi.org/10.3349/ymj.2013.54.5.1168.
21. Briasoulis E, Karavasilis V, Kostadima L, Ignatiadis M, Fountzilas G, Pavlidis N. Metastatic breast carcinoma confined to bone: portrait of a clinical entity. Cancer. 2004;101(7):1524–8. https://doi.org/10.1002/cncr.20545.
22. Sherry MM, Greco FA, Johnson DH, Hainsworth JD. Metastatic breast cancer confined to the skeletal system. An indolent disease. Am J Med. 1986;81(3):381–6. https://doi.org/10.1016/0002-9343(86)90286-x.
23. Leone BA, Romero A, Rabinovich MG, et al. Stage IV breast cancer: clinical course and survival of patients with osseous versus extraosseous metastases at initial diagnosis. The GOCS (Grupo Oncológico Cooperativo del Sur) experience. Am J Clin Oncol. 1988;11(6):618–22. https://www.ncbi.nlm.nih.gov/pubmed/3055932
24. Ahmad A. Pathways to breast cancer recurrence. ISRN Oncol. 2013;2013:290568. https://doi.org/10.1155/2013/290568.
25. Lafourcade A, His M, Baglietto L, Boutron-Ruault M-C, Dossus L, Rondeau V. Factors associated with breast cancer recurrences or mortality and dynamic prediction of death using history of cancer recurrences: the French E3N cohort. BMC

Cancer. 2018;18(1):171. https://doi.org/10.1186/s12885-018-4076-4.
26. Greenberg PA, Hortobagyi GN, Smith TL, Ziegler LD, Frye DK, Buzdar AU. Long-term follow-up of patients with complete remission following combination chemotherapy for metastatic breast cancer. J Clin Oncol. 1996;14(8):2197–205. https://doi.org/10.1200/JCO.1996.14.8.2197.
27. Hortobagyi GN. Can we cure limited metastatic breast cancer? J Clin Oncol. 2002;20(3):620–3. https://doi.org/10.1200/JCO.2002.20.3.620.
28. Sun Y-S, Zhao Z, Yang Z-N, et al. Risk factors and preventions of breast cancer. Int J Biol Sci. 2017;13(11):1387–97. https://doi.org/10.7150/ijbs.21635.
29. Landreneau FE, Landreneau RJ, Keenan RJ, Ferson PF. Diagnosis and management of spinal metastases from breast cancer. J Neuro-Oncol. 1995;23(2):121–34. https://doi.org/10.1007/bf01053417.
30. Levack P, Graham J, Collie D, et al. Don't wait for a sensory level--listen to the symptoms: a prospective audit of the delays in diagnosis of malignant cord compression. Clin Oncol (R Coll Radiol). 2002;14(6):472–80. https://doi.org/10.1053/clon.2002.0098.
31. Purushothamdas S, Quraishi N, Giannoulis K. Results of surgical management of metastatic spinal tumors based on an epidural spinal cord compression scale. Spine J. 2011;11(10):S79. https://doi.org/10.1016/j.spinee.2011.08.197.
32. Ju DG, Yurter A, Gokaslan ZL, Sciubba DM. Diagnosis and surgical management of breast cancer metastatic to the spine. World J Clin Oncol. 2014;5(3):263–71. https://doi.org/10.5306/wjco.v5.i3.263.
33. Schirrmeister H. Detection of bone metastases in breast cancer by positron emission tomography. PET Clin. 2006;1(1):25–32. https://doi.org/10.1016/j.cpet.2005.09.005.
34. Kawaguchi T, Koh Y, Ando M, et al. Prospective analysis of oncogenic driver mutations and environmental factors: Japan molecular epidemiology for lung cancer study. J Clin Oncol. 2016;34(19):2247–57. https://doi.org/10.1200/JCO.2015.64.2322.
35. Shi Y, Au JS-K, Thongprasert S, et al. A prospective, molecular epidemiology study of EGFR mutations in Asian patients with advanced non-small-cell lung cancer of adenocarcinoma histology (PIONEER). J Thorac Oncol. 2014;9(2):154–62. https://doi.org/10.1097/JTO.0000000000000033.
36. Bergethon K, Shaw AT, Ou S-HI, et al. ROS1 rearrangements define a unique molecular class of lung cancers. J Clin Oncol. 2012;30(8):863–70. https://doi.org/10.1200/JCO.2011.35.6345.
37. Chin LP, Soo RA, Soong R, Ou S-HI. Targeting ROS1 with anaplastic lymphoma kinase inhibitors: a promising therapeutic strategy for a newly defined molecular subset of non-small-cell lung cancer. J Thorac Oncol. 2012;7(11):1625–30. https://doi.org/10.1097/JTO.0b013e31826baf83.
38. Rimkunas VM, Crosby KE, Li D, et al. Analysis of receptor tyrosine kinase ROS1-positive tumors in non-small cell lung cancer: identification of a FIG-ROS1 fusion. Clin Cancer Res. 2012;18(16):4449–57. https://doi.org/10.1158/1078-0432.CCR-11-3351.
39. Shaw AT, Ou S-HI, Bang Y-J, et al. Crizotinib in ROS1-rearranged non-small-cell lung cancer. N Engl J Med. 2014;371(21):1963–71. https://doi.org/10.1056/NEJMoa1406766.
40. Drilon A, Somwar R, Wagner JP, et al. A novel crizotinib-resistant solvent-front mutation responsive to cabozantinib therapy in a patient with ROS1-rearranged lung cancer. Clin Cancer Res. 2016;22(10):2351–8. https://doi.org/10.1158/1078-0432.CCR-15-2013.
41. Kinno T, Tsuta K, Shiraishi K, et al. Clinicopathological features of nonsmall cell lung carcinomas with BRAF mutations. Ann Oncol Off J Eur Soc Med Oncol. 2014;25(1):138–42. https://doi.org/10.1093/annonc/mdt495.
42. Sequist LV, Heist RS, Shaw AT, et al. Implementing multiplexed genotyping of non-small-cell lung cancers into routine clinical practice. Ann Oncol Off J Eur Soc Med Oncol. 2011;22(12):2616–24. https://doi.org/10.1093/annonc/mdr489.
43. Paik PK, Arcila ME, Fara M, et al. Clinical characteristics of patients with lung adenocarcinomas harboring BRAF mutations. J Clin Oncol. 2011;29(15):2046–51. https://doi.org/10.1200/JCO.2010.33.1280.
44. Uei H, Tokuhashi Y, Maseda M. Treatment outcome of metastatic spine tumor in lung cancer patients: did the treatments improve their outcomes? Spine (Phila Pa 1976). 2017;42(24):E1446–51. https://doi.org/10.1097/BRS.0000000000002382.
45. Niu Y-J, Wen Y-T, Shen W-W, Deng L, Liu L-L, Zhang H-L. Risk factors for bone metastasis in patients with primary lung cancer: study protocol for a systematic review. BMJ Open. 2014;4(7):e005202. https://doi.org/10.1136/bmjopen-2014-005202.
46. al-Kattan K, Sepsas E, Fountain SW, Townsend ER. Disease recurrence after resection for stage I lung cancer. Eur J Cardiothorac Surg. 1997;12(3):380–4. https://doi.org/10.1016/s1010-7940(97)00198-x.
47. Carnio S, Novello S, Papotti M, Loiacono M, Scagliotti GV. Prognostic and predictive biomarkers in early stage non-small cell lung cancer: tumor based approaches including gene signatures. Transl Lung Cancer Res. 2013;2(5):372–81. https://doi.org/10.3978/j.issn.2218-6751.2013.10.05.
48. Cruz C, Afonso M, Oliveiros B, Pêgo A. Recurrence and risk factors for relapse in patients with non-small cell lung cancer treated by surgery with curative intent. Oncology. 2017;92(6):347–52. https://doi.org/10.1159/000458533.
49. Nakagawa M, Uramoto H, Oka S, et al. Clinical significance of IGF1R expression in non-small-cell lung cancer. Clin Lung Cancer. 2012;13(2):136–42. https://doi.org/10.1016/j.cllc.2011.10.006.

50. Oka S, Uramoto H, Chikaishi Y, et al. Abstract 1149: The expression of Ki-67, but not IGF1R, predicts a poor disease-free survival in patients with adenocarcinoma of the lung. Cancer Res. 2012;72(8 Supplement):1149 LP–1149. https://doi.org/10.1158/1538-7445.AM2012-1149.
51. Yoshino I, Yohena T, Kitajima M, et al. Survival of non-small cell lung cancer patients with post-operative recurrence at distant organs. Ann Thorac Cardiovasc Surg. 2001;7(4):204–9. https://www.ncbi.nlm.nih.gov/pubmed/11578260
52. Blandin Knight S, Crosbie PA, Balata H, Chudziak J, Hussell T, Dive C. Progress and prospects of early detection in lung cancer. Open Biol. 2017;7(9):170070. https://doi.org/10.1098/rsob.170070.
53. Milovanovic IS, Stjepanovic M, Mitrovic D. Distribution patterns of the metastases of the lung carcinoma in relation to histological type of the primary tumor: an autopsy study. Ann Thorac Med. 2017;12(3):191–8. https://doi.org/10.4103/atm.ATM_276_16.
54. da Cunha SG, Shepherd FA, Tsao MS. EGFR mutations and lung cancer. Annu Rev Pathol. 2011;6:49–69. https://doi.org/10.1146/annurev-pathol-011110-130206.
55. Chia PL, Mitchell P, Dobrovic A, John T. Prevalence and natural history of ALK positive non-small-cell lung cancer and the clinical impact of targeted therapy with ALK inhibitors. Clin Epidemiol. 2014;6:423–32. https://doi.org/10.2147/CLEP.S69718.
56. Davies KD, Doebele RC. Molecular pathways: ROS1 fusion proteins in cancer. Clin Cancer Res. 2013;19(15):4040–5. https://doi.org/10.1158/1078-0432.CCR-12-2851.
57. Boyle P, Chapman CJ, Holdenrieder S, et al. Clinical validation of an autoantibody test for lung cancer. Ann Oncol Off J Eur Soc Med Oncol. 2011;22(2):383–9. https://doi.org/10.1093/annonc/mdq361.
58. Chapman CJ, Healey GF, Murray A, et al. EarlyCDT®-Lung test: improved clinical utility through additional autoantibody assays. Tumour Biol. 2012;33(5):1319–26. https://doi.org/10.1007/s13277-012-0379-2.
59. James ND, de Bono JS, Spears MR, et al. Abiraterone for prostate cancer not previously treated with hormone therapy. N Engl J Med. 2017;377(4):338–51. https://doi.org/10.1056/NEJMoa1702900.
60. Fizazi K, Tran N, Fein L, et al. Abiraterone plus prednisone in metastatic, castration-sensitive prostate cancer. N Engl J Med. 2017;377(4):352–60. https://doi.org/10.1056/NEJMoa1704174.
61. Sweeney CJ, Chen Y-H, Carducci M, et al. Chemohormonal therapy in metastatic hormone-sensitive prostate cancer. N Engl J Med. 2015;373(8):737–46. https://doi.org/10.1056/NEJMoa1503747.
62. Kyriakopoulos CE, Chen Y-H, Carducci MA, et al. Chemohormonal therapy in metastatic hormone-sensitive prostate cancer: long-term survival analysis of the randomized phase III E3805 CHAARTED trial. J Clin Oncol. 2018;36(11):1080–7. https://doi.org/10.1200/JCO.2017.75.3657.
63. Kantoff PW, Higano CS, Shore ND, et al. Sipuleucel-T immunotherapy for castration-resistant prostate cancer. N Engl J Med. 2010;363(5):411–22. https://doi.org/10.1056/nejmoa1001294.
64. Parker C, Nilsson S, Heinrich D, et al. Alpha emitter radium-223 and survival in metastatic prostate cancer. N Engl J Med. 2013;369(3):213–23. https://doi.org/10.1056/nejmoa1213755.
65. Mahal BA, Butler S, Franco I, et al. Use of active surveillance or watchful waiting for low-risk prostate cancer and management trends across risk groups in the United States, 2010–2015. JAMA. 2019;321(7):704. https://doi.org/10.1001/jama.2018.19941.
66. Meng T, Chen R, Zhong N, et al. Factors associated with improved survival following surgical treatment for metastatic prostate cancer in the spine: retrospective analysis of 29 patients in a single center. World J Surg Oncol. 2016;14(1). https://doi.org/10.1186/s12957-016-0961-y.
67. Drzymalski DM, Oh WK, Werner L, Regan MM, Kantoff P, Tuli S. Predictors of survival in patients with prostate cancer and spinal metastasis. J Neurosurg Spine. 2010;13(6):789–94. https://doi.org/10.3171/2010.6.spine10167.
68. Robson M, Dawson N. How is androgen-dependent metastatic prostate cancer best treated? Hematol Oncol Clin North Am. 1996;10(3):727–47. https://doi.org/10.1016/s0889-8588(05)70364-6.
69. Ginzburg S, Nevers T, Staff I, et al. Prostate cancer biochemical recurrence rates after robotic-assisted laparoscopic radical prostatectomy. JSLS J Soc Laparoendosc Surg. 2012;16(3):443–50. https://doi.org/10.4293/108680812x13462882736538.
70. McCormick BZ, Mahmoud AM, Williams SB, Davis JW. Biochemical recurrence after radical prostatectomy: current status of its use as a treatment endpoint and early management strategies. Indian J Urol. 2019;35(1):6–17. https://doi.org/10.4103/iju.IJU_355_18.
71. Jeffers A, Sochat V, Kattan MW, et al. Predicting prostate cancer recurrence after radical prostatectomy. Prostate. 2016;77(3):291–8. https://doi.org/10.1002/pros.23268.
72. Sridharan S, Macias V, Tangella K, et al. Prediction of prostate cancer recurrence using quantitative phase imaging: Validation on a general population. Sci Rep. 2016;6(1). https://doi.org/10.1038/srep33818.
73. Cereceda LE, Flechon A, Droz J-P. Management of vertebral metastases in prostate cancer: a retrospective analysis in 119 patients. Clin Prostate Cancer. 2003;2(1):34–40. https://doi.org/10.3816/cgc.2003.n.010.

74. Sarkar S, Das S. A review of imaging methods for prostate cancer detection. Biomed Eng Comput Biol. 2016;7s1:BECB.S34255. https://doi.org/10.4137/becb.s34255.
75. Fottner A, Szalantzy M, Wirthmann L, et al. Bone metastases from renal cell carcinoma: patient survival after surgical treatment. BMC Musculoskelet Disord. 2010;11(1). https://doi.org/10.1186/1471-2474-11-145.
76. Angelov L, Chao S, Heng DY, Djemil T, Kolar M, Suh J. Stereotactic spine radiosurgery (SRS) for pain and tumor control in patients with spinal metastases from renal cell carcinoma: a prospective study. Int J Radiat Oncol. 2008;72(1):S489. https://doi.org/10.1016/j.ijrobp.2008.06.1437.
77. Motzer RJ. Prognostic factors for survival of patients with stage IV renal cell carcinoma: Memorial Sloan-Kettering Cancer Center experience. Clin Cancer Res. 2004;10(18):6302S–3S. https://doi.org/10.1158/1078-0432.ccr-040031.
78. Jonasch E, Gao J, Rathmell WK. Renal cell carcinoma. BMJ. 2014;349(nov10 11):g4797. https://doi.org/10.1136/bmj.g4797.
79. Fuchs B, Trousdale RT, Rock MG. Solitary bony metastasis from renal cell carcinoma. Clin Orthop Relat Res. 2005;NA;(431):187–192. https://doi.org/10.1097/01.blo.0000149820.65137.b4.
80. Flanigan RC, Salmon SE, Blumenstein BA, et al. Nephrectomy followed by interferon Alfa-2b compared with interferon Alfa-2b alone for metastatic renal-cell cancer. N Engl J Med. 2001;345(23):1655–9. https://doi.org/10.1056/nejmoa003013.
81. Mickisch GHJ, Garin A, van Poppel H, de Prijck L, Sylvester R. Radical nephrectomy plus interferon-alfa-based immunotherapy compared with interferon alfa alone in metastatic renal-cell carcinoma: a randomised trial. Lancet. 2001;358(9286):966–70. https://doi.org/10.1016/s0140-6736(01)06103-7.
82. Motzer RJ, Penkov K, Haanen J, et al. Avelumab plus Axitinib versus Sunitinib for advanced renal-cell carcinoma. N Engl J Med. 2019;380(12):1103–15. https://doi.org/10.1056/nejmoa1816047.
83. Rini BI, Plimack ER, Stus V, et al. Pembrolizumab plus Axitinib versus Sunitinib for advanced renal-cell carcinoma. N Engl J Med. 2019;380(12):1116–27. https://doi.org/10.1056/nejmoa1816714.
84. Janzen NK, Kim HL, Figlin RA, Belldegrun AS. Surveillance after radical or partial nephrectomy for localized renal cell carcinoma and management of recurrent disease. Urol Clin North Am. 2003;30(4):843–52. https://doi.org/10.1016/s0094-0143(03)00056-9.
85. Ljungberg A, Rasmuson R. Follow-up guidelines for nonmetastatic renal cell carcinoma based on the occurrence of metastases after radical nephrectomy. BJU Int. 2001;84(4):405–11. https://doi.org/10.1046/j.1464-410x.1999.00202.x.
86. Hafez KS, Novick AC, Campbell SC. Patterns of tumor recurrence and guidelines for followup after nephron sparing surgery for sporadic renal cell carcinoma. J Urol. 1997:2067–70. https://doi.org/10.1097/00005392-199706000-00008.
87. Sandock DS, Seftel AD, Resnick MI. A new protocol for the followup of renal cell carcinoma based on pathological stage. J Urol. 1995:28–31. https://doi.org/10.1097/00005392-199507000-00011.
88. Kroeger N, Choueiri TK, Lee J-L, et al. Survival outcome and treatment response of patients with late relapse from renal cell carcinoma in the era of targeted therapy. Eur Urol. 2014;65(6):1086–92. https://doi.org/10.1016/j.eururo.2013.07.031.
89. Bilsky MH, Laufer I, Fourney DR, et al. Reliability analysis of the epidural spinal cord compression scale. J Neurosurg Spine. 2010;13(3):324–8. https://doi.org/10.3171/2010.3.spine09459.
90. Manke C, Bretschneider T, Lenhart M, et al. Spinal metastases from renal cell carcinoma: effect of preoperative particle embolization on intraoperative blood loss. AJNR Am J Neuroradiol. 2001;22(5):997–1003. https://www.ncbi.nlm.nih.gov/pubmed/11337348
91. Woodward E, Jagdev S, McParland L, et al. Skeletal complications and survival in renal cancer patients with bone metastases. Bone. 2011;48(1):160–6. https://doi.org/10.1016/j.bone.2010.09.008.
92. Louie PK, Sayari AJ, Frank RM, An HS, Colman MW. Metastatic renal cell carcinoma to the spine and the extremities. JBJS Rev. 2019;7(9):e7. https://doi.org/10.2106/jbjs.rvw.19.00002.
93. Eeles RA, O'Brien P, Horwich A, Brada M. Non-Hodgkin's lymphoma presenting with extradural spinal cord compression: functional outcome and survival. Br J Cancer. 1991;63(1):126–9. https://doi.org/10.1038/bjc.1991.25.
94. Dürr H, Müller P, Hiller E, et al. Malignant lymphoma of bone. Arch Orthop Trauma Surg. 2001;122(1):10–6. https://doi.org/10.1007/s004020100316.
95. Perry JR, Deodhare SS, Bilbao JM, Murray D, Muller P. The significance of spinal cord compression as the initial manifestation of lymphoma. Neurosurgery. 1993;32(2):157–62. https://doi.org/10.1097/00006123-199302000-00001.
96. Flanagan EP, O'Neill BP, Porter AB, Lanzino G, Haberman TM, Keegan BM. Primary intramedullary spinal cord lymphoma. Neurology. 2011;77(8):784–91. https://doi.org/10.1212/wnl.0b013e31822b00b9.
97. Hashi S, Goodwin CR, Ahmed AK, Sciubba DM. Management of extranodal lymphoma of the spine: a study of 30 patients. CNS Oncol. 2018;7(2):CNS11. https://doi.org/10.2217/cns-2017-0033.
98. Vela D, Ribera JM, Florensa R, et al. Spinal cord compression in non-Hodgkin's lymphoma. A study of 10 patients TT – compresión medular en los linfomas no hodgkinianos. Estudio de 10 pacientes. Med Clin (Barc). 1997;109(10):375–7. https://www.ncbi.nlm.nih.gov/pubmed/9379720
99. Ferreri AJM, Blay J-Y, Reni M, et al. Prognostic scoring system for primary CNS lymphomas: the

International Extranodal Lymphoma Study Group experience. J Clin Oncol. 2003;21(2):266–72. https://doi.org/10.1200/jco.2003.09.139.
100. Epelbaum R, Haim N, Ben-Shahar M, Ben-Arie Y, Feinsod M, Cohen Y. Non-Hodgkin's lymphoma presenting with spinal epidural involvement. Cancer. 1986;58(9):2120–4. https://doi.org/10.1002/1097-0142(19861101)58:9<2120::aid-cncr2820580926>3.0.co;2-a.
101. Uehara M, Takahashi J, Hirabayashi H, et al. Hodgkin's disease of the thoracic vertebrae. Spine J. 2013;13(8):e59–63. https://doi.org/10.1016/j.spinee.2013.03.026.
102. Moussaly E, Nazha B, Zaarour M, Atallah JP. Primary non-Hodgkin's lymphoma of the spine: a case report and literature review. World J Oncol. 2015;6(5):459–63. https://doi.org/10.14740/wjon947w.
103. Durie BGM, Hoering A, Abidi MH, et al. Bortezomib with lenalidomide and dexamethasone versus lenalidomide and dexamethasone alone in patients with newly diagnosed myeloma without intent for immediate autologous stem-cell transplant (SWOG S0777): a randomised, open-label, phase 3 trial. Lancet. 2017;389(10068):519–27. https://doi.org/10.1016/s0140-6736(16)31594-x.
104. Facon T, Lee JH, Moreau P, et al. Carfilzomib or bortezomib with melphalan-prednisone for transplant-ineligible patients with newly diagnosed multiple myeloma. Blood. 2019;133(18):1953–63. https://doi.org/10.1182/blood-2018-09-874396.
105. Moreau P, Attal M, Hulin C, et al. Bortezomib, thalidomide, and dexamethasone with or without daratumumab before and after autologous stem-cell transplantation for newly diagnosed multiple myeloma (CASSIOPEIA): a randomised, open-label, phase 3 study. Lancet (London, England). 2019;394(10192):29–38. https://doi.org/10.1016/S0140-6736(19)31240-1.
106. Conyers R, Young S, Thomas DM. Liposarcoma: molecular genetics and therapeutics. Sarcoma. 2011;2011:1–13. https://doi.org/10.1155/2011/483154.
107. Kyle RA, Rajkumar SV. Multiple myeloma. N Engl J Med. 2004;351(18):1860–73. https://doi.org/10.1056/nejmra041875.
108. Fonseca R, Bergsagel PL, Drach J, et al. International Myeloma Working Group molecular classification of multiple myeloma: spotlight review. Leukemia. 2009;23(12):2210–21. https://doi.org/10.1038/leu.2009.174.
109. Narita T, Inagaki A, Kobayashi T, et al. t(14;16)-positive multiple myeloma shows negativity for CD56 expression and unfavorable outcome even in the era of novel drugs. Blood Cancer J. 2015;5(2):e285. https://doi.org/10.1038/bcj.2015.6.
110. Rajkumar SV, Dimopoulos MA, Palumbo A, et al. International Myeloma Working Group updated criteria for the diagnosis of multiple myeloma. Lancet Oncol. 2014;15(12):e538–48. https://doi.org/10.1016/s1470-2045(14)70442-5.
111. Siegel RL, Miller KD, Jemal A. Cancer statistics, 2016. CA Cancer J Clin. 2016;66(1):7–30. https://doi.org/10.3322/caac.21332.
112. Thorsteinsdottir S, Dickman PW, Landgren O, et al. Dramatically improved survival in multiple myeloma patients in the recent decade: results from a Swedish population-based study. Haematologica. 2018;103(9):e412–5. https://doi.org/10.3324/haematol.2017.183475.
113. Watanabe Y, Endou A, Ooi S, Matsushima E, Shimisu Y, Nakashima K. Extraosseous epidural IgD myeloma presenting with compression myelopathy. Psychiatry Clin Neurosci. 2000;54(6):665–7. https://doi.org/10.1046/j.1440-1819.2000.00767.x.
114. Lasocki A, Gaillard F, Harrison SJ. Multiple myeloma of the spine. Neuroradiol J. 2017;30(3):259–68. https://doi.org/10.1177/1971400917699426.
115. Edelstyn GA, Gillespie PJ, Grebbell FS. The radiological demonstration of osseous metastases. Experimental observations. Clin Radiol. 1967;18(2):158–62. https://doi.org/10.1016/s0009-9260(67)80010-2.
116. Regelink JC, Minnema MC, Terpos E, et al. Comparison of modern and conventional imaging techniques in establishing multiple myeloma-related bone disease: a systematic review. Br J Haematol. 2013;162(1):50–61. https://doi.org/10.1111/bjh.12346.
117. Stäbler A, Baur A, Bartl R, Munker R, Lamerz R, Reiser MF. Contrast enhancement and quantitative signal analysis in MR imaging of multiple myeloma: assessment of focal and diffuse growth patterns in marrow correlated with biopsies and survival rates. Am J Roentgenol. 1996;167(4):1029–36. https://doi.org/10.2214/ajr.167.4.8819407.
118. Dutoit JC, Verstraete KL. Whole-body MRI, dynamic contrast-enhanced MRI, and diffusion-weighted imaging for the staging of multiple myeloma. Skelet Radiol. 2017;46(6):733–50. https://doi.org/10.1007/s00256-017-2609-6.
119. Sachpekidis C, Hillengass J, Goldschmidt H, et al. Comparison of (18)F-FDG PET/CT and PET/MRI in patients with multiple myeloma. Am J Nucl Med Mol Imaging. 2015;5(5):469–78. https://www.ncbi.nlm.nih.gov/pubmed/26550538
120. Shah SN, Oldan JD. PET/MR imaging of multiple myeloma. Magn Reson Imaging Clin N Am. 2017;25(2):351–65. https://doi.org/10.1016/j.mric.2017.01.003.
121. Jones RL, Fisher C, Al-Muderis O, Judson IR. Differential sensitivity of liposarcoma subtypes to chemotherapy. Eur J Cancer. 2005;41(18):2853–60. https://doi.org/10.1016/j.ejca.2005.07.023.
122. Groves ML, Zadnik PL, Kaloostian P, et al. Epidemiologic, functional, and oncologic outcome analysis of spinal sarcomas treated surgi-

cally at a single institution over 10 years. Spine J. 2015;15(1):110–4. https://doi.org/10.1016/j.spinee.2014.07.005.
123. Schwab J, Gasbarrini A, Bandiera S, et al. Osteosarcoma of the mobile spine. Spine (Phila Pa 1976). 2012;37(6):E381–6. https://doi.org/10.1097/brs.0b013e31822fb1a7.
124. Bekiesinska-Figatowska M, Duczkowska A, Duczkowski M, et al. CNS metastases from bone and soft tissue sarcomas in children, adolescents, and young adults: are they really so rare? Biomed Res Int. 2017;2017:1–9. https://doi.org/10.1155/2017/1456473.
125. Raciborska A, Bilska K, Drabko K, et al. Validation of a multi-modal treatment protocol for Ewing sarcoma-A report from the polish pediatric oncology group. Pediatr Blood Cancer. 2014;61(12):2170–4. https://doi.org/10.1002/pbc.25167.
126. Rao G, Suki D, Chakrabarti I, et al. Surgical management of primary and metastatic sarcoma of the mobile spine. J Neurosurg Spine. 2008;9(2):120–8. https://doi.org/10.3171/spi/2008/9/8/120.
127. Woll PJ, Reichardt P, Le Cesne A, et al. Adjuvant chemotherapy with doxorubicin, ifosfamide, and lenograstim for resected soft-tissue sarcoma (EORTC 62931): a multicentre randomised controlled trial. Lancet Oncol. 2012;13(10):1045–54. https://doi.org/10.1016/s1470-2045(12)70346-7.
128. Merimsky O, Kollender Y, Bokstein F, et al. Radiotherapy for spinal cord compression in patients with soft-tissue sarcoma. Int J Radiat Oncol. 2004;58(5):1468–73. https://doi.org/10.1016/j.ijrobp.2003.09.026.
129. Sakellaridis N, Mahera H, Pomonis S. Hemangiopericytoma-like synovial sarcoma of the lumbar spine. J Neurosurg Spine. 2006;4(2):179–82. https://doi.org/10.3171/spi.2006.4.2.179.
130. Schwab JH, Boland P, Guo T, et al. Skeletal metastases in myxoid liposarcoma: an unusual pattern of distant spread. Ann Surg Oncol. 2007;14(4):1507–14. https://doi.org/10.1245/s10434-006-9306-3.
131. Dürr HR, Rauh J, Baur-Melnyk A, et al. Myxoid liposarcoma: local relapse and metastatic pattern in 43 patients. BMC Cancer. 2018;18(1). https://doi.org/10.1186/s12885-018-4226-8.
132. Ciftdemir M, Kaya M, Selcuk E, Yalniz E. Tumors of the spine. World J Orthop. 2016;7(2):109. https://doi.org/10.5312/wjo.v7.i2.109.
133. Schwab JH, Boland PJ, Antonescu C, Bilsky MH, Healey JH. Spinal metastases from myxoid liposarcoma warrant screening with magnetic resonance imaging. Cancer. 2007;110(8):1815–22. https://doi.org/10.1002/cncr.22992.
134. Nakanishi K, Kobayashi M, Nakaguchi K, et al. Whole-body MRI for detecting metastatic bone tumor: diagnostic value of diffusion-weighted images. Magn Reson Med Sci. 2007;6(3):147–55. https://doi.org/10.2463/mrms.6.147.

Modern Technical Concepts in Surgical Metastatic Disease

15

Michiel E. R. Bongers and Joseph H. Schwab

Introduction

Metastatic disease to the spine is generally not considered curable, and so treatment is intended to be palliative. Indications for surgery include symptomatic spinal cord compression in otherwise radioresistant tumors, as well as mechanical instability. The greatest advances in the technical application of surgery in the last few years have focused on less invasive techniques. These techniques have the theoretical advantage of less morbidity for the patient and presumed faster recovery. Another major advance has been in the more widespread acceptance of ablative technology in the management of bone tumors, which is now being used more commonly in the spine. The following section will review some of the modern techniques being employed in the management of spinal tumors.

M. E. R. Bongers · J. H. Schwab (✉)
Department of Orthopaedic Surgery, Orthopaedic Oncology Service, Massachusetts General Hospital – Harvard Medical School, Boston, MA, USA
e-mail: jhschwab@mgh.harvard.edu

A Brief History

Posterior decompression using laminectomies was the first choice of treatment for metastatic spinal disease prior to the 1980s. This procedure aimed to create space and alleviate pressure of the spinal cord, regardless of the location of the tumor [1, 2]. The surgical procedure, however, suffered from a low success rate, due to disappointing numbers of neurological improvement [1–6]. Radiotherapy became the main treatment for metastatic spinal disease after the finding that there is no gross difference in efficacy between treatment with laminectomy alone, laminectomy combined with radiotherapy, or radiotherapy alone [1, 2]. The introduction of new surgical approaches in the early 1990s, enabling surgeons to perform ventral vertebral body resections at the site of the spinal cord compression with subsequent stabilization, improved neurological status and quality of life [7, 8]. In 2005, Patchell et al. [9] demonstrated superiority of immediate circumferential decompression of the spinal cord and stabilization of the spine plus postoperative radiotherapy over a radiotherapy-only treatment in a randomized controlled trial. In the following years, the need for decompression and stabilization was repeatedly confirmed in patients with metastatic spinal disease in need for surgery [10, 11]. Aside from spinal cord compression, mechanical spinal instability is another important indication for which patients might need surgical correction. In 2010,

K. Singh, M. Colman (eds.), *Surgical Spinal Oncology*,
https://doi.org/10.1007/978-3-030-50722-0_15

the criteria for the Spinal Instability Neoplastic Score (SINS) were developed to guide physicians in the assessment of the relative stability of the neoplastic spine, which can aid in determining when to refer for surgical consultation [12]. The SINS criteria are based on six variables: location, pain, bone lesion quality, radiographic spinal alignment, amount of vertebral body collapse, and posterolateral involvement of the spinal elements [10, 12]. However, since the treatment of patients with metastatic spine disease progressively grew to a multidisciplinary approach, it could not be dictated by only the neurologic and mechanical considerations. Thus, the NOMS decision framework was introduced, in which Neurologic, Oncologic, Mechanical, and Systemic considerations together determine the optimal combination of treatments [13]. Through advancements in surgical techniques joined by its decreased morbidity, neurologic and mechanical issues are increasingly more manageable by minimally invasive surgery (MIS), while open procedures are often undesirable in view of oncologic and systemic considerations [14].

Minimally Invasive Surgery

Percutaneous Pedicle Screw Fixation

Percutaneous pedicle screw fixation (PPSF) is a minimally invasive technique that can be considered for patients with symptomatic spinal metastases suffering from instability without spinal cord compression. During the procedure, the patient is placed in the prone position, tending to preserve the sagittal alignment of the spine. Percutaneous screws can be inserted using image guidance either in the form of fluoroscopy or CT guidance. CT guidance includes the use of preoperative CT images or images obtained with CT at the time of surgery. The principle theoretical advantage of percutaneous screws is that they require less muscle dissection. This may lead to less postoperative pain. Screws can be placed with or without guidewires depending on the method one utilizes. If fluoroscopy is used, Jamshidi needles are used to develop a pilot hole in the pedicle through which the guidewire is placed. After the guidewire is placed, the Jamshidi is removed. If navigation is utilized with preoperative or intraoperative CT, guidewires may not be necessary. From a technical perspective, it is important to pay close attention to the trajectory of one's screw placement. This is particularly true at the most cephalad and caudal screws. One must avoid "hubbing" the screw directly on the cephalad adjacent facet joint. If the adjacent joint is incarcerated by the tulip of the screw, patients may experience chronic discomfort with extension. If one is using guidewires to place these screws, one must pay attention to avoid advancing the guidewire when passing the screw over the wire. This can occur when blood coats the guidewire and dries, which can lead to the screw "sticking" to the wire. The wire can then be inadvertently advanced through the vertebrae placing anterior structures at risk. Although there are no controlled studies, percutaneous screw placement has been associated with decreased postoperative pain and a high number of patients are ambulatory within three days after surgery [15–18]. In addition, the level IV evidence suggests that percutaneous screw placement may be associated with fewer complications than open placement.

Cement-Augmented Screws

Bone quality is often poor in patients with spinal metastases due to the metastases, comorbidities, and the deleterious effect on bone that some chemotherapeutic agents have such as doxorubicin as well as radiation. In addition, many patients with cancer have osteoporosis unrelated to their diagnosis of cancer. Revision surgery for instrumentation failure is a potential major burden for these patients. Optimal fixation of these constructs in the compromised spine is therefore crucial. The application of methyl methacrylate has long been used as a means to gain purchase in otherwise compromised bone. More recently, specialized screws have been developed that allow the injection of methyl methacrylate through the screws [19, 20]. More recent studies have suggested that the revision rate due to screw failure is decreased using these specialized screws [21].

Minimal Invasive Surgical Decompression

Patients with spinal cord compression - either due to propulsion of bony fragments secondary to vertebral collapse or by direct tumor extension - often require decompression surgery, especially when a neurologic deficit exists [22]. Surgery may be needed in these cases particularly if the tumor is not sensitive to conventional radiation, and there is insufficient space between the tumor and the spinal cord to allow for safe application of stereotactic radiosurgery. If the bony fragments are causing the pain, or the pain is otherwise related to instability, then radiation will not alleviate the symptoms since it will not improve the stability of the spine. Historically, one may approach the spine anteriorly. However, the anterior approach has been shown to be associated with increased blood loss, a longer surgical time, and increased morbidity [23]. Similarly, a posterior laminectomy without instrumentation was often found to be inadequate due to the introduction of kyphosis or inadequate anterior decompression. More recently, the use of a posterior only approach with instrumentation has gained in popularity. This approach allows 360-degree decompression of the spinal cord without the morbidity of an anterior approach [24]. In some cases, a less invasive or "minimally invasive" approach can be utilized. A smaller incision or use of a tubular retractor system is included in this category. The chief theoretical advantage of these approaches is that they involve less muscle dissection and therefore may be associated with less blood loss and less patient morbidity. These approaches are often combined with percutaneous pedicle screws. In some cases, less invasive approaches can be facilitated by using intraoperative navigation, which allows one to identify their anatomic location using the navigation.

Case Description

A 58-year-old male patient with non-small-cell lung carcinoma metastasized to T6 presented with increasing thoracic radiculopathy (Fig. 15.1).

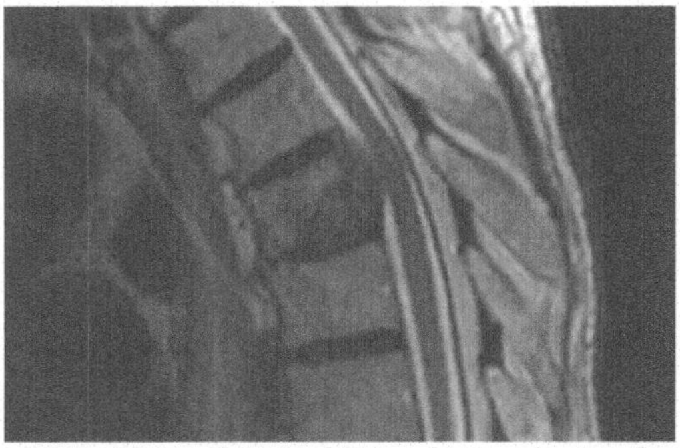

Fig. 15.1 Sagittal MRI image of lytic lesion to T6 compressing the spinal cord

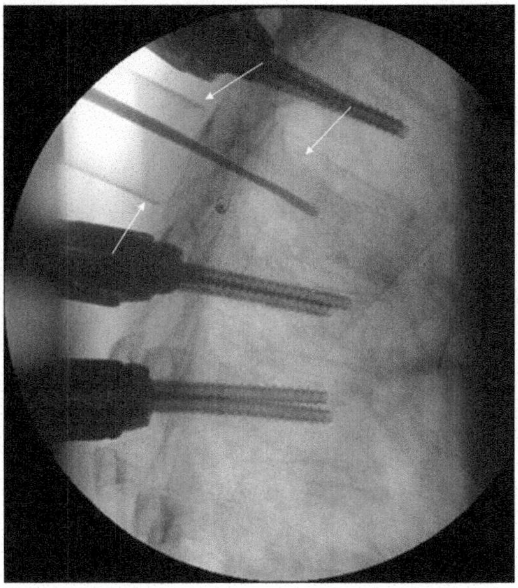

Fig. 15.2 Tubular decompression of thoracic spine (white arrows). Placement of percutaneous pedicle screw fixation

He underwent minimal invasive decompression through a tube (Fig. 15.2). Following decompression, percutaneous instrumentation was performed (Fig. 15.3).

Robot-Assisted Surgery

Robotic-assisted surgery is beginning to gain acceptance with its principle usage focused on instrumentation. It is likely that use of robotic-assisted instrumentation will be used to manage instrumentation needs in patients with metastasis. The principle disadvantage of robotic-assisted

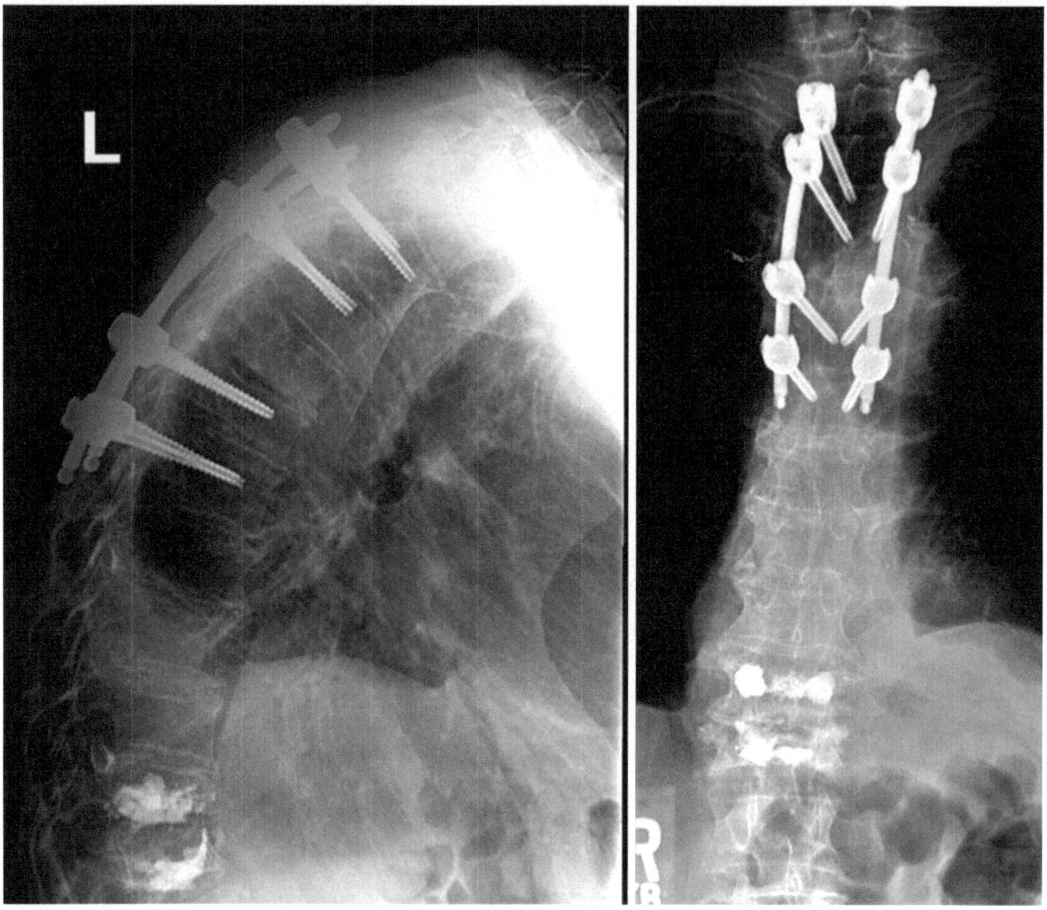

Fig. 15.3 Ultimate fixation using percutaneous pedicle screws

surgery is the high initial costs of the robot and the costs associated with developing a new operative workflow. The promise of robotic-assisted surgery lies in the marriage of preoperative planning with intraoperative navigation with a robotic arm that keeps these two entities dovetailed. While the initial attraction for surgeons will focus on instrumentation, it is likely that machine learning algorithms will develop, and other applications such as tumor resection will emerge. Capacity far beyond screw insertion is likely.

Ablative Technologies

Radiofrequency Ablation

Radiofrequency ablation (RFA) therapy can be a satisfying palliative alternative for the treatment of pain for patients with spinal metastases who have contraindications or are nonresponsive for radiation therapy. The principles of RFA rely on using the heat generated by a high-frequency alternating current that passes through a needle electrode into the tumor. The rapid fluctuation of the electromagnetic current causes water molecules to rapid change directions under the influence of the current. This leads to friction and ultimately tissue necrosis. This can be followed by the injection of bone cement to reestablish spinal stability depending on the tumor size. Retrospective analysis showed reduction in pain which was seen over multiple time points [25, 26]. Due to the fact that this procedure is percutaneous, it is usually not necessary to interrupt other ongoing systemic therapy as with open surgical approaches [27]. Reported complication rates differ from 0% to 7% and vary from puncture site hematoma to neurovascular injury [26, 27].

Cryoablation

Cryoablation is another form of thermal ablation. This technique uses extreme cold to cause tumor cell death. Insulated cryoprobes are inserted into the vertebral body tumor followed by the introduction of high-pressure argon gas through the probe. The quick expansion of the gas in the tip of the probe causes temperatures as low as −100° Celsius [28]. The margin of the treated area can be visualized by CT and MRI making this technique useful in metastases with critical surrounding structures – an advantage RFA lacks [28–30]. The cooling effect can penetrate deeper into bone than RFA, potentially affecting a larger tumor volume. Upon completion of the cooling phase and thus the ice-ball, helium is introduced generating heat into the tip of the cryoprobe. This causes an osmotic gradient and the cell absorbs an exceeding amount of extracellular fluid, ultimately bursting the tumor cell. When the procedure is completed and the tip is recovered to an appropriate temperature - guarding for iatrogenic damage to the healthy tissue - the cryoprobe is removed safely from the patient. Also in cryoablation, sometimes, cementoplasty or vertebroplasty is warranted to reestablish structural support. Retrospective studies have reported favorable pain reduction at different time points following the procedure, with decreased analgesics dosage. No postprocedural transient pain was seen, and there was no evidence of tumor progression in 96.7% [26, 30].

Microwave Ablation

The principles of microwave ablation (MWA) rely on the polarity of water molecules in cells. As the side of the two hydrogen molecules is charged positive and the oxygen side is charged negative, the oscillating microwave radiation causes the molecule to turn when passed through the tissue. Due to the fact that the microwaves have an extremely high frequency (9.2×10^8 Hz), the molecules turn around 2–5 billion times a second. The friction created by agitating the water molecules causes heat, which promotes coagulation necrosis in the cell [31]. There are multiple ways to administer MWA, but percutaneous is the least invasive. The microwave antenna is introduced using guided CT into the tumor, and through the not insulated, exposed part of the antenna, an electromagnetic microwave is radiated. Advantages of this procedure are that no grounding pads are required, higher intertumoral temperatures can be reached, larger tumor volumes can be ablated in quicker intervals, and it is possible to use multiple antennas simultaneously. However, due to the large defect left in the tissue after treatment, some form of stabilization such as with cement may be indicated. A disadvantage is that real-time visualization is not possible as in cryoablation. One study reported results on the use of MWA on painful extraspinal osseous metastases and states that 64 of the 65 patient (98%) had immediate pain relief, and local control was seen in 65% of the survivors after 20–24 weeks [32]. Another study with 17 patients with metastatic spine disease showed a significant decrease of pain immediately following the procedure, which was durable after 6 months of follow-up with all patients discontinuing opioid agents [33].

Future

The future of metastatic spine disease management will likely include a growing use of ablative technologies with less invasive operative techniques. Machine learning algorithms will also likely assist surgeons intraoperatively with and without the use of robotic arms.

The ablative technologies may be in the form of injectable radiation sensitizers. There is a growing interest in the use of systemic agents that by themselves do not have effective oncologic capacity; yet, they do seem to sensitize tumors to radiation. Ongoing preclinical work involving the injection of these radiation sensitizers suggests that the local delivery of these agents will help mitigate systemic side effects. These agents would be most useful in combination with stereotactic radiation.

Robot-assisted surgery will likely continue to gain acceptance particularly as other technologies marry with machine learning algorithms. For instance, preclinical probes are being developed that effectively identify tissue type based on electrochemical differences within tissue types. These probes will likely help robotic arms, which will use them in combination with embedded MRI or CT images to help guide surgical techniques. These same probes will prove to be useful to minimally invasive and/or endoscopic approaches in helping surgeons identify nerve tissues versus disc tissues, for example.

Machine learning algorithms will likely continue to help surgeons as decision aids. Several machine learning algorithms have been used to predict survival in spinal metastasis. These studies are now being validated in other patient populations, and they are available online (www.SORG-AI.com). These types of machine-learning-based decision aids will assist in decision-making, as they will provide more reliable probabilities of adverse events, survival, and overall outcomes [34–38].

References

1. Klimo PJ, Schmidt MH. Surgical management of spinal metastases. Oncologist. 2004;9:188–96.
2. Findlay G. Occasional review adverse effects of the management of malignant spinal cord compression. J Neurol Neurosurg Psychiatry. 1984;47:761–8.
3. Perese DM. Treatment of metastatic extradural spinal cord tumors. A series of 30 cases. Cancer. 1958;11(1):214–21.
4. Arseni CN, Simionescu MD, Horwath L. Tumors of the spine. A follow-up study of 350 patients with neurosurgical considerations. Acta Psychiatr Scand. 1959;34(4):398–410.
5. Black P. Spinal metastasis. Neurosurgery. 1979;5(6):726–46.
6. Young RF, Post EM, King GA. Treatment of spinal epidural metastases. Randomized prospective comparison of laminectomy and radiotherapy. J Neurosurg. 1980;53(6):741–8.
7. Gokaslan ZL, York JE, Walsh GL, et al. Transthoracic vertebrectomy for metastatic spinal tumors. J Neurosurg. 1998;89(4):599–609.
8. Hosono N, Yonenobu K, Fuji T, Ebara S, Yamashita K, Ono K. Orthopaedic management of spinal metastases. Clin Orthop Relat Res. 1995;312:148–59.
9. Patchell RA, Tibbs PA, Regine WF, et al. Direct decompressive surgical resection in the treatment of spinal cord compression caused by metastatic cancer: a randomised trial. Lancet (London, England). 366(9486):643–8.
10. Fourney DR, Frangou EM, Ryken TC, et al. Spinal instability neoplastic score: an analysis of reliability and validity from the Spine Oncology Study Group. J Clin Oncol. 2011;29:3072–7.
11. Sciubba DM, Petteys RJ, Dekutoski MB, et al. Diagnosis and management of metastatic spine disease. A review. J Neurosurg Spine. 2010;13(1):94–108.
12. Fisher CG, Dipaola CP, Ryken TC, et al. A novel classification system for spinal instability in neoplastic disease: an evidence-based approach and expert consensus from the spine oncology study group. Spine (Phila Pa 1976). 2010;35(22):E1221–9.
13. Laufer I, Rubin DG, Lis E, et al. The NOMS framework: approach to the treatment of spinal metastatic tumors. Oncologist. 2013;18(6):744–51.
14. Molina CA, Gokaslan ZL, Sciubba DM. A systematic review of the current role of minimally invasive spine surgery in the management of metastatic spine disease. Int J Surg Oncol. 2011;2011:598148.
15. Schwab JH, Gasbarrini A, Cappuccio M, et al. Clinical study minimally invasive posterior stabilization improved ambulation and pain scores in patients with plasmacytomas and/or metastases of the spine. Int J Surg Oncol. 2011;2011:239230.
16. Versteeg AL, Verlaan JJ, de Baat P, et al. Complications after percutaneous pedicle screw fixation for the treatment of unstable spinal metastases. Ann Surg Oncol. 2016;23(7):2343–9.
17. Hamad A, Vachtsevanos L, Cattell A, Ockendon M, Balain B. Minimally invasive spinal surgery for the management of symptomatic spinal metastasis. Br J Neurosurg. 2017;31(5):526–30.
18. Uei H, Tokuhashi Y, Maseda M, et al. Comparison between minimally invasive spine stabilization with and without posterior decompression for the management of spinal metastases: a retrospective cohort study. J Orthop Surg Res. 2018;13(1):87.
19. Elder BD, Lo S-FL, Holmes C, et al. The biomechanics of pedicle screw augmentation with cement. Spine J. 2015;15(6):1432–45.
20. Frankel BM, Jones T, Wang C. Segmental polymethylmethacrylate-augmented pedicle screw fixation in patients with bone softening caused by osteoporosis and metastatic tumor involvement: a clinical evaluation. Neurosurgery. 2007;61:531–7.
21. Barzilai O, McLaughlin L, Lis E, Reiner AS, Bilsky MH, Laufer I. Utility of cement augmentation via percutaneous fenestrated pedicle screws for stabilization of cancer-related spinal instability. Oper Neurosurg (Hagerstown, Md). 2019;16(5):593–9.
22. Cameron Hatrick N, Lucas JD, Timothy AR, Smith MA. The surgical treatment of metastatic disease of the spine. Radiother Oncol. 2000;56(3):335–9.

23. Donnelly DJ, Abd-El-Barr MM, Lu Y. Minimally invasive muscle sparing posterior-only approach for lumbar circumferential decompression and stabilization to treat spine metastasis--technical report. World Neurosurg. 2015;84(5):1484–90.
24. Saigal R, Wadhwa R, Mummaneni PV, Chou D. Minimally invasive extracavitary transpedicular corpectomy for the management of spinal tumors introduction: nature of the problem. Neurosurg Clin N Am. 2014;25(2):305–15.
25. Goetz MP, Callstrom MR, Charboneau JW, et al. Percutaneous image-guided radiofrequency ablation of painful metastases involving bone: a multicenter study. J Clin Oncol. 2004;22:300–6.
26. Lee S-K, Weiss B, Yanamadala V, Brook A. Percutaneous interventional management of spinal metastasis goals and treatment options for spinal metastatic lesion. Semin Interv Radiol. 2019;36:249–54.
27. Wallace XAN, Tomasian XA, Vaswani XD, Vyhmeister XR, Chang XRO, Jennings XJW. Radiographic local control of spinal metastases with percutaneous radiofrequency ablation and vertebral augmentation. AJNR Am J Neuroradiol. 2016;37(4):759–65.
28. Kurup AN, Callstrom MR. Ablation of skeletal metastases: current status. J Vasc Interv Radiol. 2010;21(8 Suppl):S242–50.
29. Saliken JC, McKinnon JG, Gray R. CT for monitoring cryotherapy. Am J Roentgenol. 1996;166(4):853–5.
30. Tomasian XA, Wallace XA, Northrup XB, Hillen TJ, Jennings XJW. Spine cryoablation: pain palliation and local tumor control for vertebral metastases. AJNR Am J Neuroradiol. 2016;37(1):189–95.
31. Simon CJ, Dupuy DE, Mayo-Smith WW. Oncologic interventions microwave ablation: principles and applications. Radiographics. 2005;25(Suppl 1):S69–83.
32. Deib G, Deldar B, Hui F, Barr JS, Khan MA. Percutaneous Microwave Ablation and Cementoplasty: Clinical Utility in the Treatment of Painful Extraspinal Osseous Metastatic Disease and Myeloma. Am J Roentgenol. 2019;212(6):1377–84.
33. Kastler A, Alnassan H, Aubry S, Kastler B. Microwave thermal ablation of spinal metastatic bone tumors. J Vasc Interv Radiol. 2014;25(9):1470–5.
34. Karhade AV, Thio QCBS, Ogink PT, et al. Predicting 90-day and 1-year mortality in spinal metastatic disease: development and internal validation. Neurosurgery. 2019;85(4):E671–81.
35. Karhade AV, Ahmed AK, Pennington Z, et al. External validation of the SORG 90-day and one-year machine learning algorithms for survival in spinal metastatic disease. Spine J. 2020;20(1):14–21.
36. Karhade AV, Shin JH, Schwab JH. Prognostic models for spinal metastatic disease: evolution of methodologies, limitations, and future opportunities. Ann Transl Med. 2019;7(10):219.
37. Karhade AV, Thio QCBS, Kuverji M, Ogink PT, Ferrone ML, Schwab JH. Prognostic value of serum alkaline phosphatase in spinal metastatic disease. Br J Cancer. 2019;120(6):640–6.
38. Karhade AV, Thio QCBS, Ogink PT, et al. Development of machine learning algorithms for prediction of 30-day mortality after surgery for spinal metastasis. Neurosurgery. 2019;85(1):E83–91.

Radiotherapy in Metastatic Spinal Disease

16

Mehee Choi, Dian Wang, and Aidnag Z. Diaz

Introduction

Spinal metastases occur in 30–40% of all cancer patients [1, 2]. Certain cancers, such as prostate, breast, and melanoma, display predilection for bone involvement, with more than one-half of patients with these cancers developing spinal metastases over the course of their illness [3]. Metastatic disease in the spine leads to spinal instability, neurological deficits, and pain. Metastatic epidural spinal cord compression (ESCC) affects 5–10% of all cancer patients and up to 40% of those with other bony metastases [4–6]. Approximately 20,000 patients present each year with spinal cord compression at the time of cancer diagnosis in the United States [7, 8], with the Inpatient Sample database reporting more than 8000 annual admissions for malignant spinal cord compression [9].

Therapeutic intervention can alleviate pain, preserve or improve neurologic function, achieve mechanical stability, optimize local tumor control, and improve quality of life. In addition to medical treatment for the systemic burden of disease, numerous surgical and radiotherapeutic strategies have been employed. In a randomized controlled study of surgical decompression with conventional radiotherapy (30 Gy in ten fractions) compared with radiotherapy alone for metastatic ESCC secondary to solid malignancies, Patchell et al. [10] demonstrated superiority of a combined surgical and radiotherapeutic approach for the maintenance and recovery of ambulation, duration of ambulation, functional ability, maintenance of continence, and survival. Since the time of this landmark study, therapeutic modalities and treatment strategies have continued to evolve.

Presentation

Early diagnosis of metastatic spinal disease is important because functional outcome depends on neurologic and mechanical condition at the time of presentation. Back pain, the most common presenting symptom in patients with metastatic tumor to the bone or epidural space, often precedes the development of other neurologic symptoms by weeks or months. Two distinct types of back pain are encountered in patients

M. Choi
Department of Radiation Oncology, Rush Copley, Chicago, IL, USA

D. Wang
Department of Radiation Oncology, Rush University Medical Center, Chicago, IL, USA
e-mail: Dian_Wang@rush.edu

A. Z. Diaz (✉)
Department of Radiation Medicine, University of Arizona Cancer Center at Dignity Health, Phoenix, AZ, USA
e-mail: Aidnag.Diaz@dignityhealth.org

K. Singh, M. Colman (eds.), *Surgical Spinal Oncology*,
https://doi.org/10.1007/978-3-030-50722-0_16

with spinal tumors: tumor-related and mechanical. Tumor-related pain is predominantly nocturnal or early morning pain and generally improves with activity during the day. This pain may be caused by inflammatory mediators or tumor stretching the periosteum of the vertebral body [11]. Tumor-related pain generally responds to administration of low-dose steroids. Definitive treatment of the underlying tumor with radiation or surgery often relieves tumor-related pain. Recurrence of pain following treatment may be a harbinger of locally recurrent tumor. Mechanical pain results from a structural abnormality of the spine, such as a pathologic compression fracture resulting in instability. This pain is movement-related and may be exacerbated by sitting or standing, which increases the axial load on the spine. Mechanical pain does not typically respond to steroids, and while it may be ameliorated with narcotics or bracing, often surgical intervention is required to improve mechanical stability.

Pathologic compression fractures often present with acute pain, which typically resolves slowly with or without bracing, unless progressive mechanical deformity occurs. Neurologic symptoms and signs often manifest with radiculopathy (nerve root symptoms) or myelopathy (spinal cord compression) depending on the extent and location of compression. Radiculopathy in the cervical or lumbar spine causes pain or weakness in the upper or lower extremity, respectively, while in the thoracic spine, radiculopathy occurs as a band-like pain at a segmental level. Some patients develop a mechanical radiculopathy resulting from instability and neuroforaminal compression by tumor. This pain occurs when bearing weight and is relieved by lying down. It is often accompanied by mechanical back pain. Myelopathy may manifest subtly, with discoordination and reflex finding such as hyperreflexia, a Babinski reflex, or clonus. More severe variants can include weakness, proprioceptive sensory loss, and loss of pain and temperature below the level of the spinal cord compression. Autonomic dysfunction may result from spinal cord compression or cauda equina compression. Painless urinary retention may suggest a neurologic cause, but obstructive GU system abnormalities can also be an explanation [12]. Specific spinal cord syndromes such as conus medullaris syndrome may present with minimal pain and with isolated loss of bowel and bladder function. Additionally, isolated sacral involvement, especially of the low sacral nerve roots, may present without pain.

Evaluation

Imaging

Advances in imaging have improved the sensitivity of detecting spinal metastases and the specificity of differentiating from other processes that involve the spine. Magnetic resonance imaging (MRI) has revolutionized assessment of metastatic spinal tumor, but other imaging modalities, including plain radiographs, bone scan, computerized tomography (CT) scan, myelogram, and positron emission topography (PET), still play a role in evaluating patients. The goal of imaging is to be as sensitive and specific as possible in identifying tumor, give precise anatomic detail, identify distant metastases, and show recurrent tumor following the placement of instrumentation.

Until MRI became widely available, myelogram and CT scan were the best diagnostic modalities for assessing acute spinal cord compression. MRI is the most sensitive and specific modality for imaging spinal metastases. Sagittal screening images of the entire spine reveal bone, epidural, and paraspinal tumor. The extent and degree of spinal cord compression can be readily appreciated [13].

Imaging sequences used to evaluate spinal metastases typically are T1- and T2-weighted. Tumor on a T1-weighted image is hypointense relative to the normal marrow signal. The ports from prior spinal radiation can be discerned on T1-weighted images as hyperintense signal change and may assist in making acute therapeutic decisions when radiation port films are not available. Tumor is hyperintense relative to marrow on standard T2-weighted imaging and produces a myelogram effect with cerebrospinal fluid appearing hyperintense. STIR images show enhanced contrast between the lipid marrow (hypointense) and tumor (hyperintense) [14–16]. Short tau inversion recovery (STIR) technique images may be the most sensitive screening modality for tumor, but give less anatomic detail than standard T1 or fast spin echo T2 images [17].

NOMS

The ESCC scale provides a common vocabulary to describe and stratify patients on the basis of the degree of epidural tumor extension [18]. Tumors confined to bone (stage 0) and tumors with minor epidural extension without abutment or compression of the spinal cord (stages Ia and Ib) have the requisite separation from the spinal cord to be safely treated with stereotactic radiosurgery (SRS). These tumors are classified as low-grade ESCC. In contrast, tumors displacing or compressing the spinal cord (stages II and III, respectively) are classified as high-grade ESCC and require resection of the epidural component to separate the tumor from the spinal cord prior to SRS. The ESCC scale has good-to-excellent intra- and inter-rater reliability scores. The ESCC scale represents 1 of the 4 considerations in the neurological, oncological, mechanical, and systemic (NOMS) algorithm. Bilsky and Smith [19] published the NOMS system, which incorporates multiple factors, including (1) neurological examination, degree of spinal cord compression on imaging; (2) tumor sensitivity to radiation (oncological); (3) presence or absence of spinal instability; and (4) systemic burden of metastatic disease.

The NOMS framework allows the determination of the optimal combination and type of treatment modalities for each patient by integrating neurological (N), oncological (O), mechanical (M), and systemic (S) considerations [20]. The neurological consideration includes the degree of radiographic ESCC and a clinical determination of neurological symptomatology attributable to spinal cord or nerve root compression, while the oncological consideration relies on tumor histology to classify tumors into either radioresistant or radiosensitive pathology. Breast, prostate, ovarian, and neuroendocrine tumors are generally considered radiosensitive, while renal, thyroid, hepatocellular, colon, non-small-cell lung carcinoma, sarcoma, and melanoma tend to be more radioresistant. Patients with radiosensitive tumors are generally treated with cEBRT regardless of ESCC, achieving good local control. By contrast, radioresistant tumors benefit from stereotactic radiosurgery (SRS) for local control if not diffusely disseminated.

The mechanical consideration serves as an independent surgical indication. In 2010, the Spine Oncology Study Group published the Spinal Instability Neoplasia Score (SINS) [21]. This system has been shown to be reliable among surgical and nonsurgical oncologic specialists [22–24]. Patients with mechanical instability often require stabilization. The spinal column may be stabilized using open or percutaneously placed instrumentation in addition to cement augmentation. The Spinal Instability Neoplastic Score is a validated decision-making tool that facilitates the diagnosis of instability [25, 26]. Factors reflecting and governing stability – including tumor-level biomechanics (with increased instability with junctional or mobile spine disease over semi-rigid thoracic or rigid sacral involvement), the presence of pain, bony lysis, vertebral body collapse, posterolateral element involvement, or frank misalignment – are tallied and weighted to provide a score classified into stable, unstable, or indeterminate categories. For patients with an indeterminate or unstable score, surgical referral is indicated.

Under the NOMS framework, patients who should be considered for surgery are those who have high-grade spinal cord compression and/or spinal instability. For very radiosensitive histologies such as lymphoma, myeloma, or seminoma, even high-grade compression may be treated with radiotherapy alone in many centers. The need for urgent surgery in other settings along with the knowledge of a high rate of local tumor control with SRS led to the concept of "separation surgery" in patients with high-grade metastatic epidural spinal cord compression [27]. The goal of separation surgery is to limit the amount of tumor resection needed by creating a tumor-free margin around the thecal sac in order to reconstitute its normal shape and the CSF interval between the cord and sac. Postoperative SRS is then used to treat the remaining spinal tumor.

Treatment

Mechanical Stabilization

Currently, the two main indications for primary surgical intervention are decompression of the spinal cord and stabilization of the spine if there is evidence of instability. There are a range of options for vertebral column reconstruction after tumor resection that have been developed over the last several decades, with many viable solutions. Relatively newer methods of providing vertebral column support for pathologic vertebral body fractures are vertebroplasty and kyphoplasty. Vertebroplasty was first described in the late 1980s [28] followed by kyphoplasty a decade later [29, 30]. For each procedure, polymethylmethacrylate is injected into the fractured vertebral body via a percutaneous transpedicular approach. Kyphoplasty has the additional step of inflating a balloon in the vertebral body to create a cavity prior to cement injection, which can theoretically help reduce kyphotic deformity and increase the overall cement volume injected without extravasation. These benefits are controversial and have not necessarily been borne out by data. Both procedures have been shown to improve pain scores (visual analog scale), reduce narcotic usage, and improve quality of life [31]. These procedures can be particularly useful as an adjunct prior to SRS [32], both to relieve mechanical back pain and to provide mechanical stability.

Radiation Therapy

Radiation therapy (RT) is a well-established treatment for metastases to the spine. Local radiation is delivered with the goal of palliation of pain, prevention of disease progression, and stopping or reversing neurological compromise. Radiation Therapy Oncology Group (RTOG) 9714 compared protracted (30 Gy per ten fractions) versus single fraction (8 Gy) standard radiation regimens and reported that the 3-month pain response was only 66%, with no significant difference in pain relief, which begs the question whether that can be improved upon and, if so, whether stereotactic body radiotherapy (SBRT) could be the treatment to do so [33].

Pain from spinal metastasis can be alleviated by radiation therapy through a combination of various mechanisms. Radiation can mechanically improve pain by decreasing pressure on the spinal cord, bone, and spinal nerves as the tumor shrinks. It can also decrease pain by reducing the inflammation caused by the growing tumor's interaction with the bone matrix. Lastly, it can improve pain by allowing the bone-healing processes to proceed unimpeded by active tumor cells.

Single-Fraction Stereotactic Radiation Therapy

SBRT involves the precise delivery of high dose per fraction RT to extracranial tumors. Its predecessor, stereotactic radiosurgery (SRS) to the brain, was first described by Leksell in 1951 and utilized a collimator helmet rigidly fixed to the skull for precise target localization accuracy in order to deliver a single high dose of radiation to the brain [34, 35]. Although the spine shares some advantages with the brain as a treatment target, SBRT did not emerge until around 40 years later due to limitations in immobilization and localization outside the cranium, as well as treatment planning technology [36]. CyberKnife system was the first advanced SRS platform applied to the treatment of spine tumors [37]. There have been many iterations of this technology since then, with impressive local tumor control rates of over 90% when used as the primary treatment modality for metastatic spine tumors. In 2007, Gerszten et al. [38] published the results of a series of 500 metastases to the spine in 393 patients who underwent spinal radiosurgery; they excluded patients with neurological deficits or spinal instability. The results were particularly encouraging, with high rates of long-term pain control (86%) and long-term tumor control (90%).

The efficacy of SRS and SBRT lies in the ability to deliver highly ablative doses to the spine while limiting normal tissue radiation exposure with the help of image-guided technology. Recent studies of survivors with metastatic disease living longer than 5 years report local tumor control rates of over 80% following high-dose, single-fraction RT. [39] At the present time, there are no randomized trials confirming the superiority of single-fraction radiosurgery to SBRT. However, it is posited that exposing tumors to a dose per fraction of at least 8 Gy may active radiobiological pathways leading to tumor cell death through mechanisms apart from mitotic catastrophe and apoptosis [40]. The dominant form of cell death when irradiated with conventional methods is apoptosis. Proposed mechanisms of increased cell death with SBRT include radiation-induced tumor antigen-specific immune response, endothelial/vascular injury, or increased cell kill secondary to higher delivered dose [41–49]. Preclinical studies support the hypothesis that radiation-induced immunogenic tumor cell death contributes to an in situ vaccine [50, 51]. This idea has been further expanded with evidence showing radiation induces an immunogenic tumor cell death and alters the tumor microenvironment to enhance recruitment of antitumor T cells [52–54].

Single-fraction treatment is often used for patients with early-stage disease who have either radioresistant histology or favorable prognosis or both that is, those likely to live long enough to experience the benefits of an ablative treatment over a conventionally fractionated palliative one. Good candidates would typically not have high-grade epidural cord compression and have not received prior RT to the same region because spinal cord integrity may be further endangered either from short-term tumor swelling or from the radiation itself. In cases that do not fit these criteria, hypofractionated or conventional treatment is generally more appropriate.

Memorial Sloan Kettering Cancer Center (MSKCC) currently utilizes 24 Gy as the standard single-fraction spine SBRT dose [55]. Their most recent outcomes reported by Yamada et al. consisted of 811 spine metastases in 657 patients, treated to a median of 24 Gy (range 16–26 Gy). With a median follow-up of 26.9 months, local failure was <1% and 3.1% at 12 and 48 months, respectively. With subgroup analysis of lesions receiving lower (median 17.09 Gy to the gross tumor volume [GTV]) and higher doses (median 23.56 Gy to the GTV), local failure rates were 14% and 2.1% at 12 and 48 months, respectively, suggesting a benefit of higher doses that was independent of histology [55].

Another large institutional experience from University of Pittsburgh Medical Center (UPMC) was reported in 2007 and consisted of 500 spinal metastases treated with single-fraction radiation doses ranging from 12.5 to 25 Gy (mean 20 Gy, median 19 Gy). Eighty-six percent experienced long-term pain control, and long-term tumor control was achieved in 90% of lesions treated upfront and 88% of lesions that had been previously irradiated [38]. A phase I/II study from University of Texas MD Anderson Cancer Center (MDACC) consisted of 61 patients treated with single-fraction doses of 16 of 18 Gy to the clinical target volume (CTV)/GTV for nonrenal cell histologies (30 lesions) and 16 of 24 Gy to the CTV/GTV for renal cell histology (33 lesions). At a mean follow-up of 20 months, they found 88% and 64% 18-month local control (LC) and overall survival (OS), respectively, with only two patients experiencing grade 2 or higher side effects [56].

Fractionated Stereotactic Radiation Therapy

Intensity-modulated radiation therapy (IMRT), developed in the 1980s to 1990s, and more recently volumetric-modulated arc therapy (VMAT) in particular have allowed for more conformal dose planning than was previously possible with conventional linear accelerator-based treatment, allowing safe delivery of ablative doses while sparing the spinal cord and other neighboring structures [57]. As a result, high-dose treatment can be delivered to the spine in short courses of 1–5 fractions, that is, SBRT and is now used in a variety of clinical settings including for metastatic disease and primary tumors of the spine.

The most common application of spine SBRT is for metastatic disease, which represents over 90% of all spinal tumors [58]. The utilization of spine SBRT for metastatic disease has increased significantly since the early 2000s [59]. As noted earlier, there are radiobiological advantages to higher dose per fraction and shorter overall treatment times, in that tumors are more likely to be ablated. This may result in more sustained pain control and less likelihood of the need for retreatment, which is especially important as new therapies continue to increase the life expectancy of patients with certain metastatic cancers [33, 60–63].

While the clinical use of SBRT continues to expand, it is important to point out that not every spinal metastasis is amenable to spine SBRT, and for some it is simply not necessary when conventional fractionation would be sufficiently effective [20, 59]. The Spinal Instability Neoplastic Score (SINS) is a validated tool to help assess the degree of mechanical instability [25]. Systemic disease is also assessed, taking into account projected survival and likelihood of tolerating the treatment.

Postoperative Radiosurgery

If a cord compression has been relieved and a greater distance has been created between the vertebral body and the cord itself, hypofractionation or even single-fraction treatment may become feasible when it had not been previously. The largest study of postoperative SBRT to the spine is the retrospective report by Laufer et al. of 186 patients treated with 24 Gy in a single fraction, 27–30 Gy in three fractions, termed "high-dose hypofractionation," or 18–26 Gy in five to six fractions, termed "low-dose hypofractionation." Overall rate of local progression was 16.4% at 1 year for SRS, 4.1% in the high-dose hypofractionation group and 22.6% in the low-dose hypofractionation group ($P = 0.04$) [20]. A review by Redmond et al. estimated the crude LC following postoperative SBRT to be 88.6% (range 70–100%) based on a combined 426 patients [64]. Tao et al. also evaluated the postoperative patients treated on the phase I/II trials at MDACC, not included in the prior review, and found 85% LC and 74% OS at 1 year [65]. Massicotte et al. described ten patients treated using a minimal access spine surgery followed by SBRT, which resulted in 70% LC and 80% OS at a median of 13 months [66].

Separation Surgery

The goals of separation surgery include epidural decompression and spinal stabilization without gross total or en bloc tumor resection [67]. This is most useful if the patient is a candidate for SBRT since a minimum physical separation of between 3 and 5 mm between the cord and the tumor is needed to allow for adequate dose falloff, particularly in those patients that have received prior radiotherapy to the spinal cord. Generally, instrumented stabilization is performed prior to decompression in order to avoid the manipulation of hardware across an open spinal canal. Partial corpectomy may be performed to facilitate decompression without aggressive attempts for gross total tumor or vertebral body resection. As a result, anterior constructs are rarely required. In cases with severe vertebral body destruction, anterior reconstruction may be carried out using polymethylmethacrylate with Steinmann pins; alternatively, polyether ether ketone or titanium cage placement can also be used with this posterolateral approach [67].

Reirradiation

In the aforementioned study of 500 patients treated at UPMC, 69% were undergoing reirradiation, and in that subgroup, LC remained high at 88% with long-term pain control of 86% [38]. Damast et al. evaluated 94 patients who had experienced in-field recurrences after 30 Gy delivered in ten fractions. These patients were then treated with either a more traditional 20 Gy in five fractions or a more aggressive 30 Gy in five fractions. Local failure was significantly reduced with the higher doses, 45% versus 26% at 1 year ($P = 0.04$), and no patients developed myelopathy [68]. Another study of reirradiation in 215 patients at seven institutions incorporated a heterogeneous mix of prior treatment and retreatment regimes. The median prior dosing was 30 Gy in ten fractions with a median retreatment dosing of 18 Gy in one fraction, given at a median of 13.1 months after prior RT. At 6 and 12 months, LC remained high at 93% and 83%, respectively [69]. A prospective study of reirradiation was performed at MDACC including 59 patients and utilized dosing of 30 Gy in five fractions or 27 Gy in three fractions. At a mean follow-up of 17.6 months, 1-year LC and survival were both 76% and freedom from neurologic deterioration was 92% at 1 year [70]. Considering that patients undergoing reirradiation are a generally less favorable group than those undergoing de novo treatment, a median LC rate of 76% (range 66–90%) in retreated patients reported by one review paper as well as improvement in pain scores from 65% to 81% are certainly encouraging [71].

Toxicity

There are several potential complications that can occur with SRS and SBRT, which are often dependent on the location of the lesion treated. Acute toxicities can include nausea, fatigue, dermatitis, esophagitis, and myelitis. Late toxicities are more significant and can include esophageal stenosis, fistula, ulcer formation, vertebral compression fracture (VCF), as well as spinal cord injury. Of these, VCF and spinal cord injury have been well characterized and extensively reported in the literature. Sahgal et al. reported pooled outcomes from 410 spine segments that were treated with spine SBRT. The 1- and 2-year VCF incidence rates were 12.35% and 13.49%, respectively, with median time to fracture of 2.46 months [72]. Significant predictors for compression fracture were dose per fraction >19 Gy, lytic tumors, baseline spinal misalignment, and baseline presence of a compression fracture. In another study, the 5-year cumulative incidence rate of symptomatic compression fractures requiring interventions was <10% among patients who received SRS to 24 Gy [73]. The experience from MSKCC of single-fraction spinal SRS with 24 Gy revealed a radiographic VCF rate of 36% of which 14% became symptomatic and required intervention [39]. Treatment of VCFs after SBRT for spinal metastases includes percutaneous cement augmentation with vertebroplasty and kyphoplasty as they provide pain relief and mechanical support; however, preventative strategies are still under investigation [74]. Spinal cord injury, or more specifically, radiation-induced myelopathy (RM), is the most potentially debilitating complication, and the risk is accepted to be less than 1% with care treatment planning and delivery. A dosimetric analysis conducted by Sahgal et al. examined 19 patients who underwent reirradiation after conventional treatment. The mean total P (max) nBED in the no-RM group was 62.3 Gy(2/2), which was significantly lower than the corresponding 105.8 Gy(2/2) in the RM group. The biologic effective dose (BED) from the initial course of radiation with conventional RT was not significantly different between the two groups. The recommended dose constraints based on this analysis were to limit the cumulative BED to <70 Gy (2/2) for the thecal sac point dose maximum and limit the maximum SBRT BED to 25 Gy (2/2) for the thecal sac point dose maximum. Furthermore, a 5-month period between radiation treatment courses was considered safe [75]. Recommendations from a retrospective study by Saghal et al. modeling nine patients who had RM following SBRT to the spine to 66 patients who did not have RM were to limit the thecal sac maximum point volume–dose to 12.4 Gy in one fraction, 20.3 Gy in three fractions, and 25.3 Gy in five fractions in order to reduce the risk of RM to less than 5% [76]. A comprehensive study examining dose–volume data for de novo SBRT spine cases found the risk of spinal cord injury to be 1% with 13 Gy in a single fraction and 20 Gy in three fractions. In the reirradiation setting, the estimated risk level was 0.4% for 10 Gy and 0.6% for 14 Gy in five fractions [77]. With regard to esophageal toxicity, Cox et al. reported on 204 patients treated to a median dose of 24 Gy in one fraction, of whom 31 (15%) patients experienced acute and 24 (12%) patients experienced late esophageal toxicity. Overall, 14 patients (6.8%) had grade 3 or higher esophageal toxicity according to CTCAE 4.0 [78]. In the secondary analysis of the MDACC phase I/II studies, esophageal toxicity rates were also low. Ten (15%) patients and eight (12%) patients had GI toxicities including esophagitis, as well as dysphagia, nausea, vomiting, anorexia, and diarrhea. There were no cases of grade 3 or higher GI toxicity [65].

Conclusion

The diagnosis and treatment of spinal metastases require multidisciplinary review. Regardless of the treatment, diagnosis and intervention before the development of significant neurologic and functional deficits would improve outcomes. Back pain is generally the earliest sign of metastatic tumor. Proper use of imaging greatly assists in screening for tumor and may help distinguish tumor from other spinal pathology. RT remains a mainstay of therapy for metastatic spinal tumors. Advances in stereotactic radiotherapy delivery techniques such as SRS and SBRT continue to improve tumor control. The role of RT, surgery, and chemotherapy is still being defined. Continued advances in imaging, chemotherapy, RT, and surgery combined with increased physician awareness may continue to help improve the quality of life for these patients.

References

1. Wong DA, Fornasier VL, MacNab I. Spinal metastases: the obvious, the occult, and the impostors. Spine (Phila Pa 1976). 1990;15(1):1–4.
2. Ortiz Gómez JA. The incidence of vertebral body metastases. Int Orthop. 1995;19(5):309–11.
3. Sutcliffe P, Connock M, Shyangdan D, et al. A systematic review of evidence on malignant spinal metastases: natural history and technologies for identifying patients at high risk of vertebral fracture and spinal cord compression. Health Technol Assess. 2013;17(42):1–274.
4. Gilbert RW, Kim JH, Posner JB. Epidural spinal cord compression from metastatic tumor: diagnosis and treatment. Ann Neurol. 1978;3(1):40–51.
5. Gerszten PC, Welch WC. Current surgical management of metastatic spinal disease. Oncology (Williston Park). 2000;14(7):1013–24, 1029-1030
6. Sciubba DM, Petteys RJ, Dekutoski MB, et al. Diagnosis and management of metastatic spine disease. A review. J Neurosurg Spine. 2010;13(1):94–108.
7. Schiff D. Spinal cord compression. Neurol Clin. 2003;21(1):67–86.
8. Ecker RD, Endo T, Wetjen NM, et al. Diagnosis and treatment of vertebral column metastases. Mayo Clin Proc. 2005;80(9):1177–86.
9. Mak KS, Lee LK, Mak RH, et al. Incidence and treatment patterns in hospitalizations for malignant spinal cord compression in the United States, 1998–2006. Int J Radiat Oncol Biol Phys. 2011;80(3):824–31.
10. Patchell RA, Tibbs PA, Regine WF, et al. Direct decompressive surgical resection in the treatment of spinal cord compression caused by metastatic cancer: a randomised trial. Lancet. 2005;366(9486):643–8.
11. Gokaslan ZL, York JE, et al. Transthoracic vertebrectomy for metastatic spinal tumors. J Neurosurg. 1998;89:599–609.
12. Graham GP, Dent CM, Burgess N, et al. Urinary retention in prostatic carcinoma: obstructive or neurogenic? Br J Hosp Med. 1993;49:733–4.
13. Schiff D, O'Neill BP, Wang CH, et al. Neuroimaging and treatment implications of patients with multiple epidural spinal metastases. Cancer. 1998;83:1593–601.
14. Traill Z, Richards MA, Moore NR. Magnetic resonance imaging of metastatic bone disease. Clin Orthop. 1995;312:76–88.
15. Jones KM, Schwartz RB, Mantello MT, et al. Fast spin-echo MR in the detection of vertebral metastases: comparison of three sequences. Am J Neuroradiol. 1994;15:401–7.
16. Mehta RC, Marks MP, Hinks RS, et al. MR evaluation of vertebral metastases: T1-weighted, short-inversion-time inversion recovery, fast spin-echo, and inversion-recovery fast spin-echo sequences. Am J Neuroradiol. 1995;16:281–8.
17. Dwyer AJ, Frank JA, Sank VJ, et al. Short T1 inversion recovery pulse sequence: analysis and initial experience in cancer imaging. Radiology. 1988;168:827–36.
18. Bilsky MH, Laufer I, Fourney DR, et al. Reliability analysis of the epidural spinal cord compression scale. J Neurosurg Spine. 2010;13(3):324–8.
19. Bilsky M, Smith M. Surgical approach to epidural spinal cord compression. Hematol Oncol Clin North Am. 2006;20:1307–17.

20. Laufer I, Rubin DG, Lis E, et al. The NOMS framework: approach to the treatment of spinal metastatic tumors. Oncologist. 2013;18(6):744–51.
21. Fisher CG, DiPaola CP, Ryken TC, Bilsky MH, Shaffrey CI, Berven SH, et al. A novel classification system for spinal instability in neoplastic disease: an evidence-based approach and expert consensus from the Spine Oncology Study Group. Spine (Phila Pa 1976). 2010;35:E1221–9.
22. Arana E, Kovacs FM, Royuela A, Asenjo B, Pérez-Ramírez Ú, Zamora J. Spine instability neoplastic score: agreement across different medical and surgical specialties. Spine J. 2016;16:591–9.
23. Campos M, Urrutia J, Zamora T, Román J, Canessa V, Borghero Y, et al. The spine instability neoplastic score: an independent reliability and reproducibility analysis. Spine J. 2014;14:1466–9.
24. Fourney DR, Frangou EM, Ryken TC, Dipaola CP, Shaffrey CI, Berven SH, et al. Spinal instability neoplastic score: an analysis of reliability and validity from the spine oncology study group. J Clin Oncol. 2011;29:3072–7.
25. Fourney DR, Frangou EM, Ryken TC, et al. Spinal instability neoplastic score: an analysis of reliability and validity from the spine oncology study group. J Clin Oncol. 2011;29(22):3072–7.
26. Campos M, Urrutia J, Zamora T, et al. The spine instability neoplastic score: an independent reliability and reproducibility analysis. Spine J. 2013;pii:S1529-9430(13)01492-7.
27. Moussazadeh N, Laufer I, Yamada Y, Bilsky MH. Separation surgery for spinal metastases: effect of spinal radiosurgery on surgical treatment goals. Cancer Control. 2014;21:168–74.
28. Galibert P, Deramond H, Rosat P, Le Gars D. Preliminary note on the treatment of vertebral angioma by percutaneous acrylic vertebroplasty. Neurochirurgie. 1987(Fr);33:166–168.
29. Belkoff SM, Mathis JM, Deramond H, Jasper LE. An ex vivo biomechanical evaluation of a hydroxyapatite cement for use with kyphoplasty. AJNR Am J Neuroradiol. 2001;22:1212–6.
30. Theodorou DJ, Theodorou SJ, Duncan TD, Garfin SR, Wong WH. Percutaneous balloon kyphoplasty for the correction of spinal deformity in painful vertebral body compression fractures. Clin Imaging. 2002;26:1–5.
31. Chi JH, Gokaslan ZL. Vertebroplasty and kyphoplasty for spinal metastases. Curr Opin Support Palliat Care. 2008;2:9–13.
32. Gerszten PC, Germanwala A, Burton SA, Welch WC, Ozhasoglu C, Vogel WJ. Combination kyphoplasty and spinal radiosurgery: a new treatment paradigm for pathological fractures. J Neurosurg Spine. 2005;3:296–301.
33. Hartsell WF, Scott CB, Bruner DW, et al. Randomized trial of short- versus long-course radiotherapy for palliation of painful bone metastases. J Natl Cancer Inst. 2005;97(11):798–804.
34. Leksell L. The stereotaxic method and radiosurgery of the brain. Acta Chir Scand. 1951;102(4):316–9.
35. Leksell L. Stereotactic radiosurgery. J Neurol Neurosurg Psychiatry. 1983;46(9):797–803.
36. Blomgren H, Lax I, Naslund I, Svanstrom R. Stereotactic high dose fraction radiation therapy of extracranial tumors using an accelerator. Clinical experience of the first thirty-one patients. Acta Oncol. 1995;34(6):861–70.
37. Ryu SI, Chang SD, Kim DH, Murphy MJ, Le QT, Martin DP, et al. Image-guided hypo-fractionated stereotactic radiosurgery to spinal lesions. Neurosurgery. 2001;49:838–46.
38. Gerszten PC, Burton SA, Ozhasoglu C, Welch WC. Radiosurgery for spinal metastases: clinical experience in 500 cases from a single institution. Spine (Phila Pa 1976). 2007;32:193–9.
39. Moussazadeh N, Lis E, Katsoulakis E, et al. Five-year outcomes of high-dose single-fraction spinal stereotactic radiosurgery. Int J Radiat Oncol Biol Phys. 2015;93(2):361–7.
40. Tseng CL, Eppinga W, Charest-Morin R, et al. Spine stereotactic body radiotherapy: indications, outcomes, and points of caution. Global Spine J. 2017;7(2):179–97.
41. Brown JM, Carlson DJ, Brenner DJ. The tumor radiobiology of SRS and SBRT: are more than the 5 Rs involved? Int J Radiat Oncol Biol Phys. 2014;88(2):254–62.
42. Dewan MZ, Galloway AE, Kawashima N, et al. Fractionated but not single-dose radiotherapy induces an immune-mediated abscopal effect when combined with anti-CTLA-4 antibody. Clin Cancer Res. 2009;15(17):5379–88.
43. Fuks Z, Kolesnick R. Engaging the vascular component of the tumor response. Cancer Cell. 2005;8(2):89–91.
44. Garcia-Barros M, Paris F, Cordon-Cardo C, et al. Tumor response to radiotherapy regulated by endothelial cell apoptosis. Science. 2003; 300(5622):1155–9.
45. Kirkpatrick JP, Meyer JJ, Marks LB. The linear-quadratic model is inappropriate to model high dose per fraction effects in radiosurgery. Semin Radiat Oncol. 2008;18(4):240–3.
46. Kocher M, Treuer H, Voges J, Hoevels M, Sturm V, Muller RP. Computer simulation of cytotoxic and vascular effects of radiosurgery in solid and necrotic brain metastases. Radiother Oncol. 2000;54(2):149–56.
47. Lugade AA, Moran JP, Gerber SA, Rose RC, Frelinger JG, Lord EM. Local radiation therapy of B16 melanoma tumors increases the generation of tumor antigen-specific effector cells that traffic to the tumor. J Immunol. 2005;174(12):7516–23.
48. Park HJ, Griffin RJ, Hui S, Levitt SH, Song CW. Radiationinduced vascular damage in tumors: implications of vascular damage in ablative hypofractionated radiotherapy (SBRT and SRS). Radiat Res. 2012;177(3):311–27.
49. Postow MA, Callahan MK, Barker CA, et al. Immunologic correlates of the abscopal effect in a patient with melanoma. N Engl J Med. 2012;366(10):925–31.

50. Formenti SC, Demaria S. Local control by radiotherapy: is that all there is? Breast Cancer Res. 2008;10(6):215.
51. Obeid M, Panaretakis T, Joza N, et al. Calreticulin exposure is required for the immunogenicity of gamma-irradiation and UVC light-induced apoptosis. Cell Death Differ. 2007;14(10):1848–50.
52. Apetoh L, Ghiringhelli F, Tesniere A, et al. Toll-like receptor 4dependent contribution of the immune system to anticancer chemotherapy and radiotherapy. Nat Med. 2007;13(9):1050–9.
53. Demaria S, Formenti SC. Sensors of ionizing radiation effects on the immunological microenvironment of cancer. Int J Radiat Biol. 2007;83(11–12):819–25.
54. Matsumura S, Wang B, Kawashima N, et al. Radiation-induced CXCL16 release by breast cancer cells attracts effector T cells. J Immunol. 2008;181(5):3099–107.
55. Yamada Y, Katsoulakis E, Laufer I, et al. The impact of histology and delivered dose on local control of spinal metastases treated with stereotactic radiosurgery. Neurosurg Focus. 2017;42(1):E6.
56. Garg AK, Shiu AS, Yang J, et al. Phase 1/2 trial of single-session stereotactic body radiotherapy for previously unirradiated spinal metastases. Cancer. 2012;118(20):5069–77.
57. Brahme A, Roos JE, Lax I. Solution of an integral equation encountered in rotation therapy. Phys Med Biol. 1982;27(10):1221–9.
58. Simmons ED, Zheng Y. Vertebral tumors: surgical versus nonsurgical treatment. Clin Orthop Relat Res. 2006;443:233–47.
59. McClelland S, Kim E III, Passias PG, Murphy JD, Attia A, Jaboin JJ. Spinal stereotactic body radiotherapy in the United States: a decade-long nationwide analysis of patient demographics, practice patterns, and trends over time. J Clin Neurosci. 2017;46:109–12.
60. Parker C, Nilsson S, Heinrich D, et al. Alpha emitter radium-223 and survival in metastatic prostate cancer. N Engl J Med. 2013;369(3):213–23.
61. Reck M, Rodriguez-Abreu D, Robinson AG, et al. Pembrolizumab versus chemotherapy for PD-L1-positive non-small-cell lung cancer. N Engl J Med. 2016;375(19):1823–33.
62. Swain SM, Kim SB, Cortes J, et al. Pertuzumab, trastuzumab, and docetaxel for HER2-positive metastatic breast cancer (CLEOPATRA study): overall survival results from a randomised, doubleblind, placebo-controlled, phase 3 study. Lancet Oncol. 2013;14(6):461–71.
63. Topalian SL, Sznol M, McDermott DF, et al. Survival, durable tumor remission, and long-term safety in patients with advanced melanoma receiving nivolumab. J Clin Oncol. 2014;32(10):1020–30.
64. Redmond KJ, Lo SS, Fisher C, Sahgal A. Postoperative stereotactic body radiation therapy (SBRT) for spine metastases: a critical review to guide practice. Int J Radiat Oncol Biol Phys. 2016;95(5):1414–28.
65. Tao R, Bishop AJ, Brownlee Z, et al. Stereotactic body radiation therapy for spinal metastases in the postoperative setting: a secondary analysis of mature phase 1-2 trials. Int J Radiat Oncol Biol Phys. 2016;95(5):1405–13.
66. Massicotte E, Foote M, Reddy R, Sahgal A. Minimal access spine surgery (MASS) for decompression and stabilization performed as an out-patient procedure for metastatic spinal tumours followed by spine stereotactic body radiotherapy (SBRT): first report of technique and preliminary outcomes. Technol Cancer Res Treat. 2012;11(1):15–25.
67. Wang JC, Boland P, Mitra N, et al. Single-stage posterolateral transpedicular approach for resection of epidural metastatic spine tumors involving the vertebral body with circumferential reconstruction: results in 140 patients. J Neurosurg Spine. 2004;1(3):287–98.
68. Damast S, Wright J, Bilsky M, et al. Impact of dose on local failure rates after image-guided reirradiation of recurrent paraspinal metastases. Int J Radiat Oncol Biol Phys. 2011;81(3):819–26.
69. Hashmi A, Guckenberger M, Kersh R, et al. Re-irradiation stereotactic body radiotherapy for spinal metastases: a multiinstitutional outcome analysis. J Neurosurg Spine. 2016;25(5):646–53.
70. Garg AK, Wang XS, Shiu AS, et al. Prospective evaluation of spinal reirradiation by using stereotactic body radiation therapy: the University of Texas MD Anderson Cancer Center experience. Cancer. 2011;117(15):3509–16.
71. Myrehaug S, Sahgal A, Hayashi M, et al. Reirradiation spine stereotactic body radiation therapy for spinal metastases: systematic review. J Neurosurg Spine. 2017;27(4):428–35.
72. Sahgal A, Atenafu EG, Chao S, et al. Vertebral compression fracture after spine stereotactic body radiotherapy: a multiinstitutional analysis with a focus on radiation dose and the spinal instability neoplastic score. J Clin Oncol. 2013;31(27):3426–31.
73. Virk MS, Han JE, Reiner AS, et al. Frequency of symptomatic vertebral body compression fractures requiring intervention following single-fraction stereotactic radiosurgery for spinal metastases. Neurosurg Focus. 2017;42(1):E8.
74. Sahgal A, Whyne CM, Ma L, Larson DA, Fehlings MG. Vertebral compression fracture after stereotactic body radiotherapy for spinal metastases. Lancet Oncol. 2013;14(8):e310–20.
75. Sahgal A, Ma L, Weinberg V, et al. Reirradiation human spinal cord tolerance for stereotactic body radiotherapy. Int J Radiat Oncol Biol Phys. 2012;82(1):107–16.
76. Sahgal A, Weinberg V, Ma L, et al. Probabilities of radiation myelopathy specific to stereotactic body radiation therapy to guide safe practice. Int J Radiat Oncol Biol Phys. 2013;85(2):341–7.
77. Grimm J, Sahgal A, Soltys SG, et al. Estimated risk level of unified stereotactic body radiation therapy dose tolerance limits for spinal cord. Semin Radiat Oncol. 2016;26(2):165–71.
78. Cox BW, Jackson A, Hunt M, Bilsky M, Yamada Y. Esophageal toxicity from high-dose, single-fraction paraspinal stereotactic radiosurgery. Int J Radiat Oncol Biol Phys. 2012;83(5):e661–7.

Part IV

Minimally Invasive Approach and Current Technology

Dan Sciubba

17 Percutaneous Modalities

Sreekumar Madassery, Bulent Arslan,
and David M. Tabriz

Spinal Bone Biopsy

David Tabriz

History, Indications, and Contraindications

Percutaneous spine biopsy was first described in the early 1930s, with radiologic guided biopsy first described in the later portion of that decade [1]. Image-guided biopsy today offers a rapid, cost-effective biopsy approach with fewer complications compared to open surgical biopsy. General indications and contraindications for percutaneous spine and bone biopsy are listed in Table 17.1 [2].

Preprocedure Evaluation

When the decision to biopsy is made, it is imperative that multidisciplinary discussion occurs regarding placement of the biopsy in light of possible planned surgical approach, since tract seeding for spine lesions (particularly sarcomas) is of concern [3]. As such, if core needle biopsies are obtained outside of the planned incision plane, the surgical procedure must be changed to now consider the potentially contaminated tissue plane.

Table 17.1 Indications and contraindications for percutaneous bone biopsy

Indications for percutaneous bone biopsy
Confirm metastatic disease
Primary lesion evaluation
Pathologic fracture assessment
Infection
Chemotherapy effectiveness
Flow cytometric analysis of myelodysplastic conditions
General contraindications to percutaneous bone biopsy
Coagulopathy or bleeding diathesis
Suspected vascular lesion
Suspected infection in overlying skin or soft tissue path to lesion
Severe allergy to required sedoanalgesia for procedure
Pregnancy

Prior to consideration for spine biopsy, a focused medical history and physical is obtained and any available preprocedural imaging reviewed. Major procedural-related items to discuss are current medications (e.g., anticoagulants or antibiotics), allergies, tolerance of procedural anesthetics, and any potential skin or tissue infections in the planned biopsy trajectory. Pertinent laboratory values include evaluation for

The authors have no financial conflicts of interest regarding the content included in this chapter.

S. Madassery (✉) · B. Arslan · D. M. Tabriz
Rush University Medical Center, Rush Oak Park Hospital, Chicago, IL, USA
e-mail: sreekumar_madassery@rush.edu

K. Singh, M. Colman (eds.), *Surgical Spinal Oncology*,
https://doi.org/10.1007/978-3-030-50722-0_17

coagulopathy (e.g., PT/INR, platelet count) and for any laboratory values that may interfere with safe procedural analgesia and sedation (e.g., basic metabolic profile).

Tools

Current imaging modalities considered for spine biopsies include ultrasound (US), fluoroscopy, computed tomography (CT), CT fluoroscopy (CTF), and magnetic resonance imaging (MRI). The current standard is CT.

When a safe percutaneous path to a spinal lesion is planned, decision to perform fine needle aspiration (FNA) versus a core needle biopsy (CNB) is made. The diagnostic yield of FNA versus CNB has been studied, with CNB providing a greater success rate [4, 5]. FNA is reserved for difficult locations where nodal diagnosis of metastatic disease is required. Osseous lesion biopsies typically require larger core samples for adequate sampling compared to non-osseous lesions.

In general, a coaxial technique is used to allow multiple samples to be obtained. If the lesion is beneath intact cortex, a trephine tip needle is used to obtain access to the lesion with both manual- and drill-insertion devices commercially available. Once access to the lesion is obtained, the density characteristic determine the coaxially inserted lesion-sampling needle, with (1) tru-cut spring-loaded needles providing better samples of soft-tissue or cystic tumors and (2) trephine tip needles increasing the likelihood of obtaining a cylindrical core of tissue for mineralized lesions. The outer cannula is typically 11- or 13-gauge, with the inner biopsy needle being 14- or 16-gauge, respectively.

Biopsy Approach Technique

Percutaneous bone biopsy should be performed with knowledge of the potential surgery required for treatment depending on the differential diagnosis. This is particularly important for sarcomas and other malignancies where needle tract seeding along the biopsy path is of concern. Like appendicular bone lesion biopsies, CT guidance is the main imaging modality used for focal osseous lesions in the axial skeleton. An exception is bone lesions involving the entire vertebral body, in which case a fluoroscopic approach can be considered, since the precise cutting pathway after transpedicular cannulation is less important. The benefit of fluoroscopic guidance is real-time imaging and monitoring of the biopsy needle as it extends toward the area of interest. Soft tissue or more superficial lesions may be approached with ultrasound guidance. Occasionally, a lesion may be so superficial and easily palpable that an in-office percutaneous biopsy without imaging guidance can be considered.

Specific Anatomic Areas (Cervical, Thoracic, Lumbar, Sacral)

Cervical Spine (Fig. 17.1/Case 17.1)

For high-cervical (C1–C3) vertebral body lesions, an anterolateral, transoral, or

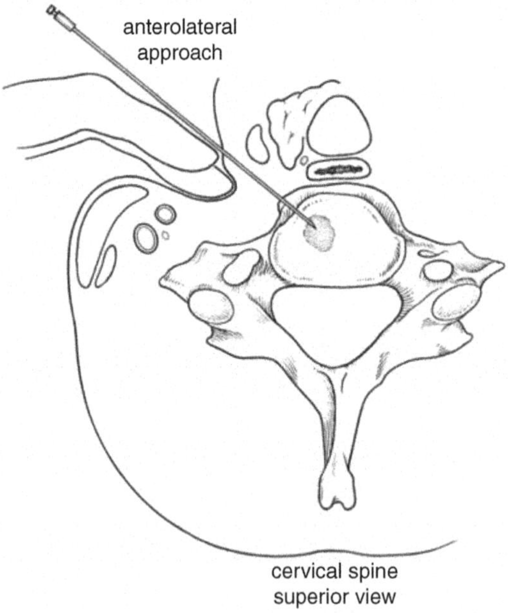

Fig. 17.1 Anterolateral technique for cervical vertebral body spine lesions. The needle passes between the carotid sheath and esophagus [2]. (Reproduced with permission from author, T Jamshid)

pharyngeal approach can be performed. Upper cervical lesions are better suited for a transoral route, whereas mid-cervical lesions are better suited for an anterolateral route (Fig. 17.1). Of note, if chordoma is suspected, transpharyngeal biopsies should be avoided due to the high-risk of tract seeding causing local recurrence in a markedly difficult surgical resection site. For posterior lesions, the comparatively larger posterior elements of the lower cervical spine (C4–7) allow for posterior access to lesions (Case 17.1).

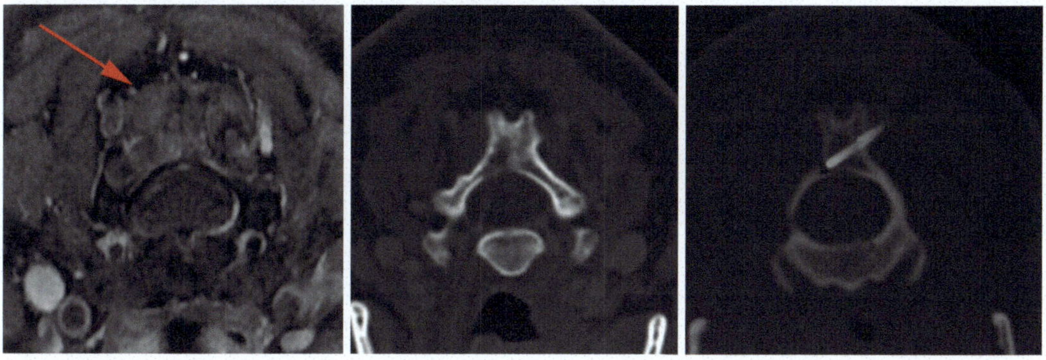

Case 17.1 A 58-year-old woman with history of invasive ductal breast carcinoma with enhancing lesion on T1 fat-suppressed postcontrast MRI within the left paramedian lamina and spinous process of C2 (red arrow). Surgical biopsy was initially requested; however, image-guided percutaneous biopsy attempt was performed. C2 lesion pathology confirmed metastatic spread consistent with patient's breast primary

Thoracic Spine (Fig. 17.2/Case 17.2)

The mediastinal structures make anterior vertebral body of the thoracic spine difficult to target; however, transpedicular, transforaminal, and paraspinal approaches exist. The pedicle provides a safe pathway to the vertebral body and is the preferred route if possible.

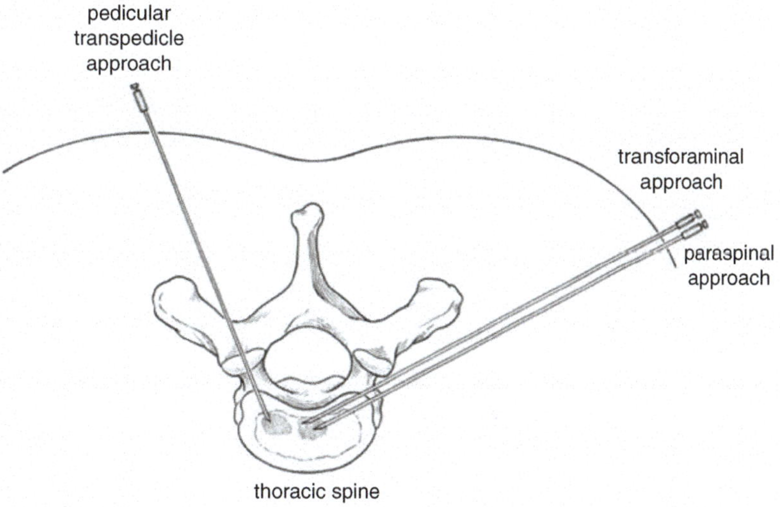

Fig. 17.2 Technique for thoracic vertebral body lesions [2]. (Reproduced with permission from author, T Jamshid)

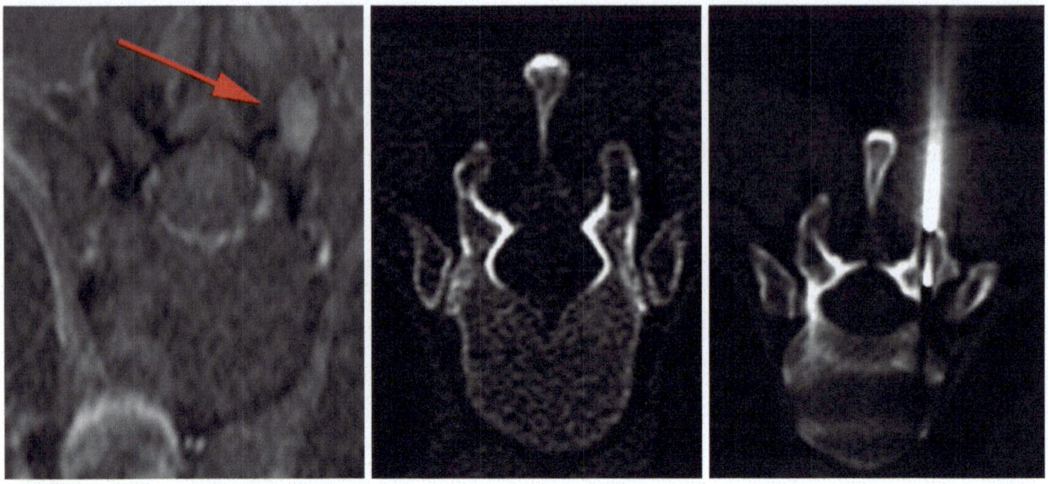

Case 17.2 A 57-year-old man with history of L3 plasmacytoma status post-L3 corpectomy, L2–L4 percutaneous pedicle screw fixation, and adjuvant radiation with follow-up imaging demonstrating an enhancing FDG-avid, lytic, T1 fat-suppressed postcontrast MRI enhancing lesion (red arrow) in the right posterior process of T12. CT-guided biopsy yielded a new focus of plasmacytoma

Lumbar Spine (Fig. 17.3/Case 17.3)
The larger posterior elements of the lumbar spine and lack of surrounding vital anatomic structures make it substantially easier for percutaneous biopsy compared to the cervical and thoracic spine. Transpedicular and posterolateral approaches exist.

Fig. 17.3 Technique for lumbar vertebral body lesions [2]. (Reproduced with permission from author, T Jamshid)

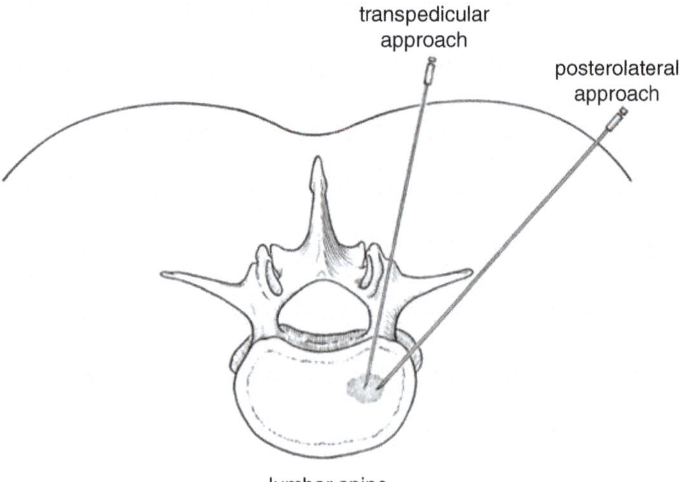

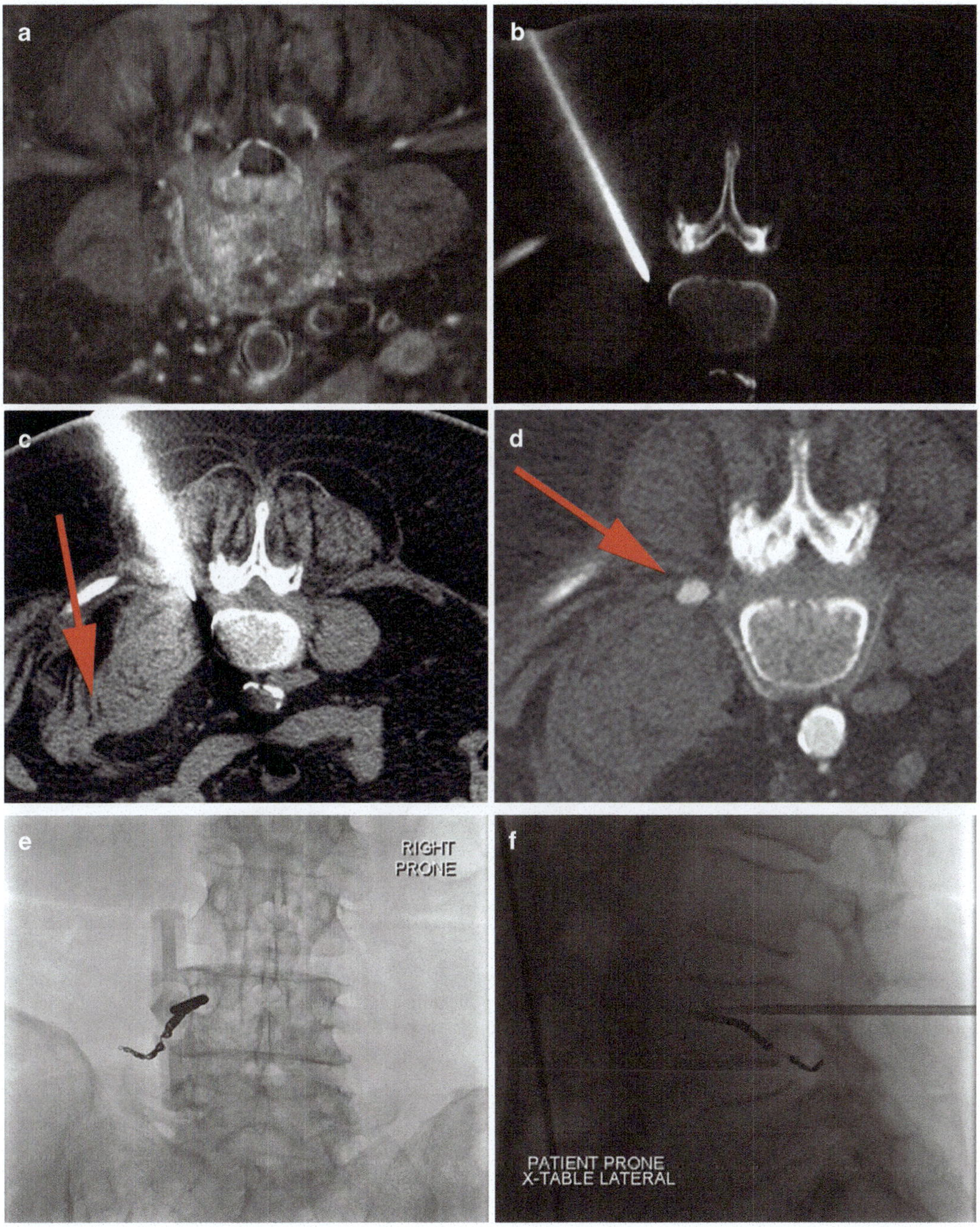

Case 17.3 82 year old woman with history of breast cancer and follicular lymphoma, with diffuse enhancement of the L4 vertebral body concerning for disease recurrence. Initial CT-guided posterolateral approach biopsy attempt (**a**–**c**) was aborted after brisk development of an intra-procedural hematoma (red arrow, **c**), which was found to be traumatic development of a lumbar artery pseudoaneurysm (red arrow, **d**). After coil embolization, transpedicular approach under fluoroscopic guidance was successful performed (**e**, **f**) with results yielding follicular lymphoma recurrence

Sacrum (Case 17.4)

Percutaneous biopsy of sacral lesions typically involves steep angulations and avoidance of the existing sacral plexus/nerve roots; however, osseous bridging between foramen usually allow for safe percutaneous paths. Posterior approaches to lesions are the standard. Transrectal or transabdominal approaches should be avoided due to concern for tract seeding in common sacral disease such as chordoma.

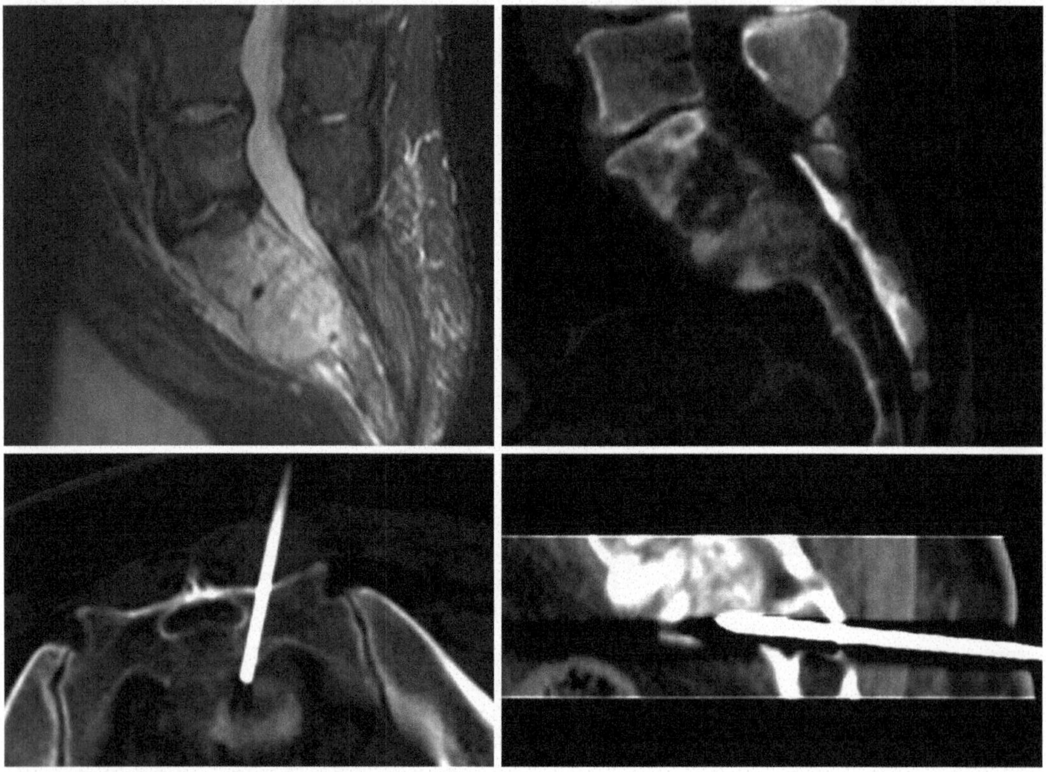

Case 17.4 A 63-year-old man who initially presented with generalized weakness was found to have an expansile sacral mass that demonstrated enhancement on T1 fat-suppressed postcontrast MRI. Percutaneous biopsy avoiding the sacral foramina was performed and yielded a diagnosis of poorly differentiated carcinoma of unknown origin

Sample Handling and Postprocedural Care

In addition to sending samples for pathologic analysis, additional testing should be performed if concern for infection (e.g., culture and sensitivity) or lymphoma (flow cytometry) is present. If a lesion is primarily cystic, aspirate samples are sent for cytopathology analysis, and ideally, the nodular/solid or MRI-enhancing component of the lesion should be targeted for core biopsy to increase diagnostic yield.

Postprocedural care predominantly focused on monitoring patients for any signs of complication, namely, bleeding or neurologic changes from preprocedural baseline. When obtaining biopsy of vertebral lesions, direct nerve or spinal cord injury is generally much less common than compressive effects of adjacent hematoma formation. As such, any neurologic symptoms or decline should be taken seriously and further clinical investigation initiated.

Vertebral Augmentation

Sreekumar Madassery

Vertebral augmentation (VA) is a minimally invasive percutaneous intervention intended to decrease pain and potentially restore height in patients with spinal compression fractures. Underlying pathology within the bony matrix, whether benign etiologies such as osteoporosis, or malignancies such as hematopoietic maladies or metastatic tumors, can dictate the structural integrity of the vertebral body. Historically, percutaneous vertebral augmentation has been utilized in cases where conservative medical management has failed to alleviate patients' symptoms resulting in decline in daily activities and overall quality of life. In the tumor setting specifically, the choice to use percutaneous augmentation must be made in the multidisciplinary setting after careful consideration of tumor histology, neurologic status, structural integrity of the bony elements, and patient preferences/comorbidities. Many augmentation techniques have been developed and utilized over the years. The choice of intervention is additionally based on fracture appearance, pathology, and operator experience.

The two common forms of VA include vertebroplasty (VP), where polymethylmethacrylate (PMMA) cement is injected through transpedicular cannulas from a posterior approach into the affected vertebral body, and kyphoplasty (KP), in which PMMA is injected after cavity creation has been performed. Once vertebral fractures occur, there tends to be intense pain due to inflammation and the instability of bone during movement. The sequelae of immobility secondary to pain causes increased rates of thromboembolism, respiratory disorders, and contributes to opioid dependence [6]. The goal of percutaneous cementation in osteoporotic insufficiency fractures is to infiltrate the porous and fractured cancellous bone, thus strengthening the overall spinal segment and ultimately reducing pain. The goals with pathologic vertebral fractures are similar, although there are specific technical concerns that arise in the setting of a spinal neoplasm. As opposed to VP, the established benefits of KP are increased height restoration and decreased cement leakage. However, similar quality of life and pain improvement are seen compared to VP [7]. Additionally, it is known that fractures cause disruption of the spinal structural integrity, which can result in adjacent vertebral fractures, particularly due to the biomechanical changes that are experienced as patients attempt ambulation in the presence of fracture-related pain. Part of the proposition of VA is to attain faster spinal stability and less perception of fracture-related pain in an attempt to reduce medical morbidity of immobilization, pathologic motion, and future fractures. KP has, generally speaking, been more successful than VP [8] with regard to these goals. This is presumed to be due to benefits of increased height restoration, which can reduce the stress on adjacent levels. However, it is also important to consider that the underlying bony disease is an important variable in this process, which can be influenced by multidisciplinary consultation with endocrinology and oncologic specialists.

There has been significant controversy over time regarding the efficacy of vertebral augmentation. This includes studies which have tried to compare VA procedures to conservative medical management, as well as to "sham" procedures in which patients undergo simulated procedures. Conservative medical management is traditionally accepted as use of nonsteroidal anti-inflammatory drugs (NSAIDs), opioids, bone-stimulating medications, and brace support, followed by possible physical therapy for 8–12 weeks. For tumor-related fractures, in addition to the above, treatments may also include radiation or systemic therapy. Farrokhi et al. in 2011 in a randomized study of VP versus medical management for osteoporotic compression fractures found statistically significant early pain improvement and quality of life in patients undergoing VP [9]. This was in contrast to earlier major controversial studies such as the 2009 Buchbinder et al. study [10] reported in the New

England Journal of Medicine, in which no statistical difference in pain was found at 6 months between treatment with VP and a sham procedure. This was further confirmed by the authors at 2 years. Other double-blinded sham-controlled studies, such as the VERTOS IV study, also showed no significant difference between VP and a sham procedure [11]. Conversely, the 2016 VAPOUR trial showed improved pain and decreased disability in VP patients compared to sham procedures in those with acute nonneoplastic compression fractures [10]. What is seen in evaluating these studies is that there are significant differences in the chronicity of the fractures included, the blinding factors, and imaging criteria used. Many operators currently choose to offer augmentation when optimal conservative medical management has failed, with persistent pain, lack of healing on imaging, and debilitation.

Moreover, there has been evolution of newer techniques and devices, with increased focus on decreasing cement leakage potential and increasing height restoration. The addition of radiofrequency energy to PMMA delivery in one system has provided the ability to deliver higher viscosity cement, resulting in potentially less cement leakage when compared to standard KP [12]. The KIVA system utilizes temporary coil insertion, with a permanent biopolymer (PEEK-OPTIMA) that goes over the coil, followed by removal of the coil and subsequent PMMA cement instillation within the polymer construct. While studies are limited, there are reports of decreased cement usage with this system, along with non-inferior pain resolution, and slightly increased height restoration compared to KP [13, 14]. Further in the extremes of maximized height restoration is the SpineJack system, recently introduced in the US market (present in Europe for over a decade), which incorporates bi-pedicular insertion of titanium expandable implants, followed by PMMA interdigitation. This system demonstrated superior height restoration and kyphosis correction evaluated up to 3 years compared to KP in the recently published SAKOS trial [15]. This system has significant promise in preventing adjacent fractures and improvement in the kyphosis-associated sequelae that many patients experience.

VA for pathologic vertebral compression fractures has also been utilized for palliative pain management in patients with metastatic spread and myeloma. Most common metastases include breast, prostate, lung, and thyroid carcinomas. The pain experienced is thought to come from mass-related periosteal, nocireceptor activation, and inflammatory cytokines [16]. Radiation therapy is primarily used in many nonoperative patients, especially when there is adjacent extra-axial disease. While this form of therapy helps to treat the tumor, this does not specifically provide increased bone stabilization, particularly with osteolytic lesions which can make patients at risk for worsening compression and debility. Lim et al. [17] reported 12-month follow-up of >100 patients that underwent VA for pathologic osteolytic VB compression fractures, showing that spine stabilization was maintained, with marked improvement symptomatically in the early follow-up period and slightly increased Visual Analog Score (VAS) at 1 year. Erdem et al. [18] in 2013 reviewed nearly 2700 VA procedures in 792 patients with multiple myeloma in the early 2000s and showed an average decrease of 4 points in their VAS, a significant reduction/cessation of narcotic requirement, and an increase in activity levels. They also reported 0.3% complications, which required antibiotics for management. A significant limitation in this review was that detailed data were only available for approximately 50% of the total patients reviewed. The Cancer Patient Fracture Evaluation (CAFÉ) study is a prospective, randomized, control trial that evaluated KP with conservative management, with 134 patients, and demonstrated significant pain improvement, quality of life, pain medication requirements, and activity for the patients that underwent VA [19]. The only major complication was an intraoperative myocardial infarction, which resolved and was attributed by the authors to anesthesia reaction. Overall, VA for pathologic compression fractures has improved pain, mobility, and quality of life while reducing narcotic medication use, with minimal adverse events.

As reported by multispecialty consensus statement, indications for VA include painful vertebral compression fractures that can be localized and is refractory to medical management, patients with vertebral bodies at risk of fracture due to malignancy, and symptomatic microfractures of vertebral bodies noted on MRI despite no height loss. The absolute contraindications for VA include septicemia, uncorrectable coagulopathy, or documented allergy to PMMA. Some of the pertinent relative contraindications include retropulsed fracture fragments resulting in neurological compromise, epidural tumor extensions into the canal, and cauda equina syndrome starting at the level of the fracture [20]. Operators tend to avoid interventions with significant posterior wall defects and sometimes with hypervasular tumors due to concerns for intra-/postprocedure bleeding complications. In general practice, patients are ideally deemed appropriate for VA when presenting with subacute, nonmedically controlled thoracolumbar (<16 weeks after incident or diagnosis) fractures, MRI fluid signal imaging showing active inflammatory changes, and pain that can be localized on exam to the level of fracture. CT is of particular help in patients with pathologic fractures, as this is allowed detailed evaluation of the cortical integrity. It has been shown that disrupted posterolateral elements can lead to early failure post VA and may at times require operative management if cord compromise develops [21]. The overall major complications (spinal cord compression, nerve root compression, cardiovascular collapse, following cement pulmonary embolism) for VA are noted to be <1% for osteoporotic fractures and <5% for neoplastic fractures [20]. The majority of reported complications are related to cement leakage, seen in the intra-disc space, prevertebral venous plxexi and sometimes in the pulmonary arteries or spinal canal if there are posterior wall defects [22]. Reported cement leakage ranged between 2–27%, and most often required no further intervention, often seen in the intra-disc space, prevertebral venous pelxi, and sometimes in the pulmonary arteries or spinal canal if there are posterior wall defects [22].

Special consideration is also given to sacroplasty, which can have a significant impact in the quality of life for patients suffering from osteoporotic or neoplastic sacral insufficiency fractures. The severe pain and immobile/recumbent positions that these patients experience can result in significant morbidity due to pressure ulcers, pulmonary compromise, and other infectious ailments. The injection of cement under fluoroscopic or CT guidance in the prone position is a fast and simple palliative procedure, which also stabilizes the fractures. The 2017 prospective review by Frey et al. that evaluated sacroplasty compared to nonsurgical management followed up for 10 years showed significant decreases in medication dependence and increases in pain relief and mobility [23]. This increases the armamentarium of palliative procedures in a cancer-surviving population that continues to grow.

In summary, vertebral augmentation offers the ability to improve the increased morbidity and mortality sequelae seen with benign and malignant spinal compression and sacral insufficiency fractures. While conflicting results from studies over the years have resulted in lack of both uniform understanding and widespread adoption of this minimally invasive approach to improve quality of life for spine tumor patients, there is increasing body of evidence supporting the benefits of VA in patients failing conservative therapy. Emerging technology and techniques have reduced prior complication concerns and have shown to decrease subsequent adjacent spinal fractures and opioid dependence. With more education and patient selection, this approach can help accelerate recovery and return to quality of life in these patients. Effective and high-quality patient care results from working with multidisciplinary specialist teams.

Cases

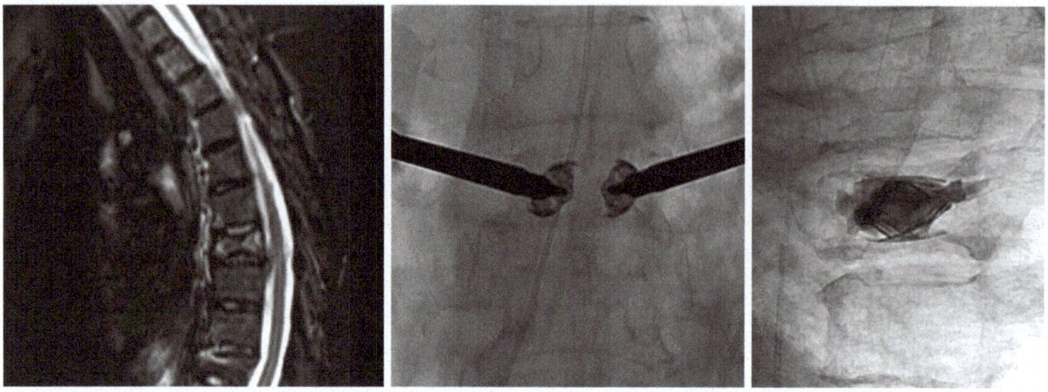

Sagittal MRI fluid signal sequence demonstrates moderate compression fracture of the T10 vertebral body. AP and Sagittal spot images demonstrate bipedicular access of the Spinejack cannulas followed by implant expansion and PMMA cement injection. Note significant height restoration.

Case 17.5 A 58-year-old male with severe compression fracture of the T10 vertebral body status post fall-induced compression fracture, with unrelenting pain despite conservative medical management

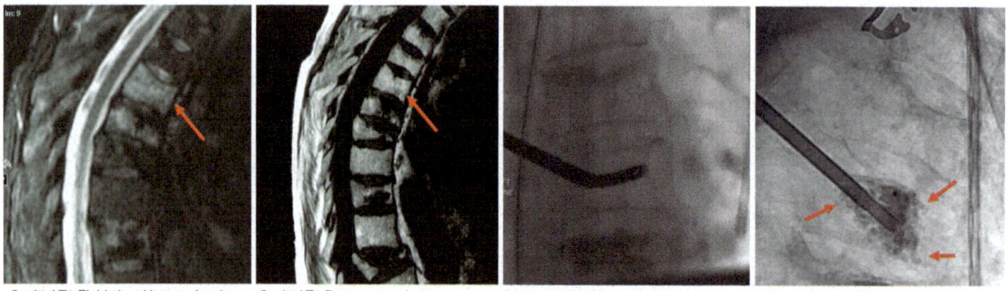

Sagittal T2 Fluid signal image showing Hyperintense T6 VCF with height loss (red arrow)

Sagittal T1 Post contrast image with gadolinium uptake in the T6 VCF (red arrow)

Intraprocedural images of unipedicular vertebroplasty of T6 VCF in the AP view with curved cannula in place

Lateral view showing instillation of PMMA cement through delivery cannula. Visualization of cement "interdigitation" (red arrows) into areas of cancellous (weak) bone.

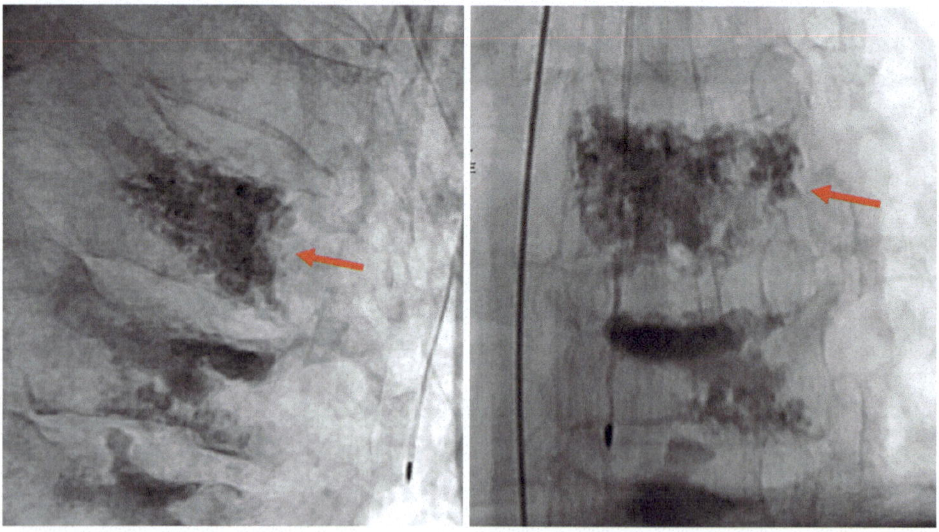

Completion Lateral (left image) and AP projection (right image) spot images demonstrating adequate distribution of cement into T6 VCF (red arrows) with no cement extravasation. Prior T7/T8 VA changes present as well.

Case 17.6 A 58-year-old female with history of breast cancer with known spinal metastases and prior treated thoracolumbar vertebral compression fractures, presented with new nontraumatic T6 fracture, biopsy proved to be pathologic

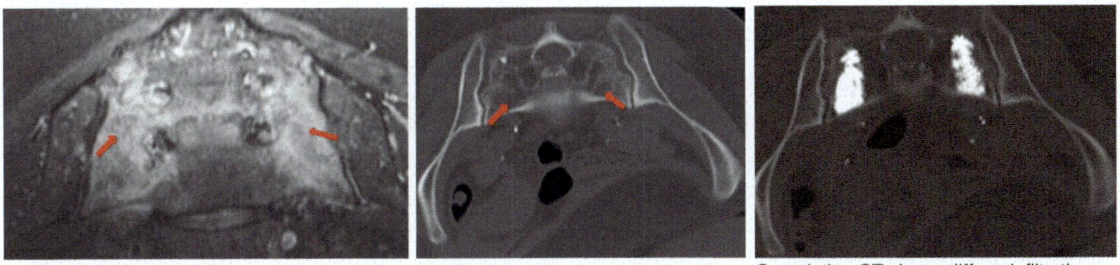

MRI Fluid sensitive sequence showing bilateral sacral insufficiency fractures

CT planning scan during at time of interventin shows area of hypodensity, consistent with fracture areas.

Completion CT shows diffuse infiltration of the cement into areas of weak bone. No non-targer cement extravasation.

Case 17.7 A 76-year-old female with history of radiation-induced sacral fractures, with severe recumbent position related pain

Spinal Ablation

Sreekumar Madassery

Pathologic vertebral compression fractures can result in similar or more pain, debilitation, quality of life decrease, and morbidities compared with nonpathologic fractures. Pain in spinal metastatic lesions may be even worse, since tumor growth in the confined vertebral body can cause pressure-mediated pain, in addition to the release of nociceptive tumor-related factors. After nonsurgical medical management of the fractures is started, helpful adjunctive treatments may include systemic chemotherapy and/or external fractionated radiation therapy. While radiotherapy may provide symptomatic relief, the effectiveness may be temporary and partial, with some studies reporting recurrent pain in almost 60% of patients around 2 weeks, with less effectiveness and potentially more complications with repeat treatments [24]. Although radiotherapy can be repeated, other palliative approaches should also be considered. Vertebral augmentation with simultaneous focal tumor ablative interventions can have several benefits in these patients including additive stability of the afflicted level, pain palliation, and tumor kill. Anecdotal experience has shown that non-radiated bone tends to be more amenable to VA and ablation. Additionally, radiation after VA can still be performed if needed.

The longest evaluated thermal ablative approach has been radio frequency ablation (RFA). While specific differences of the propriety devices in this category are beyond the scope of this chapter, the unifying aspect of all technologies is high temperature ablation to achieve tumor destruction. This is accomplished with either a single articulating probe or simultaneous bi-pedicular probes with water cooling to mitigate the charring effect that can occur, depending on the case specifics. Tomasian et al. demonstrated that bi-pedicular RFA with VA resulted in safe local tumor control in a review of 33 tumors evaluated for 1 month [25]. Other studies with up to 55 patients also showed similar significant pain relief in this patient population, including 23% of patients that had already received radiotherapy [26]. As mentioned, combining VA with RFA for spinal metastases, which can be performed from the same access, provides combined benefits of pain palliation, tumor ablation, and stabilization of the fractured vertebrae. Both RFA energy and the mechanics of PMMA cement demonstrate a synergistic effect for pain relief. Wallace et al. evaluated 55 radiotherapy naïve patients and found 89% local tumor control at 3 months and 70% control at 1 year [27]. A prospective study in 2017 by Reyes et al. reviewed 72 spinal metastases treated with RFA and VA combination, with significant pain relief, improved functional status, and tumor control without major complications [28]. What can be taken from these studies is that there is great utility in this treatment modality, and it may be offered as effective palliative treatment in a multidisciplinary approach. However, further randomized and blinded studies would be beneficial.

Freezing thermal ablation using Argon gas, termed cryoablation (CA), has been utilized in spinal tumors as well. This technique demonstrates good visibility on CT imaging and results in decreased associated pain when compared to RFA [29]. Cryoablation with VA versus VA alone was evaluated in 46 patients in a double-arm study, showing significant sustained improvement in pain scores and quality of life in the combination arm evaluated out to 6 months [30].

Microwave ablation that is used in other interventional oncologic procedures tends to have benefits compared to other ablative methods, mainly in fewer number of probes required for comparable ablation volumes, higher intratumoral temperatures, and faster procedure times. Utilizing these qualities with VA has been evaluated by Khan MA et al., in which 69 patients with spinal metastases were treated, and showed 94% of patients with immediate pain relief that was sustained to 6 months. In addition, local tumor control was also noted [31].

One of the downsides for ablative technologies currently being used in the spine is that the far posterior aspects of the vertebral body or posterior elements are not ideal targets due to potential adjacent nerve or spinal cord damage that can occur. Some technologies have mitigated this effect with spinal temperature probes for monitoring. Although currently used only in animal studies for evaluation, irreversible electroporation (IRE) is a potential tool that may benefit patients with painful osseous metastases and lesions in the posterior aspects/elements of the spine [32]. This technology causes irreversible depolarization of cell membranes, which does not affect nerve integrity.

Although there is a lack of abundant solid randomized and blinded data, combining thermal ablation with vertebral augmentation appears to be a safe and effective method of achieving rapid and sustained pain relief while simultaneously stabilizing fractured vertebra with good local tumor control. Choice of ablative method presently is operator dependent; however, radiofrequency energy has been the longest utilized approach. As a palliative treatment, this warrants further consideration and trials. This also requires well-functioning multidisciplinary efforts which are important in the ever-growing oncologic population.

Cases

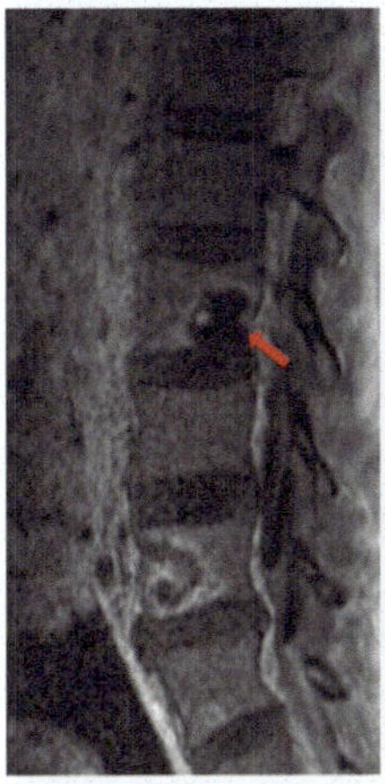

Sagittal contrast enhanced MRI shows enhancing lesion posteriorly at L2 (red arrow).

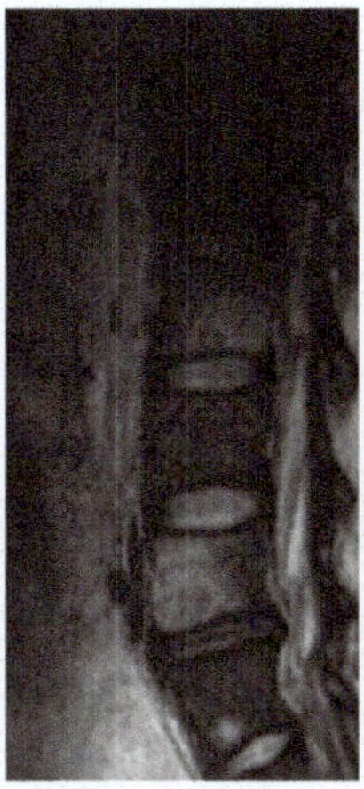

Sagittal fluid signal MRI sequence shows fluid signal in the vertebral body of L2.

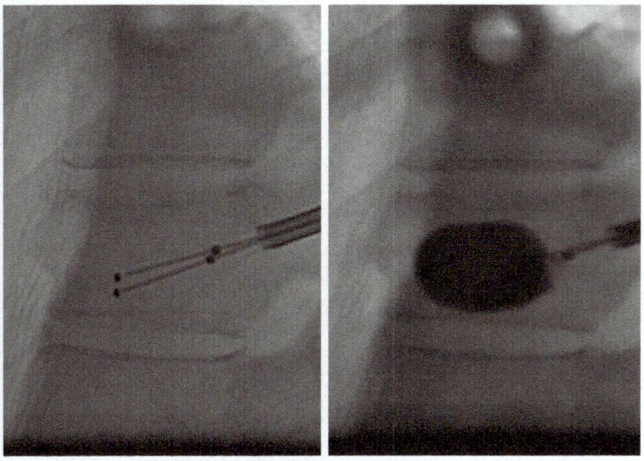

Bipedicular probes from the Osteocool™ (Medtronic, Minneapolis MN), Ablation system followed by balloon kyphoplasty.

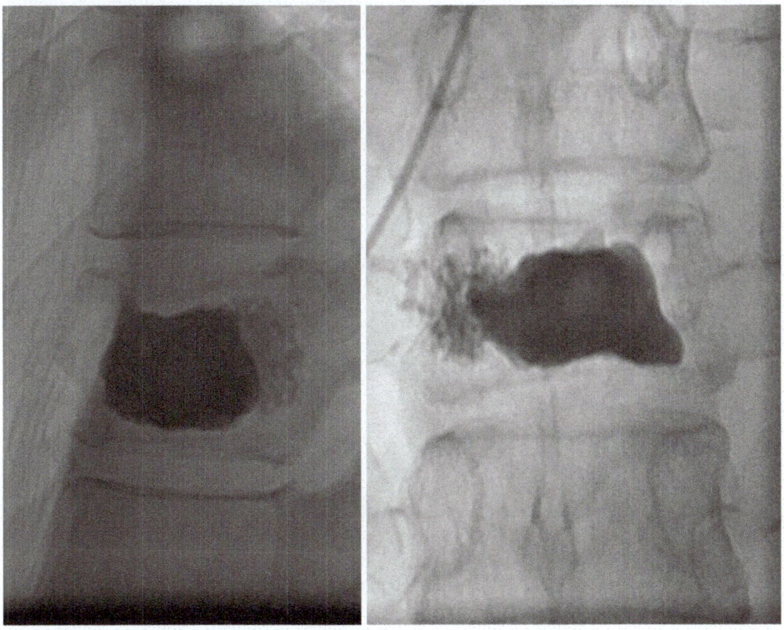

Post ablation and kyphoplasty images show cement filling the balloon created cavities as well as interdigitation of vulnerable bone.

Case 17.8 A 65-year-old female with multiple enhancing spine metastases on imaging, with mild height loss; however, severe pain is observed at the L2 level

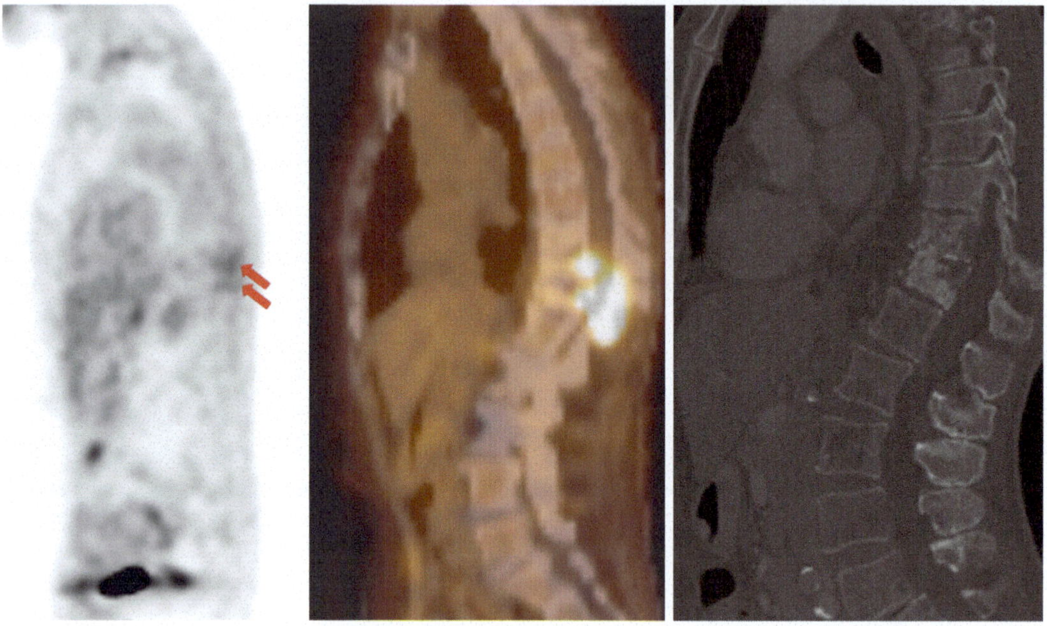

Attenuation corrected images from PET-CT shows activity T11 and T12

Fused PET-CT images shows intense activity within and surrounding the T11-T12 levels.

CT images shows areas of sclerosis and osseous destruction at the same levels.

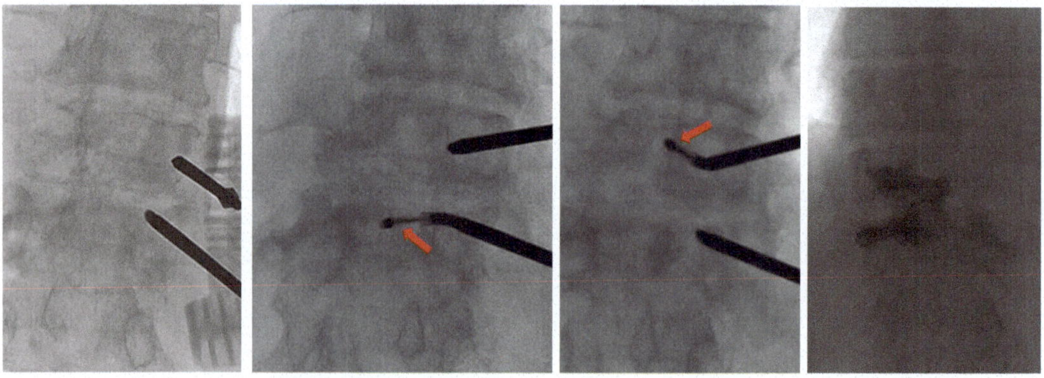

Unipedicular access obtained into both T11- and T12 levels. Middle and third image shows STAR™ (Merit, Jordan UT) RFA probes (red arrows) extended within the vertebral bodies in order to perform radiofrequency ablation.

Post ablation and vertebroplasty cementing image shows adequate coverage.

Case 17.9 A 74-year-old male with history of prostate cancer with focal moderate-to-severe pain of the lower thoracic spine, with imaging findings suggestive of metastases, proven on biopsy

Embolotherapy in Spine Oncology

Bulent Arslan

Introduction

There are several indications for embolization to manage spinal disorders. The most common indication is preoperative embolization of vascular tumors to minimize bleeding during surgical interventions. The second common indication for spinal embolization is for symptomatic hemangiomas. Arteriovenous malformations (AVMs) and bleeding are also rare indications for spinal embolization and, however, are not within the scope of this chapter. This chapter will review preoperative embolization of hypervascular tumors and symptomatic hemangiomas of the spine.

Embolotherapy has evolved significantly during the past 40 years. The first successful intra-arterial embolization was performed in 1970s and since then the development of multiple embolic agents as well as access and support catheters including ultra-small microcatheters now allow interventional radiologists to treat lesions that are in challenging locations. As much as the field has evolved, we have also become more familiar with embolization-related complications. A rare but potentially devastating complication is "nontarget" embolization.

The chapter reviews common use of spinal embolization procedures, clinical indications, techniques, and complications.

Embolization Technique

Embolization is performed in a wide variety of clinical settings, such as aneurysm management, active or impending bleeding, flow diversion, tumor treatment, and other indications. Every clinical scenario involves different techniques and approaches. Each embolization procedure involves obtaining a detailed percutaneous angiogram. Our focus will be on embolization of spinal pathology. In most procedures, the eventual goal is to occlude target blood vessels to diminish vascularity in the setting of a hypervascular tumor or AVM.

Arterial supply to the spinal cord is via the anterior spinal artery through vertebral, thoracic segmental, and lumbar branches of the aorta. There are extensive collateral branches allowing interconnections and supply overlap. Although watershed areas do exist, closure of several branches will be usually tolerated by the spinal cord, as long as the collateral circulation can compensate or flow dynamics self-regulate. There are a few important technical considerations when embolizing structures involving the spine. First and foremost is avoidance of the artery of Adamkiewicz (key thoracolumbar radiculomedullary feeder of the anterior spinal artery). Direct embolization of this branch or other non-collateralized feeders of the anterior spinal artery runs a significant risk of spinal ischemia/infarct. The thoracic and thoracolumbar areas are the most likely locations for the artery of Adamkiewicz and have the worst collateral supply. The second most important consideration is the size of the embolic agent. If the embolic agent is small enough, it can traverse to the spinal cord level and can cause intraparenchymal infarction. In general, when particles are used, a particle that is 300 micron or larger in size is generally considered safe. These are typically large enough to not travel too distally. When liquid embolics are used (i.e., Onyx or Glue), it is crucial to assess the arterial anatomy carefully to ensure the branches feeding the spine are avoided. Alcohol is one of the most effective embolic/sclerosant agent used in AVMs throughout the peripheral system, but its utilization in the spine can be devastating. When coils or even microvascular plugs are used, generally the risks are significantly less. Coils and plugs are commonly used in the proximal segment (segmental) arteries, and they will not result in ischemia or infect of the spine as long as anterior spinal artery is avoided.

In most cases, a common femoral artery access will be obtained into the arterial system. Radial artery access is gaining popularity in some centers due to faster recovery and discharge times but currently the majority of available tools are designed for common femoral artery. A 5 French (inner lumen diameter) sheath is standard, and through this a 5 French (outer diameter) catheter is advanced to select the target artery. There are variety of selective catheters with different shapes, and catheter selection is usually based on operator experience and preference. A common catheter used in our institution is a Sos-2 catheter (AngioDynamics, Latham, NY) for initial vessel selection. An angiogram performed through this catheter can be obtained to identify the target (tumor, AVM). More distal approach toward the target is usually performed coaxially with a micro-catheter (1.7 Fr to 2.8 Fr) with the assistance of a 0.014- or 0.018-inch guidewire. From this location, additional selective angiograms are obtained to confirm proper vessel selection and position, with focused evaluation for nontarget branches. The embolization is then performed with the preferred agent (microsphere, particle, or liquid embolic). Some operators will prefer to use coils or plugs more proximally as they feel necessary. In certain cases, microsphere or liquid embolic may not be safe due to proximity of the target to the aorta and/or spine, which may lead the operator to use micro coils and micro plugs only. Coils and plugs will diminish the blood flow to the target area, but they will not devascularize the target itself. The main goal of microspheres and liquid embolics is better devascularization of the target, although carries with it a slightly higher procedural risk.

In general, particles and microspheres are preferred for hypervascular tumor embolization, while liquid embolics, especially Onyx, are reserved for AVMs of the spine. Both can be used with or without accompanying micro coils or micro plugs.

Preoperative Embolization of Hypervascular Spinal Metastatic Tumors

The tumors that metastasize to the spine are usually hypervascular. Renal cell carcinoma (RCC) is the most common metastatic culprit, although thyroid carcinoma may also be hypervascular. Naturally, the more rare vascular-based malignant entities such as angiosarcoma are also extremely vascular. Symptoms may include pain in the area, instability of the spine, and neurologic deficits. Treatment options include external radiation, vertebral augmentation, and surgical resection with spinal stabilization [33]. Due to hypervascularity of the tumors, surgery (especially intralesional surgery) carries a high risk for significant blood loss, and embolization of the tumor or the arteries feeding the tumor region may help in significant reduction of blood loss. Manke and his colleagues demonstrated that particle embolization can decrease surgical blood loss from 5000 to 1500 ccs [34].

For preoperative embolization of spinal tumors, many agents have been used as an embolic agent. Today, medium-sized (300–700 micron) particles/microspheres are recognized as the most safe and effective practice (see Case 17.10). In addition, embolization may be used as stand-alone therapy or combined with other minimally invasive modalities. Two studies reported direct embolization or ablation of the tumor combined with vertebroplasty as an effective alternative to traditional approaches [34, 35].

After small-particle embolization is performed, coil and/or plug embolization of the main proximal branch will further diminish blood flow to the tumor and may also serve as localizing tool under fluoroscopy for subsequent surgery (see Case 17.10). Upstream coil or plug use is generally not recommended if repeat embolization of the target is a possibility, as these tools will prevent re-accessing the branch. However, in the setting of preoperative embolization, repeat embolization is rarely necessary since the surgeon will remove the tumor directly.

As mentioned above, the most devastating complication of a spinal embolization procedure is spinal cord ischemia and infarction. It is important to perform a pre-embolization angiogram to identify anterior spinal artery, which classically has a downward coursing hairpin appearance, and if embolization cannot be performed without risk to the anterior spinal artery, it should be either aborted or performed partially. Even incomplete embolization has been shown to reduce intraoperative blood loss [34, 36]. Lastly, other less significant complications are skin and/or muscle necrosis, dissection of blood vessels, bleeding from access site, allergy to contrast agent, and others.

Embolization of Symptomatic Vertebral Hemangiomas

Vertebral hemangiomas are seen in about 10% of the population with a predilection to young female patients. Although they are mostly benign, aggressive lesions can result in expansion of the vertebral body, pain, neurologic deficits, and may require treatment. Primary treatment has been surgical and may result in significant blood loss. One of the first articles published to assess the role of embolization in the treatment of symptomatic vertebral hemangiomas demonstrated that embolization was a promising therapeutic option when used alone [37]. However, it was safe and effective if used as an adjunctive procedure to surgery [35]. Later, Hurley and his colleagues showed that Onyx can perform better in preoperative embolization of aggressive vertebral hemangiomas compared to microspheres [38]. In two cases, after failing to achieve satisfactory embolization with microspheres, they were able to achieve very good end result with Onyx embolization of these hemangiomas (see Case 17.11) [38]. Current practice involves utilization of both particles and liquid embolic agents in preoperative embolization of hemangiomas. The embolization needs to be performed within 24–48 hours prior to surgery to obtain the maximum benefit of embolization. Especially with particles and microspheres, recanalization is possible and if the time between embolization and surgery is too long, potential blood loss benefit of the embolization procedure may diminish.

Conclusion

Embolization has been shown to provide significant benefit in preoperative management of metastatic lesions and hemangiomas of the spine. In both settings, significant reduction in blood loss has been shown. This practice is most important for renal cell carcinoma, thyroid carcinoma, and any entity that originates from a vascular precursor cell. As a standalone therapy, no significant benefit has been thus far shown, likely due to the intrinsic neovascularization ability of malignancies, but this theoretical use remains an option. Nonsurgical options for hemangiomas include ablation and/or cementoplasty of the vertebral bodies. Direct liquid embolic injection to the lesion has also been studied with promising results.

The most important complication of embolization is spinal infarction. Other complications include skin and muscle necrosis, bleeding, as well as injury to the arteries. Meticulous technique and choosing the optimal embolic material in the correct anatomical setting will minimize complications.

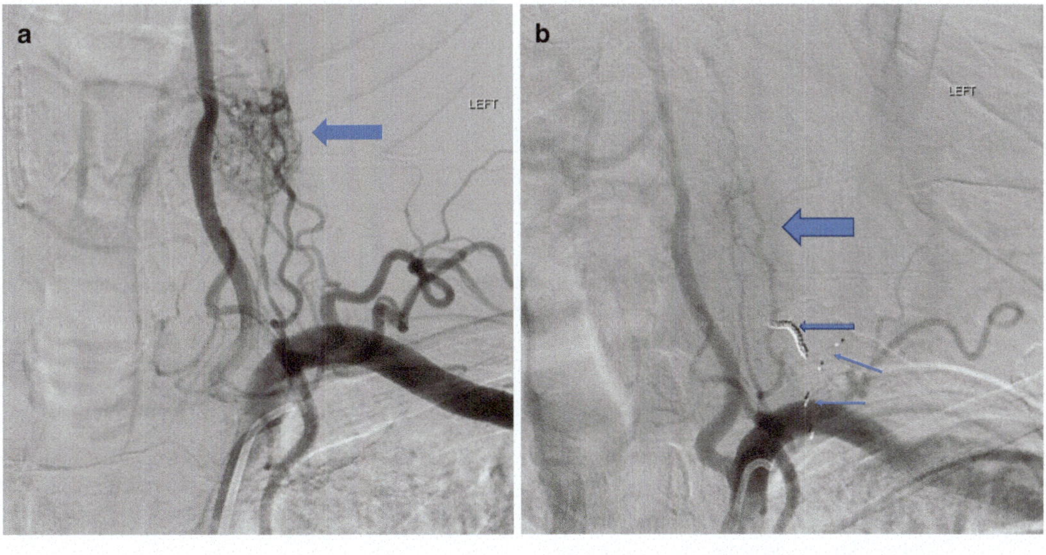

Case 17.10 (**a**) Renal cell cancer metastasis to cervical spine (large bold arrow). Patient planned for resection and spinal fusion. (Image property of coauthor B. Arslan). (**b**) Microsphere embolization with 300–500 micron spheres (large bold arrow). Additional embolization of the feeding branches with coils (small bold arrow) and microvascular plugs (thin arrows). (Image property of coauthor B. Arslan)

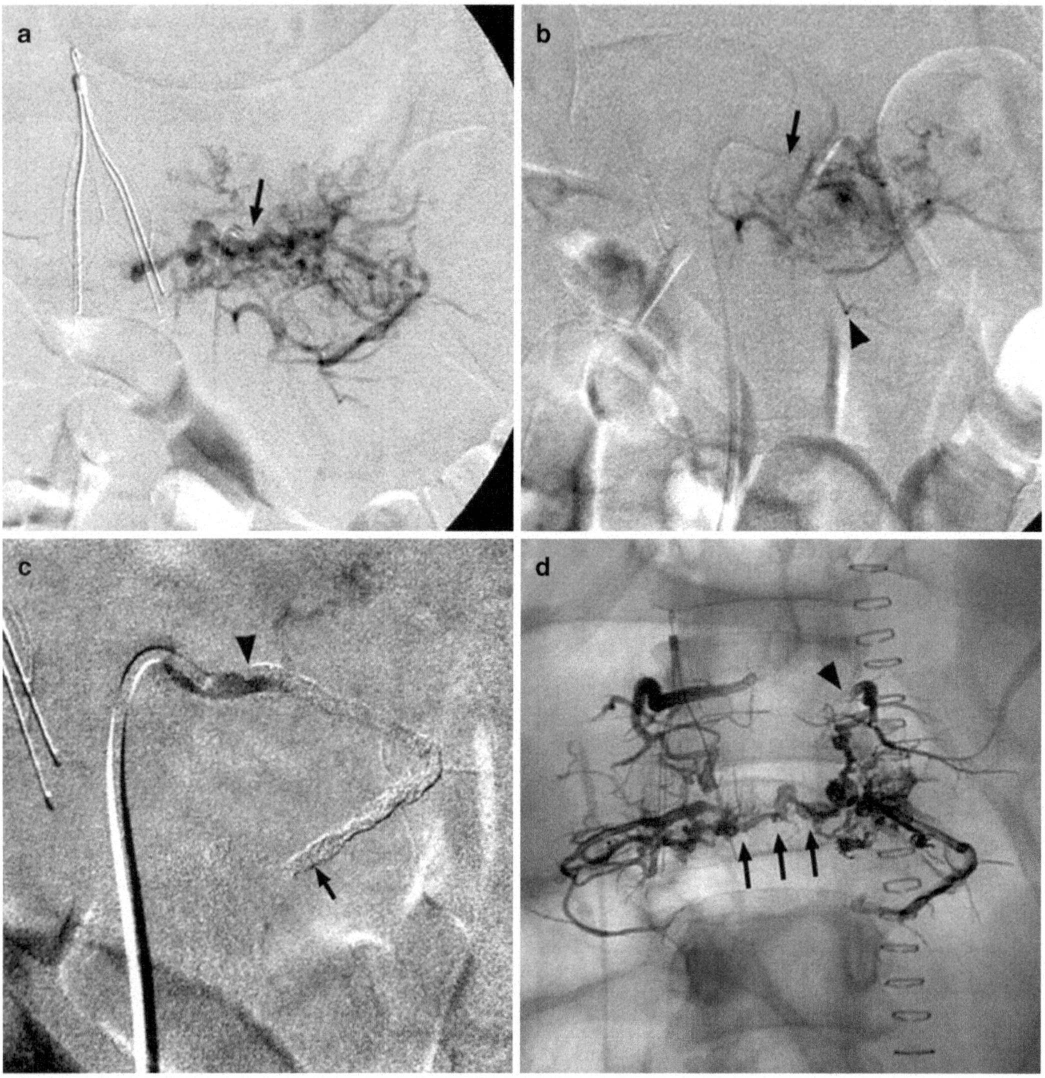

Case 17.11 (**a**) Selective angiography of the left L2 lumbar artery shows prominent tumor vascularity. No spinal anastomoses were identified. Note inferior venacava filter and diagnostic catheter in situ (arrow). (**b**) Post-embosphere-embolization angiography via the Prowler microcatheter (Cordis) (arrowhead) reveals persistent tumor enhancement. (**c**) Note the guide catheter (arrow) after Onyx embolization, where the artery is occluded, but the agent is largely restricted to the main artery (extending from arrowhead to arrow). (**d**) Plain anterior/posterior radiograph shows distribution of the 4 Onyx embolizations. Note extension of Onyx from the proximal left L1 lumbar artery (arrowhead) inferior to L2 and then across the midline (arrows). (Reproduced with permission from AJNR)

References

1. Murphy WA, Destouet JM, Gilula LA. Percutaneous skeletal biopsy 1981: a procedure for radiologists--results, review, and recommendations. Radiology. 1981;139(3):545–9. https://doi.org/10.1148/radiology.139.3.7232719.
2. Tehranzadeh J, Tao C, Browning CA. Percutaneous needle biopsy of the spine. Acta Radiol. 2007;48(8):860–8. https://doi.org/10.1080/02841850701459783.
3. Roberts CC, Beauchamp CP. Guidelines for core needle biopsy of bone tumors: implications for limb-sparing. Radiographics. 2007;27:189–206.

4. Rekhi B. Core needle biopsy versus fine needle aspiration cytology in bone and soft tissue tumors. J Cytol. 2019;36(2):118. https://doi.org/10.4103/JOC.JOC_125_18.
5. Yang YJ, Damron TA. Comparison of needle core biopsy and fine-needle aspiration for diagnostic accuracy in musculoskeletal lesions. Arch Pathol Lab Med. 2004;128(7):759–64. https://doi.org/10.1043/1543-2165(2004)128<759:CONCBA>2.0.CO;2.
6. Winking M, Stahl JP, Oertel M, Schnettler R, Böker DK. Treatment of pain from osteoporotic vertebral collapse by percutaneous PMMA vertebroplasty. Acta Neurochir. 2004;146(5):469–76. https://doi.org/10.1007/s00701-004-0259-7.
7. Wang B, Zhao C-P, Song L-X, Zhu L. Balloon kyphoplasty versus percutaneous vertebroplasty for osteoporotic vertebral compression fracture: a meta-analysis and systematic review. J Orthop Surg Res. 2018;13(1):264. https://doi.org/10.1186/s13018-018-0952-5.
8. Boonen S, Van Meirhaeghe J, Bastian L, et al. Balloon kyphoplasty for the treatment of acute vertebral compression fractures: 2-year results from a randomized trial. J Bone Miner Res. 2011;26(7):1627–37. https://doi.org/10.1002/jbmr.364.
9. Farrokhi MR, Alibai E, Maghami Z. Randomized controlled trial of percutaneous vertebroplasty versus optimal medical management for the relief of pain and disability in acute osteoporotic vertebral compression fractures. J Neurosurg Spine. 2011;14(5):561–9. https://doi.org/10.3171/2010.12.SPINE10286.
10. Clark W, Bird P, Gonski P, et al. Safety and efficacy of vertebroplasty for acute painful osteoporotic fractures (VAPOUR): a multicentre, randomised, double-blind, placebo-controlled trial. Lancet. 2016;388(10052):1408–16. https://doi.org/10.1016/S0140-6736(16)31341-1.
11. Firanescu CE, de Vries J, Lodder P, et al. Vertebroplasty versus sham procedure for painful acute osteoporotic vertebral compression fractures (VERTOS IV): randomised sham controlled clinical trial. BMJ. 2018:k1551. https://doi.org/10.1136/bmj.k1551.
12. Bornemann R, Jansen TR, Kabir K, et al. Comparison of radiofrequency-targeted vertebral augmentation with balloon kyphoplasty for the treatment of vertebral compression fractures. Clin Spine Surg. 2017;30(3):E247–51. https://doi.org/10.1097/BSD.0000000000000050.
13. Tutton SM, Pflugmacher R, Davidian M, Beall DP, Facchini FR, Garfin SR. KAST study. Spine (Phila Pa 1976). 2015;40(12):865–75. https://doi.org/10.1097/BRS.0000000000000906.
14. Korovessis P, Vardakastanis K, Repantis T, Vitsas V. Balloon kyphoplasty versus KIVA vertebral augmentation—Comparison of 2 techniques for osteoporotic vertebral body fractures. Spine (Phila Pa 1976). 2013;38(4):292–9. https://doi.org/10.1097/BRS.0b013e31826b3aef.
15. Noriega DC, Rodríguez-Monsalve F, Ramajo R, Sánchez-Lite I, Toribio B, Ardura F. Long-term safety and clinical performance of kyphoplasty and SpineJack® procedures in the treatment of osteoporotic vertebral compression fractures: a pilot, monocentric, investigator-initiated study. Osteoporos Int. 2019;30(3):637–45. https://doi.org/10.1007/s00198-018-4773-5.
16. Witham TF, Khavkin YA, Gallia GL, Wolinsky J-P, Gokaslan ZL. Surgery insight: current management of epidural spinal cord compression from metastatic spine disease. Nat Clin Pract Neurol. 2006;2(2):87–94; quiz 116. https://doi.org/10.1038/ncpneuro0116.
17. Lim B-S, Chang U-K, Youn S-M. Clinical outcomes after percutaneous vertebroplasty for pathologic compression fractures in osteolytic metastatic spinal disease. J Korean Neurosurg Soc. 2009;45(6):369–74. https://doi.org/10.3340/jkns.2009.45.6.369.
18. Erdem E, Samant R, Malak SF, et al. Vertebral augmentation in the treatment of pathologic compression fractures in 792 patients with multiple myeloma. Leukemia. 2013;27(12):2391–3. https://doi.org/10.1038/leu.2013.162.
19. Berenson J, Pflugmacher R, Jarzem P, et al. Balloon kyphoplasty versus non-surgical fracture management for treatment of painful vertebral body compression fractures in patients with cancer: a multicentre, randomised controlled trial. Lancet Oncol. 2011;12(3):225–35. https://doi.org/10.1016/S1470-2045(11)70008-0.
20. ACR; ASNR; ASSR; SIR; SNIS. Acr – Asnr – Assr – Sir – Snis Practice parameter for the performance of vertebral augmentation. 2017;1076:1–18. https://www.acr.org/-/media/ACR/Files/Practice-Parameters/verebralaug.pdf
21. Rajah G, Altshuler D, Sadiq O, Nyame VK, Eltahawy H, Szerlip N. Predictors of delayed failure of structural kyphoplasty for pathological compression fractures in cancer patients. J Neurosurg Spine. 2015;23(2):228–32. https://doi.org/10.3171/2014.11.SPINE14909.
22. Papanastassiou ID, Phillips FM, Van Meirhaeghe J, et al. Comparing effects of kyphoplasty, vertebroplasty, and non-surgical management in a systematic review of randomized and non-randomized controlled studies. Eur Spine J. 2012;21(9):1826–43. https://doi.org/10.1007/s00586-012-2314-z.
23. Frey ME, Warner C, Thomas SM, et al. Sacroplasty: a ten-year analysis of prospective patients treated with percutaneous sacroplasty: literature review and technical considerations. Pain Physician. 2017;20(7):E1063–72. http://www.ncbi.nlm.nih.gov/pubmed/29149151
24. Tong D, Gillick L, Hendrickson FR. The palliation of symptomatic osseous metastases final results of the study by the radiation therapy oncology group. Cancer. 1982;50(5):893–9. https://doi.org/10.1002/1097-0142(19820901)50:5<893::AID-CNCR2820500515>3.0.CO;2-Y.
25. Tomasian A, Hillen TJ, Chang RO, Jennings JW. Simultaneous bipedicular radiofrequency ablation

combined with vertebral augmentation for local tumor control of spinal metastases. Am J Neuroradiol. 2018;39(9):1768–73. https://doi.org/10.3174/ajnr.A5752.
26. Dupuy DE, Liu D, Hartfeil D, et al. Percutaneous radiofrequency ablation of painful osseous metastases. Cancer. 2010;116(4):989–97. https://doi.org/10.1002/cncr.24837.
27. Wallace AN, Tomasian A, Vaswani D, Vyhmeister R, Chang RO, Jennings JW. Radiographic local control of spinal metastases with percutaneous radiofrequency ablation and vertebral augmentation. Am J Neuroradiol. 2016;37(4):759–65. https://doi.org/10.3174/ajnr.A4595.
28. Reyes M, Georgy M, Brook L, et al. Multicenter clinical and imaging evaluation of targeted radiofrequency ablation (t-RFA) and cement augmentation of neoplastic vertebral lesions. J Neurointerv Surg. 2018;10(2):176–82. https://doi.org/10.1136/neurintsurg-2016-012908.
29. Tomasian A, Wallace A, Northrup B, Hillen TJ, Jennings JW. Spine cryoablation: pain palliation and local tumor control for vertebral metastases. Am J Neuroradiol. 2016;37(1):189–95. https://doi.org/10.3174/ajnr.A4521.
30. Masala S, Chiocchi M, Taglieri A, et al. Combined use of percutaneous cryoablation and vertebroplasty with 3D rotational angiograph in treatment of single vertebral metastasis: comparison with vertebroplasty. Neuroradiology. 2013;55(2):193–200. https://doi.org/10.1007/s00234-012-1096-7.
31. Khan MA, Deib G, Deldar B, Patel AM, Barr JS. Efficacy and safety of percutaneous microwave ablation and cementoplasty in the treatment of painful spinal metastases and myeloma. Am J Neuroradiol. 2018;39(7):1376–83. https://doi.org/10.3174/ajnr.A5680.
32. Tschon M, Salamanna F, Ronchetti M, et al. Feasibility of electroporation in bone and in the surrounding clinically relevant structures. Technol Cancer Res Treat. 2016;15(6):737–48. https://doi.org/10.1177/1533034615604454.
33. Prince E, Ahn S. Interventional management of vertebral body metastases. Semin Intervent Radiol. 2013;30(03):278–81. https://doi.org/10.1055/s-0033-1353480.
34. Manke C, Bretschneider T, Lenhart M, et al. Spinal metastases from renal cell carcinoma: effect of preoperative particle embolization on intraoperative blood loss. AJNR Am J Neuroradiol. 2001;22(5):997–1003. http://www.ncbi.nlm.nih.gov/pubmed/11337348
35. Schirmer CM, Malek AM, Kwan ES, Hoit DA, Weller SJ. Preoperative embolization of hypervascular spinal metastases using percutaneous direct injection with n-butyl cyanoacrylate. Neurosurgery. 2006;59(2):E431–2. https://doi.org/10.1227/01.NEU.0000223503.92392.CE.
36. Mendel E, Bourekas E, Gerszten P, Golan JD. Percutaneous techniques in the treatment of spine tumors. Spine (Phila Pa 1976). 2009;34(Supplement):S93–S100. https://doi.org/10.1097/BRS.0b013e3181b77895.
37. Smith TP, Koci T, Mehringer CM, et al. Transarterial embolization of vertebral hemangioma. J Vasc Interv Radiol. 1993;4(5):681–5. https://doi.org/10.1016/S1051-0443(93)71948-X.
38. Hurley MC, Gross BA, Surdell D, et al. Preoperative onyx embolization of aggressive vertebral hemangiomas. Am J Neuroradiol. 2008;29(6):1095–7. https://doi.org/10.3174/ajnr.A1010.

Lateral Corpectomy for Spinal Neoplasms

18

Philip Louie and Matthew Colman

Introduction and Concept

Direct lateral approaches to the thoracolumbar spine were born out of the trauma setting [10, 16], but are of importance when considering local control and reconstruction of both benign and malignant neoplasms. This technique offers full anatomic access to the anterior and middle columns of nearly the entire thoracolumbar spine. Further, it is performed through a minimal-access exposure, which facilitates both rapid recovery and mobilization of a frequently frail or ill patient population. While this technique and its variations are not appropriate for all clinical situations, it has emerged as a useful tool for the modern spine tumor surgeon, especially considering the morbidity associated with transthoracic, open retroperitoneal, or even posterior extracavitary approaches [5, 11, 23].

The Weinstein-Boriani-Biagnini classification describes the anatomic extent and axial depth of spinal neoplasms [7]. This framework is useful when considering a direct lateral approach to spinal neoplasms, which is most useful for tumors in radial zones 4 through 9. Intrabody (depth modifier B/C) or unilateral lateral or anterolateral extraosseous extension (depth modifier A) is the most easily treated tumor distribution using this technique. While ventral intracanal (depth modifier D) and unilateral intrapedicular (radial modifier 10/3) tumors are technically accessible using a direct lateral approach, advanced maneuvers are required for these areas and most intracanal or dorsal disease should be accessed using dorsal-based approaches.

P. Louie
Department of Orthopaedics and Neurosurgery, Virginia Mason Neuroscience Institute, Seattle, WA, USA

M. Colman (✉)
Department of Orthopaedic Surgery, Rush University Medical Center, Chicago, IL, USA
e-mail: matthew.colman@rushortho.com

Indications and Contraindications (Table 18.1)

The histology of a tumor is important to consider when choosing a lateral approach for oncologic control. Although en bloc techniques are possible through a lateral exposure [19], most procedures performed via direct lateral corpectomy will be intralesional. Thus, this technique is best used for radio/chemoresponsive tumors such as myeloma, lymphoma, or breast carcinoma, which require intralesional resection but respond to postoperative adjuvants for local control. Likewise, malignant surgical diseases which require wide margins and do not respond well to adjuvant treatments, such as chondrosarcoma or chordoma, would generally not be approached through a direct lateral strategy. Benign aggressive disease (aneurysmal bone cyst, giant cell

K. Singh, M. Colman (eds.), *Surgical Spinal Oncology*,
https://doi.org/10.1007/978-3-030-50722-0_18

Table 18.1 Indications and contraindications for direct lateral thoracolumbar tumor surgery

Indications	Relative contraindications
Anatomic extent	*Anatomic extent*
Vertebral body Unilateral lateral or anterolateral extraosseous extension Select ventral canal involvement Select unilateral pedicle involvement L4-mid thoracic levels	Intracanal tumor Dorsal tumor Bilateral extraosseous extension L5/S1 levels Anatomic variations such as high-riding ileum or retroperitoneal neurovascular anatomy High thoracic levels blocked by axillary contents or great vessel anatomy
Histology	*Histology*
Very radioresponsive (myeloma, lymphoma, small cell lung, germ cell)	Primary malignant (chordoma, chondrosarcoma, other bone sarcomas)
Moderately responsive (breast, thyroid)	Aggressive benign with inaccessible extent (osteoblastoma, ABC, GCTB)
Radioinsensitive tumors if R1 resection is possible	Radioinsensitive with inaccessible extent (renal cell, soft tissue sarcoma, melanoma, non-small-cell lung)
Clinical	*Clinical*
Pathologic compression/ burst fracture requiring anterior column reconstruction Impending pathologic fracture of the vertebral body	Requirement for direct circumferential or bilateral neural decompression

tumor of bone) or intermediate to low-radiation responders such as lung carcinoma or renal cell carcinoma, if using intralesional margins, must be thoroughly excised via gross total resection. This is because the quality of the resection has a direct impact on the risk of local recurrence. Thus, when choosing direct lateral surgery, the surgeon must be confident that all aspects of the disease can be accessed.

Tumor locations involving the spinal canal, dorsal tumor, or tumor which extends in an extraosseus manner to involve the great vessels or both segmental vessels of a given spinal segment are generally not appropriate for direct lateral surgery given the risk of injury to poorly visualized neurologic or vascular structures. Likewise, situations which require extensive direct canal-level neurologic decompression are not approached using the direct lateral corridor given the difficulty in obtaining circumferential decompression. Lastly, traditional contraindications for direct lateral disc surgery such as pathology at L5/S1 or high thoracic levels blocked by a great vessel or axillary anatomy also apply to direct lateral corpectomy procedures.

Naturally, in some situations, the goal of surgery is not purely based on oncologic control, but rather reconstruction and palliation of pain. In these situations, the direct lateral approach provides arguably the most thorough and robust reconstruction of the anterior column. This is because the exposure provides a full and direct view of the column, and facilitates the use of reconstruction hardware which spans the apophyseal ring of the vertebral bodies for maximum support.

Technique

Preoperative

Preoperative optimization is critical for success using the direct lateral technique. An estimated lifespan greater than 3 months, lack of acute hypercalcemia or other metabolic abnormality, ability to preserve performance status, and lack of major cardiopulmonary comorbidities are important considerations. The T1 MRI should be carefully scrutinized for great vessel or segmental vascular aberration or other anatomic structures, which may block the lateral access corridor. Preservation of spinal cord blood supply is another important consideration. For segmental vessel division in the thoracic spine involving more than 3–4 levels, the authors recommend a preoperative angiogram to identify potential key radiculomedullary vessels supplying the spinal cord via the anterior spinal artery. If divided, these key vessels may lead to spinal cord ischemia [3]. Lastly, hypervascular tumors such as renal cell carcinoma, thyroid carcinoma, and other vascular origin sarcomas should be preoperatively embolized to minimize intraoperative blood loss.

Intraoperative

The patient is positioned in the familiar right lateral decubitus position, with enough operative table flexion to allow presentation of the desired levels. The mid to high thoracic level approach may be facilitated by using an arm positioner for the ipsilateral arm. As in traditional direct lateral disc surgery, the left-sided approach is generally preferred due to the distant anatomic location of the vena cava, but may be converted safely to a right-sided approach depending on the tumor extent and individual patient anatomy. Neuromonitoring with electromyography (EMG) and other modalities facilitates the initial docking and neural navigation steps, and so muscle paralytics should be avoided on anesthesia induction. An axillary roll is used and extremities are well padded and protected.

Perfect AP and lateral fluoroscopy images are obtained by manipulation of the bed itself with the fluoroscopy machine locked in neutral position with no rotation or tilt. The desired disc spaces above and below the corpectomy extent are marked on the skin, and an oblique incision in line with the rib cage is used to access the exposure extent (Fig. 18.1).

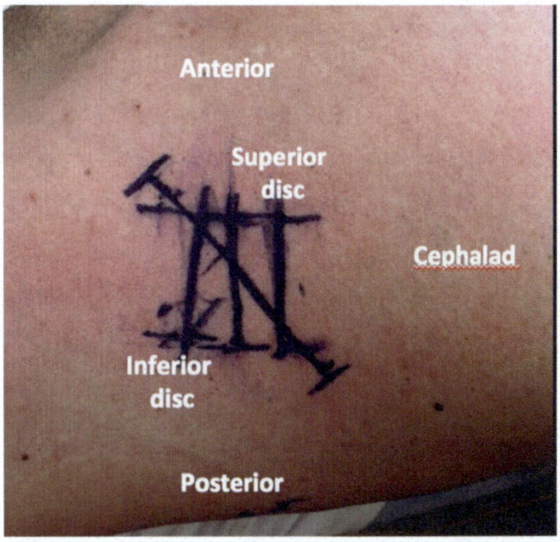

Fig. 18.1 The typical skin incision for a single-level lateral lumbar corpectomy procedure, with the cephalad and caudad disc levels accessed via an oblique incision in line with the rib cage

Dissection is carried out down to the abdominal wall, and a meticulous division of the fascia in line with the external oblique fibers is accomplished. In cases where one or more ribs impede the operative exposure, the intervening rib has its corresponding neurovascular bundle controlled and is osteotomized or resected to allow retractor opening. Resected ribs are useful as autograft later in the procedure. The retroperitoneal contents are cleared by blunt sweeping with a finger. Diaphragmatic insertional fibers may impede the corridor from T10-L3, and need to be carefully released in a blunt fashion.

Initial docking, transpsoas dilatation, and retractor placement at the supra- and subadjacent disc spaces are sequentially performed under direct neuromonitoring guidance. Discectomy, endplate preparation, and far-annulus transection using a Cobb elevator are sequentially accomplished above and below the corpectomy extent. In the lower lumbar spine, the authors prefer this stepwise method to one longer retractor "episode", and allow 5–7 minutes of "rest" time in between retractor series. The individual disc/endplate preparation retractor episodes should last less than 15–20 minutes, especially in the low lumbar spine to minimize risk of retractor-related lumbar plexopathy.

At each spinal segment included in the corpectomy, the instrumentation is gently re-docked, psoas dilated, and retractor opened at the midbody. A gauze dissector is used to locate the segmental artery and vein, which may be cauterized or ligated and divided. Division of these vessels as far posteriorly as possible allows easy identification and visualization of the remnant stump; division too far anteriorly risks self-retraction or avulsion of the vessel, which can then be difficult to control close to the aorta.

Final retractor placement is accomplished from cephalad to caudad spanning the prior discectomy sites (Fig. 18.2). A basket retractor may be placed anteriorly to retract retroperitoneal or thoracic contents from the exposure. A high-speed

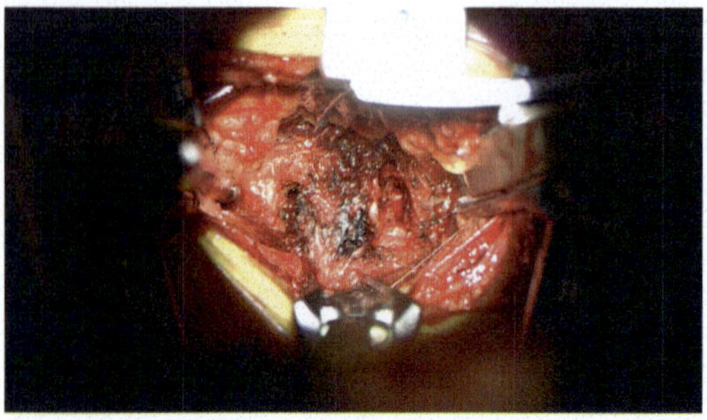

Fig. 18.2 The typical intraoperative exposure for the vertebral body to be resected following cephalad and caudad discectomy and final retractor placement

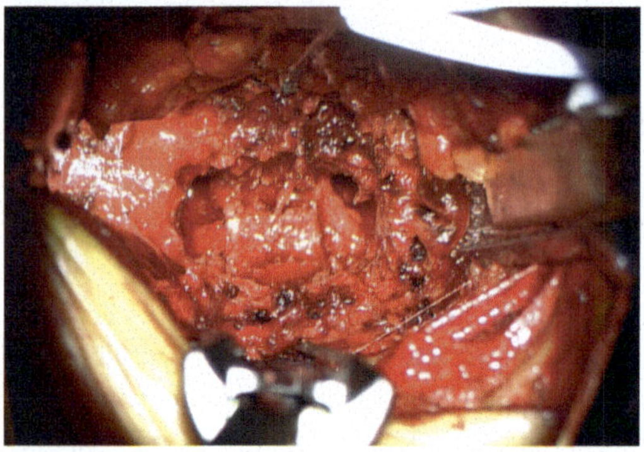

Fig. 18.3 The typical intraoperative exposure following vertebral body resection

drill is used to cut posterior and anterior troughs, and the corpectomy is carried out down to the far lateral vertebral wall using the drill, currettes, or rongeurs. It is very important to preserve the far lateral wall, since bleeding from the far-side segmental vessels (which lie directly deep to the lateral wall at the mid-waist) can be difficult to control. Generally, the anterior wall is also preserved for protection of the great vessels (Fig. 18.3).

The retractor can be manipulated or angled either anteriorly or posteriorly toward the canal to accomplish the full extent of desired resection. The operator can remain oriented to position using fluoroscopy or simple palpation of the transverse process and pedicle posteriorly. For direct canal decompression, the near-sided pedicle should be resected (along with its overlying rib head if in the thoracic zones) and used as a landmark to the canal, exiting root, and thecal sac. The posterior longitudinal ligament provides an excellent barrier to tumor and can usually be left intact as a protective pre-dural layer in this technique.

The technique can be tailored to the anatomic zone or individual anatomy. For example, the technique for lateral corpectomy is feasible in the thoracic spine, with several modifications. First, the approach is done with greater care, so as to preserve the parietal pleura and avoid pneumothorax. After rib resection, gauze dissectors are used to gently access the retropleural plane, close to the inner chest wall, and the pleura is preserved and stripped all the way to the costotransverse junction. An anterior basket retractor can then be used to retract the lung and great vessels anteriorly to facilitate exposure of the lateral vertebral bodies. If the pleura is violated, direct repair is attempted, with chest tube insertion required only when the pleural vacuum cannot be reconstituted.

Oblique anterior-to-psoas versions of this technique are also possible, with the theoretical advantage being less lumbar plexus retraction and less psoas-related postoperative morbidity. Although data are lacking for lateral corpectomy, in the field of direct lateral interbody fusion, the reported rates of transient hip flexor weakness or sensory disturbance are significantly lower than for the transpsoas approach, but with a reciprocal increase in risk for sympathetic chain or major vascular injuries [22]. This is likely because the pre-psoas approach requires direct visualization and blunt dissection of the vasculature. Nevertheless, the pre-psoas technique for corpectomy is feasible in a similar way to the transpsoas technique described above using specialized retractors and implants.

Lastly, the lateral corpectomy technique need not be used for complete corpectomy resections, but may be utilized according to the WBB extent of the tumor. Partial corpectomy resections, which spare the anatomy and avoid the requirement of fusion, are possible in select cases. Figures 18.4, 18.5, and 18.6 demonstrate a case of a 42-year-old female

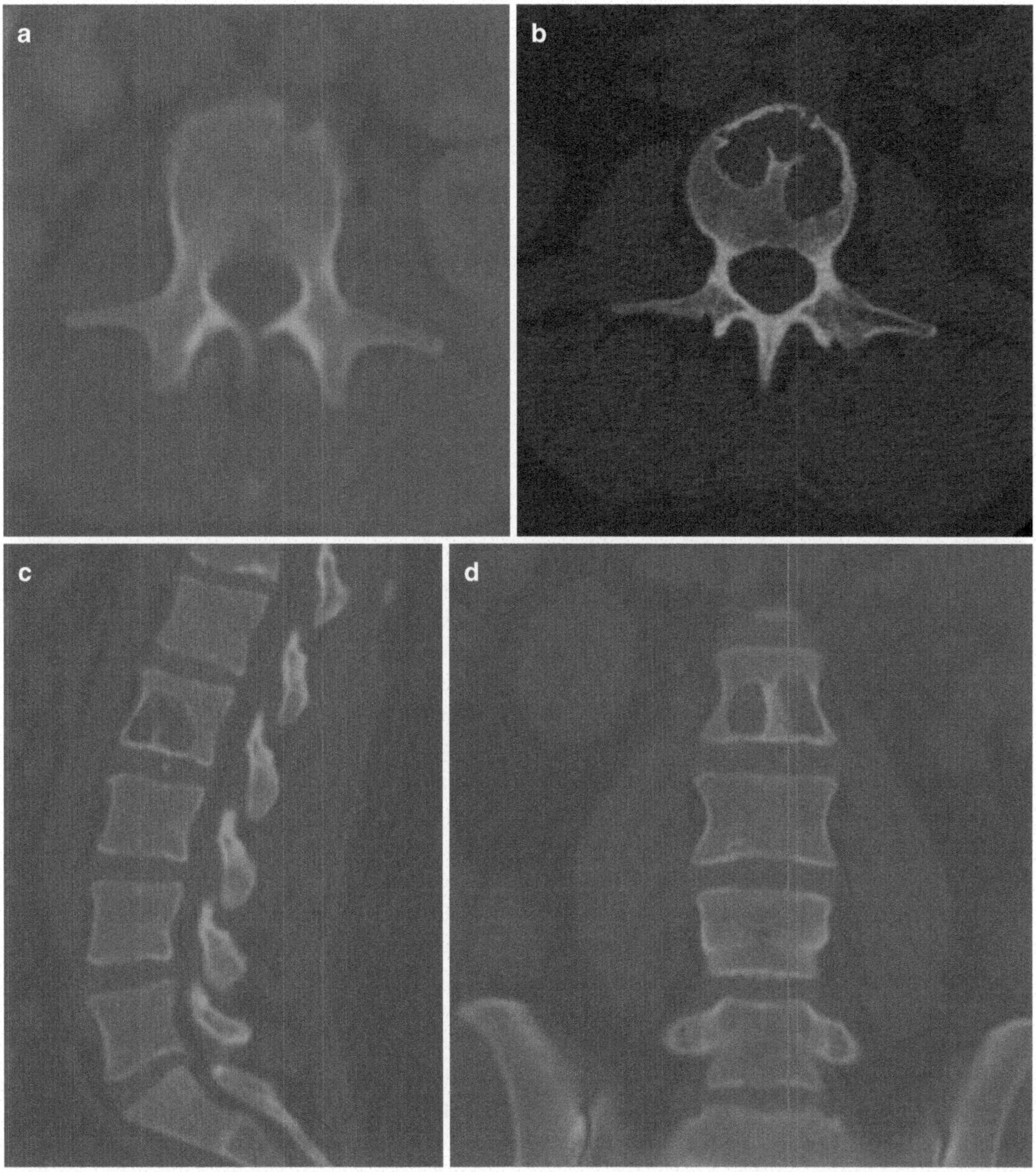

Fig. 18.4 The CT scan images of the L2 vertebral 6 years prior to presentation (**a**; axial) and at the time of presentation (**b**; axial, **c**; sagittal, **d**; coronal)

patient with a biopsy-proven benign fibrous lesion, which progressed over 6 years, causing pain and impending fracture in the L2 vertebra. Given the health of the endplates and the discs above and below, a limited direct lateral corpectomy and cementation was performed, without violation of the endplates or discs and without metallic reconstruction.

Reconstruction

Reconstruction can be performed using any number of static or expandable implants including radiolucent or metal cages, pins, and cement, or structural allograft bone. The authors favor a lateral-based expandable reconstruction cage, whose modular endplates are similar in design to

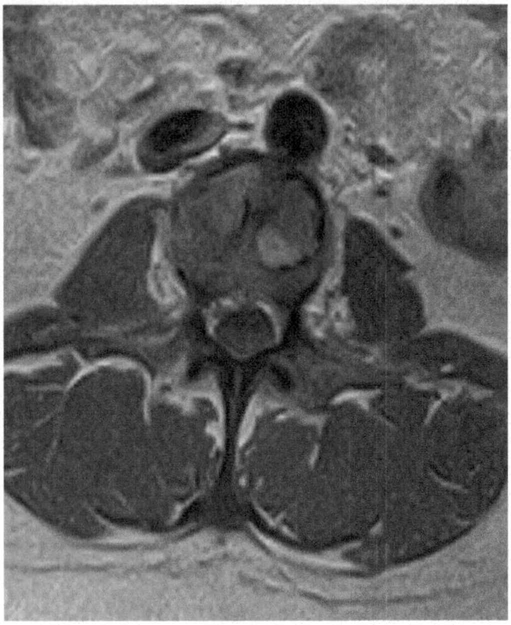

Fig. 18.5 The axial T1 post-gadolinium MRI of the tumor at the time of presentation

a direct-lateral interbody spacer, spanning the vertebral body apophysis and expanding to fit via a smaller expandable core. Figures 18.7 and 18.8 demonstrate a case of a 63-year-old man with biopsy-proven multiple myeloma and a pathologic fracture of L3. The tumor was approached via direct lateral transpsoas technique, resected, and reconstructed using the XLIF corpectomy device (Nuvasive, Inc, San Diego, CA).

The corpectomy defect is sized and trialed using calipers and/or trial instrumentation (Fig. 18.9). When using an expandable cage, the device is inserted from a direct lateral position, ensuring that the endplates pass through the previously completed discectomy defects across the endplate apophysis. The far lateral wall is not violated. The cage is then expanded to fit, taking care not to over-distract the defect space (Fig. 18.10).

Posterior segmental instrumentation is recommended when performing destabilizing lateral corpectomy. Where direct neural decompression and intraspinal canal tumor excision is required, the authors use a traditional same-day staged open posterior approach, or, for select cases, a prone-position lateral corpectomy approach to facilitate single-position, dual-approach surgery. When the canal does not require direct access, the authors favor minimally invasive percutaneous pedicle screw instrumentation. To save fusion levels, the lumbar spine may be an appropriate anatomic zone to consider one level of screws above and below the defect, but this should be based on excellent stability of the anterior column reconstruction, excellent bone quality, and other individualized factors. For most thoracic or thoracolumbar reconstructions, or any multilevel corpectomy, the authors favor two levels of segmental instrumentation above and below the defect.

For long-term good tumor prognosis, it is also important to consider the sagittal balance and deformity correction when performing this procedure. In patients who present with global sagittal imbalance, often due to a focal kyphotic deformity at the level of the tumor, restoration of sagittal alignment is critical in this patient population. Spinal deformity literature has described an association between pelvic incidence (PI), lumbar lordosis (LL), and health-related quality of life (HRQOL) outcomes [14, 16]. Thus, a focus on restoring a PI-LL mismatch to the patient's age-adjusted goal can provide the patient with the optimal balance to recover from surgery and return to their activities [9]. Upon completion of the reconstruction, the authors recommend obtaining an intraoperative full-length spine 36″ cassette plain radiograph to immediately evaluate the global sagittal correction obtained during surgery. Naturally, the concept of sagittal balance is most relevant in rare cases of long-term survival with metastatic spinal disease. However, these cases are becoming more common given the evolution of more effective adjuvant therapies. Additionally, immediate postoperative reconstruction failure, while multifactorial, may be at least partially related to sagittal imbalance and increased biomechanical stresses on the implant–host interface.

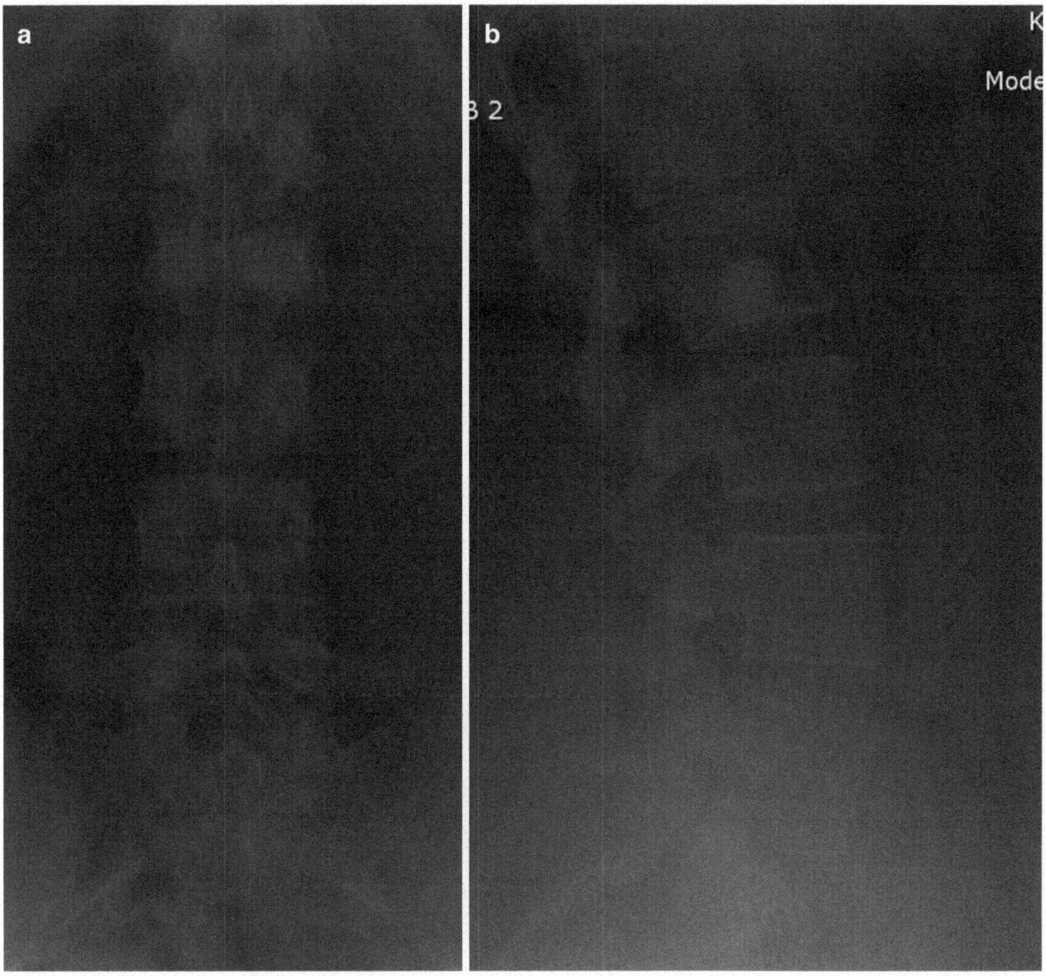

Fig. 18.6 The postoperative standing lumbar radiographs following tumor excision and cementation (**a**; anteroposterior, **b**; lateral)

Perioperative Care

Principles of aftercare following lateral corpectomy include rapid mobilization and return to ambulation. Walking and activities of daily living are permitted with no lifting over 10 pounds and no strenuous activity for 6 weeks. Bracing is rarely used by the authors and is indicated on a case-by-case basis depending on bone quality and stability of the implants. Physical therapy for muscle strength rebuilding, gait training, and stretching is often necessary at the 6-week postoperative point. Standing radiographs are obtained prior to hospital discharge and at 6 weeks for comparison.

Complications

The direct lateral transpsoas corpectomy procedure is subject to a similar neurologic complication profile compared with traditional direct-lateral interbody fusion, which includes transient hip flexor weakness (~20%), transient ipsilateral sensory disturbance (~20%), or permanent neurologic weakness (<3%) [22]. It makes intuitive sense that since retractor time appears to be a driver of these neurologic disturbances following direct lateral surgery, the complication rates would be higher in the corpectomy procedures. Robust data on neurologic complications following direct lateral corpectomy are lacking, how-

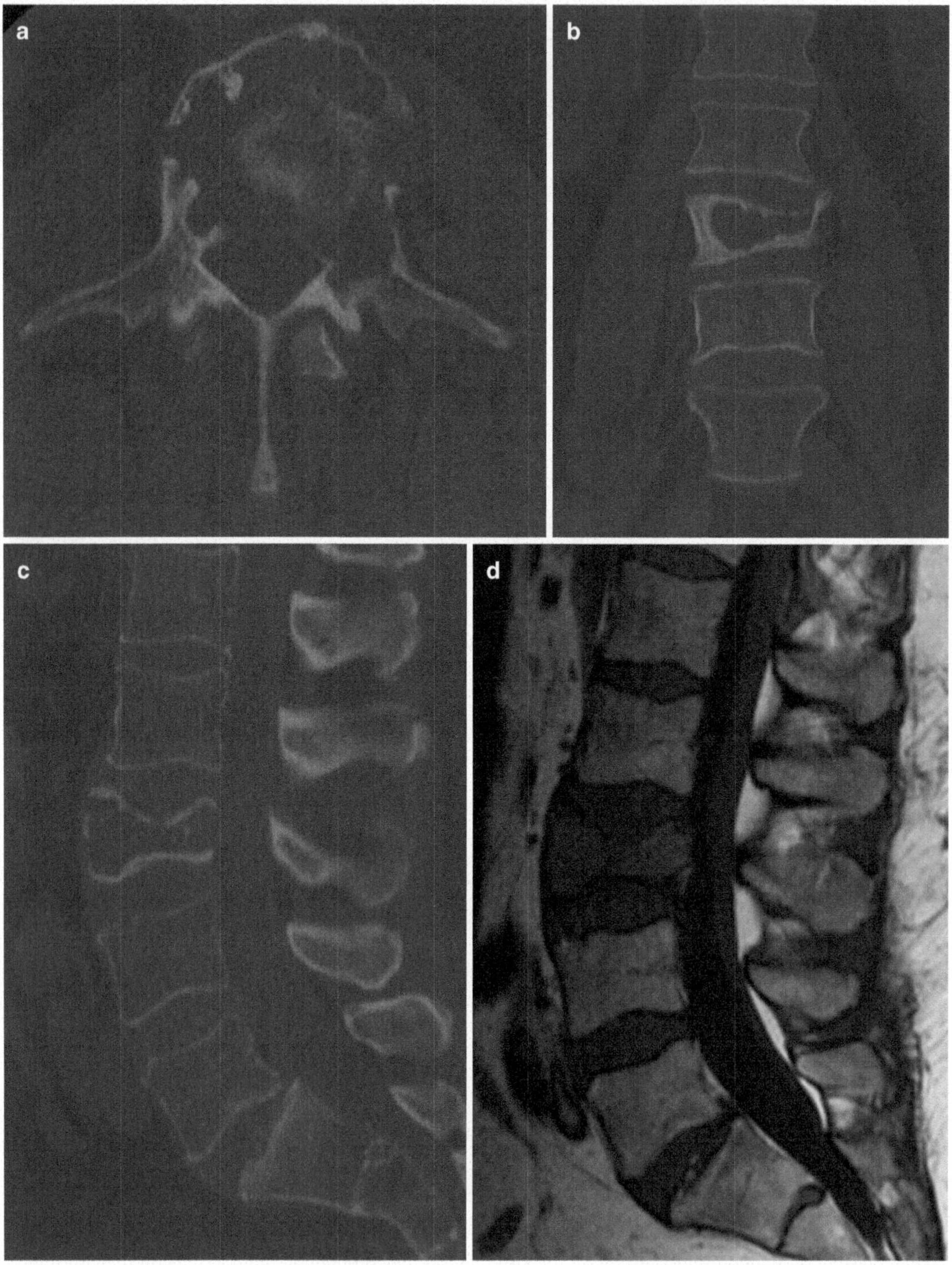

Fig. 18.7 The axial CT (**a**), coronal CT (**b**), sagittal CT (**c**), sagittal T1 MRI (**d**), and axial T2 MRI (**e**) of a 63-year-old man presenting with a biopsy-proven plasma cell lesion in the L3 vertebral body causing pathologic fracture

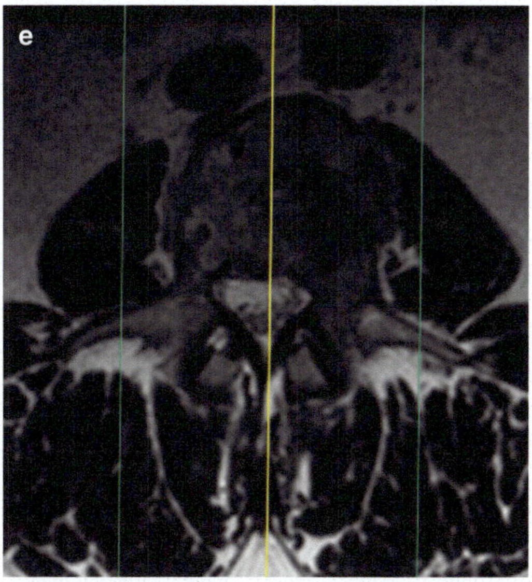

Fig. 18.7 (continued)

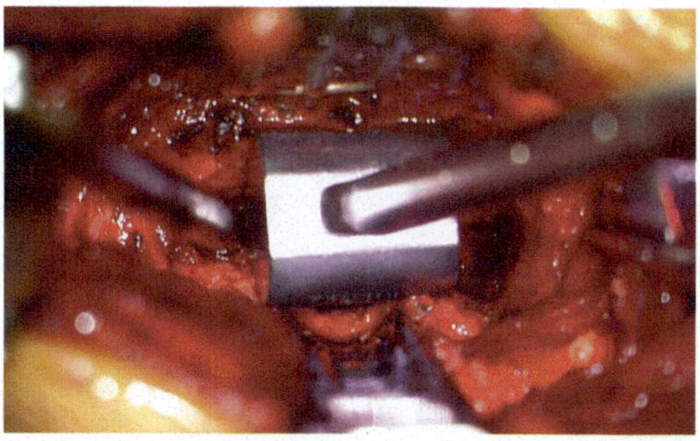

Fig. 18.9 Typical cage trailing using a template to ensure adequate vertebral body resection prior to cage insertion

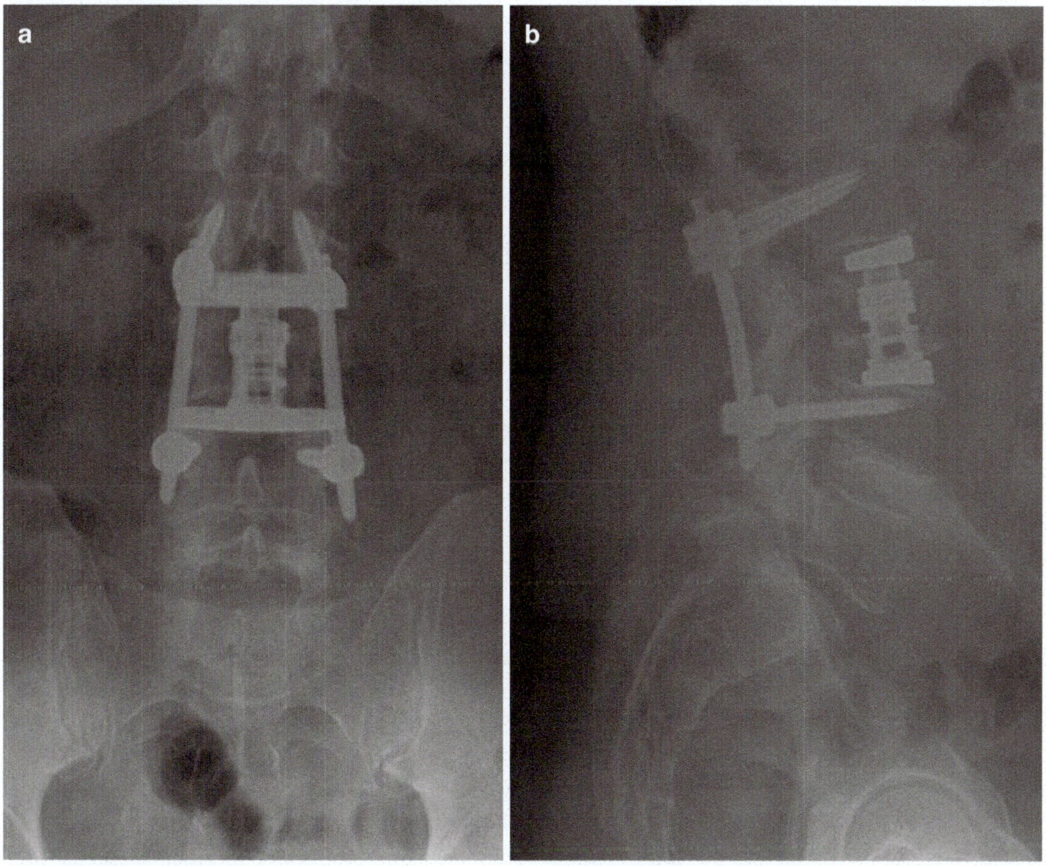

Fig. 18.8 The anteroposterior (**a**) and lateral (**b**) postoperative radiographs of the patient from Fig. 18.7 following direct lateral corpectomy and reconstruction

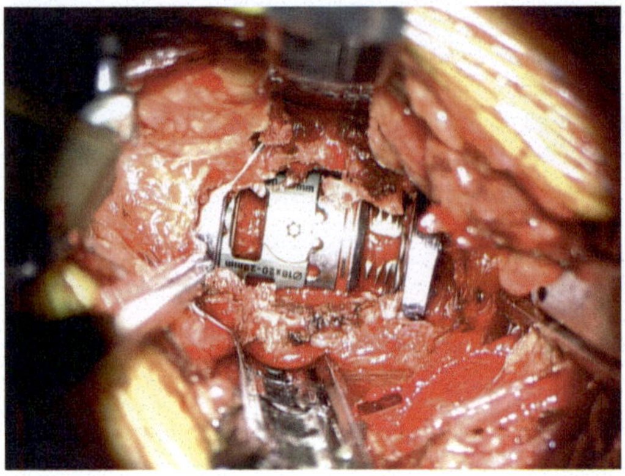

Fig. 18.10 Typical intraoperative exposure following cage insertion following lumbar corpectomy

ever, and most series report minimal neurologic events [15, 17]. Baaj et al. reported on 80 direct lateral corpectomy procedures and described no incidences of postoperative neurologic complications. The overall complication rate was 12.5% due to rare isolated events such as hardware failure, DVT, dural tear, and infection [1]. In two other series of direct lateral corpectomy for traumatic injuries [16] and tumors [20], the neurologic status was improved or maintained, and overall complication profiles were 5–15%, again due to isolated events such as pneumonia, hardware failure, hemothorax, and other events. Regardless, as discussed in the technique above, we recommend shortest possible retractor times, retractor rest/repositioning, direct EMG neuromonitoring, and direct visualization of the surgical field to minimize neurologic complications.

Other complications are rare. The great vessels are at a higher risk with pre-psoas approaches, right-sided approaches, and any surgical maneuver, which results in violation of the anterior longitudinal ligament or involves migration of implants, trials, or instruments anterior to the vertebral body. Visceral injury is minimized by using an accessory incision and ensuring that the thoracoabdominal wall is digitally cleared of contents, which are then swept anteriorly during the exposure. Significant bleeding from the segmental vessels may be avoided by preservation of the far lateral vertebral body wall and by careful control of the near sided segmental vessel so as to avoid retraction or avulsion from the aorta. Abdominal wall hernia has been reported [2], and is likely due to intercostal nerve disruption and flank musculature paralysis rather than failure of fascial repair; thus abdominal wall division should occur in line with the external oblique fibers and/or rib. Lastly, pleural rent or trauma to the thoracic cavity can result in pneumothorax or hemothorax [17, 21]. Liberal use of water-suction drainage is recommended when chest cavity negative pressure or hemostasis cannot be re-established with direct repair.

Reoperation rates appear to be very low for direct lateral corpectomy. While true successful arthrodesis rates are not well reported, Smith et al. reported only one case of reoperation for construct failure in the series of 52 patients (2%), while noting that traditional methods of performing anterior corpectomy in the traumatic setting have reoperation rates as high as 19% [16]. Another series reported one of 12 patients where a nonapophyseal cage subsidence was observed in the setting of single level posterior segmental fixation. This required revision and was revised to posterior instrumentation three segments above and two segments below the corpectomy defect [18].

Outcomes

Traditional benefits of minimally invasive or minimal exposure surgery such as shorter hospital stays and less intraoperative blood loss are also realized with lateral corpectomy. The largest series performed for traumatic or tumor applications have reported operative times in the 2-hour range and estimated intraoperative blood loss in the 300–400 mL range, with hospital stays of 3–4 days [16, 20]. This is in comparison to other techniques, both traditional and minimally invasive, which report much higher operative times and blood losses for corpectomy procedures [5, 8, 12, 13]. It should be noted that the direct lateral series have been reported by authors who are very experienced with traditional lateral lumbar surgery in the degenerative setting, and these numbers may not apply to other surgeons who are at different stages in the learning curve of lateral surgery.

Neurologic decline is rare after performing lateral corpectomy for tumors or trauma, and the technique appears to be effective for direct canal decompression despite the technical demands of this maneuver [4, 17]. In a series of 19 patients undergoing direct lateral corpectomy for metastatic epidural cord compression, 32% of patients improved by one or more Frankel grades, and with no incidence of neurologic decline [17].

Patient reported outcomes have been favorably reported following this technique. Uribe, et al. reported on their series of 21 patients undergoing direct lateral corpectomy for tumors, with an improvement in visual analogue scale (VAS) scores from 7.7 to 2.9, and mean Oswestry index score improvement from 53% to 25%. The mean final postoperative Oswestry index in another series of 12 patients improved to 20% [18].

The ability of the transpsoas direct lateral technique to correct alignment and deformity has also been assessed. In the traumatic setting for single-level burst fractures, the previously mentioned series reported a segmental lordosis improvement of 22 degrees and an overall lumbar lordosis improvement of 15 degrees, with only minimal deterioration at the final follow-up [18]. In the tumor setting, Tan et al. reported an average of 8 mm of vertebral height restoration and 8 degrees of lordosis correction [17].

Summary

In conclusion, the direct lateral corpectomy procedure is a safe, reliable, minimally invasive technique, which allows full access to the anterior column for tumor resection, neural decompression, and alignment/deformity correction. It enables transapophyseal reconstructions and short segment posterior fixation, which may be of benefit in functional restoration and early postoperative recovery. These benefits are especially apropos for oncology patients who tend to be more frail and can expect shortened overall lifespans. It should be used with some caution, however, since the procedure carries a slow learning curve, and favorable results have been reported predominantly by groups who have significant underlying experience with lateral surgery in the degenerative setting.

References

1. Baaj AA, Dakwar E, Le TV, et al. Complications of the mini-open anterolateral approach to the thoracolumbar spine. J Clin Neurosci. 2012;19(9):1265–7.
2. Choi JH, Jang JS, Jang IT. Abdominal flank bulging after lateral retroperitoneal approach: a case report. NMC Case Rep J. 2016;4(1):23–6.
3. Colman MW, Hornicek FJ, Schwab JH. Spinal cord blood supply and its surgical implications. J Am Acad Orthop Surg. 2015;23(10):581–91.
4. Gandhoke GS, Tempel ZJ, Bonfield CM, Madhok R, Okonkwo DO, Kanter AS. Technical nuances of the minimally invasive extreme lateral approach to treat thoracolumbar burst fractures. Eur Spine J. 2015;24(Suppl 3):353–60.
5. Gokaslan ZL, York JE, Walsh GL, et al. Transthoracic vertebrectomy for metastatic spinal tumors. J Neurosurg. 1998;89:599–609.
6. Justin SS, Christopher IS, Steven DG, et al. Clinical and radiographic parameters that distinguish between the best and worst outcomes of scoliosis surgery for adults. Eur Spine J. 2013;22(2):402–10.
7. Hart RA, Boriani S, Biagini R, Currier B, Weinstein JN. A system for surgical staging and management of spine tumors: a clinical outcome study of giant cell tumors of the spine. Spine. 1997;22(15):1773–82.
8. Kossman T, Jacobi D, Trentz O. The use of a retractor system (SynFrame) for open, minimal invasive reconstruction of the anterior column of the thoracic and lumbar spine. Eur Spine J. 2001;10:396–402.
9. Lafage R, Schwab F, Glassman S, et al. Age-adjusted alignment goals have the potential to reduce PJK. Spine. 2017;17(42)1275–82.
10. Malham GM. Minimally invasive direct lateral corpectomy for the treatment of a thoracolumbar fracture. J Neurol Surg A Cent Eur Neurosurg. 2015;76(3):240–3.
11. Park MS, Deukmedjian AR, Uribe JS. Minimally invasive anterolateral corpectomy for spinal tumors. Neurosurg Clin N Am. 2014;25:317–25.
12. Payer M, Sottas C. Mini-open anterior approach for corpectomy in the thoracolumbar spine. Surg Neurol. 2008;69:25–32. 51.
13. Ragel BT, Kan P, Schmidt MH. Blood transfusions after thoracoscopic anterior thoracolumbar vertebrectomy. Acta Neurochir. 2010;152:597–603.
14. Schwab F, Lafage V, Patel A, Farcy JP. Sagittal plane considerations and the pelvis in the adult patient. Spine. 2009;34(17):1828–33.
15. Serak J, Vanni S, Levi AD. The extreme lateral approach for treatment of thoracic and lumbar vertebral body metastases. J Neurosurg Sci. 2019;63(4):473–8.

16. Smith WD, Dakwar E, Le TV, Christian G, Serrano S, Uribe JS. Minimally invasive surgery for traumatic spinal pathologies: a mini-open, lateral approach in the thoracic and lumbar spine. Spine. 2010;35(26 Suppl):S338–46.
17. Tan T, Chu J, Thien C, Wang YY. Minimally invasive direct lateral corpectomy of the thoracolumbar spine for metastatic spinal cord compression. J Neurol Surg A Cent Eur Neurosurg. 2017;78(4):358–67.
18. Theologis AA, Tabaraee E, Toogood P, Kennedy A, Birk H, McClellan RT, et al. Anterior corpectomy via the mini-open, extreme lateral, transpsoas approach combined with short-segment posterior fixation for single-level traumatic lumbar burst fractures: analysis of health-related quality of life outcomes and patient satisfaction. J Neurosurg Spine. 2016;24(1):60–8.
19. Turner JD, Zaidi HA, Godzik J, Albuquerque FC, Uribe JS. Mini-open lateral en bloc corpectomy: cadaveric feasibility and early clinical experience. Clin Spine Surg. 2019;32(4):143–9.
20. Uribe JS, Dakwar E, Le TV, Christian G, Serrano S, Smith WD. Minimally invasive surgery treatment for thoracic spine tumor removal: a mini-open, lateral approach. Spine. 2010;35(26 Suppl):S347–54.
21. Uribe JS, Dakwar E, Cardona RF, Vale FL. Minimally invasive lateral retropleural thoracolumbar approach: cadaveric feasibility study and report of 4 clinical cases. Neurosurgery. 2011;68(1 Suppl Operative):32–9.
22. Walker CT, Farber SH, Cole TS, Xu DS, Godzik J, Whiting AC, Hartman C, Porter RW, Turner JD, Uribe J. Complications for minimally invasive lateral interbody arthrodesis: a systematic review and meta-analysis comparing prepsoas and transpsoas approaches. J Neurosurg Spine. 2019:1–15.
23. Zuckerman SL, Laufer I, Sahgal A, et al. When less is more: the indications for MIS techniques and separation surgery in metastatic spine disease. Spine. 2016;41(suppl 20):S246–53.

Minimally Invasive Approaches to Thoracic and Lumbar Metastatic Spine Disease

19

Eric Vess, Bowen Qui, and Addisu Mesfin

Introduction

Spinal metastases are the most common malignant tumors of the axial spine. Following the lung and the liver, the skeletal system is the most common site of metastases. Within the skeletal system, the spine is the number one sissete of metastases. Primary spine tumors are rare. Compression of neural elements and destabilization via osseous destruction are significant contributors to pain and morbidity. Open surgical treatment of these lesions is well established in patients with spinal instability and/or symptomatic neural element compression [1, 2]. However, open surgical techniques with large dissection fields can be physiologically stressful to patients with an already increased morbidity profile. Minimally invasive surgery (MIS) is a promising solution for treating patients with neoplastic spinal disease by decreasing the soft tissue exposure and decreasing blood loss.

Minimally invasive surgery (MIS) or minimal access spine technique (MALT) represents a wide range of therapies including video-assisted thoracoscopy, mini-open, and percutaneous techniques. MIS is a set of principles with the priority of respecting natural tissue architecture and minimizing tissue dissection while still achieving the same goals of traditional techniques. The common misbelief is that Minimally Invasive Spinal Surgery (MISS) is a modern concept partially driven by marketing but in actuality has been evolving since the 1960s with the adaptation of the operating microscope for lumbar discectomy [3]. With further advancements in illumination, magnification, and specialized instrumentation, MIS techniques continue to evolve [4].

Oncological patients pose surgical challenges due to the complexity of their condition and associated comorbidities. MISS within this critical patient population is particularly appealing given the established association with reduced intraoperative blood loss, decreased postoperative pain, and shorter hospital stays [5–8]. Additionally, earlier initiation of adjuvants such as postoperative radiation or systemic therapies can be achieved with less concern for wound complications.

Principles of MISS in Tumor

The basic oncologic principles of MISS as applied to tumor surgery are identical to the same principles in open surgery. It is critical that utilization of MISS techniques does not influence the treatment strategy of the target site and that basic oncologic principles are observed. In other

E. Vess · B. Qui · A. Mesfin (✉)
Department of Orthopaedics & Rehabilitation, University of Rochester School of Medicine & Dentistry, Rochester, NY, USA

K. Singh, M. Colman (eds.), *Surgical Spinal Oncology*,
https://doi.org/10.1007/978-3-030-50722-0_19

words, these principles can be universally applied to all patients, and the surgeon must ensure that any MISS technique accomplishes the appropriate goals [9].

The treatment of metastatic disease is palliative. With this in mind, en-bloc resection of a tumor is rarely indicated. The main indication for applying surgical treatment to spinal tumors is for decompression of the neural elements and stabilization of the spine. Metastatic lesions can cause de-novo spinal deformity in the coronal and sagittal planes. The Spinal Instability Neoplastic Score (SINS) can help guide treatment (nonoperative, observation, operative) in the setting of spinal instability [10]. MISS techniques can be used in the same manner as traditional open techniques in achieving these goals through a wide range of procedures. The focus of this chapter will be on decompression and stabilization as these are the most common reasons for operative intervention in the oncology patient.

Limitations of MISS

The indications for MISS are the same as for open techniques as long as the same principles are followed. The limitations of MIS surgery include limited exposures and increased exposure to intraoperative radiation for the surgeon and patient. While MIS can allow for some access to the anterior spinal column and canal, it can be difficult to achieve sufficient exposure. Some cases that require multiple levels of anterior or circumferential decompression may be more suited for open techniques. In the thoracic spine, lateral-based decompression may be feasible. Tumor characteristics must also be considered; some vascularized tumor histologies such as renal cell or thyroid carcinoma which are associated with excessive bleeding might best be approached using open techniques if preoperative embolization was not feasible or performed. Finally, the learning curve associated with MIS can be steep and surgeon experience should play a factor when choosing a surgical approach. The highest complication rate for MIS surgery and longest operative times occur within a surgeon's first 30 cases and plateaus thereafter [11, 12].

MIS Spinal Decompression

Originally, spinal cord decompression completed via an open posterior laminectomy was shown clinically to be equivalent to radiation therapy [13]. This technique at best offered indirect decompression for anterior lesions. As the majority of metastatic lesions lie within the anterior elements or in the anterior epidural space, anterior-based approaches became popularized and demonstrated superiority compared to posterior laminectomy alone [14, 15]. Bridwell et al. were one of the first to report on an open posterolateral spinal cord decompression for spinal metastases through a transpedicular approach, which addressed ventral spinal cord compression and improved neurological outcomes [16]. Posterior-only thoracic corpectomies (costotransversectomy, lateral extracavitary) were subsequently popularized and thought to be associated with less morbidity and did not require an access surgeon compared to anterior approaches [17–19]. However, even novel posterior approaches such as costotransversectomy still required large fascial dissections and carry substantial recovery time and morbidity [19, 20]. Thus, minimally invasive approaches to neural element decompression were developed to provide an approach that offered decreased morbidity in a population that already has a high rate of comorbidities, frailty, and risk of wound complications.

Although minimally invasive anterior thoracoscopic and extreme lateral minithoracotomy techniques have been described, most of the focus surrounding minimally invasive decompression of metastatic spinal disease has been on posterior or lateral-based approaches [21, 22]. These techniques can be accomplished using either percutaneous tubular retractors or through a mini-open incision where the skin is incised completely but the fascia is preserved except over the immediate area of interest. Although mini-open approaches still utilize a larger skin

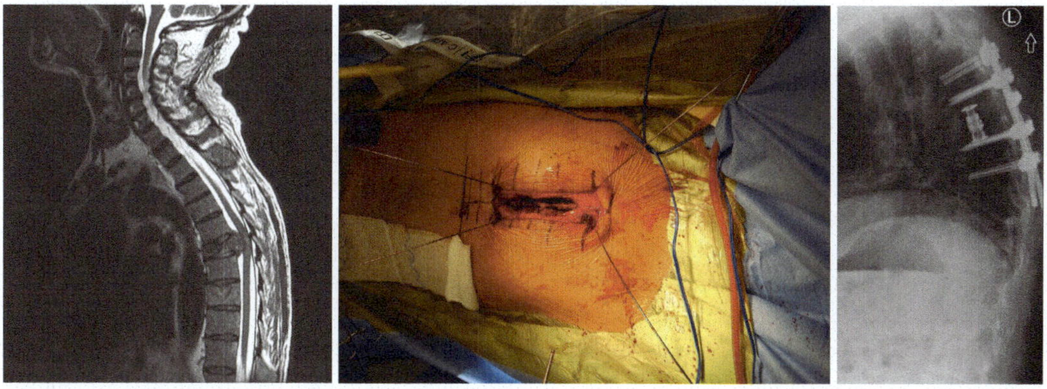

Fig. 19.1 A 59-year-old male with metastatic prostate cancer and epidural spinal cord compression with SINS of 16 managed with mini-open fascia incision, percutaneous screws at the bottom and top of the construct, transpedicular decompression, and expandable cage placement

incision, minimally invasive instrumentation, visualization, and surgical techniques are still utilized deep to the fascia (Fig. 19.1).

It is important to recognize the interdependent relationship between spinal cord decompression and stabilization. The integrity of the metastatic spine is already violated, and decompression often results in further iatrogenic destabilization. With few exceptions (lumbar spine epidural compression, compression dorsal to the thecal sac), decompression of the spinal cord should be accompanied by some form of stabilization. Percutaneous posterior stabilization can be performed universally, but depending on the degree of anterior destabilization, anterior supplementation might also be necessary.

Minimally invasive techniques can be technically demanding and for the most part, the techniques that have been developed thus far are variations of the established open technique. Thus, knowledge of the open technique is an initial prerequisite. Intraoperatively, the surgeon must be comfortable converting to the open approach if visualization is unsuitable or complications (durotomies, excessive bleeding) arise.

Transpedicular Approach

Transpedicular decompression provides direct access to 25% of the ventral spinal canal and indirect access to up to 75% for posterolateral

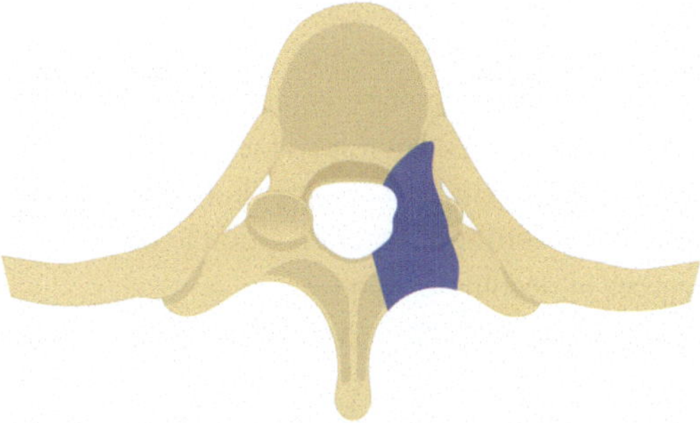

Fig. 19.2 Depiction of the surgical corridor of transpedicular decompression. The zone of direct visualization is highlighted in purple

decompression (Fig. 19.2). Deutsch et al. originally described this technique and there have been multiple technical adaptations that have expanded the utility of the approach [23–25]. The hallmark of the technique is rib head preservation, which theoretically avoids the morbidity associated with pleural dissection. Other advantages include a direct midline incision, which can provide access to both sides of the spinal cord from the same mini-open incision. Transpedicular decompression can be accomplished through a mini-open or percutaneously through tubular retractors; however, the use of tubular retractors might preclude cage placement. In most lytic lesions, the vertebral body resection can be easily performed due to the soft nature of the bone, although there will be increased bleeding.

In brief, the approach begins with laminectomy and complete removal of the superior articulating process at the level of interest. The pedicle is identified and, using a high-speed burr, the posterior cortex is breached. If needed, in the thoracic spine the exiting nerve is ligated and cut. The tie on the exiting nerve root can be used to gently retract the spinal cord to allow for further ventral decompression. The senior author's preference is to use a combination of angled curettes and a high-speed burr to decancellate the pedicle and vertebral body. A woodson periosteal elevator is used to sweep and remove any epidural lesion ventral to the spinal cord. The posterior longitudinal ligament is cut and the dorsal cavity created in the vertebral body can be backfilled with allograft. A unilateral or bilateral transpedicular decompression is performed as needed. There have been reports combining unilateral transpedicular decompression with contralateral costotransversectomy for complete circumferential decompression and expandable cage insertion as another option to obtain 360 degrees of decompression [26].

There have been several published series regarding minimally invasive transpedicular decompression within the thoracic and lumbar spine [7, 9, 23]. Deutsch et al. initially reported on a series of eight patients undergoing transpedicular decompression without stabilization with neurologic improvement and decreased pain reported in five of the eight patients [23]. Zairi et al. reported on ten patients undergoing transpedicular spinal cord decompression with posterior stabilization using tubular retractors and reported no complications and improved neurological function [8]. Of note, the goal of decompression in this study was to obtain a 2–3 mm zone of debulking with early postoperative stereotactic radiotherapy (separation surgery algorithm) and no recurrence or spinal cord compression was noted at the 1-year follow-up [8]. Chou et al. reported on a retrospective study of 49 patients comparing mini-open versus open transpedicular corpectomy with anterior cage reconstruction and posterior stabilization, and reported a lower blood loss and shorter hospital stay in the mini-open group [6]. Mean operative time was comparable between the groups (413 minutes in the open versus 452 minutes in the mini-open). However, this was substantially greater compared to the 170 minutes average reported by Zairi et al. [6] Overall, minimally invasive transpedicular decompression is a viable therapeutic option in patients with symptomatic spinal cord compression and is at least comparable to conventional techniques with regards to short-term efficacy and complication rates. Further investigations would be needed to completely elucidate superiority in overall morbidity rates and recurrence rate but initial investigations have shown promise.

Costrotransversectomy/Lateral Extracavitary Approach

These approaches provide an oblique approach to the vertebral body and spinal canal without entering the pleural cavity. The traditional open approach is associated with extensive muscular dissection and elevation of the erector spinae off the ribs, making minimally invasive techniques particularly appealing. The approach provides increased exposure to the anterior structures, which allows for almost complete ventral decompression and corpectomy as seen in Fig. 19.3. Kim et al. first described a minimally invasive technique using tubular retractors and an average of 93% of the ventral canal was decompressed and a total of 80% of the vertebral body was removed [24].

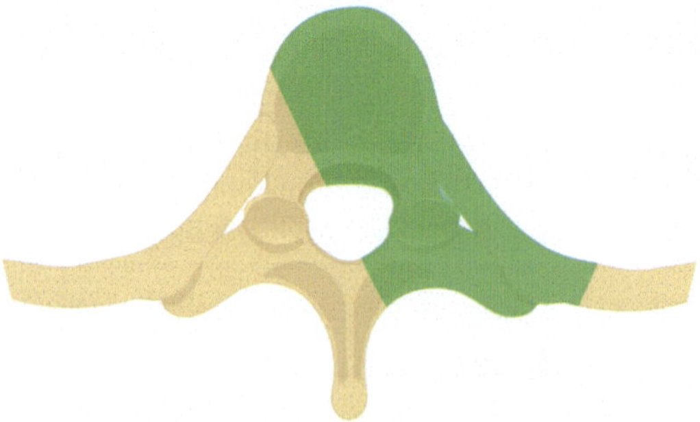

Fig. 19.3 Depiction of the surgical corridor of a posterolateral approach with the zone of direct visualization highlighted in green

The procedure is based over a lateral skin incision of varying degrees from the midline depending on the desired trajectory. A Kirschner wire is then introduced and docked on the ipsilateral facet near the pedicle for a costotransversectomy approach. The track is sequentially dilated and a tubular retractor or expandable retractor is introduced. The transverse process, proximal rib, and pedicle are then carefully removed with a high-speed burr or Kerrison. The adjacent nerve root is often sacrificed. The periosteum of the proximal rib and ventral vertebral body directly adjacent to the pleura are carefully preserved to protect the lungs. Once adequate access to the spinal cord is obtained, decompression and corpectomy are performed and generally, an expandable cage is placed to restore the anterior column stability. There are reports of combining a lateral approach with a contralateral transpedicular approach for more complete circumferential decompression [25, 26].

Compared to transpedicular decompression, the literature surrounding minimally invasive costotransversectomy is sparse. There have been several cadaveric feasibility reports associated with small clinical case series but the focus was not solely for tumor decompression [26–28]. Kim et al. were the first to describe the technique in a series of four patients, two of which involved the decompression of metastatic disease, using a costotransversectomy approach with anterior cage placement and posterior percutaneous stabilization [24]. Mild neurologic improvement was reported in these patients but it is unclear if their pain was decreased and no neurologic or dural violation was reported. Smith et al. described a similar study on three patients, one of which was the decompression of multiple myeloma with postoperative neurologic improvement but there was a breach of the pleura requiring temporary chest tube placement [28]. Although more research is necessary, minimally invasive costotransversectomy and corpectomy has been shown to provide adequate decompression especially over the ventral spinal cord with likely equivalent outcomes compared to open approaches. Long-term outcomes and larger patient cohorts will provide further clinical data regarding the potential for decreased morbidity in comparison to traditional techniques.

MIS Spinal Stabilization

Spinal tumors can be destructive to the osseous spine and often result in pathologic fractures and instability causing mechanical pain. Deformity as a result of vertebral body collapse can be progressive and increase segmental force at adjacent levels, thereby increasing the risk of further fracture and instability [29, 30]. For all of these reasons, stabilization of the spine is an important aspect of management both as a stand-alone adjunct and in combination with neural element decompression if deficits are present. Percutaneous pedicle screws and, if needed, anterior column support remain the hallmarks of minimally invasive stabilization (MIS).

There are some unique stabilization considerations regarding the oncology patient. Compared to other pathologies, osseous fusion is often not the goal nor feasible especially with solely percutaneous posterior stabilization. The healing capacity of the bone and ability to reliably fuse is oftentimes reduced as a result of chemotherapy, radiation therapy, and poor nutritional status. Life expectancy can also be unpredictable, and tumor pathology and prognosis play important roles when selecting a construct. Rao et al. presented a small series that focused on minimizing the surgical insult of stabilization and decompression based on a modified Tokuhashi score and advocated for robust stabilization with anterior reconstruction for patients with a prognosis greater than 12 months [31]. In another series reporting on 50 patients undergoing percutaneous pedicle screws, with/without minimally invasive decompression, a single instrumentation failure in a patient with a Tomita score of 4 and a survival of 51 months was reported [32]. Metastatic patients may sustain pedicle screw pull-out due to poor bone quality from lytic lesions, prior radiation, and osteoporosis. Although some have advocated for cement augmentation, which has been shown to increase pull-out strength in osteoporotic patients, there are few studies regarding this in oncology patients [33–35]. Overall, the approach to stabilization in the oncology patient must include consideration of life expectancy and prognosis, since osseous fusion cannot be achieved with some minimally invasive techniques. Patients who exhibit long-term survival and who do not achieve arthrodesis by definition may be exposed to implant failure.

Posterior stabilization through percutaneous pedicle screw fixation (PPSF) was first described in 2001 and since has been used with success in the treatment of a multitude of pathologies [36]. It can be performed independently of the decompression approach with minimal posterior tissue disruption or through a mini-open incision if performing a posterior decompression. There have been many reports in the literature for metastatic disease with minimal complications [6, 8, 23–25, 27, 37]. There are multiple commercial systems available, and the technique is well described in the literature. If treating one affected vertebrae the senior author's preference is to percutaneously instrument one level above and one level below the affected level. A mini-open incision is performed for a transpedicular decompression. (Fig. 19.4).

Although technically more challenging, longer constructs can be created if multicentric disease is present and reports of ultralong constructs up to 15 levels have been reported (Fig. 19.5) [38]. Posterior MIS instrumentation without decompression can help with intractable pain and has been shown to have a significant effect on pain as measured by VAS, ambulation status, as well as ability to manage activities of daily living [39, 40]. The senior author's preference is to trial a hyperextension brace first and if there is minimal relief of symptoms then to consider MIS instrumentation depending on the patient's life expectancy and ability to withstand surgery. Overall, percutaneous posterior pedicle screw stabilization has demonstrated decreased risks of infection and instrumentation failure. Mesfin et al., in a systematic review article on methods to decrease wound complications in metastatic spine surgery, gave MIS instrumentation a weak recommendation [41]. As more prospective multicenter data are collected and reported, a stronger recommendation to use MIS instrumentation in order to decrease wound complications may emerge [42, 43].

MIS access and reconstruction of the anterior spinal column through anterior column support is sometimes a necessary adjunct to posterior stabilization if significant anterior destruction is present or the patient has a favorable prognosis that could threaten the long-term survivorship of a posterior-only construct. There are many commercially available cage systems with expansion technology that are well suited for placement through an MIS approach. Static mesh cages and fibula strut graft are also options. Posterior cage placement can be accomplished through a variety of described techniques including percutaneous transpedicular interbody fusion and lateral extracavitary interbody fusion. Anterior options include anterior thoracoscopic and extreme lateral minithoractomy techniques but are far less common [20, 21]. In the setting of metastatic epidural spinal cord compression, we would not recommend stand-alone anterior instrumentation and prefer a circumferential approach.

Radiotherapy and MISS

Earlier initiation of postoperative radiotherapy is a major drawback of MISS owing to the reduced soft tissue dissection and theoretical lower wound complications compared to open surgery. In general, most surgeons are comfortable with initiating radiotherapy 2–3 weeks after MISS, and there are even reports of initiating radiation 3 days post-op [44]. Meanwhile, with open surgery, a recent consensus amongst surgeons indicated that 33% routinely wait 4–6 weeks before initiating conventional radiotherapy [45]. Patients who may have previously received radiotherapy may also benefit from the decreased tissue dissection compared to traditional surgery as well.

The concept of separation surgery (SS) deserves attention when discussing minimally invasive tumor surgery. Introduced in 2010, SS combines surgical neural element-tumor separation with postoperative tumor control via Stereotactic Body Radiation Therapy (SBRT)

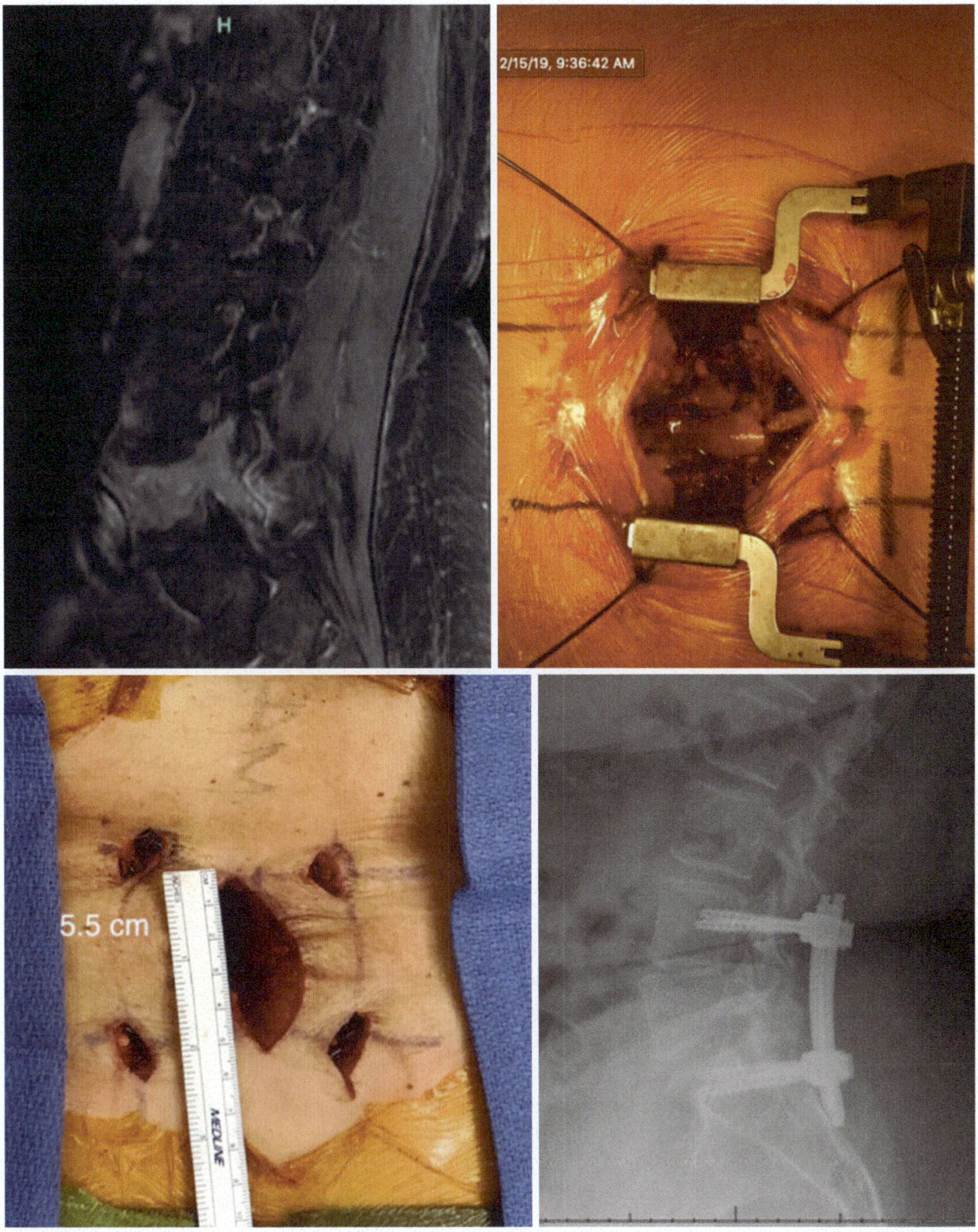

Fig. 19.4 A 67-year-old female with metastatic breast cancer to L5 and associated radicular symptoms treated with Percutaneous screws at L4 and S1 and transpedicular decompression with L5

[46]. Originally described using open surgical techniques, interest in applications in MISS have recently emerged. Given the modified surgical goal of a limited 2–3 mm circumferential decompression, the degree of tumor resection is significantly reduced and conceivably can be achieved through smaller corridors. There have been multiple reports of separation surgery using MIS and even reports of outpatient surgery, which is very promising in a population where the focus

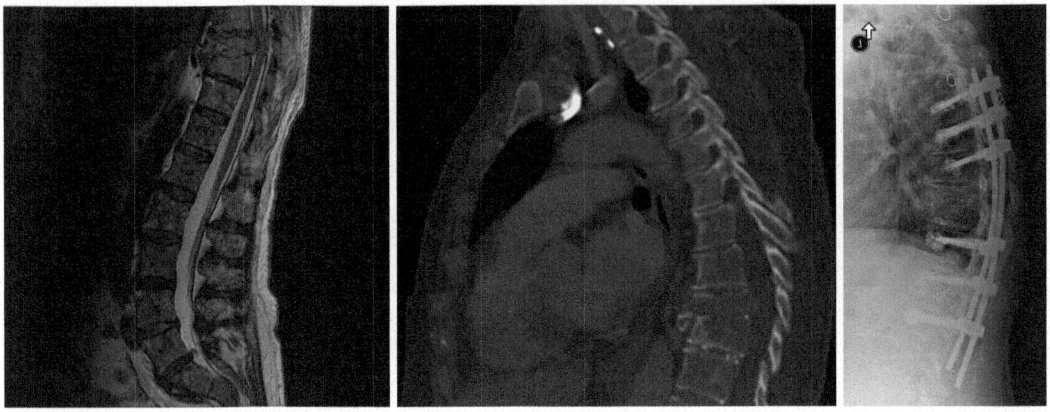

Fig. 19.5 A 63-year-old female with pathologic fractures of T9 and T10 with associated spinal cord compression as the first manifestation of multiple myeloma. The patient was treated with T6 – L1 percutaneous screws (8 levels) with mini-open transpedicular decompression of T9 and T10 without anterior column support. The MIS pedicle screws were also augmented with cement

is palliative care [47, 48]. Although the full clinical advantages have yet to be elucidated, this is a promising technique.

Future Directions

As techniques are refined and minimally invasive training becomes more commonplace, undoubtedly the application of minimally invasive techniques for spine tumors will expand. Specifically, there have been recent advancements in the field of endoscopic spine surgery that might have promise for the treatment of metastatic disease. Early case reports have described the use of a transforaminal endoscopic decompression technique within the lumbar spine with some success [49]. Further advancements in video technology, robotics, and specialized instrumentation will undoubtedly play a role in further advancement as well.

Conclusions

Minimally invasive spinal cord/thecal sac decompression and stabilization are a suitable and safe option for patients with metastatic spine disease. Compared to open surgery, there is less blood loss, shorter length of hospital stays, and lower risk of wound complications. Radiation therapy can also be initiated faster. Longer-term outcomes are still needed, but 1-year follow-up results appear to be at least equivalent to traditional open surgery. Patient considerations are important and certain scenarios including vascularized tumor pathologies, significant deformity, and certain cases of circumferential decompression might not be suited for MIS. Many viable techniques have been successfully described and overall are a good alternative to conventional open surgery in a population with an already elevated comorbidity profile.

References

1. Bilsky MH, Boland P, Lis E, Raizer J, Healey JH. Single-stage posterolateral transpedicle approach for spondylectomy, epidural decompression, and circumferential fusion of spinal metastases. Spine. 2000;25(17):2240–50.
2. Patchell RA, Tibbs PA, Regine WF, et al. Direct decompressive surgical resection in the treatment of spinal cord compression caused by metastatic cancer: a randomized trial. Lancet. 2005;366(9486):643–8.
3. Yaşargil MG. Microsurgical operation of herniated lumbar disc. Adv Neurosurg. 1977;4:81.
4. Oppenheimer JH, DeCastro I, McDonnell DE. Minimally invasive spine technology and minimally invasive spine surgery: a historical review. Neurosurg Focus. 2009;27:E9.
5. Holly LT, Schwender JD, Rouben DP, Foley KT. Minimally invasive transforaminal lumbar inter-

body fusion: indications, technique, and complications. Neurosurg Focus. 2006;20(3):E6.
6. Lau D, Chou D. Posterior thoracic corpectomy with cage reconstruction for metastatic spinal tumors: comparing the mini-open approach to the open approach. J Neurosurg Spine. 2015;23:217–27.
7. Selznick LA, Shamji MF, Isaacs RE. Minimally invasive interbody fusion for revision lumbar surgery: technical feasibility and safety. J Spinal Disord Tech. 2009;22:207–13.
8. Zairi F, Arikat A, Allaoui M, Marinho P, Assaker R. Minimally invasive decompression and stabilization for the management of thoracolumbar spine metastasis. J Neurosurg Spine. 2012;17:19–23.
9. Hartl R, Korge A. Minimally invasive spine surgery – techniques, evidence, and controversies. New York, NY: Thieme Publishers; 2013.
10. Fourney DR, et al. Spinal instability neoplastic score: an analysis of reliability and validity from the spine oncology study group. J Clin Oncol. 2011;29(22):3072–7.
11. Sclafani JA, Kim CW. Complications associated with the initial learning curve of minimally invasive spine surgery: a systematic review. Clin Orthop Relat Res. 2014;472:1711–7.
12. Nomura K, Yoshida M. Assessment of the learning curve for microendoscopic decompression surgery for lumbar spinal canal stenosis through an analysis of 480 cases involving a single surgeon. Global Spine J. 2017;7:54–8.
13. Grant R, Papadopoulos SM, Greenberg HS. Metastatic epidural spinal cord compression. Neurol Clin. 1991;9:825–41.
14. Sundaresan N, Galicich JH, Lane JM, et al. Treatment of neoplastic epidural cord compression by vertebral body resection and stabilization. J Neurosurg. 1985;63(5):676–84.
15. Harrington KD. Anterior cord decompression and spinal stabilization for patients with metastatic lesions of the spine. J Neurosurg. 1984;61:107–17.
16. Bridwell KH, Jenny AB, Saul T, et al. Posterior segmental spinal instrumentation (PSSI) with posterolateral decompression and debulking for metastatic thoracic and lumbar spine disease. Limitations of the technique. Spine. 1988;13:1383–94.
17. Han SJ, Lau D, Lu DC, Theodore P, Chou D. Anterior thoracolumbar corpectomies: approach morbidity with and with- out an access surgeon. Neurosurgery. 2011;68(5):1220–5.
18. Jarrett CD, Heller JG, Tsai L. Anterior exposure of the lumbar spine with and without an "access surgeon": morbidity analysis of 265 consecutive cases. J Spinal Disord Tech. 2009;22:559–64.
19. Lau D, Song Y, Guan Z, Sullivan S, La Marca F, Park P. Perioperative characteristics, complications, and outcomes of single-level versus multilevel thoracic corpectomies via modified costotransversectomy approach. Spine (Phila Pa 1976). 2013;38:523–30.
20. Lu DC, Lau D, Lee JG, Chou D. The transpedicular approach compared with the anterior approach: an analysis of 80 thoracolumbar corpectomies. J Neurosurg Spine. 2010;12:583–91.
21. Meredith DS, Kepler CK, Huang RC, Hegde VV. Extreme lateral interbody fusion (XLIF) in the thoracic and thoracolumbar spine: technical report and early outcomes. HSS J. 2013;9(1):25–31.
22. Kan P, Schmidt M. Minimally invasive thoracoscopic approach for anterior decompression and stabilization of metastatic spine disease. Neurosurg Focus. 2008;25:E8.
23. Deutsch H, Boco T, Lobel J. Minimally invasive transpedicular vertebrectomy for metastatic disease to the thoracic spine. J Spinal Disord Tech. 2008;21:101–5.
24. Kim DH, O'Toole JE, Ogden AT, et al. Minimally invasive posterolateral thoracic corpectomy: cadaveric feasibility study and report of four clinical cases. Neurosurgery. 2009;64(4):746–53.
25. Taghva A, Li KW, Liu JC, Gokaslan ZL, Hsieh PC. Minimally invasive circumferential spinal decompression and stabilization for symptomatic metastatic spine tumor: technical case report. Neurosurgery. 2010;66:E620–2.
26. Musacchio M, Patel N, Bagan B, Deutsch H, Vaccaro AR, Ratliff J. Minimally invasive thoracolumbar costotransversectomy and corpectomy via a dual-tube technique: evaluation in a cadaver model. Surg Technol Int. 2007;16:221–5.
27. Khoo LT, Smith ZA, Asgarzadie F, et al. Minimally invasive extracavitary approach for thoracic discectomy and interbody fusion: 1-year clinical and radiographic outcomes in 13 patients compared with a cohort of traditional anterior transthoracic approaches. J Neurosurg. 2011;14(2):250–60.
28. Smith ZA, Li Z, Chen NF, Raphael D, Khoo LT. Minimally invasive lateral extracavitary corpectomy: cadaveric evaluation model and report of 3 clinical cases. J Neurosurg. 2012;16(5):463–70.
29. Lindsay R, Silverman SL, Cooper C. Risk of new vertebral fracture in the year following a fracture. JAMA. 2001;285:320–3. https://doi.org/10.1001/jama.285.3.320.
30. Costa L, Badia X, Chow E, Lipton A, Wardley A. Impact of skeletal complications on patients' quality of life, mobility, and functional independence. Support Care Cancer. 2008;16:879–89. https://doi.org/10.1007/s00520-008-0418-0.
31. Rao PJ, Thayaparan GK, Fairhall JM, et al. Minimally invasive percutaneous fixation techniques for metastatic spinal disease. Orthop Surg. 2014;6:187–95.
32. Kwan MK, Lee CK, Chan CY. Minimally invasive spinal stabilization using fluoroscopic-guided percutaneous screws as a form of palliative surgery in patients with spinal metastasis. Asian Spine J. 2016;10:99–110.
33. Burval DJ, McLain RF, Milks R, Inceoglu S. Primary pedicle screw augmentation in osteoporotic lumbar vertebrae: biomechanical analysis of pedicle fixation strength. Spine (Phila Pa 1976). 2007;32:1077–83.
34. Sawakami K, Yamazaki A, Ishikawa S, Ito T, Watanabe K, Endo N. Polymethylmethacrylate aug-

mentation of pedicle screws increases the initial fixation in osteoporotic spine patients. J Spinal Disord Tech. 2012;25:28–35.

35. Kim P, Won Kim S. Bone cement-augmented percutaneous screw fixation for malignant spinal metastases: is it feasible? J Korean Neurosurg Soc. 2017;60:189–94. https://doi.org/10.3340/jkns.2016.0909.003.
36. Foley KT, Gupta SK, Justis JR, Sherman MC. Percutaneous pedicle screw fixation of the lumbar spine. Neurosurg Focus. 2001;10(4):E10.
37. Zhao Q, Zhang H, Hao D, Guo H, Wang B, He B. Complications of percutaneous pedicle screw fixation in treating thoracolumbar and lumbar fracture. Medicine (Baltimore). 2018;97:e11560.
38. Lee CK, Chan CY, Kwan MK. Ultra long construct minimally invasive spinal stabilization using percutaneous pedicle screws in the treatment of symptomatic multicentric spinal metastasis. Asian Spine J. 2015;9:962–5.
39. Schwab JH, Gasbarrini A, Cappuccio M, Boriani L, De Iure F, Colangeli S, et al. Minimally invasive posterior stabilization improved ambulation and pain scores in patients with plasmocytomas and/or metastases of the spine. Int J Surg Oncol. 2011;2011:239230.
40. Uei H, Tokuhashi Y, Oshima M, Maseda M, Matsumoto K, Soma H, et al. Clinical results of minimally invasive spine stabilization for spinal metastases. Orthopedics. 2017;40:e693–8.
41. Mesfin A, Sciubba D, Dea N, Nater A, Bird J, Quraishi NA, et al. Changing the adverse event profile in metastatic spine surgery: an evidence based approach to target wound complications and instrumentation failure. Spine. 2016;41(Suppl 20):S262–70.
42. Mesfin A, Baldwin A, Bernstein D, Emanski E, Molinari RW, Menga EM, et al. Reducing surgical site infections in spine tumor surgery: a comparison of three methods. Spine. 2019;44(24):E1428–35.
43. Jubril A, Sherif S, Mesfin A. Clinical outcomes of percutaneous pedicle screws and open decompression in the management of thoracolumbar and lumbar spine metastases. Lumbar spine research society annual meeting. J Neurosurg Spine. 2019:103.
44. Zuckerman SL, Laufer I, Sahgal A, Yamada YJ, Schmidt MH, Chou D, et al. When less is more: the indications for MIS techniques and separation surgery in metastatic spine disease. Spine. 2016;41(Suppl 20):s246–53.
45. Lee RS, Batke J, Weir L, Dea N, Fisher CG. Timing of surgery and radiotherapy in the management of metastatic spine disease: expert opinion. J Spine Surg. 2018;4(2):368–73. https://doi.org/10.21037/jss.2018.05.05.
46. Moulding HD, Elder JB, Lis E, Lovelock DM, Zhang Z, Yamada Y, et al. Local disease control after decompressive surgery and adjuvant high-dose single-fraction radiosurgery for spine metastases. J Neurosurg Spine. 2010;13(1):87–93. [PubMed: 20594023].
47. Turel MK, Kerolus MG, O'Toole JE. Minimally invasive "separation surgery" plus adjuvant stereotactic radiotherapy in the management of spinal epidural metastases. J Craniovertebr Junction Spine. 2017;8(2):119–26. https://doi.org/10.4103/jcvjs.JCVJS_13_17.
48. Moussazadeh N, Laufer I, Yamada Y, Bilsky MH. Separation surgery for spinal metastases: effect of spinal radiosurgery on surgical treatment goals. Cancer Control. 2014;21(2):168–74.
49. Gao Z, Wu Z, Lin Y, Zhang P. Percutaneous transforaminal endoscopic decompression in the treatment of spinal metastases: a case report. Medicine. 2019;98:e14819. https://doi.org/10.1097/MD.0000000000014819.

20 Complex Reconstruction in Tumor Patients

Alexander R. Vaccaro, Srikanth N. Divi, and Waqaas A. Hassan

Introduction

Arguably, the greatest scientific accomplishment of the past century has been the increase in general human life expectancy from almost 50 years to an estimated 80 years [1]. Such progress has led to an epidemiologic transition in healthcare, especially with an increasing prevalence of cancer; hence, the annual incidence of new cases is projected to rise 70% (22–23 million/year) worldwide by the year 2030 [2–4]. The majority of cancer-related morbidity and mortality is related to metastases and not necessarily the primary tumor itself [5]. In particular, functional disability from osseous metastasis is a disastrous complication for most patients, although it may remain clinically silent until the later stages of disease.

While there have not been large-scale studies on the prevalence or incidence of bone metastasis, there have been studies on the distribution and frequency of metastatic disease. Such studies have established a strong preference for the axial skeleton, most frequently, the spine [6]. The thoracic and lumbar spines are the most frequently involved, with the cervical region being the least commonly implicated [6, 7]. Theoretically, any tumor can spread to the spine; however, the most common primary malignancies with a tendency to metastasize to the spinal column are breast (21%), lung (19%), prostate (7.5%), renal (5%), gastrointestinal (4.5%), and thyroid (2.5%) [5]. Though the vast majority of spinal metastases are usually found as bone metastasis (extradural), they are not exclusive to the vertebral column. Other much less common spinal metastases include intramedullary and extramedullary tumors. Furthermore, it is estimated that over 50% of metastatic spinal patients have multiple levels affected, with up to 38% of patients having nonadjacent segments affected [6, 7].

Complex spine reconstructive surgery is often considered a final option in the treatment of deformity, instability, or neurologic compromise from spinal metastases. The goals of reconstructive surgery generally fall into the categories of palliative pain relief, prevention of impending structural collapse, correction of deformity (due to frank pathologic fracture), or reconstruction (following iatrogenic tumor resection). Complex issues of neural decompression and local control of tumor are frequently intermingled. Spinal reconstructive surgery has provided extensive improvements in the quality of life for patients suffering from metastatic disease, along with its sequelae. Over 80% of patients with neurologic compromise caused by vertebral malignancy improve, at minimum, 1 functional grade following decompression and stabilization, and almost

A. R. Vaccaro · S. N. Divi (✉) · W. A. Hassan
Department of Orthopaedic Surgery, Rothman Institute, Thomas Jefferson University Hospital, Philadelphia, PA, USA
e-mail: srikanth.divi@rothmanortho.com

K. Singh, M. Colman (eds.), *Surgical Spinal Oncology*,
https://doi.org/10.1007/978-3-030-50722-0_20

90% experience relief from back pain and a restoration of walking ability [8].

Surgery is not without significant risks and major potential complications including permanent cord injury, life-threatening blood loss, infection, urinary tract infection (UTI), thrombosis, life-threatening blood loss, and anesthesia-related events [9, 10]. However, as reconstruction techniques have advanced, the use of revolutionary technologies such as minimally invasive surgery and intraoperative navigation has resulted in a higher safety profile and better efficiency, along with fewer intra- and postoperative complications. Indications for surgical procedures are determined not only by histology but rather by severity of the presenting disease, the patient's overall health, and other patient-related factors. This chapter will focus on the goals of complex reconstructive spine-tumor surgery including surgical methods, special considerations in tumor patients, traditional instrumentation and implant types, and state-of-the art modern tumor implants.

Goals of Tumor Surgery

The advancement of instrumentation and techniques has expanded and improved the quality and options of surgical intervention over the last few decades [11, 12]. Consequently, metastatic spinal disease can be addressed via a wide array of surgical options, and it is important to keep in mind the goals of surgery when deciding the approach for treatment [11]:

- Achieve local tumor control
- Decompress the spinal cord/neural element compression
- Stabilize the spinal column
- Improve spinal deformity

Both mechanical and neural stability of the spinal column allow patients to attain pain palliation, ambulatory mobility, and quality of life [11]. The specific operative approach is dependent upon the location of metastasis. For example, the approach is often determined by the location of the tumor, i.e., ventrally located tumors can be approached anteriorly and posteriorly located tumors can be approached posteriorly. A combination of anterior and posterior approaches is often utilized [11, 13]. However, it is clear that the choice of surgical reconstruction is made based not only on anatomic location of tumor but on myriad other factors including tumor biology, biomechanical factors, patient frailty, patient prognosis, and patient preferences.

Decompression and stabilization techniques come in many forms. Choosing the appropriate approach must consider both circumferential spinal cord decompression and biomechanical stabilization of the bony/ligamentous columns. While this may include posterior laminectomy and fusion or anterior discectomy/corpectomy and fusion using standard techniques, more extensive approaches involving vertebrectomy or other destabilizing resections may apply [10–14]. Total en bloc vertebrectomy may even be indicated in select patients presenting with a solitary metastasis, or in most patients with isolated primary malignancy [11, 13].

Once the operative approach and tumor-specific strategy have been selected, key parameters to consider include extent of reconstruction, inclusion of arthrodesis, implant materials, and selection of biologics. This chapter discusses each of these parameters with an emphasis on complex open reconstruction.

Biomechanical Considerations

Operative strategy is further influenced by the region of the spine affected by the tumor. Special considerations should be given to each region of the spine given unique anatomic features. Prior to the development of the Spinal Instability Neoplastic Score [15], few guidelines existed that aided surgeons in assessing the key components of spinal stability in the setting of neoplastic disease. As defined by the Spine Oncology Study Group, spine instability is associated with movement-related pain, symptomatic or progressive deformity, or neural compromise under physiological loads [15].

Several authors have attempted to classify spinal stability based on biomechanical concepts. Initially, a two-column model of spinal stability was proposed based upon an anterior column composed of vertebral bodies and a posterior column composed of the neural arches [16]. Expanding on this, Denis suggested a three-column model that emphasized the importance of the posterior vertebral body, posterior longitudinal ligament, and the posterior annulus fibrosus in spinal stability [17]. Most trauma classifications use injury morphology to infer stability to each spinal column. Recently developed trauma classifications for the cervical as well as thoracolumbar spine have also suggested the importance of the posterior ligamentous complex (PLC) in maintaining stability [18, 19]. Oncologic processes, however, affect local biology differently than traumatic mechanisms of injury and thus warrant further consideration in each region of the spine. Due to the presence of an extensive venous plexus, metastatic lesions preferentially affect the vertebral bodies compared to the posterior elements such as the facets or the PLC. Therefore, spinal stability may be intact in these cases unless it is further disrupted traumatically or iatrogenically.

In addition, regional variations in the spine can affect stability. For example, the rib cage confers significant stability in the thoracolumbar spine. Metastatic lesions that preferentially affect the costovertebral joint and its surrounding cortical bone rather than the cancellous core of the vertebral body may contribute more to vertebral body collapse [20]. In contrast, in the lumbar spine, involvement of the pedicle is thought to have a much higher risk of vertebral collapse due to the absence of stability provided by the rib cage. Lesions that affect key transition points in the spine necessitate long constructs to increase rigidity of fixation. For example, lesions at the cervicothoracic or thoracolumbar junction should not be managed with short-segment fixation, as this may not include enough rigidity in the construct. In addition, anterior and posterior reconstruction of the spinal column should be considered to restore overall sagittal and coronal balance.

Operative Approaches

Posterior Approaches

The posterior approach is the workhorse approach for all areas of the thoracolumbar spine. It provides decompression by directly removing posterior spinal elements, direct access for providing pedicle screw fixation, and a large area for creating a fusion mass in the posterolateral gutter.

Posterior Decompression Without Reconstruction

In the pre-modern era of spine tumor surgery, procedures involving posterior decompressive laminectomy without fusion were common [11]. However, almost one out of five adults eventually required further treatment with recurrence of symptoms due to ventral tumor progression [21, 22]. Furthermore, laminectomy alone in combination with radiation also demonstrated poor outcomes and complications including spinal deformity, instability, neurologic deficits, and wound complications [11]. Lastly, certain anatomic zones, such as the cervical spine or any junctional zone (cervicothoracic, thoracolumbar), should generally be instrumented following wide decompressive laminectomy to avoid kyphotic deformity and instability. However, there may be select cases where laminectomy alone without reconstruction is appropriate. This includes cases of epidural disease in the lumbar spine where facets and anterior column bone are relatively preserved or cases of dorsal cord-level epidural disease where the anatomic supports are similarly uninvolved.

Posterior Decompression and Fusion

Posterior decompression and fusion surgery are now the standard methods of the neural elements. Reconstruction is typically performed via posterior segmental screw instrumentation with rods [23–25]. It offers potentially fewer complications such as progression of spinal deformity with a reduction in soft tissue morbidities through the introduction of minimally invasive approaches in select cases [23–25]. In addition, many surgeons are familiar with this approach and technique, making it a more universal option. However, a notable disadvantage of this approach is its limited exposure and poor visualization of a ventrally located tumor mass [23–25]. Additionally, reconstruction of the posterior tension band may not be sufficient if significant compromise of the anterior columns has occurred.

Posterolateral Decompression and Stabilization

The posterolateral approach to the spine has allowed a direct method to circumferentially decompress cord-level neural elements and to access anatomy required for both posterior and anterior stabilizations [25]. This may include a transpedicular approach (TPA) or costotransversectomy approach, and is most commonly utilized in the thoracic spine. TPA or extra cavitary technique can also be used in the lumbar spine, although working corridors are more limited by inability to sacrifice the lumbar nerve roots. Advantages of these techniques include a single incision to achieve decompression and stability along with anterior column reconstruction [11]. This approach is particularly useful in treating lesions in the upper thoracic region and thoracolumbar junction [11].

As metastatic spinal disease disproportionately affects the elderly, the direct anterior approach is not preferred in patients with increased frailty and poor general health due to increased risk of vascular and pulmonary complications [26]. To work around this, there has been a trend towards performing circumferential decompression and fusion through these posterior only approaches. Specifically, posterolateral TPA or costotransversectomy with circumferential decompression and anterior reconstruction have shown overall excellent patient results [26, 27].

Anterior Decompression and Reconstruction

Anterior decompression and reconstruction is the best method to directly address compression in the anterior spinal column. Anterior column reconstruction can be performed using structural bone allograft (iliac crest, femur or fibula), autologous structural graft (iliac crest, fibular, rib), Steinman pins with cement, or synthetic reconstruction cages. For cervical metastases specifically, the traditional surgical approach is anterior decompression with corpectomy, vertebral body replacement, and cervical plate stabilization [13, 28, 29]. Multilevel corpectomy or the presence of posterior element tumor involvement is a relative indication to also reconstruct the posterior tension band through a separate approach. In addition, patients with thoracolumbar anterior column metastases have been found to have better outcomes after anterior reconstruction, especially when disease is isolated to 1–2 continuous segments [11, 30]. In fact, return of neurologic function has been reported in over 70% of patients after anterior decompressions [11]. A retrospective review of surgical treatment for spinal metastases of 100 patients demonstrated clinical improvement in 80% of patients at follow-up [11]. In one study detailing the anterior approach to metastatic disease in the thoracic and lumbar spine, approximately 94% of patients had stabilized or improved motor function while almost 90% were ambulatory postoperatively [31]. Alignment was maintained in all patients with no reported instrumentation failures [31].

En Bloc Spondylectomy

Patients with metastatic spinal disease who are carefully selected based on extent of disease (oligometastases), long latency since primary diagnosis, excellent performance status, and other factors may be candidates for “en bloc spondylectomy” [13, 32]. This procedure entails thorough resection of the tumor along with a layer of otherwise healthy tissue [33]. Hence, this is the treatment of choice for solitary and oligometastasis with favorable histology [13, 32]. As metastatic spinal disease often presents very late, the vast majority of patients are not candidates for this procedure [28, 34, 35].

The total en bloc spondylectomy (TES) is a modification that involves removal of the complete vertebral body and lamina, concurrently [35–37]. Surgeons will use either a staged, anterior-posterior, or solely posterior approach [36–40].

TES, especially when multilevel, demands the careful release of surrounding neurovascular structures from the tumor, followed by resection of the tumor, posterior instrumentation, and reconstruction of the defect [32, 35–38, 40, 41].

The potential instability from such a procedure does not preclude frequent and potentially debilitating complications. Such sequelae as pseudarthrosis, sepsis, neurovascular injury, cord injury, CSF leakage, sepsis, hematoma formation, and hemorrhage with subsequent myocardial infarction have been documented throughout recent medical literature [33–35, 37, 39, 42–46].

Combined Anterior/Posterior Approach

While each of the aforementioned techniques is indicated on a case-by-case basis, there has been an increasing trend toward performing circumferential fusion (combined anterior approach and posterior approach or via posterior approach only). This has been proven to increase healing rates and reduced reoperation rates when compared with traditional single-column techniques [47]. In addition, it has been shown to be more cost-effective at an average of $55,000 per case compared to $68,000 for traditional techniques [47]. However, as previously mentioned, it comes at a cost of a higher blood loss and complication rates [47].

Restoration of Mechanical Stability

Patients with metastatic spinal disease resulting in structural failure of the spine are at exceptionally high risk for cord compression [14]. While neurologic compromise due to epidural compression of the spinal cord is the most common reason for undergoing surgery, patients with treatment-resistant mechanical pain may also be offered surgery to increase mechanical stability [14]. Thus, the restoration of mechanical stability of the spine is critical to the well-being and/or palliative care of the patient. It is important to note that conventional external body radiotherapy has been shown to have negative effects on bone healing in metastatic spinal disease, specifically for the healing of pathological fractures and thus on successful achievement of mechanical stability. In fact, a 2015 study found that such patients did not experience any improvements in pain control while undergoing radiation for metastatic disease [48]. Radiation has been shown to hinder postoperative bone fusion and, therefore, most surgeons wait up to 6 weeks after surgery to commence adjuvant radiotherapy [48].

Special Considerations for Reconstruction in Tumor Patients

Unique challenges to reconstructive surgery in tumor patients include age, medical morbidities, frailty, bone quality (osteopenia/osteoporosis), concomitant chemotherapy and radiation, intraoperative bleeding, and intraoperative contamination of cancer cells.

Age

Increasing age generally carries increased surgical risks, especially in the setting of surgery for malignancy. The frequency of spinal surgery within the United States has noticeably increased in the last few decades, especially in the geriatric population [49]. An increasing prevalence of comorbidities with age (cardiopulmonary disease, diabetes, obesity, etc.) combined with increasing complexity of reconstructive spinal surgery and its demanding recovery all contribute to a substantially higher potential for complications [7]. While age itself is not a contraindication for spinal surgery, several studies have noted a higher risk for complications and mortality, especially with increasing surgical complexity [7, 50, 51].

Frailty

While not defined by chronological age itself, frailty is medically defined as a pattern of physiological decline characterized by susceptibility to adverse health outcomes [52]. Decreased bone quality in combination with decreased muscle pliability and muscle tone contribute toward an increased level of frailty [53]. Frail adults are unable to adapt to stressors, thus predisposing themselves to procedural/surgical complications, among other dangers. In fact, frailty has been found to be predictive of adverse events, mortality, in-hospital length of stay, and discharge disposition [54]. Patients with frailty also have a longer road to recovery from complex surgery. The surgical and reconstructive event is a mentally and physically demanding process often taking more than a year for full recovery. Consequently, patients with age-related health decline and comorbidities face an even longer road to recovery. While there is no current majority consensus or standardization on measuring frailty (over 70 unique measures have been proposed), it has nonetheless been implicated in an increased risk of postoperative complications, chemotherapy intolerance, disease progression, and death [53]. A recent study proposed a spine-tumor specific frailty index for patients with metastatic spinal disease [55].

Bone Quality (Osteopenia/Osteoporosis)

Osteopenia, often referred to as the midpoint between healthy bones and osteoporosis, is medically defined as the decrease in density of bone defined by a bone densitometry (T-score) of -1 to -2.5. Osteopenia patients have bones that are weaker than normal but not weak enough to fracture easily. Osteoporosis, on the other hand, is defined by a T-score of <-2.5 and signals a reduction in bone mineral density (BMD) due to an imbalance of calcium, vitamin-D, and phosphate homeostasis. This presents in the spine as decreased trabecular density in the vertebral body, thus predisposing the patient to compression fractures, as well as subsequent poor healing [56].

Poor bone quality poses additional challenges in patients undergoing tumor surgery. These patients have lower rates of bone healing/fusion due to decreased and inefficient osteoblast activity, low marrow quality, and poor vascularity [56, 57]. Nonunion rates are estimated to reach up to 35% in this population [56]. In the setting of an osteoporotic patient needing spinal fusion, certain precautions can help minimize risks. First, it is important to obtain a detailed history of any bone fractures especially in at-risk patients. These patients should then be referred for further osteoporosis screening if not already obtained. At risk is defined by the United States Preventative Services Task Force as all women over the age of 65 and postmenopausal women under 65 at increased risk for low bone mineral density [58]. Currently, there is insufficient evidence to recommend any age for screening for males [58]. Osteoporosis is currently diagnosed using dual energy X-ray absorptiometry (DXA) scans, which measures BMD at the lumbar spine and hip (total hip and femoral neck) [57]. The FRAX score additionally quantifies the 10-year risk of an osteoporotic insufficiency fracture with or without DEXA data and may be a useful proxy in the spine tumor population [59].

Several considerations of treatment options exist for patients with osteoporosis that need to undergo surgery for a neoplastic reason. Fixation is difficult in weaker bone, necessitating larger and stronger screws along with additional bone grafting. Furthermore, it is important to note that osteoporosis affects trabecular bone more than the outer cortical layer of bone, leading to higher rates of screw loosening and overall implant failure [56]. Studies have shown that screws that are longer and have a larger diameter enhance stabilization. In addition, screw positioning and angulation in higher density areas increase rigidity and subsequently, fusion rates [56]. Computer navigation may assist with precision placement of screws for this purpose. Screw augmentation with polymethyl methacrylate (PMMA) has also demonstrated favorable outcomes by increasing rigidity of the construct in weak bone [56].

Other treatment options include directly altering the bone quality with the use of osteoinductive growth factors such as bone morphogenic proteins (BMPs) or increasing osteoblastic (bone-forming) activity via exogenous administration of parathyroid hormone (PTH) [56].

However, in tumor patients, use of BMP is not properly studied for safety and efficacy and should generally be avoided for concerns over stimulation of local tumor growth. Calcium and vitamin D supplementation in combination with the use of biologic therapy to inhibit osteoclast activity and decrease bony resorption (e.g., denosumab, odanacatib) have shown some increased efficacy compared to conventional bisphosphonate therapy by increasing spine density [56]. Another treatment option may include the use of a postoperative spinal brace to further increase rigidity. Discouraging practices that may disrupt proper fusion such as smoking or the prolonged use of nonsteroidal anti-inflammatory drugs (NSAIDs) may also help increase fusion rates [56].

Deformity Considerations

Another important consideration in patients with an aging spine is the overall sagittal balance. Depending on the manner in which the lumbosacral spine is set in the pelvis, balanced lumbar lordosis and thoracic kyphosis are essential to keep one's spine and center of gravity in alignment and thus avoid excess energy expenditure. Pathologic disruption to any of the spinal zones may result in excessive strain on the cervical spine, pelvis, and lower limbs due to easily exhausted compensatory efforts. Specifically, in pathologically kyphotic thoracolumbar spines, compensation maneuvers include cervical hyperlordosis, thoracic hypokyphosis, pelvic retroversion, and/or knee flexion [60]. It is pertinent to note these physical demands often induce severe fatigue as the patient's hips, thighs, and knees are forced to endure persistent strain [60]. The resultant forward-leaning posture also has sociological and psychological implications as this disorder correlates with struggles in social interactions and self-image [61]. Furthermore, positive sagittal balance has been associated with overall worse health outcomes. The implications of a preexisting sagittal imbalance for patients, especially those with spinal malignancy, warrant special consideration and detailed evaluation. In order to avoid progression of spinal deformity, it should be directly addressed in the surgical approach, since sagittal malalignment may also contribute to early implant or bony failure [62].

Adjuvant Therapy (Radiation and Chemotherapy) Effect on Reconstruction

Radiation and chemotherapy are frequently used as an adjunct to surgery in spine tumor patients [63, 64]. Such circumstances warrant an understanding of the biologic and reconstructive implications of both therapies.

Radiation directly affects the skin and surrounding vasculature, thereby impairing or delaying wound healing, resulting in an ongoing inflammatory cycle with cell regeneration [65–67]. Surgical wound healing is normally expected within the first 2 weeks and is considered delayed healing if skin or tissue approximation is not noted by this time. The first two stages of wound healing (inflammatory and proliferative stage) are interrupted the earliest by radiation. Specific pro-inflammatory cytokines (interleukin-1 [IL-1] and IL-8) become overexpressed causing excessive inflammation and fibrosis [65]. In addition, the rebuilding and maintenance stage is left weakened due to deficient and dysfunctional collagen deposition (due to dysfunctional fibroblasts) and decreased activity of matrix metalloproteinases [65].

Radiation also has deleterious effects on the circulatory system, causing loss of vessel elasticity with subsequent dilation, sclerosis, and occlusion [67–69]. These effects result in erythema, chronic tissue hypoxia, and edema, respectively; as they progressively worsen, the patient experiences lifelong deficits in wound healing [67]. Radiation's effects on the epidermis has been widely noted, specifically damage to the basal layer [68, 69]. The classic acute presentation is that of extensive local erythema and deep ulcerations to dry desquamation and skin necrosis, with increasing radiation dosage [67–69]. While acute effects are generally self-limiting and reversible, chronic effects (seen after 6 months) are not. Chronic effects include fibrosis, loss of hair follicles, significant skin necrosis, changes in skin pigmentation, and the formation of new tumors [67–69].

Postoperative rather than preoperative radiation not only causes fewer wound complications but also has shown significant advantages in reducing residual tumor bed, specifically within 6 weeks of surgery [67]. Postoperative radiation is often indicated after surgery with negative margins or when the tumor is still adherent to surrounding tissue [70]. This is often administered in lower dosage (fractionated) form. One special consideration of the use of postoperative radiation is in the setting of structural bone grafts. The purpose of using a structural bone graft is to stimulate new bone formation and subsequent fusion by providing a framework for new bone growth and providing stability concomitantly [71–74].

Radiation on bone grafts is often accompanied by concurrent fibrosis. This diminishes vascularization and cell regulation of homeostasis/apoptosis, resulting in lower rates of successful fusion [63, 74]. Ensuing complications may also include osteonecrosis, malunion, and postoperative fracture [63, 74].

For these reasons, postoperative radiotherapy may not be ideal when using structural bone graft. Therefore, many surgeons prefer the commencement of radiation, if possible, beginning at least 6 weeks after surgical intervention.

Interestingly, while it is generally accepted that perioperative radiotherapy is also proven to hinder bone fusion, some recent studies show that low-dose radiation actually aids in the healing of fractures, via subsequent upregulation of vascular endothelial growth factor (VEGF) [63, 71]. However, varying patient outcomes and a lack of sufficient clinical studies have left outcomes on bone graft in the setting of perioperative radiation as uncertain [63]. As studies have shown that a combined regimen of surgery and radiotherapy provides better outcomes compared to radiation alone, it may be best to delay postoperative radiation from the operative date for as long as possible [63]. If radiotherapy is used as a neoadjuvant therapy, bringing vascularized tissue into the previously radiated fields via axial rib flaps or other flaps can be helpful in establishing arthrodesis. Other strategies to aid in successful bone fusion in the presence of radiotherapy include using stereotactic radiosurgery to minimize normal tissue damage, using autologous graft options instead of allogeneic, and when possible delaying postoperative radiotherapy for 6 weeks [63].

Systemic therapy regimens are often used alone or in combination with surgery and radiation in the treatment of metastatic spinal disease [63, 65, 70]. The term "chemotherapy" is often incorrectly used and should generally be reserved for classes of drugs that work via systemic cytotoxic effect. Other general classes such as targeted molecular drugs, antiangiogenesis drugs, or others may have wildly different complication profiles and recommendations on perioperative usage, especially in the setting of complex reconstruction. Chemotherapy drugs specifically target dividing cells and can affect bone healing and bone turnover, resulting in defective wound healing, decreased bone formation, and bone marrow suppression [75–78]. As metastatic spinal disease is a systemic problem that is most common in cancer patients older than 60 years, systemic therapy often eclipses local therapies as the preferred treatment modality [77]. However, it should be noted that systemic treatments carry significant complication profiles which may be additive to complications already exposed by local therapy such as radiation or surgery. Additionally, the perioperative usage of systemic chemotherapy may have profound implications on healing and arthrodesis, mandating active planning and discussion with the multidisciplinary team.

Technical Considerations and Complications of Complex Reconstruction

Spinal Column Shortening

Spinal column shortening is often necessary in aggressive benign, primary, or secondary tumors resulting in a significant spinal deformity [79]. When considering reconstruction and alignment, it is generally far more neuroprotective to allow some spinal shortening than to attempt a spinal column lengthening. However, safe limits along with resultant physiological effects of this procedure have yet to be definitively determined [80]. In a study of seven patients with angular kyphosis in the thoracolumbar spine treated by closing-opening wedge osteotomy using a single posterior approach, Kawahara et al. found that spinal shortening of approximately 20% was safe in terms of neurologic integrity [80, 81]. Studies in dog models suggest that a safe range for spinal shortening maybe up to 1/3 of the vertebral segment and a warning range between 1/3 and 2/3 of the vertebral segment [79, 82]. Alemdaroğlu et al. found that the additional removal of laminar bone avoided excessive cord kinking through all stages of shortening [79].

Atraumatic Handling of Neural Elements

As neurologic compromise is a key issue guiding intervention and disease management, it is critical to ensure adequate and nontraumatic handling of the neural elements including the spinal cord and nerve roots. Complications regardless of surgical technique can include damage to surrounding structures and further neurologic deficit and/or paralysis [11]. Physical maneuvers such as "stretch" or "compression" may further destroy already vulnerable nerve fibers. Another potential aspect of surgery that may contribute to nerve injury is patient positioning. Positioning of a patient in a manner that pathologically stretches one's neural elements may cause increased intraneural pressure leading to reduced perfusion and subsequent nerve ischemia [83–86]. Specifically, neural stretch above 15% of normal resting length has been associated with conduction defects [83]. This warrants the use of intraoperative neuromonitoring of the spinal cord, especially if instrumentation is employed [84–86].

Limiting Intraoperative Bleeding

Complex reconstructive spine surgery, especially for metastatic spinal disease, is often associated with a high perioperative blood loss [11, 87–89]. This carries the potential for significant morbidity and mortality as acute blood loss can lead to stroke, myocardial infarction, and embolic events via peripheral circulatory failure [87, 88, 90–92]. In cases where significant blood loss is expected, certain interventions may prove beneficial such as preoperative embolization, normotensive anesthesia, and the use of fibrin-glue tamponade.

Preoperative Embolization

The goal of preoperative embolization for metastatic spinal tumors is to eradicate the blood supply to the tumor in order to minimize intraoperative blood loss. Preoperative embolization has been determined as relatively safe with minimal complications for treating benign, malignant, and metastatic tumors exhibiting hypervascularity [88, 93–100]. This technique also affords benefits of pain and neurologic symptom control in patients with significantly advanced disease [101]. Notable risks stem from the inadvertent embolization of blood vessels, resulting in ischemia of the spinal cord and displaced embolic material to the intracranial blood supply [88, 97, 100, 102].

Renal cell carcinoma (RCC) and thyroid carcinoma remain the most frequently encountered origins of hypervascular metastatic tumors. As such, most existing literature on this topic has focused on RCC metastases to the spine, with satisfactory outcomes when preoperative embolization is utilized [95–100].

Normotensive Anesthesia

Normal anesthesia or "normotensive anesthesia" is the current standard for anesthesia. In this mode of anesthesia, the patient's blood pressure is kept stable and within normal limits during the operation. For nontumor patients undergoing elective spinal surgery, hip or knee arthroplasty, and other potentially volume depleting procedures, the overall blood loss can be reduced via induction of hypotension [89, 103]. However, this form of anesthesia is rarely used in the setting of cord compression from a neoplastic process since lack of adequate cord perfusion may result in a catastrophic ischemic event. Generally, mean arterial pressure goals should be in the 80–90 mm Hg range for optimal neuroprotection [104, 105].

Fibrin Glue Tamponade

While steps such as preoperative embolization and "normotensive anesthesia" are taken to prevent significant intraoperative blood loss, the surgeon may still experience significant intraoperative blood loss. In the case of such an event, the surgeon and operative team must act swiftly. If the source of bleeding is secondary to a small blood vessel, use of electrocautery or pressure-packing with gauze pads will help control bleeding. A critical hemostatic tool that can aid in formation of a stable clot is fibrin glue. A composite of cryoprecipitate and thrombin, fibrin glue is sprayed onto the affected area via a double-barrel syringe. The mechanism of action of fibrin glue is that it mimics the final stages of the coagulation cascade forming a fibrin clot [106–110]. Studies have found it to be markedly useful in instances of significant hemorrhage and blunt force trauma, regardless of the patient's coagulation status [107, 108]. It is a particularly useful maneuver to control epidural bleeding during long or tedious cord-level spinal canal decompressions where direct pressure is difficult.

Damage to Major and Segmental Vessels

Vascular injury, while rare, is a dangerous and devastating complication of spine surgery. Injuries may occur during the direct manipulation of a vessel or via tumor adherence to the vessel wall [89]. Specific risk factors include perivascular infiltration of tumor cells, bone pathologies such as osteomyelitis, migration of implant devices, and previous history of spine surgery [89, 107, 108]. Such injury may lead to the formation of pseudoaneurysm, infarction, and dissection [89, 108].

Particular attention should be paid to specific anatomy depending on the region of the spine undergoing surgery. In the setting of the cervical spine, the carotid and vertebral arteries are most vulnerable from the placement of transarticular/pedicular screws [89]. Surgery involving the thoracic spine details immediate and delayed risk to the aorta, particularly between the levels of T5-T12 [89]. Physical deformities such as scoliosis further enhance such morbidity [89, 107]. Vascular injuries involving the lumbar spine have mortality rates as high as 40%, with the abdominal aorta as well as the left common iliac vasculature most at risk [89, 107, 108].

General preventative measures include thorough preoperative assessment of tumor and vessel location, cautious handling of vasculature, and the use of hemostatic agents [89, 107, 108]. Postoperative evaluation for deep venous thrombosis is also necessary [111–113]. Successful management of such complications often necessitates consultation between the spine surgeon and a vascular surgeon, options range from endovascular methods to open exploration and repair [89, 107, 108].

Management and Opportunistic Use of Cancer Cells During Surgery

The migration of malignant cells to a remote site is a possibility during spinal cancer surgery. This transplantation is believed to be attributable to contaminated instrumentation and/or surgical gloves and poses significant threat of tumor recurrence [114–117].

Surgeons are cautioned to take necessary precautions including changing gloves and instruments when changing anatomic fields [114]. Additional methods of prevention include irrigation of wounds with saline, water, iodine/peroxide, and/or chemotherapeutics [114–117].

Naturally, local autogenous bone grafting with contaminated bone is inadvisable. Lastly, the use of systems which recycle and re-infuse packed red cells during high-blood loss procedures ("cell saver" device) is controversial due to the theoretical systemic circulation of cancer cells [118–123].

Freezing autografts via liquid nitrogen is a novel method to eradicate contamination and residual tumor cells/debris. This represents a critical step in preventing infection and recurrence of malignancy and is both convenient and efficient as it may be performed inside the operating room. Frozen autograft provides the greatest potential for successful fusion while limiting complications [124–126]. This is believed to be due to the presence of endogenous BMP and VEGF [124, 127]. The role of BMP has been well established in the initiation, promotion, and maintenance of bone and cartilage formation/repair [127–129]. Additionally, VEGF serves as the chief regulator of angiogenesis, which is critical for successful osteo- and chondrogenesis [127, 130–132].

When compared to hyperthermic methods of autograft treatment such as irradiation, frozen/hypothermic methods have yielded superior osteoinduction and osteogenesis with minimal to no tumor recurrence [124–126, 133, 134].

Traditional Material Types and Implants with Limitations in Tumor Surgery

PEEK

The past three decades have seen increasing research, development, and utilization of the polymer family known as poly-aryl-ether-ketones (PAEK). PAEK is a group of heat-resistant synthetic polymers with a backbone chain made of ether and ketone units [135]. The molecular and chemical structure of PAEK also ensures resistance to chemicals and radiation [135]. They are generally radiolucent and therefore not susceptible to imaging scatter or deflection of radiotherapeutics. In addition, they possess greater strength and durability than most metals and a high biocompatibility, allowing synergy with carbon and/or glass reinforcement modalities [135]. They have been incorporated as biomaterial in the treatment of trauma, orthopedic reconstruction, and spinal implantation [135]. Specifically, one member of this family with extensive application in orthopedic and spinal implantation is poly-ether-ether-ketone or PEEK. In fact, it can be argued that PEEK has had its greatest clinical impact in the design of spinal implants and is widely accepted as an alternative to many metallic biomaterials [135].

An initial FDA clinical trial demonstrated significant success rates in terms of clinical outcomes, fusion success, and patient satisfaction for patients undergoing posterior lumbar interbody fusion (PLIF) with the Lumbar I/F (Brantigan) cage [136]. Results were maintained at 10-year follow-up, as this trial effectively set the stage for today's extensive use of PEEK as an interbody spacer [135]. Today, PEEK is available in various preparations with varying molecular weight and may be combined with carbon fiber-reinforced polymers (CFRP).

Drawbacks of using PEEK include slow incorporation and slightly reduced fusion rate when compared to titanium implants. PEEK's hydrophobic surface has also been shown to prevent bone deposition via fibrous capsule formed in between bone and the implant [135, 137, 138]. Recent research has focused on reducing the degree of encapsulation using surface modifications [135, 138–145]. Such surface modification has involved the creation of a porous PEEK surface and/or thin (lamellar) coating of titanium. Increased porosity or roughness is believed to increase osteogenesis while simultaneously permitting tissue permeation. The resulting connection of spinal implant with bone promises superior overall fusion and stability, thus decreasing the probability of migration or non-healing [135, 145].

Titanium and Titanium Alloys

Titanium has extensive applications across the medical field, in part, due to its biocompatibility, as well as its strength, low weight, and durability [145–150]. The ability to resist corrosion, non-toxic nature, and safe indications under MRI have also contributed to its widespread use for implantation [145–147]. In addition, a high biocompatibility affords titanium and its alloys optimal status to ensure successful osseointegration [145–147].

However, it is pertinent to note that titanium is vulnerable to subsidence in the setting of osteoporosis or weakened endplates. This often occurs in the setting of a modulus of elasticity mismatch between the spinal implant and host bone. Other properties that may prove influential in subsidence include the cage shape, size, and surface architecture, as well as the patient's age, overall health, and bone mineral density [151]. Additionally, graft placement, endplate preparation, and applied distraction and compression must also be considered [151–153].

In fact, a cohort study of 300 patients undergoing 1- and 2-level anterior cervical corpectomy with titanium mesh cages reported subsidence in an estimated 80% of cases [146]. Furthermore, 20% of these subsidence cases were classified as severe (>3 mm) with associated complications of neck pain, neurologic deterioration, and instrument failure [146]. This is likely due to the sharp edges of the titanium mesh and the focused forces distributed over a relatively small surface area. Modern design evolution and improvement of titanium implants has involved porous and less stiff configurations with more force distribution over larger endplate surfaces.

Titanium alloys combine other metals to produce metals with differing mechanical properties. Similar to stainless steel cages, some titanium alloys are stiffer and more rigid than pure titanium implants, which increases susceptibility to endplate subsidence [149]. Various surface modification techniques have been explored in order to improve titanium implant osseointegration and decrease rates of subsidence [154, 155]. Specifically, the creation of a rougher surface, modification of surface topography (with macro- and nanocoating), treatment with heat or alkali, creation of porous material, and hydroxyapatite-titanium composites can all improve osseointegration and bioactivity.

Rougher surface areas have demonstrated faster bone integration and superior contact between the implant and bone [154, 155]. This facilitates shorter healing periods as a rougher surface enhances osteoblast sensitivity, via production of local growth factors (transforming growth factor (TGF)-β1 and Prostaglandin E2) [154, 155]. The osseointegration of titanium implants may also be enhanced via organic and inorganic nanocoating, which mimics the organic and inorganic components of human cortical bone, facilitating cell adhesion, proliferation, and osteoconduction, respectively [156–159].

PEEK Composite Materials

PEEK/Titanium

The addition of titanium to PEEK enhances mechanical/strength and osseointegration when compared to PEEK alone (Figs. 20.1 and 20.2) [135, 141, 147, 149, 160, 161]. Studies have demonstrated enhanced cell attachment and increased bone/tissue volume, growth factors, and direct bone-implant contact [135, 141, 147, 149, 160, 161]. In particular, a study using a sheep model evaluating PEEK-Ti composite cages against conventional PEEK cages showed that composite cages exhibited a significant reduction in the range of motion with a simultaneous increase in stiffness [161]. These findings were further reinforced by the confirmation of significantly more bone at the fusion site and ingrowth into the end plates [161]. In addition, treatments once exclusively used for titanium implants, such as "surface bioactivation modules" are currently under development for use in PEEK/titanium composites [160].

PEEK/HA

It has been reported that HA was originally added to PEEK in order to form a composite closer to natural bone (Fig. 20.3) [135, 160]. This type of composite has enhanced bioactivity compared to PEEK alone; however, this comes at the expense of mechanical strength [135]. Despite this, one study assessing the use of PEEK-HA composite cages for anterior cervical discectomy and fusion demonstrated good-to-excellent clinical outcomes in 97% of patients [143]. Successful cervical fusion rates were observed on follow-up for up to a year (16.7% at 3 months, 61.1% at 6 months, and 100% at 1 year) [143].

PEEK/Carbon Fiber Reinforced Polymer

CFRP has an elastic modulus closer to cortical bone. PEEK-CFRP has been of particular interest due to its increased mechanical strength, biocompatibility, versatility, and radiological compati-

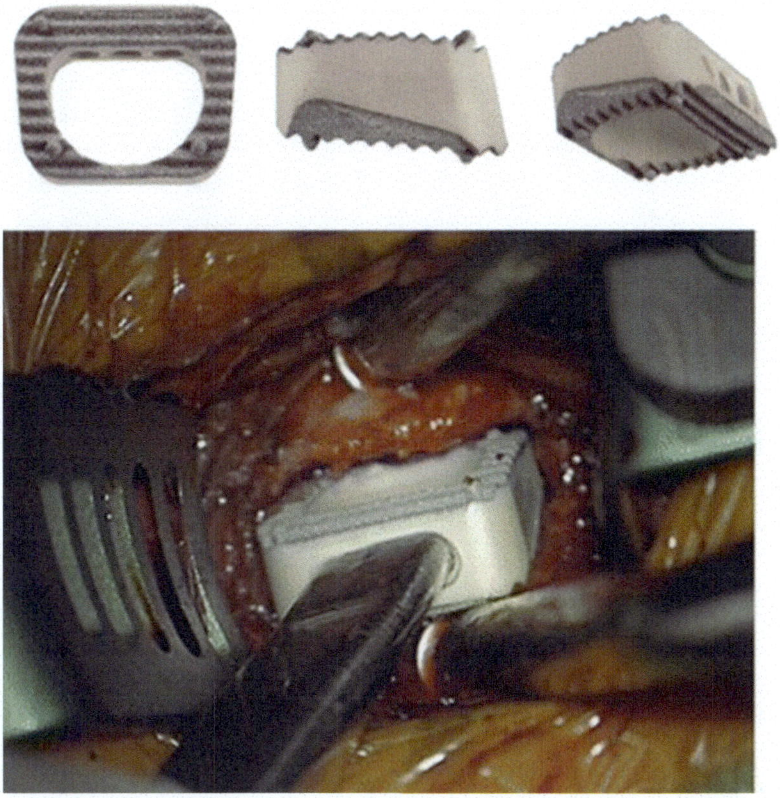

Fig. 20.1 Top image: superior, lateral, and oblique views showing the tips of the tantalum pins at each of the four corners for visualization on X-ray; Bottom image: intraoperative photograph of the spacer being implanted into a patient, showing the base PEEK implant coated with titanium on top and bottom surfaces only. (Reproduced with no changes from Kotsias et al. [270]. © CC BY 4.0 (https://creativecommons.org/licenses/by/4.0/))

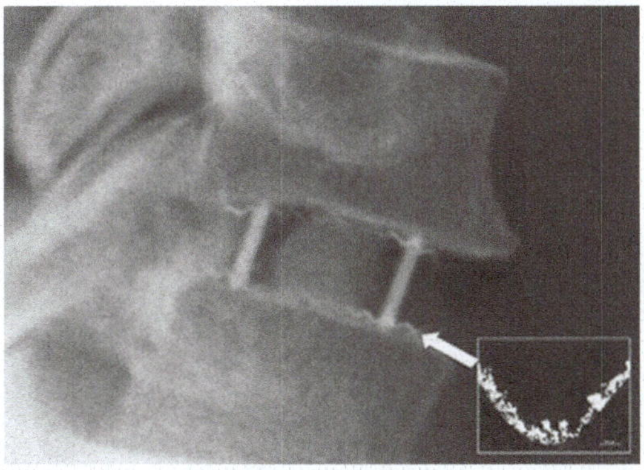

Fig. 20.2 Lateral cervical X-ray showing PEEK-Ti implant. The thin wavy line of titanium can be seen along the edges of the implant at the cervical endplates. (Reproduced with no changes from Kotsias et al. [270]. © CC BY 4.0 (https://creativecommons.org/licenses/by/4.0/))

bility; literature strongly supports PEEK-CFRP as an appropriate and promising modality for orthopedic implantation [162]. Current indications for PEEK-CFRP use include spinal cages, bone fixation screws/fracture fixation, and orthopedic implants (Fig. 20.4) [162]. The radiological compatibility allows fusion to be visualized postoperatively with any imaging modality [162]. In addition, chemical stability permits sterilization via conventional methods such as gamma radiation [162]. This is further discussed in the next section.

Poly-Methyl-Methacrylate (PMMA)

PMMA is effective for providing structural support for large defects as it helps stabilize weak or fractured vertebrae. PMMA is also effective in strengthening screw fixation [163]. This is necessary for patients with poor bone quality, malnutrition, or comorbidities such as those with metastatic spinal disease, as they are at increased risk for implantation failure.

Advantages include ease of use and reduced operative time [164]. In addition, production of the PMMA implant can be done during surgery,

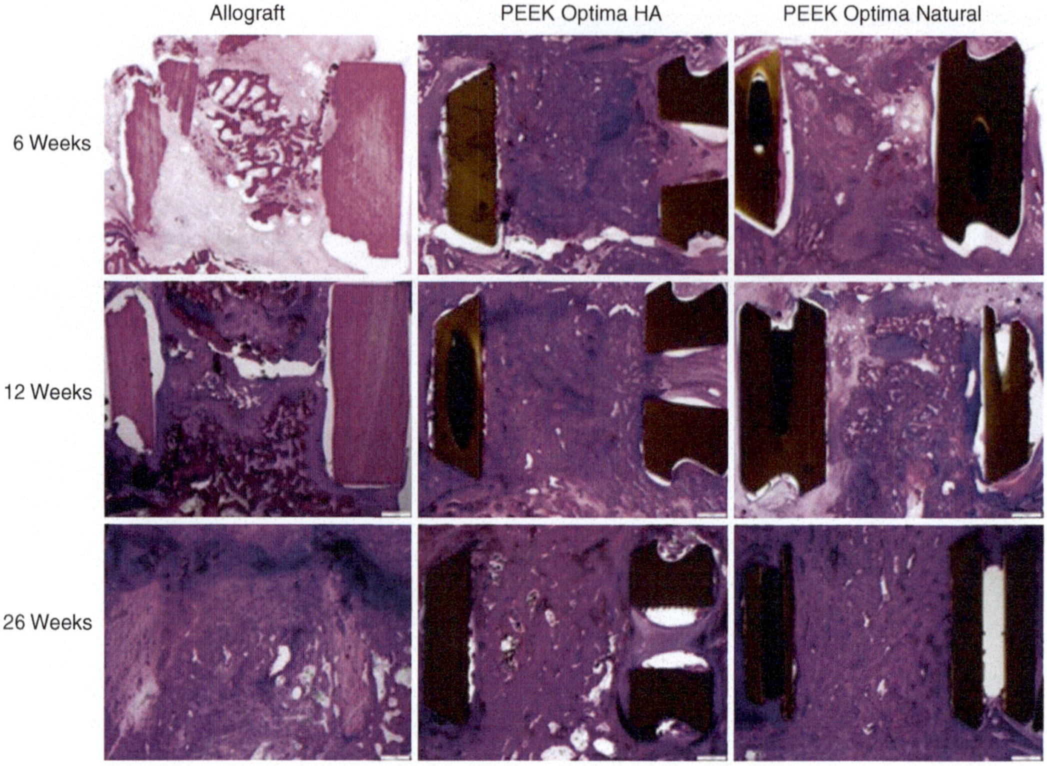

Fig. 20.3 A macroscopic overview of histology at 6, 12, and 26 weeks for allograft, PEEK-HA, and PEEK. There was a progression in fusion versus time for all groups. No observed failure in PEEK-HA or PEEK devices, whereas allograft cages fractured and resorbed with time. A fibrous tissue interface was noted for PEEK at 6 and 12 weeks, and direct bone contact was noted with PEEK-HA at 12 weeks. All fusions remodeled with time and were mature by 26 weeks. (Reproduced with no changes from Walsh et al. [271].

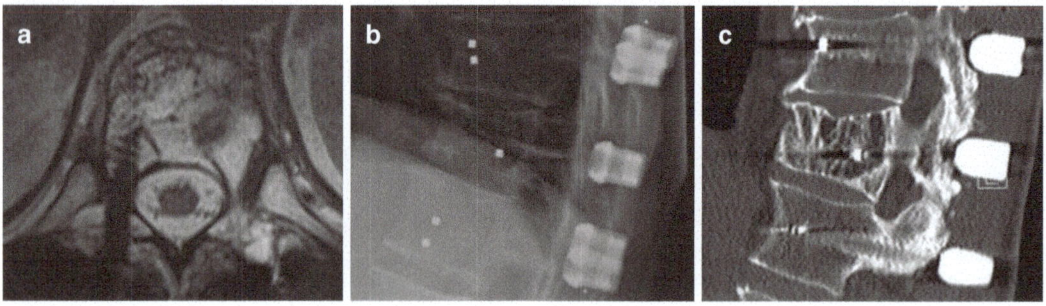

Fig. 20.4 (**a**) PEEK-CFRP are best depicted in the MRI with artifact reduction protocol. (**b**) Lateral X-ray showing carbon fiber screws that are not radiopaque. (**c**) Follow-up CT scan shows the accomplished posterolateral fusion without artifact from screws. (Reproduced with no changes from Laux et al. [179].

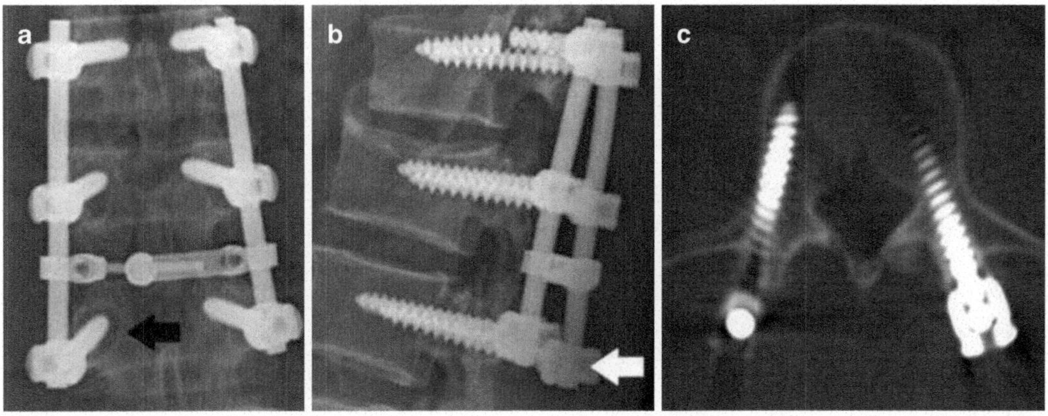

Fig. 20.5 Lumbar radiographs showing (**a**) anteroposterior X-ray with radiolucent zone and double halo around the screw (black arrow) indicating screw loosening. In addition, there is screw breakage demonstrated at the superior-most level. (**b**) Lateral X-ray demonstrating that the inferior screw has pulled out (white arrow). (**c**) CT scan in this case did not show a gap or halo around the inferior screw. (Reproduced with no changes from Wu et al. [170]. © CC BY 4.0 (https://creativecommons.org/licenses/by/4.0/))

as is often done in vertebroplasty and kyphoplasty procedures [164, 163].

Disadvantages of PMMA include wound infection, transient hypotension, loosening/displacement, allergic reaction, and thermal injury [165]. Thermal injury in particular is a result of the cement's hardening in the body and has been shown to reach temperatures as high as 86 °C [165, 166].

Whereas vertebroplasty involves direct injection of bone cement, kyphoplasty utilizes PMMA as a "filler" for structural reinforcement [163]. It is important to note, however, that there have been reports of cement leakage (extra-vertebral) associated with vertebroplasty, with conflicting reports on clinical significance [163].

Traditional Implant Failures (Rods/Screws/Cages)

Screw Loosening, Cut-Out, Pullout, and Screw/Rod Breakage

Screw loosening is a frequently reported complication of pedicle screw fixation. This can necessitate revision surgery and negatively affect overall postoperative clinical results [167, 168]. Current literature suggests a variation in rates of screw loosening, specifically, dependent upon bone quality [166–168]. Ranges of loosening have been as low as 1% and as high as 15% in those without osteoporosis, but are much higher for patients with osteoporosis, some estimates being over 50% [167, 169]. Ultimately, screw loosening, pullout, or fracture will result in pseudarthrosis (Fig. 20.5) [56, 167, 168, 170]. As mentioned in the previous section, unhealthy bone significantly complicates fixation efforts [56]. Other contributory factors include the length of fixation, number of levels fused, type of fusion, and the scope of surgical decompression [167, 168, 170].

Cage Subsidence and Failure

Cage subsidence has been linked to bone density, age, size, and surface-contact ratio, to name a few [171]. Along with age come changes in the physiological composition and curvature of the spine. Such changes precede aberrant stress bearing and weakened bone (Fig. 20.6) [171]. Increasing age, osteoporosis, and frailty are common covariates with metastatic spinal disease and further complicate successful cage implantation [172]. Additional factors include but are not limited to surgical technique, overweight/obesity, and variations of cage design [173].

Surgical technique such as aggressive endplate preparation may also contribute to the

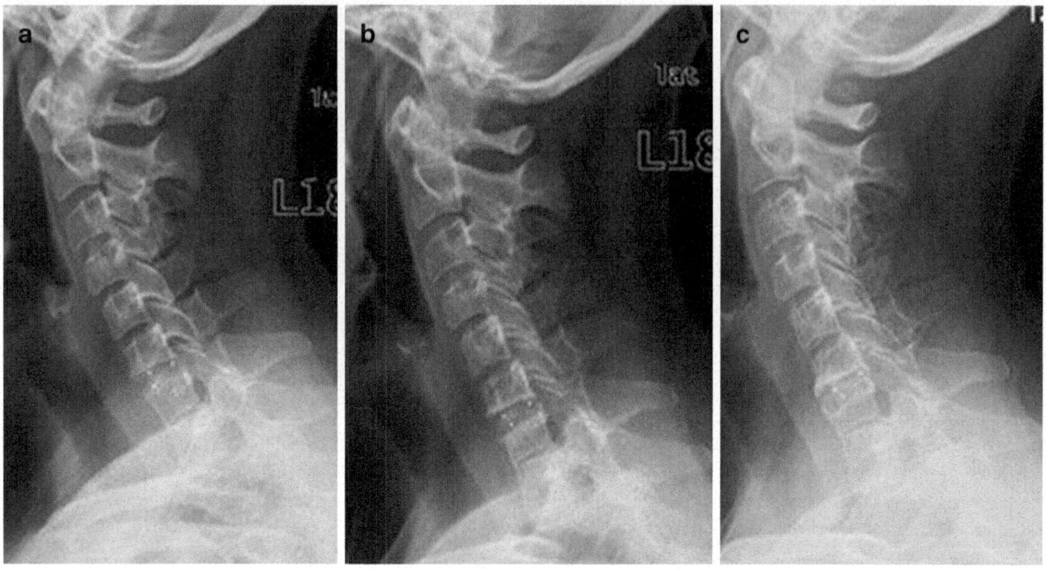

Fig. 20.6 Lateral cervical radiographs of a 59-year-old female treated with a cervical cage at C6/C7. (**a**) X-rays immediately postoperatively showing satisfactory cage placement, (**b**) 1 year after surgery with initial subsidence into the superior endplate of C7, and (**c**) 2.5 years postoperatively with advanced subsidence and osseous bridging. (Reproduced with no changes from Zajonz et al. [272]. © CC BY 4.0 (https://creativecommons.org/licenses/by/4.0/))

risk of subsidence [173]. However, it is also important to mention that studies have failed to establish significant correlation between degree of subsidence and changes in clinical outcomes [174–177]. Such studies suggest that fusion and patient-reported pain and disability were not significantly worsened by cage subsidence.

As mentioned later in this chapter, nonabsorbable/biocompatible PEEK cages are indicated in this regard, due to (mechanical and radiological) advantages of load-tolerance and accurate postoperative assessment [135, 139, 140, 173, 178–180].

Junctional Failure

Proximal junctional failure is recognized as a serious complication of spinal reconstructive surgery, entailing risk of neurologic injury, pain, gait difficulty, sagittal imbalance, and even social isolation [181, 182]. It is defined as junctional kyphosis of at least 15° along with fracture (or failure of fixation) of the uppermost instrumented vertebra (or one level above), or the need for extension of said instrumentation within 6 months of surgery [181].

Underlying pathology for proximal junctional failure is believed to be an acute postoperative structural occurrence; however, it can also include a more progressive deformity over months to years [181, 183, 184]. In fact, a multicenter-retrospective study reported that the most common mechanisms were fracture (47%) and disruption of soft tissue (44%) [181, 185]. The same study reported failure due to fracture most frequently occurred in the thoracolumbar region while failure due to soft tissue disruption (without fracture or instrumentation failure) was most commonly noted in the upper thoracic spine [185]. Furthermore, those who experienced thoracolumbar proximal junctional failure also happened to be older, have fewer levels of fusion, and have a worse postoperative sagittal imbalance than those of the other group [185]. Modifiable risk factors were found to correlate with degree of curvature correction, combined anterior-posterior fusion, incorporation of pedicle screw structures, and residual sagittal imbalance [181, 182]. Non-modifiable risk factors were found to correlate with age (over 55 years), (preoperative) sagittal imbalance, low bone mineral density, and body mass index [181, 182] [145–150].

State of the Art in Tumor Implants

Structural Titanium Mesh

With properties such as strong mechanical performance, durability, biocompatibility, relative ease of manipulation, and resistance to infection and corrosion, structural titanium mesh is a reliable modality for a wide array of surgical indications [186–188]. This includes anterior column replacement, graft control, and deformity correction [186–188]. These cages are most commonly used in cervical and thoracolumbar fusion cases due to robust mechanical performance, prolonged stability, and favorable clinical outcomes.

Structural titanium mesh also helps avoid complications from the use of autografts such as graft fracture and/or collapse [186]. This is achieved mainly via its porous metal sheets that can support onlay graft until bone mineralization occurs [186]. The incorporation of graft within the cage transforms an inactive metal cage into a biologically functional vertebral body replacement. One significant advantage of using a structural titanium mesh cage is avoiding the need to harvest ICBG and sparing the patient/donor from traditional site morbidity [186]. Avoiding the use of allograft also decreases the chances of less common implant complications such as immune response and transmission of disease [186].

The versatility of titanium mesh allows its use for defects of different sizes (Figs. 20.7 and 20.8) [186]. This is accomplished using an adaptable/moldable design in order to achieve desired length. In addition, titanium mesh can also be tailored via 3D printing [187]. It is critical to mention that despite the apparent benefits to using titanium mesh cages, complications similar to traditional titanium implants, such as subsidence, can still occur [186].

Techniques to reduce subsidence include increasing the surface area of the implant/cage-endplate interlink [189, 190]. One method that has been described is the addition of rings at the ends of the mesh cylinder, which has been shown to enhance the maximum load capacity, up to 27% [189]. Studies have demonstrated this addition facilitates a more uniform distribution of stress across the endplate [189].

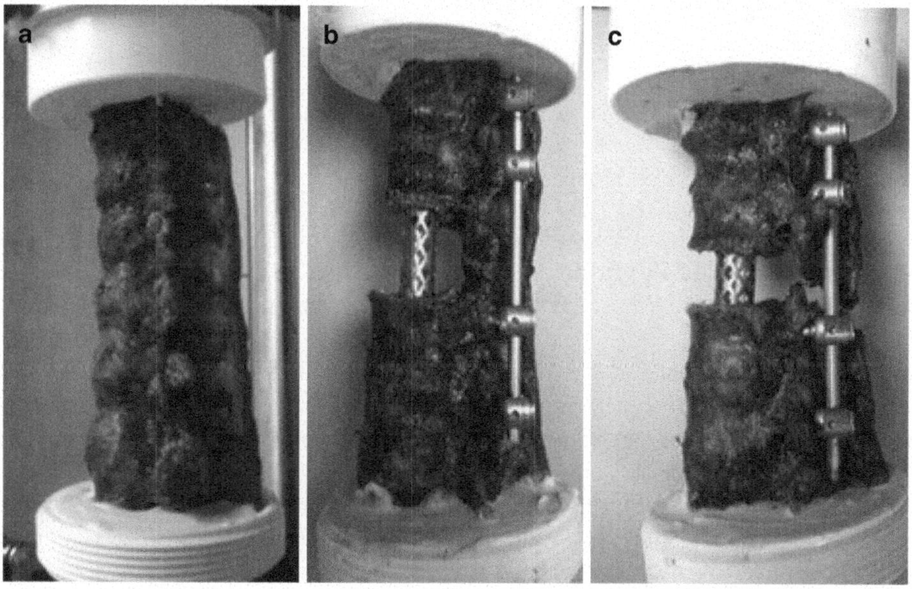

Fig. 20.7 Biomechanical model of the thoracolumbar spine depicting a Harms titanium mesh cage with two different sizes: (**a**) intact spine, (**b**) spondylectomy with 17 mm cage, and (**c**) spondylectomy with short 10 mm cage. (Reproduced with no changes from Kim et al. [273].)

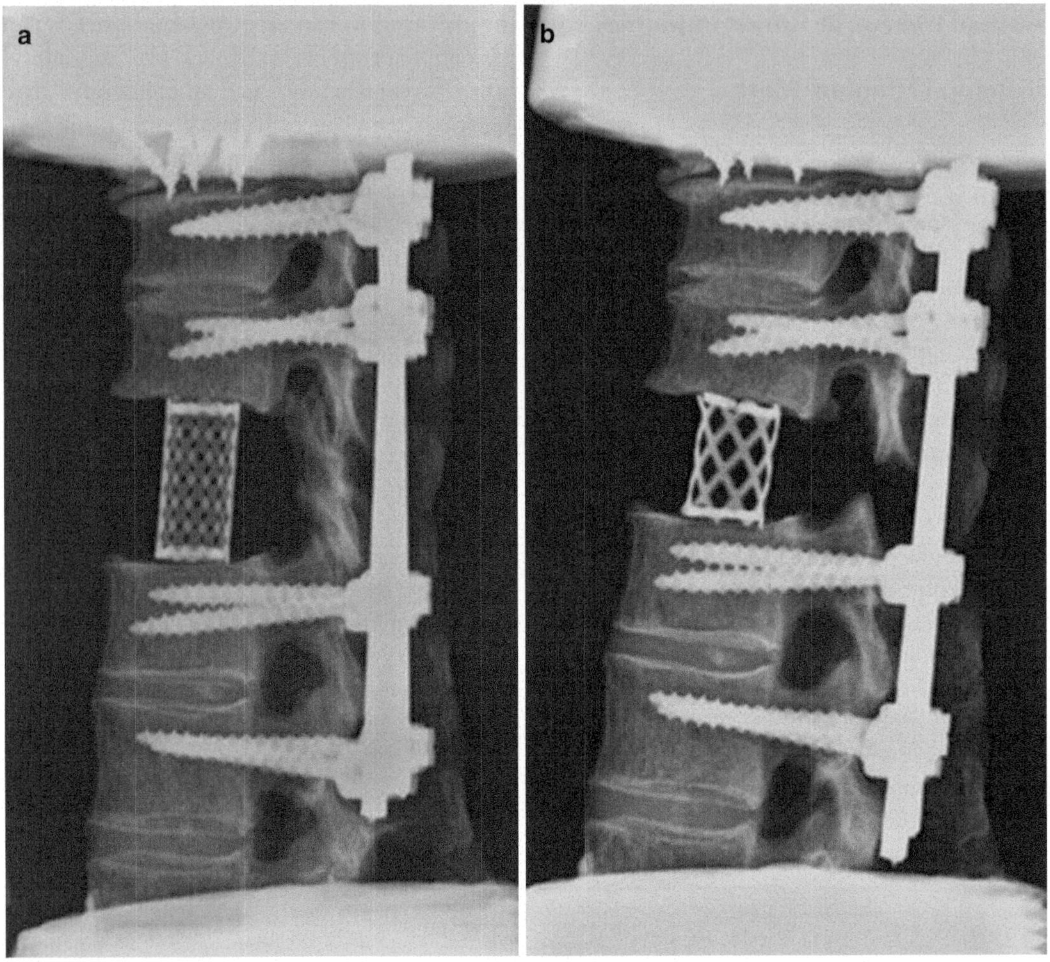

Fig. 20.8 Lateral thoracolumbar radiographs of the two reconstruction models with different size cages: (**a**) 17 mm and (**b**) 10 mm. (Reproduced with no changes from Kim et al. [273]. © CC BY 4.0 (https://creativecommons.org/licenses/by/4.0/))

Carbon Fiber-Reinforced Polymer Implants (CFRP)

CFRP has been used as implant material for over two decades. Current applications are primarily for vertebral body replacement and/or interbody fusion [190, 191]. CFRP proves advantageous in situations requiring mechanical strength, durability, biocompatibility, and radiolucency [190]. In addition, CFRPs offer functional strength and stability seen in traditional metallic implants but with significantly fewer episodes of loosening/migration and subsidence [190]. Furthermore, CFRP's radiological compatibility allows accurate postoperative assessment of fusion [162]. CFRP implants possess a modulus of elasticity similar to that of cortical bone; consequently, this affords the advantage of preventing stress shielding and end plate subsidence while offering superior fusion and complication rates compared to traditional metallic implants [190, 191]. However, CFRP cages have also demonstrated implant failure from inadequate stiffness [191].

As mentioned above, PEEK is heat-resistant, has greater strength and durability than most metals, is compatible with diagnostic imaging, and has a high biocompatibility [135]. Such advantages of PEEK are further enhanced when integrated with carbon fibers to form CFRP-PEEK. The resultant CFRP-PEEK can be altered to that of cortical or cancellous bone [192]. Furthermore, mechanical testing has shown PEEK to have low strength in tensile, bending, and compression tests; however, after the incorporation with carbon fiber, mechanical elements have shown significant improvement, analogous to those of (human) cortical bone [193].

CFRP-PEEK is predominantly utilized as a cage construct; however, pedicle screws and rods with this technology have also been developed [162]. It is highly biocompatible and can withstand prolonged fatigue/strain [162]. A 40-patient retrospective study analyzed clinical outcomes, fusion rates, and the percentage of vertebral body coverage for stackable CFRP-PEEK cages used in multilevel thoracolumbar reconstruction. Thirty-nine patients demonstrated successful fusion with exceptional clinical and radiographic results (covering an average of 60% of the vertebral body with the CFR-PEEK cage) [162, 194]. These studies suggest that stackable carbon fiber cages are indeed effective in achieving thoracolumbar fusion in large reconstructions [194].

Due to an elastic modulus close to that of a cortical bone, CFRP-PEEK implants have been shown to reduce stress and demonstrate improved longevity [179]. This is especially critical in structurally deficient bone, as healing may be delayed in spine tumor patients [179]. Current surgical management of spinal tumors involves instrumentation with pedicle screw and rod systems. As most modern pedicle screws and rods are composed of titanium alloy, they carry sufficient stiffness but also pose unique challenges to postoperative imaging and management for the patient [178, 179, 195, 196]. This has serious implications for the timely diagnosis of local recurrence.

In addition, conventional metal instrumentation often impedes the planning and administration of postoperative radiation therapy [178, 179, 195, 196]. Metal implants have been shown to absorb radiation and thereby hinder percutaneous radiation therapy [195]. Consequently, CFRP implants were developed for radiolucency (producing less artifacts and absorbing less radiation) and have proven to facilitate follow-up imaging [178, 179, 195, 196]. Furthermore, studies have also successfully established CFR-PEEK screw-rod systems as more appropriate in patients (eligible for radiotherapy) due to this very absence of image artifacts and less dose interference [178, 179, 195, 196].

Expandable Cages

Expandable cages are particularly valuable for anterior column reconstruction via minimally invasive posterior approach as they can be used in both the thoracic and the lumbar spine [197]. In addition to being available in multiple sizes, expandable cages include the ability to be inserted in a collapsed position with expansion in situ [197]. Many of the previously mentioned cage types are manufactured in such an expandable form, allowing the surgeon to modify the size as needed (Fig. 20.9). While expandable cages have been successfully used in spinal reconstruction for the treatment of infection, trauma, etc., their use in treating metastatic spinal disease is not well documented in current literature [198, 199].

The use of titanium expandable implants for reconstruction in spine tumor surgery has been reported. A 5-year review of 95 patients with thoracic and lumbar spinal malignancy (primary and metastatic) who underwent vertebral body resection and anterior column reconstruction demonstrated very positive results from the use and incorporation of an expandable titanium cage [200]. Specifically, patients demonstrated significant improvement in their numerical pain scores, as well as postoperative radiographic findings such as a median height correction of 14% (with values as high as 118%), and a median improvement in sagittal alignment of roughly 6° (with values as high as 28°) [200]. Another study reported on the use of a single posterior approach to treat 21 cases of vertebral body malignancy and reported complications directly attributable to use of the expandable cage [201]. These complications were a traction injury to a lumbar nerve root (during expansion), cage subsidence, and

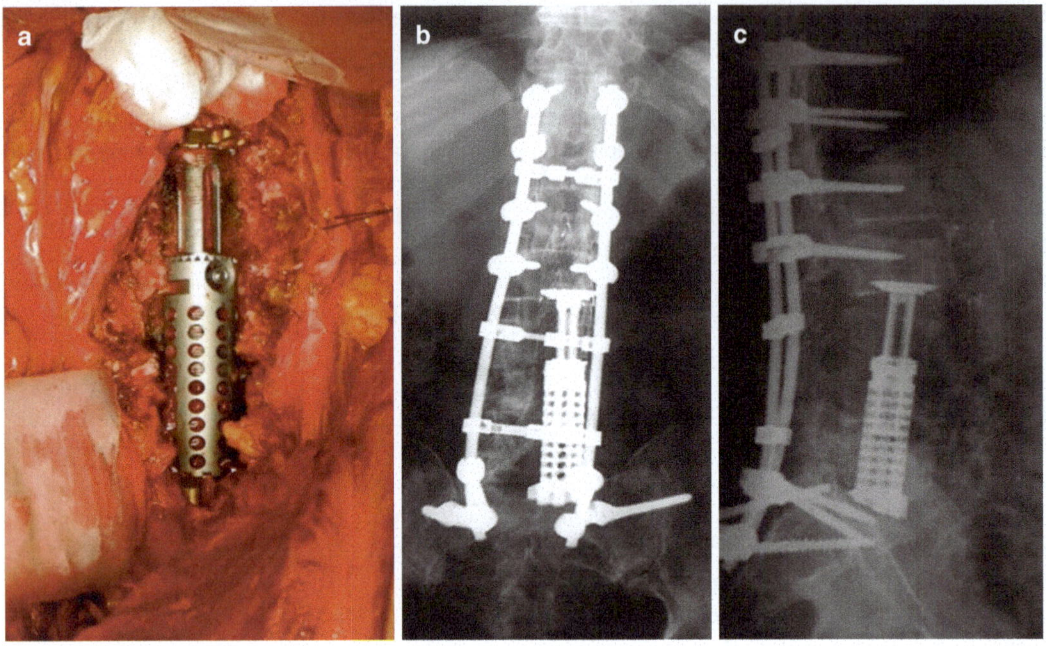

Fig. 20.9 (**a**) Intraoperative pictures depicting placement of expandable mesh cage. (**b**, **c**) 12-month postoperative AP and lateral X-rays showing slight settling of mesh cage but maintained lumbar lordosis. (Reproduced with no changes from Roberto et al. [274].)

necessary revision surgery due to oblique cage placement [201].

Additionally, a case series of five patients that underwent multilevel cervical corpectomies with the incorporation of expandable cages supplemented with anterior cervical plating and posterior instrumentation to ensure full circumferential fusion demonstrated fusion in 80% of patients, as well as correction of preoperative kyphotic deformity in all five patients and a significant decrease in preoperative pain [199]. Another retrospective study gathered and reviewed data on 24 patients with metastatic spinal disease, who were also treated with expandable cages from T5-L5. Thirteen patients exhibited significant improvements in neurologic function with no significant postoperative complications [198]. Out of the remaining patients, there was no postoperative neurological deterioration [198]. The authors of both of the above-mentioned studies concluded that expandable cages are a safe and effective modality for anterior column reconstruction and prevention of further neurologic deterioration in metastatic spinal disease [198, 199]. While such treatment is deemed palliative, it nonetheless has been shown to provide immediate stabilization in the deformed spine, as well as relief of symptoms of cord compression, radiculopathy, and/or axial pain [198, 199].

Due to their ability for providing superior correction, expandable cages provide a valuable addition to a surgeon's treatment options. Specifically, expandable cages allow a single posterior approach for circumferential decompression and stabilization of the thoracolumbar spine. One study reported using this technique in eight patients suffering from spinal malignancy, tuberculosis, and traumatic deformity [202]. The authors reported that all patients underwent complete vertebrectomy with postoperative improvement of deficits and no major neurological complications [202]. Similarly, a 17-year-old woman with a fibrous histiocytoma in the L5 segment and significant bone destruction underwent a posterior decompression and vertebral body replacement with an expandable cage and screw fixation [203]. The authors note that the expandable cage was successfully implanted (after resection) and expanded with excellent clinical results [203].

Additionally, a laboratory study compared the biomechanical stability between two similarly sized implants, via different surgical approaches: an expandable TLIF cage deployed in situ compared to a traditional fixed dimension ALIF cage [204]. The biomechanical stability of the expandable TLIF cage was found to be equivalent to the ALIF cage in coronal, axial, and sagittal planes [204]. However, authors note that the deployable and expandable TLIF cage provided advantages of a single minimally invasive approach and extensive (endplate) imprint with preservation of the anterior tension band [204].

It is important to mention that little is known about the long-term use and late complications of expandable cages. Only one study noted possible complications from using expandable cages. Liu et al. documented that patients with expandable cages had almost double the subsidence rate of those with fixed cages [205]. This observation remained beginning from the first postoperative month and was also noted at the 1-year mark [205].

Linked Cage/Screw Constructs

The aim of interbody cages is to achieve anterior column fusion, whereas posterior instrumentation and decortication with bone graft is used for posterior fusion. While interbody cages act as load-bearing devices and rely on axial compression, in cases with large segment resection, this may not be ideal [206]. As mentioned previously, catastrophic failure can occur with cage fatigue, subsidence, and loss of stability with progressive motion. This is especially true in tumor cases where a large segment is spanned by a single implant. To avoid this potential failure and increased rigidity in the model, novel anterior interbody implants have been developed that couple with posterior load-sharing instrumentation.

Traditionally, this was accomplished by placing posterior-based screws aimed anteriorly into titanium mesh cages. In addition, anteriorly based "Kaneda instrumentation" has also been used to fix interbody cages with screws [207]. This theoretically strengthens the overall construct and stiffens the motion segment preventing complications. Newer techniques have also been developed allowing posterior pedicle screws to link with anterior corpectomy cages. The cage is allowed to move parallel to the pedicle screws through this link while still undergoing axial compression. A biomechanical model was used to evaluate properties of a construct designed to maximize stiffness and minimize intervertebral cage subsidence [206]. This spondylectomy model determined that connecting the anterior column-cage to posterior instrumentation using additional pedicle screws can result in a system that is almost 40% stiffer and has 50% less subsidence compared to a traditional unconnected cage [206].

3D-Printed Implants

Reconstructive surgery is an extremely challenging endeavor even for the most experienced surgeons [208]. Anatomical complexity, uniqueness of each defect, and sensitivities of involved systems further contribute to such challenges [208]. Patient-specific implants are designed with a precise fit to defects [208]. Demand to advance such implants has led to technological advancements, most pertinently, 3D printing [208]. In fact, the United States Food and Drug Administration recently increased the approval of 3D printed implants under the "510k (premarket notification)" approval system, allowing providers to use 3D printed parts in routine and complex surgical procedures [208].

Various alloplastic implant materials including ceramics, metals, polymers, and composites are currently produced from 3D printing [208]. Among these, metals and ceramics have been most frequently used in orthopedic implants; however, both have significant drawbacks. The high mechanical strength and elastic modulus of metallic 3D implants have a modulus mismatch with vertebral bone, resulting in potential stress shielding, subsidence, and loosening [208]. Additionally, metallic nature impedes necessary radiologic tests as they have been found to cause "streak artifacts" on advanced spinal imaging.

Ceramics, while biocompatible and bioactive, have a low mechanical strength with a high modulus of elasticity and brittleness; consequently, they are susceptible to fracture [208]. More recently, the use of polymers as a sustainable 3D implant alternative has been studied using PEEK [208]. As mentioned in the previous section, PEEK has a wide range of applications due to its lightweight, strength, durability, and resistance to heat and chemical insult [208]. In the realm of spinal reconstruction, PEEK and its composites (CFRP-PEEK) have primarily been used for interbody fusion cages [208].

While the use of PEEK in 3D printing has proven challenging, recent technological advances have provided improved 3D printing via "fused filament fabrication" (FFF) technology [208]. This specialized printing permits successful creation of almost any complex construct [208].

Furthermore, the increasing availability of affordable 3D printing is expected to allow surgeons to produce tailored implants from within the healthcare setting [208]. Thus far, FFF exhibits advantages including cost control, efficient implant production, and greater individualized approach to patient care [208]. However, recent literature also notes a concurrent expansion of regulatory oversight (targeting 3D printing) that may lengthen the approval and manufacture of novel implants [208–210].

Biologics and Bone Grafts

Bone Grafts

Over 200,000 spinal fusions are performed every year in the United States, and virtually all use either autograft or allograft to help achieve successful fusion [211]. The most frequent sites of bone graft include local autograft from the operative region of the spine, iliac crest, fibula, rib, tibia, and femoral shaft [74, 211–214]. An ideal bone graft facilitates healing and fusion in a minimal amount of time with minimal complications [211–214]. Important characteristics include osteogenesis (capacity to form bone), osteoconduction (facilitate bone growth onto graft/implant), and osteoinduction (recruitment and stimulation of immature cells to develop into osteoblasts) [74, 211–214]. While both autograft and allograft exhibit osteoconductive properties, only autograft can directly facilitate osteogenesis, thanks to its biologically active bone marrow [211]. This superior biological advantage does however come with significant risks of patient-morbidity and complications [11, 74, 215]. In addition, autograft carries the risk of transmitting infectious and malignant tissue from harvest site to the donor site [11, 74, 211, 215, 216].

Iliac Crest Bone Graft

ICBG is an effective, safe, and readily harvested source of autograft. In fact, it is still the most frequently used site to harvest bone graft [212, 213, 217]. Unique features include a reliable structural integrity (due to its cortical components) and osteoinductive, as well as osteogenic properties (due to its cancellous components) [212, 213, 217]. It is also advantageous as a larger size graft and can be harvested without excessive damage to the structure or function of the ilium. However, in recent years, concern regarding donor site morbidity/pain has caused a sharp decline in the utilization of this method [212, 213, 216]. Less common complications such as infection are rare, yet prevalent [216, 218]. Additional drawbacks of ICBG harvest include excessive loss of blood, subsequent weakness/fractures at the harvest site, and (tender) scar formation [11, 212, 213, 219–222].

Vascularized Autografts

Vascularized autografts have unique advantages exclusively attributable to the preservation of blood supply. This directly expedites ideal incorporation of cortical bone and matrix remodeling [211, 212, 223]. The avoidance of necrosis preserves and facilitates osteocytes and osteoblast/progenitor cells, culminating in superior strength, fusion, and overall reliability, especially in those with concurrent or anticipated large defects (>6 cm) [211, 212, 223–227]. In addition to documented success rates of up to 90%, vascularized grafts also exhibit shorter fusion times compared to nonvascularized grafts in spine tumor reconstruction [223–225].

Disadvantages to vascularized autografts stem from the degree of invasiveness, namely, the high rate of complications. As such, this modality should only be considered if simple reconstructive modalities are not deemed appropriate [225]. Medical literature currently reports complications including excessive operative time, difficulties with anastomosis, neurovascular injury, pain, instability, and fracture [223, 225, 227–230]. This can be further complicated by the presence of a poor recipient vascular bed, which has been proven to hinder absorption and revascularization of the graft [217, 224, 231].

Free vascularized fibula grafts (FVFG) are currently the most commonly used free vascularized bone grafts [227, 230, 232, 233]. FVFGs were initially reserved exclusively for posttraumatic bony defects; however, modern indications have since expanded to include deformity from infection, malignancy, and congenital causes, as well as failed arthrodesis, large segment defects, and poor bone quality [217, 230, 232, 233]. FVFGs have unique features such as advantageous length, exceptional bone mass, and exclusive blood supply [217, 230, 232]. Complications of vascularized fibular grafts include hemorrhage at the anastomosis site with/without thrombosis, muscle weakness, compartment syndrome, nonunion, infection, and fracture [230, 232, 234].

Vascularized rib grafts are a more convenient option than vascularized fibular grafts due to their proximity to the spine, lack of significant donor site morbidity, and relative ease of harvesting [72, 228, 235]. Pedicle rib grafts have historically been limited in spinal surgery to the correction of kyphotic deformity, as well as infective/necrotic lesions of the spine [228, 235]. Clinical outcomes postimplementation of vascularized rib grafts in complex spinal reconstruction have not been widely studied; however, limited studies have found fusion rates similar to those of ICBG [72]. The same studies also reported significantly fewer major complications and donor site morbidity in the rib autograft compared to the ICBG [72, 235]. One disadvantage is that rib grafts do not have the structural integrity of ICBG. In addition, for very large defects, vascularized rib grafts may not be appropriate for use and FVFG should be considered instead. However, they are much more flexible and can thus be contoured in specific areas such as the posterior cervical spine [228].

Structural Allograft

Structural allografts have also played an important role in spinal reconstruction as they provide relatively high rates of fusion without additional donor site morbidity. Although autogenous bone grafting is still the standard for spine fusion, current literature demonstrates that allograft is a valuable alternative [11, 71, 74, 211–213, 215, 222]. Depending on the preparation of allograft (fresh-frozen vs. freeze-dried), there is little to no immunogenicity [11, 74, 215]. This has previously been thought to result in a higher complication and failure rates compared to autografts overall, yet recent studies have demonstrated similar fusion rates between allo- and autograft [222, 236–238]. In addition, no significant differences have been noted with regard to infection, bleeding, neurovascular compromise, need for revision surgery, or patient satisfaction [222, 237, 238]. However, for multilevel and complex cases, autograft continues to outperform allograft [11, 222]. A unique risk of allograft is the risk for transmission of infection from the donor [212, 213, 215, 239]. Specifically, the risk of transmission of viral diseases such as HIV and hepatitis has been estimated at between 1/200,000 and 1/1,600,000 [11, 212]. However, with freeze-dried allograft (lyophilization), there has never been a documented transmission of virus [11, 213].

When a strut allograft is incorporated, the immediate immunological response from the host is with the initiation of osteogenesis via rapid mobilization of mesenchymal tissue [240]. The healing process includes inflammation, graft resorption, neo/revascularization, and new bone formation [74, 213, 240–242]. Current strut allografts used in clinical practice include femur, tibia, or fibula [74, 240, 243]. While not as extensively used in spinal reconstruction, tibial struts are used in revision arthroplasty of the hip for cortical repair, bone stock restoration, and periprosthetic fracture stabilization [74, 240–242, 244].

Femoral shaft allografts lack osteoinductive properties due to an empty medullary space [11, 29, 74, 215]. Unique advantages include resistance to or avoidance of vertebral collapse due to their diameter and large contact surface [29]. In addition, femoral shaft allografts are able to avoid stress shielding, thanks in part to functional similarities with autologous bone [29]. Structural femoral shaft allografts have mostly been utilized in spinal reconstruction post resection of compromised bone, as they produce clinically sound fusion results [29, 245, 246]. Recent retrospective analyses have also shown satisfactory outcomes with improved kyphosis and minimal subsidence when used in the osteoporotic spine [29].

Fibular strut allografts are highly versatile and are indicated in cases of structural damage/instability [247, 248]. Additionally, they may prove beneficial in achieving necessary fixation in those with compromised bone quality [247].

Studies have highlighted positive results of fibular allograft use in cervical reconstruction, with fusion rates reaching as high as over 90%, without significant complications [248–250]. These patients also experienced shorter duration of (hospital) stays when compared to those who had ICBG [250].

However, conflicting studies have noted fibular allograft cases with failed union rates as high as 41% [248, 251]. The overall reduced surface contact area of the vertebral body with the ends of the graft may also subject this region to excessive "shear stress" and subsequent nonunion [248, 252, 253]. In addition, multilevel cervical cases often exhibit decreased stability, which may place the graft at further risk for dislodgment [248, 252, 253].

Bone Graft Substitutes and Extenders

Bone graft substitutes and extenders help avoid harvesting the patient's own bone and thus facilitate recovery with minimal morbidity [211, 212, 239]. In general, bone graft substitutes and extenders may be synthetic or organic [211–213]. They are classified as ceramics (HA, β-tricalcium phosphate [β-TCP], calcium sulfate), growth factors (demineralized bone matrix [DBM], platelet-rich plasma [PRP], or bone morphogenetic proteins [BMPs]) [215].

DBM is the final product after allograft bone is processed to separate osteogenic and osteoinductive proteins (collagens, non-collagenous proteins, and growth factors such as insulin-like growth factor, transforming growth factor, and fibroblast growth factor) [74, 215]. This collection of material is then made available for surgical use in various forms such as powder, chips, and putty [74, 212, 215, 254]. Advantages of DBM include that it is readily obtainable, off-the-shelf, and easy to apply [211–213, 254]. Examples of carriers include calcium sulfate, lecithin, hyaluronic acid, and glycerol [254]. Lecithin, in particular, has been shown to significantly improve osteoinduction in fusion sites [254–256]. In addition to using carriers, an effective delivery system (i.e., syringes) aids in ease of use [255]. Specific handling requirements such as mandatory temperature levels and storage restrictions should be noted [255, 257]. Unique disadvantages of DBM include a variation in efficacy/osteogenic activity due to different preparations and demineralization methods [255].

Ceramic grafts have become increasingly utilized as an alternative to traditional bone grafts [211–213] [33]. The main subtypes of ceramics include HA, β-TCP, silicate-substituted calcium phosphate, calcium sulfate, and/or a combination of the above [72, 215, 258]. Ceramics enhance fusion rates by providing sound support yet are unable to stimulate bone growth. Consequently, ceramics must be paired with osteoinductive modalities such as autograft/allograft and/or growth factors in order to be effective [72, 258]. They are physically versatile and abundant in supply, hence providing cost-efficiency [72, 215].

Calcium Phosphate Bone Cement

Polymethyl methacrylate (PMMA) traditional bone cement has a storied history being indicated in implant fixation [165]. Its main function was to occupy space in order to press the implant against the bone. However, a toxic composition and lack of bioresorption have proven clinically burdensome. Specifically, its toxicity, hypovolemia, hypotension, inflammation, infection, abnormal cardiac conduction, etc. culminate in "bone cement implantation syndrome" [165]. In addition, the lack of biodegradability leaves PMMA susceptible to excessive heat production [165]. As such, attention has turned toward a more biocompatible alternative that does not exhibit such toxicity, calcium phosphate bone cement.

In addition to being biologically resorbable and biocompatible, calcium phosphate bone cement also contributes to structural integrity via promotion of osteogenesis and remodeling [259–261]. This represents a stark contrast to traditional PMMA, which influences neither the former nor the latter [165].

In fact, studies involving vertebral models (sheep) can only demonstrate superior stiffness with PMMA immediately postimplantation, while calcium phosphate cement displays far superior tolerance, tissue response, osteogenesis, and osteointegration [259, 260]. Furthermore, a study comparing both variates on the reinforcement of vertebral screw fixation of osteoporotic human spines (cadavers) found significantly greater rigidity and pull out strength in the calcium phosphate group [261].

Current literature for the use of HA in spinal fusion surgery has shown variation in efficacy [72, 258]. In cervical interbody spine fusion, one level I study showed HA to be structurally deficient compared to traditional ICBG, resulting in a fragmentation rate of nearly 90% compared to 10% with ICBG, despite similar clinical results and fusion rates [258]. In addition, four level IV studies reported positive overall results with cervical interbody fusion rates from almost 93% to 100%, suggesting that HA is also an effective alternative to iliac crest autograft [258]. In the setting of lumbar fusion surgery, however, HA has not shown to be a significantly better alternative to iliac crest autograft [258]. One level III retrospective study and three level IV studies concluded that "porous hydroxyapatite" was valuable as a graft extender in posterolateral fusion but only when used with other bone substitutes such as auto/allografts [258].

Current literature for the use of β-TCP also shows conflicting results depending on its use [211–213]. Evidence for its use for lumbar spine fusion has been inconclusive; however, good fusion and clinical outcomes have been noted in its application in the cervical spine and management of scoliosis [258]. Silicate-substitute calcium phosphate is another type of ceramics-based material used in spinal fusion. Silicate is thought to facilitate osteoconduction and osteoinduction by bringing osteoblasts to the material's surface via its negative charge [258].Level IV retrospective studies in cervical and lumbar fusion have shown fusion rates ranging from 76% to 90%; however, there are insufficient high-level studies (level I and II) comparing this ceramic alternative to conventional autologous bone grafts [258].

Calcium sulfate ceramics have been limited to use in mainly lumbar fusions with conflicting results regarding their efficacy. Specifically, a level I prospective, randomized study of single-level lumbar fusions compared fusion rates between ICBG and calcium sulfate chips mixed with bone marrow aspirate. The calcium sulfate group was found to have significantly lower fusion rates compared to ICBG [258]. Contrarily, a level II and level III prospective study in patients that underwent single level or multilevel lumbar fusion procedures showed almost equal fusion rates between calcium sulfate "pellets" with local autograft compared to conventional ICBG, at 87% vs. 89% (for one-level lumbar fusion) and 83% vs. 85% (for two-level lumbar fusion), respectively [258]. These studies potentially establish efficiency and benefits of calcium sulfate ceramics when used with local autologous bone [258].

Biologics

Biologics are currently an expanding category in the search for the most reliable substances to aid in achieving fusion. The demand for biologics in spinal fusions is expected to increase, in part, because of the morbidity associated with current autograft methods. In addition, as the science and technology of BMPs, stem cells, and other biologics advance, their use for non-fusion procedures is also expected to increase.

Bone Morphogenetic Protein

BMPs are growth factors that regulate bone and cartilage formation from stem cells [72, 211–213, 258]. Current literature has established BMP as the most effective family of growth factors for osteogenesis [62, 211–213, 239, 256]. Numerous subtypes of BMPs play a role in bone formation (2, 4, 6, 7, 9, and 14) [72]. BMPs that are used in patients are often manufactured through recombinant expression and administered as recombinant BMPs (rhBMP) [262]. Currently, rhBMP-2 is currently the only FDA-approved BMP for use in the spine (anterior lumbar interbody fusion) with off-label indications also in practice [72, 212, 213, 262].

However, in the context of spinal oncology, the use of BMP is controversial. Because of its effects on cancer growth, the use of BMP to promote spinal fusion in patients with existing malignancy is contraindicated [263, 264]. Interestingly, biological function studies have discovered BMP roles in both the development and suppression of such malignancy [263]. In fact, a study performed to evaluate the risk of new malignancy in patients with degenerative lumbar spinal pathologies undergoing instrumented arthrodesis (receiving high-dose rhBMP-2) found 15 new cancer events in 11 patients (in the rhBMP-2 group) compared with only two new malignancies in the control group (treated with autogenous bone graft) at 2 years follow-up [265]. A significantly greater incidence of cancer was still observed in the same (rhBMP-2) group at 5 years follow-up [265]. There have also been studies demonstrating that BMPs are safe to use in the general population. Specifically, a retrospective 5-year analysis examining the incidence of new cancer cases in just under 470,000 Medicare patients (who underwent spinal arthrodesis) determined that the clinical use of BMPs was not associated with a detectable increase in the risk of cancer [266]. This study had an average follow-up period of approximately 3 years [266]. Additionally, a longitudinal case-cohort study of Medicare beneficiaries within Surveillance, Epidemiology, and End Results (SEER) Program-Medicare cohort (almost 7300 individuals) also found that BMP usage during lumbar arthrodesis was not associated with cancer risk or mortality [264]. Such lack of association between BMP usage and subsequent cancer risk and mortality has been reported consistently among a wide array of cancers for individuals who received high doses of BMPs [264].

Mesenchymal Stem Cells

Mesenchymal stem cells (MSCs) can differentiate into three cell lines: osteoblasts, adipocytes, and chondrocytes. Their primary role is to replace damaged cells and stimulate tissue regeneration [212, 213, 267]. MSCs that are harvested from adipose tissue, bone marrow, periosteum, and/or skeletal muscle have all demonstrated the capacity to differentiate into osteoblasts and thus induce osteogenesis [267]. It is worth mentioning that the most common source of MSCs is bone marrow aspirate (BMA) [268]. Harvesting BMA is typically done percutaneously from the posterior ilium intraoperatively and has a significantly less local morbidity than traditional ICBG harvest [267, 268].

Preclinical studies on animal models have demonstrated similar fusion success rates to those achieved by traditional autograft [267, 269]. However, inconsistencies are noted in existent literature. Some studies demonstrate that fusion rates with MSCs are far superior to autograft; however, others have demonstrated the exact opposite [267, 269]. The clinical study and subsequent application/usage of stem cells is currently limited due to scarcity and variability in cells that can be harvested [267, 269]. While promising, there is still uncertainty as to whether the use of these cells can directly translate to success clinically.

References

1. Xu J, Murphy SL, Kochanek KD, Bastian B, Arias E. Deaths: final data for 2016. Natl Vital Stat Rep Cent Dis Control Prev Natl Cent Health Stat Natl Vital Stat Syst. 2018;67(5):1–76.
2. Franceschi S, Wild CP. Meeting the global demands of epidemiologic transition — the indispensable role of cancer prevention. Mol Oncol. 2013;7(1):1–13. https://doi.org/10.1016/j.molonc.2012.10.010.
3. Fitzmaurice C, Akinyemiju TF, Al Lami FH, et al. Global, regional, and national cancer incidence, mortality, years of life lost, years lived with disability, and disability-adjusted life-years for 29 cancer groups, 1990 to 2016. JAMA Oncol. 2018;4(11) https://doi.org/10.1001/jamaoncol.2018.2706.
4. Bray F, Jemal A, Grey N, Ferlay J, Forman D. Global cancer transitions according to the Human Development Index (2008–2030): a population-based study. Lancet Oncol. 2012;13(8):790–801. https://doi.org/10.1016/S1470-2045(12)70211-5.
5. Budczies J, von Winterfeld M, Klauschen F, et al. The landscape of metastatic progression patterns across major human cancers. Oncotarget. 2014;6(1):570–83.
6. Maccauro G, Spinelli MS, Mauro S, Perisano C, Graci C, Rosa MA. Physiopathology of spine metastasis. Int J Surg Oncol. 2011;2011:107969. https://doi.org/10.1155/2011/107969.
7. Ziu E, Mesfin FB. Cancer, spinal metastasis. In: StatPearls. Treasure Island (FL): StatPearls Publishing; 2020. http://www.ncbi.nlm.nih.gov/books/NBK441950/. Accessed 9 Feb 2020.
8. Harrington KD. Orthopedic surgical management of skeletal complications of malignancy. Cancer. 1997;80(8 Suppl):1614–27. https://doi.org/10.1002/(sici)1097-0142(19971015)80:8+<1614::aid-cncr12>3.3.co;2-0.
9. Deyo RA, Mirza SK, Martin BI, Kreuter W, Goodman DC, Jarvik JG. Trends, major medical complications, and charges associated with surgery for lumbar spinal stenosis in older adults. JAMA J Am Med Assoc. 2010;303(13):1259–65. https://doi.org/10.1001/jama.2010.338.
10. Sobottke R, Csécsei G, Kaulhausen T, et al. Spinal surgery in the elderly: does age have an influence on the complication rate? Orthopade. 2008;37(4):367–73. https://doi.org/10.1007/s00132-008-1233-5.
11. Dunning EC, Butler JS, Morris S. Complications in the management of metastatic spinal disease. World J Orthop. 2012;3(8):114–21. https://doi.org/10.5312/wjo.v3.i8.114.
12. Riskin DJ, Longaker MT, Gertner M, Krummel TM. Innovation in surgery. Ann Surg. 2006;244(5):686–93. https://doi.org/10.1097/01.sla.0000242706.91771.ce.
13. Delank K-S, Wendtner C, Eich HT, Eysel P. The treatment of spinal metastases. Dtsch Ärztebl Int. 2011;108(5):71–80. https://doi.org/10.3238/arztebl.2011.0071.
14. National Collaborating Centre for Cancer (UK). Metastatic spinal cord compression: diagnosis and management of patients at risk of or with metastatic spinal cord compression. Cardiff (UK): National Collaborating Centre for Cancer (UK); 2008. http://www.ncbi.nlm.nih.gov/books/NBK55007/. Accessed 9 Feb 2020.
15. Fisher CG, DiPaola CP, Ryken TC, et al. A novel classification system for spinal instability in neoplastic disease: an evidence-based approach and expert consensus from the Spine Oncology Study Group. Spine. 2010;35(22):E1221–9. https://doi.org/10.1097/BRS.0b013e3181e16ae2.
16. Kelly RP, Whitesides TE. Treatment of lumbodorsal fracture-dislocations. Ann Surg. 1968;167(5):705–17.
17. Denis F. The three column spine and its significance in the classification of acute thoracolumbar spinal injuries. Spine. 1983;8(8):817–31. https://doi.org/10.1097/00007632-198311000-00003.
18. Vaccaro AR, Lehman RA, Hurlbert RJ, et al. A new classification of thoracolumbar injuries: the importance of injury morphology, the integrity of the posterior ligamentous complex, and neurologic status. Spine. 2005;30(20):2325–33. https://doi.org/10.1097/01.brs.0000182986.43345.cb.
19. Vaccaro AR, Hulbert RJ, Patel AA, et al. The subaxial cervical spine injury classification system: a novel approach to recognize the importance of morphology, neurology, and integrity of the disco-ligamentous complex. Spine. 2007;32(21):2365–74. https://doi.org/10.1097/BRS.0b013e3181557b92.
20. Taneichi H, Kaneda K, Takeda N, Abumi K, Satoh S. Risk factors and probability of vertebral body collapse in metastases of the thoracic and lumbar spine. Spine. 1997;22(3):239–45. https://doi.org/10.1097/00007632-199702010-00002.
21. Turner JA, Ersek M, Herron L, Deyo R. Surgery for lumbar spinal stenosis. Attempted meta-analysis of the literature. Spine. 1992;17(1):1–8. https://doi.org/10.1097/00007632-199201000-00001.
22. Katz JN, Lipson SJ, Lew RA, et al. Lumbar laminectomy alone or with instrumented or noninstrumented arthrodesis in degenerative lumbar spinal stenosis. Patient selection, costs, and surgical outcomes. Spine. 1997;22(10):1123–31. https://doi.org/10.1097/00007632-199705150-00012.
23. Voulgaris S, Alexiou GA, Mihos E, et al. Posterior approach to ventrally located spinal meningiomas. Eur Spine J. 2010;19(7):1195–9. https://doi.org/10.1007/s00586-010-1295-z.
24. Steck JC, Dietze DD, Fessler RG. Posterolateral approach to intradural extramedullary thoracic tumors. J Neurosurg. 1994;81(2):202–5. https://doi.org/10.3171/jns.1994.81.2.0202.
25. St Clair SF, McLain RF. Posterolateral spinal cord decompression in patients with metastasis: an

endoscopic assisted approach. Surg Technol Int. 2006;15:257–63.
26. Chiu Y-C, Yang S-C, Kao Y-H, Tu Y-K. Single posterior approach for circumferential decompression and anterior reconstruction using cervical trabecular metal mesh cage in patients with metastatic spinal tumour. World J Surg Oncol. 2015;13:256. https://doi.org/10.1186/s12957-015-0685-4.
27. Lau D, Chou D. Posterior thoracic corpectomy with cage reconstruction for metastatic spinal tumors: comparing the mini-open approach to the open approach. J Neurosurg Spine. 2015;23(2):217–27. https://doi.org/10.3171/2014.12.SPINE14543.
28. Zeng H, Shen X, Luo C, et al. Comparison of three surgical approaches for cervicothoracic spinal tuberculosis: a retrospective case–control study. J Orthop Surg. 2015;10:100. https://doi.org/10.1186/s13018-015-0238-0.
29. Chang B-S, Jung J-H, Park S-M, Lee SH, Lee C-K, Kim H. Structural femoral shaft allografts for anterior spinal column reconstruction in osteoporotic spines. Biomed Res Int. 2016;2016:8681957. https://doi.org/10.1155/2016/8681957.
30. Harrington KD. Anterior cord decompression and spinal stabilization for patients with metastatic lesions of the spine. J Neurosurg. 1984;61(1):107–17. https://doi.org/10.3171/jns.1984.61.1.0107.
31. Cooper PR, Errico TJ, Martin R, Crawford B, DiBartolo T. A systematic approach to spinal reconstruction after anterior decompression for neoplastic disease of the thoracic and lumbar spine. Neurosurgery. 1993;32(1):1–8. https://doi.org/10.1227/00006123-199301000-00001.
32. Yao KC, Boriani S, Gokaslan ZL, Sundaresan N. En bloc spondylectomy for spinal metastases: a review of techniques. Neurosurg Focus. 2003;15(5):E6. https://doi.org/10.3171/foc.2003.15.5.6.
33. Kim K, Miller D, de Gonzalez A, et al. Occupational radiation doses to operators performing fluoroscopically-guided procedures. Health Phys. 2012;103(1):80–99. https://doi.org/10.1097/HP.0b013e31824dae76.
34. Luzzati AD, Shah S, Gagliano F, Perrucchini G, Scotto G, Alloisio M. Multilevel en bloc spondylectomy for tumors of the thoracic and lumbar spine is challenging but rewarding. Clin Orthop. 2015;473(3):858–67. https://doi.org/10.1007/s11999-014-3578-x.
35. Amendola L, Cappuccio M, De Iure F, Bandiera S, Gasbarrini A, Boriani S. En bloc resections for primary spinal tumors in 20 years of experience: effectiveness and safety. Spine J Off J North Am Spine Soc. 2014;14(11):2608–17. https://doi.org/10.1016/j.spinee.2014.02.030.
36. Huang W, Wei H, Cai W, et al. Total en bloc spondylectomy for solitary metastatic tumors of the fourth lumbar spine in a posterior-only approach. World Neurosurg. 2018;120:e8–e16. https://doi.org/10.1016/j.wneu.2018.06.251.
37. Jones M, Holton J, Hughes S, Czyz M. Total en bloc spondylectomy. J Spine Surg. 2018;4(3):663–5. https://doi.org/10.21037/jss.2018.06.12.
38. Shimizu T, Murakami H, Demura S, et al. Total en bloc spondylectomy for primary tumors of the lumbar spine. Medicine (Baltimore). 2018;97(37):e12366. https://doi.org/10.1097/MD.0000000000012366.
39. Zaidi HA, Awad A-W, Dickman CA. Complete spondylectomy using orthogonal spinal fixation and combined anterior and posterior approaches for thoracolumbar spinal reconstruction: technical nuances and clinical results. Clin Spine Surg. 2017;30(4):E466–74. https://doi.org/10.1097/BSD.0000000000000292.
40. Sciubba DM, De la Garza RR, Goodwin CR, et al. Total en bloc spondylectomy for locally aggressive and primary malignant tumors of the lumbar spine. Eur Spine J Off Publ Eur Spine Soc Eur Spinal Deform Soc Eur Sect Cerv Spine Res Soc. 2016;25(12):4080–7. https://doi.org/10.1007/s00586-016-4641-y.
41. Tomita K, Kawahara N, Murakami H, Demura S. Total en bloc spondylectomy for spinal tumors: improvement of the technique and its associated basic background. J Orthop Sci. 2006;11(1):3–12. https://doi.org/10.1007/s00776-005-0964-y.
42. Zoccali C, Scotto G, Cannavò L, Baldi J, Scaffidi-Argentina U, Luzzati A. En bloc spondylectomy in patients older than 60 years: indications, results and complications in a series of 37 patients. Eur Spine J. 2019;28(6):1512–9. https://doi.org/10.1007/s00586-019-05970-x.
43. Neves RPM, Oliveira VC, Costa LMD, et al. Major complications following total en bloc spondylectomy for giant-cell tumor. J Surg Case Rep. 2014;2014(1):rjt131. https://doi.org/10.1093/jscr/rjt131.
44. Zeng H, Zhang P, Shen X, et al. One-stage posterior-only approach in surgical treatment of single-segment thoracic spinal tuberculosis with neurological deficits in adults: a retrospective study of 34 cases. BMC Musculoskelet Disord. 2015;16:186. https://doi.org/10.1186/s12891-015-0640-0.
45. Huang L, Chen K, Ye J, et al. Modified total en bloc spondylectomy for thoracolumbar spinal tumors via a single posterior approach. Eur Spine J. 2013;22(3):556–64. https://doi.org/10.1007/s00586-012-2460-3.
46. Yokogawa N, Murakami H, Demura S, et al. Perioperative complications of total en bloc spondylectomy: adverse effects of preoperative irradiation. PLoS One. 2014;9(6):e98797. https://doi.org/10.1371/journal.pone.0098797.
47. Han X, Zhu Y, Cui C, Wu Y. A meta-analysis of circumferential fusion versus instrumented posterolateral fusion in the lumbar spine. Centre for Reviews and Dissemination (UK); 2009. https://www.ncbi.nlm.nih.gov/books/NBK78128/. Accessed 9 Feb 2020.

48. Cho JH, Ha J-K, Hwang CJ, Lee D-H, Lee CS. Patterns of treatment for metastatic pathological fractures of the spine: the efficacy of each treatment modality. Clin Orthop Surg. 2015;7(4):476–82. https://doi.org/10.4055/cios.2015.7.4.476.
49. Epstein NE. Spine surgery in geriatric patients: sometimes unnecessary, too much, or too little. Surg Neurol Int. 2011;2:188. https://doi.org/10.4103/2152-7806.91408.
50. Cloyd JM, Acosta FL, Cloyd C, Ames CP. Effects of age on perioperative complications of extensive multilevel thoracolumbar spinal fusion surgery: clinical article. J Neurosurg Spine. 2010;12(4):402–8. https://doi.org/10.3171/2009.10.SPINE08741.
51. POORMAN GW, MOON JY, WANG C, et al. Rates of mortality in lumbar spine surgery and factors associated with its occurrence over a 10-year period: a study of 803,949 patients in the nationwide inpatient sample. Int J Spine Surg. 2018;12(5):617–23. https://doi.org/10.14444/5076.
52. Chen X, Mao G, Leng SX. Frailty syndrome: an overview. Clin Interv Aging. 2014;9:433–41. https://doi.org/10.2147/CIA.S45300.
53. Ethun CG, Bilen MA, Jani AB, Maithel SK, Ogan K, Master VA. Frailty and cancer: implications for oncology surgery, medical oncology, and radiation oncology. CA Cancer J Clin. 2017;67(5):362–77. https://doi.org/10.3322/caac.21406.
54. Moskven E, Bourassa-Moreau É, Charest-Morin R, Flexman A, Street J. The impact of frailty and sarcopenia on postoperative outcomes in adult spine surgery. A systematic review of the literature. Spine J Off J North Am Spine Soc. 2018;18(12):2354–69. https://doi.org/10.1016/j.spinee.2018.07.008.
55. De la Garza RR, Goodwin CR, Jain A, et al. Development of a metastatic spinal tumor frailty index (MSTFI) using a nationwide database and its association with inpatient morbidity, mortality, and length of stay after spine surgery. World Neurosurg. 2016;95:548–555.e4. https://doi.org/10.1016/j.wneu.2016.08.029.
56. Park SB, Chung CK. Strategies of spinal fusion on osteoporotic spine. J Korean Neurosurg Soc. 2011;49(6):317–22. https://doi.org/10.3340/jkns.2011.49.6.317.
57. Camacho PM, Petak SM, Binkley N, et al. American Association of Clinical Endocrinologists and American College of Endocrinology Clinical Practice Guidelines for the diagnosis and treatment of postmenopausal osteoporosis — 2016. Endocr Pract. 2016;22(Supplement 4):1–42. https://doi.org/10.4158/EP161435.GL.
58. Final recommendation statement: osteoporosis to prevent fractures: screeningâ US Preventive Services Task Force. https://www.uspreventiveservicestaskforce.org/Page/Document/RecommendationStatementFinal/osteoporosis-screening1. Accessed 9 Feb 2020.
59. Kanis JA, Johnell O, Oden A, Johansson H, McCloskey E. FRAX and the assessment of fracture probability in men and women from the UK. Osteoporos Int J Establ Result Coop Eur Found Osteoporos Natl Osteoporos Found USA. 2008;19(4):385–97. https://doi.org/10.1007/s00198-007-0543-5.
60. Kim D, Menger RP. Spine sagittal balance. In: StatPearls. Treasure Island (FL): StatPearls Publishing; 2020. http://www.ncbi.nlm.nih.gov/books/NBK534858/. Accessed 9 Feb 2020.
61. Roussouly P, Nnadi C. Sagittal plane deformity: an overview of interpretation and management. Eur Spine J. 2010;19(11):1824–36. https://doi.org/10.1007/s00586-010-1476-9.
62. Makhni MC, Shillingford JN, Laratta JL, Hyun S-J, Kim YJ. Restoration of sagittal balance in spinal deformity surgery. J Korean Neurosurg Soc. 2018;61(2):167–79. https://doi.org/10.3340/jkns.2017.0404.013.
63. Kim T-K, Cho W, Youn SM, Chang U-K. The effect of perioperative radiation therapy on spinal bone fusion following spine tumor surgery. J Korean Neurosurg Soc. 2016;59(6):597–603. https://doi.org/10.3340/jkns.2016.59.6.597.
64. Heidecke V, Rainov NG, Burkert W. Results and outcome of neurosurgical treatment for extradural metastases in the cervical spine. Acta Neurochir. 2003;145(10):873–80; discussion 880-881. https://doi.org/10.1007/s00701-003-0107-1.
65. Wound healing after radiation therapy: review of the literature | Radiation Oncology | Full Text. https://ro-journal.biomedcentral.com/articles/10.1186/1748-717X-7-162. Accessed 9 Feb 2020.
66. Wallace HA, Basehore BM, Zito PM. Wound healing phases. In: StatPearls. Treasure Island (FL): StatPearls Publishing; 2020. http://www.ncbi.nlm.nih.gov/books/NBK470443/. Accessed 9 Feb 2020.
67. Payne WG, Naidu DK, Wheeler CK, et al. Wound healing in patients with cancer. Eplasty. 2008;8:e9.
68. Bray FN, Simmons BJ, Wolfson AH, Nouri K. Acute and chronic cutaneous reactions to ionizing radiation therapy. Dermatol Ther. 2016;6(2):185–206. https://doi.org/10.1007/s13555-016-0120-y.
69. Ryan JL. Ionizing radiation: the good, the bad, and the ugly. J Invest Dermatol. 2012;132(3 Pt 2):985–93. https://doi.org/10.1038/jid.2011.411.
70. Park H-Y, Lee S-H, Park S-J, Kim E S, Lee C-S, Eoh W. Surgical management with radiation therapy for metastatic spinal tumors located on cervicothoracic junction: a single center study. J Korean Neurosurg Soc. 2015;57(1):42–9. https://doi.org/10.3340/jkns.2015.57.1.42.
71. Gupta A, Kukkar N, Sharif K, Main BJ, Albers CE, El-Amin SF III. Bone graft substitutes for spine fusion: a brief review. World J Orthop. 2015;6(6):449–56. https://doi.org/10.5312/wjo.v6.i6.449.
72. Vaz K, Verma K, Protopsaltis T, Schwab F, Lonner B, Errico T. Bone grafting options for lumbar spine surgery: a review examining clinical efficacy and

complications. SAS J. 2010;4(3):75–86. https://doi.org/10.1016/j.esas.2010.01.004.
73. Polo-Corrales L, Latorre-Esteves M, Ramirez-Vick JE. Scaffold design for bone regeneration. J Nanosci Nanotechnol. 2014;14(1):15–56.
74. Roberts TT, Rosenbaum AJ. Bone grafts, bone substitutes and orthobiologics. Organogenesis. 2012;8(4):114–24. https://doi.org/10.4161/org.23306.
75. Morcuende JA, Gomez P, Stack J, et al. Effect of chemotherapy on segmental bone healing enhanced by rhBMP-2. Iowa Orthop J. 2004;24:36–42.
76. Baskar R, Lee KA, Yeo R, Yeoh K-W. Cancer and radiation therapy: current advances and future directions. Int J Med Sci. 2012;9(3):193–9. https://doi.org/10.7150/ijms.3635.
77. Liang T, Wan Y, Zou X, Peng X, Liu S. Is surgery for spine metastasis reasonable in patients older than 60 years? Clin Orthop. 2013;471(2):628–39. https://doi.org/10.1007/s11999-012-2699-3.
78. Kaliberov SA, Buchsbaum DJ. Chapter Sevenâ "Cancer treatment with gene therapy and radiation therapy". In: Curiel DT, Fisher PB, editors. Advances in cancer research. Vol 115. Applications of viruses for cancer therapy. Academic Press; 2012. p. 221–63. https://doi.org/10.1016/B978-0-12-398342-8.00007-0.
79. Alemdaroğlu KB, Atlıhan D, Çimen O, Kılınç CY, İltar S. Morphometric effects of acute shortening of the spine: the kinking and the sliding of the cord, response of the spinal nerves. Eur Spine J. 2007;16(9):1451–7. https://doi.org/10.1007/s00586-007-0325-y.
80. Moon M-S, Lee B-J, Kim S-S. Spinal deformity. Indian J Orthop. 2010;44(2):123. https://doi.org/10.4103/0019-5413.61725.
81. Kawahara N, Tomita K, Baba H, Kobayashi T, Fujita T, Murakami H. Closing-opening wedge osteotomy to correct angular kyphotic deformity by a single posterior approach. Spine. 2001;26(4):391–402. https://doi.org/10.1097/00007632-200102150-00016.
82. Kawahara N, Tomita K, Kobayashi T, Abdel-Wanis ME, Murakami H, Akamaru T. Influence of acute shortening on the spinal cord: an experimental study. Spine. 2005;30(6):613–20. https://doi.org/10.1097/01.brs.0000155407.87439.a2.
83. Kamel I, Barnette R. Positioning patients for spine surgery: avoiding uncommon position-related complications. World J Orthop. 2014;5(4):425–43. https://doi.org/10.5312/wjo.v5.i4.425.
84. Stecker MM. A review of intraoperative monitoring for spinal surgery. Surg Neurol Int. 2012;3(Suppl 3):S174–87. https://doi.org/10.4103/2152-7806.98579.
85. Ibrahim T, Mrowczynski O, Zalatimo O, et al. The impact of neurophysiological intraoperative monitoring during spinal cord and spine surgery: a critical analysis of 121 cases. Cureus. 2017;9(11):e1861. https://doi.org/10.7759/cureus.1861.
86. Hadley MN, Shank CD, Rozzelle CJ, Walters BC. Guidelines for the use of electrophysiological monitoring for surgery of the human spinal column and spinal cord. Neurosurgery. 2017;81(5):713–32. https://doi.org/10.1093/neuros/nyx466.
87. Lyaker MR, Tulman DB, Dimitrova GT, Pin RH, Papadimos TJ. Arterial embolism. Int J Crit Illn Inj Sci. 2013;3(1):77. https://doi.org/10.4103/2229-5151.109429.
88. Patsalides A, Leng LZ, Kimball D, et al. Preoperative catheter spinal angiography and embolization of cervical spinal tumors: outcomes from a single center. Interv Neuroradiol. 2016;22(4):457–65. https://doi.org/10.1177/1591019916637360.
89. Hu SS. Blood loss in adult spinal surgery. Eur Spine J. 2004;13(Suppl 1):S3–5. https://doi.org/10.1007/s00586-004-0753-x.
90. Irita K. Risk and crisis management in intraoperative hemorrhage: human factors in hemorrhagic critical events. Korean J Anesthesiol. 2011;60(3):151–60. https://doi.org/10.4097/kjae.2011.60.3.151.
91. Casualties I of M (US) C on FR for C, Pope A, French G, Longnecker DE. Pathophysiology of Acute Hemorrhagic Shock. National Academies Press (US); 1999. https://www.ncbi.nlm.nih.gov/books/NBK224592/. Accessed 10 Feb 2020.
92. Gupta RK, Fahim M. Regulation of cardiovascular functions during acute blood loss. Indian J Physiol Pharmacol. 2005;49(2):213–9.
93. Kobayashi K, Ozkan E, Tam A, Ensor J, Wallace MJ, Gupta S. Preoperative embolization of spinal tumors: variables affecting intraoperative blood loss after embolization. Acta Radiol Stockh Swed 1987. 2012;53(8):935–42. https://doi.org/10.1258/ar.2012.120314.
94. Awad A-W, Almefty KK, Ducruet AF, et al. The efficacy and risks of preoperative embolization of spinal tumors. J Neurointerv Surg. 2016;8(8):859–64. https://doi.org/10.1136/neurintsurg-2015-011833.
95. Wilson MA, Cooke DL, Ghodke B, Mirza SK. Retrospective analysis of preoperative embolization of spinal tumors. Am J Neuroradiol. 2010;31(4):656–60. https://doi.org/10.3174/ajnr.A1899.
96. Griessenauer CJ, Salem M, Hendrix P, Foreman PM, Ogilvy CS, Thomas AJ. Preoperative embolization of spinal tumors: a systematic review and meta-analysis. World Neurosurg. 2016;87:362–71. https://doi.org/10.1016/j.wneu.2015.11.064.
97. Shi HB, Suh DC, Lee HK, et al. Preoperative transarterial embolization of spinal tumor: embolization techniques and results. AJNR Am J Neuroradiol. 1999;20(10):2009–15.
98. Nair S, Gobin YP, Leng LZ, et al. Preoperative embolization of hypervascular thoracic, lumbar, and sacral spinal column tumors: technique and outcomes from a single center. Interv Neuroradiol. 2013;19(3):377–85.
99. Hong CG, Cho JH, Suh DC, Hwang CJ, Lee D-H, Lee CS. Preoperative embolization in patients with

metastatic spinal cord compression: mandatory or optional? World J Surg Oncol. 2017;15(1):45. https://doi.org/10.1186/s12957-017-1118-3.
100. Berkefeld J, Scale D, Kirchner J, Heinrich T, Kollath J. Hypervascular spinal tumors: influence of the embolization technique on perioperative hemorrhage. Am J Neuroradiol. 1999;20(5):757–63.
101. Breslau J, Eskridge JM. Preoperative embolization of spinal tumors. J Vasc Interv Radiol JVIR. 1995;6(6):871–5. https://doi.org/10.1016/s1051-0443(95)71205-2.
102. Prince EA, Ahn SH. Interventional management of vertebral body metastases. Semin Interv Radiol. 2013;30(3):278–81. https://doi.org/10.1055/s-0033-1353480.
103. Barak M, Yoav L, Abu el-Naaj I. Hypotensive anesthesia versus normotensive anesthesia during major maxillofacial surgery: a review of the literature. ScientificWorldJournal. 2015;2015:480728. https://doi.org/10.1155/2015/480728.
104. Kiabi FH, Soleimani A, Habibi MR. Neuroprotective effect of low mean arterial pressure on postoperative cognitive deficit attenuated by prolonged coronary artery bypass time: a meta-analysis. Braz J Cardiovasc Surg. 2019;34(6):739–48. https://doi.org/10.21470/1678-9741-2018-0263.
105. Leone M, Asfar P, Radermacher P, Vincent J-L, Martin C. Optimizing mean arterial pressure in septic shock: a critical reappraisal of the literature. Crit Care. 2015;19(1):101. https://doi.org/10.1186/s13054-015-0794-z.
106. Martinowitz U, Saltz R. Fibrin sealant. Curr Opin Hematol. 1996;3(5):395–402. https://doi.org/10.1097/00062752-199603050-00011.
107. Hauser CJ. Hemostasis of solid viscus trauma by intraparenchymal injection of fibrin glue. Arch Surg Chic Ill 1960. 1989;124(3):291–3. https://doi.org/10.1001/archsurg.1989.01410030037006.
108. Chiara O, Cimbanassi S, Bellanova G, et al. A systematic review on the use of topical hemostats in trauma and emergency surgery. BMC Surg. 2018;18(1):68. https://doi.org/10.1186/s12893-018-0398-z.
109. Mankad PS, Codispoti M. The role of fibrin sealants in hemostasis. Am J Surg. 2001;182(2 Suppl):21S–8S. https://doi.org/10.1016/s0002-9610(01)00773-5.
110. Jackson MR. Fibrin sealants in surgical practice: an overview. Am J Surg. 2001;182(2 Suppl):1S–7S. https://doi.org/10.1016/s0002-9610(01)00770-x.
111. Tominaga H, Setoguchi T, Tanabe F, et al. Risk factors for venous thromboembolism after spine surgery. Medicine (Baltimore). 2015;94(5):e466. https://doi.org/10.1097/MD.0000000000000466.
112. Yang S-D, Liu H, Sun Y-P, et al. Prevalence and risk factors of deep vein thrombosis in patients after spine surgery: a retrospective case-cohort study. Sci Rep. 2015;5:11834. https://doi.org/10.1038/srep11834.
113. Al-Dujaili TM, Majer CN, Madhoun TE, Kassis SZ, Saleh AA. Deep venous thrombosis in spine surgery patients: incidence and hematoma formation. Int Surg. 2012;97(2):150–4. https://doi.org/10.9738/CC71.1.
114. Berger-Richardson D, Xu RS, Gladdy RA, McCart JA, Govindarajan A, Swallow CJ. Glove and instrument changing to prevent tumour seeding in cancer surgery: a survey of surgeons' beliefs and practices. Curr Oncol. 2018;25(3):e200–8. https://doi.org/10.3747/co.25.3924.
115. Moran B, Wynne B, Thomas S, Griffin M, McMenamin M, Ormond P. Malignant cytology in washings of mohs micrographic surgery instruments. Dermatol Surg. 2013;39(1pt1):133–5. https://doi.org/10.1111/j.1524-4725.2012.02517.x.
116. Lu Z, Wang J, Wientjes MG, Au JL-S. Intraperitoneal therapy for peritoneal cancer. Future Oncol Lond Engl. 2010;6(10):1625–41. https://doi.org/10.2217/fon.10.100.
117. Muraoka M, Oka T, Akamine S, et al. Modified intrapleural cisplatin treatment for lung cancer with positive pleural lavage cytology or malignant effusion. J Surg Oncol. 2006;93(4):323–9. https://doi.org/10.1002/jso.20470.
118. Kumar N, Zaw AS, Kantharajanna SB, Khoo BL, Lim CT, Thiery JP. Metastatic efficiency of tumour cells can be impaired by intraoperative cell salvage process: truth or conjecture? Transfus Med Oxf Engl. 2017;27(Suppl 5):327–34. https://doi.org/10.1111/tme.12453.
119. Kumar N, Zaw AS, Khoo BL, et al. Intraoperative cell salvage in metastatic spine tumour surgery reduces potential for reinfusion of viable cancer cells. Eur Spine J Off Publ Eur Spine Soc Eur Spinal Deform Soc Eur Sect Cerv Spine Res Soc. 2016;25(12):4008–15. https://doi.org/10.1007/s00586-016-4478-4.
120. Goubran HA, Elemary M, Radosevich M, Seghatchian J, El-Ekiaby M, Burnouf T. Impact of transfusion on cancer growth and outcome. Cancer Growth Metastasis. 2016;9:1–8. https://doi.org/10.4137/CGM.S32797.
121. Cata JP, Gottumukkala V. Blood transfusion practices in cancer surgery. Indian J Anaesth. 2014;58(5):637–42. https://doi.org/10.4103/0019-5049.144675.
122. Trudeau JD, Waters T, Chipperfield K. Should intraoperative cell-salvaged blood be used in patients with suspected or known malignancy? Can J Anesth Can Anesth. 2012;59(11):1058–70. https://doi.org/10.1007/s12630-012-9781-x.
123. Esper SA, Waters JH. Intra-operative cell salvage: a fresh look at the indications and contraindications. Blood Transfus. 2011;9(2):139–47. https://doi.org/10.2450/2011.0081-10.
124. Wu P-K, Chen C-F, Chen C-M, et al. Intraoperative extracorporeal irradiation and frozen treatment on tumor-bearing autografts show equivalent outcomes for biologic reconstruction. Clin Orthop. 2018;476(4):877–89. https://doi.org/10.1007/s11999.0000000000000022.
125. Sangsin A, Murakami H, Shimizu T, Kato S, Tsuchiya H. Four-year survival of a patient with

spinal metastatic acinic cell carcinoma after a total en bloc spondylectomy and reconstruction with a frozen tumor-bearing bone graft. Orthopedics. 2018;41(5):e727–30. https://doi.org/10.3928/01477447-20180613-05.
126. Igarashi K, Yamamoto N, Shirai T, et al. The long-term outcome following the use of frozen autograft treated with liquid nitrogen in the management of bone and soft-tissue sarcomas. Bone Joint J. 2014;96-B(4):555–61. https://doi.org/10.1302/0301-620X.96B4.32629.
127. Kakudo N, Kusumoto K, Wang YB, Iguchi Y, Ogawa Y. Immunolocalization of vascular endothelial growth factor on intramuscular ectopic osteoinduction by bone morphogenetic protein-2. Life Sci. 2006;79(19):1847–55. https://doi.org/10.1016/j.lfs.2006.06.033.
128. Knippenberg M, Helder MN, Zandieh Doulabi B, Wuisman PIJM, Klein-Nulend J. Osteogenesis versus chondrogenesis by BMP-2 and BMP-7 in adipose stem cells. Biochem Biophys Res Commun. 2006;342(3):902–8. https://doi.org/10.1016/j.bbrc.2006.02.052.
129. Taşlı PN, Aydın S, Yalvaç ME, Sahin F. Bmp 2 and bmp 7 induce odonto- and osteogenesis of human tooth germ stem cells. Appl Biochem Biotechnol. 2014;172(6):3016–25. https://doi.org/10.1007/s12010-013-0706-0.
130. Roldán JC, Detsch R, Schaefer S, et al. Bone formation and degradation of a highly porous biphasic calcium phosphate ceramic in presence of BMP-7, VEGF and mesenchymal stem cells in an ectopic mouse model. J Cranio Maxillo fac Surg Off Publ Eur Assoc Cranio Maxillo fac Surg. 2010;38(6):423–30. https://doi.org/10.1016/j.jcms.2010.01.003.
131. Hu K, Olsen BR. The roles of vascular endothelial growth factor in bone repair and regeneration. Bone. 2016;91:30–8. https://doi.org/10.1016/j.bone.2016.06.013.
132. Clarkin CE, Gerstenfeld LC. VEGF and bone cell signalling: an essential vessel for communication? Cell Biochem Funct. 2013;31(1):1–11. https://doi.org/10.1002/cbf.2911.
133. Yonezawa N, Murakami H, Sangsin A, Mizukoshi E, Tsuchiya H. Lung metastases regression with increased CD8+T lymphocyte infiltration following preoperative spinal embolization and total en bloc spondylectomy using tumor-bearing frozen autograft in a patient with spinal metastatic leiomyosarcoma. Eur Spine J Off Publ Eur Spine Soc Eur Spinal Deform Soc Eur Sect Cerv Spine Res Soc. 2019;28(Suppl 2):41–50. https://doi.org/10.1007/s00586-018-5831-6.
134. Takata M, Sugimoto N, Yamamoto N, et al. Activity of bone morphogenetic protein-7 after treatment at various temperatures: freezing vs. pasteurization vs. allograft. Cryobiology. 2011;63(3):235–9. https://doi.org/10.1016/j.cryobiol.2011.09.001.
135. Kurtz SM, Devine JN. PEEK biomaterials in trauma, orthopedic, and spinal implants. Biomaterials. 2007;28(32):4845–69. https://doi.org/10.1016/j.biomaterials.2007.07.013.
136. Brantigan JW, Neidre A, Toohey JS. The lumbar I/F cage for posterior lumbar interbody fusion with the variable screw placement system: 10-year results of a Food and Drug Administration clinical trial. Spine J. 2004;4(6):681–8. https://doi.org/10.1016/j.spinee.2004.05.253.
137. Gittens RA, Olivares-Navarrete R, Schwartz Z, Boyan BD. Implant osseointegration and the role of microroughness and nanostructures: lessons for spine implants. Acta Biomater. 2014;10(8):3363–71. https://doi.org/10.1016/j.actbio.2014.03.037.
138. Zou Q, Zhou Q, Liu L, Dai H. A highly hydrophilic and biodegradable novel Poly(amide-imide) for biomedical applications. Polymers. 2016;8(12):441. https://doi.org/10.3390/polym8120441.
139. Jockisch KA, Brown SA, Bauer TW, Merritt K. Biological response to chopped-carbon-fiber-reinforced peek. J Biomed Mater Res. 1992;26(2):133–46. https://doi.org/10.1002/jbm.820260202.
140. Ha S-W, Mayer J, Koch B, Wintermantel E. Plasma-sprayed hydroxylapatite coating on carbon fibre reinforced thermoplastic composite materials. J Mater Sci Mater Med. 1994;5(6):481–4. https://doi.org/10.1007/BF00058987.
141. Cook SD, Rust-Dawicki AM. Preliminary evaluation of titanium-coated PEEK dental implants. J Oral Implantol. 1995;21(3):176–81.
142. Cho D-Y, Lee W-Y, Sheu P-C, Chen C-C. Cage containing a biphasic calcium phosphate ceramic (Triosite) for the treatment of cervical spondylosis. Surg Neurol. 2005;63(6):497–503; discussion 503-504. https://doi.org/10.1016/j.surneu.2004.10.016.
143. Mastronardi L, Ducati A, Ferrante L. Anterior cervical fusion with polyetheretherketone (PEEK) cages in the treatment of degenerative disc disease. Preliminary observations in 36 consecutive cases with a minimum 12-month follow-up. Acta Neurochir. 2006;148(3):307–12; discussion 312. https://doi.org/10.1007/s00701-005-0657-5.
144. S-W HA, GISEP A, MAYER J, WINTERMANTEL E, GRUNER H, WIELAND M. Topographical characterization and microstructural interface analysis of vacuum-plasma-sprayed titanium and hydroxyapatite coatings on carbon fibre-reinforced poly(etheretherketone). J Mater Sci Mater Med. 1997;8(12):891–6. https://doi.org/10.1023/A:1018562023599.
145. Torstrick FB, Safranski DL, Burkus JK, et al. Getting PEEK to stick to bone: the development of porous PEEK for interbody fusion devices. Tech Orthop Rockv Md. 2017;32(3):158–66. https://doi.org/10.1097/BTO.0000000000000242.
146. Chen Y, Chen D, Guo Y, et al. Subsidence of titanium mesh cage: a study based on 300 cases. J Spinal Disord Tech. 2008;21(7):489–92. https://doi.org/10.1097/BSD.0b013e318158de22.

147. Li Z-J, Wang Y, Xu G-J, Tian P. Is PEEK cage better than titanium cage in anterior cervical discectomy and fusion surgery? A meta-analysis. BMC Musculoskelet Disord. 2016;17:379. https://doi.org/10.1186/s12891-016-1234-1.
148. Rousseau M-A, Lazennec JY, Saillant G. Circumferential arthrodesis using PEEK cages at the lumbar spine. J Spinal Disord Tech. 2007;20:278–81. https://doi.org/10.1097/01.bsd.0000211284.14143.63.
149. Seaman S, Kerezoudis P, Bydon M, Torner JC, Hitchon PW. Titanium vs. polyetheretherketone (PEEK) interbody fusion: meta-analysis and review of the literature. J Clin Neurosci Off J Neurosurg Soc Australas. 2017;44:23–9. https://doi.org/10.1016/j.jocn.2017.06.062.
150. Junaid M, Rashid MU, Bukhari SS, Ahmed M. Radiological and clinical outcomes in patients undergoing anterior cervical discectomy and fusion: comparing titanium and PEEK (polyetheretherketone) cages. Pak J Med Sci. 2018;34(6):1412–7. https://doi.org/10.12669/pjms.346.15833.
151. Cabraja M, Oezdemir S, Koeppen D, Kroppenstedt S. Anterior cervical discectomy and fusion: comparison of titanium and polyetheretherketone cages. BMC Musculoskelet Disord. 2012;13:172. https://doi.org/10.1186/1471-2474-13-172.
152. Barsa P, Suchomel P. Factors affecting sagittal malalignment due to cage subsidence in standalone cage assisted anterior cervical fusion. Eur Spine J. 2007;16(9):1395–400. https://doi.org/10.1007/s00586-006-0284-8.
153. Effects of cervical cages on load distribution of cancellous core: a finite element analysis. Abstractâ Europe PMC. https://europepmc.org/article/med/15167339. Accessed 9 Feb 2020.
154. Nasatzky E, Gultchin J, Schwartz Z. The role of surface roughness in promoting osteointegration. Refuat Ha-Peh Veha-Shinayim 1993. 2003;20(3):8–19, 98
155. Rizo-Gorrita M, Luna-Oliva I, Serrera-Figallo M-A, Torres-Lagares D. Superficial characteristics of titanium after treatment of chorreated surface, passive acid, and decontamination with argon plasma. J Funct Biomater. 2018;9(4):71. https://doi.org/10.3390/jfb9040071.
156. Gurzawska K, Svava R, Jørgensen NR, Gotfredsen K. Nanocoating of titanium implant surfaces with organic molecules. Polysaccharides including glycosaminoglycans. J Biomed Nanotechnol. 2012;8:1012–24. https://doi.org/10.1166/jbn.2012.1457.
157. Gurzawska K, Svava R, Yihua Y, et al. Osteoblastic response to pectin nanocoating on titanium surfaces. Mater Sci Eng C Mater Biol Appl. 2014;43:117–25. https://doi.org/10.1016/j.msec.2014.06.028.
158. de Jonge LT, Leeuwenburgh SCG, Wolke JGC, Jansen JA. Organic–inorganic surface modifications for titanium implant surfaces. Pharm Res. 2008;25(10):2357–69. https://doi.org/10.1007/s11095-008-9617-0.
159. Søballe K, Overgaard S. The current status of hydroxyapatite coating of prostheses. J Bone Joint Surg Br. 1996;78(5):689–91.
160. Rao PJ, Pelletier MH, Walsh WR, Mobbs RJ. Spine interbody implants: material selection and modification, functionalization and bioactivation of surfaces to improve osseointegration. Orthop Surg. 2014;6(2):81–9. https://doi.org/10.1111/os.12098.
161. McGilvray KC, Waldorff EI, Easley J, et al. Evaluation of a polyetheretherketone (PEEK) titanium composite interbody spacer in an ovine lumbar interbody fusion model: biomechanical, microcomputed tomographic, and histologic analyses. Spine J Off J North Am Spine Soc. 2017;17(12):1907–16. https://doi.org/10.1016/j.spinee.2017.06.034.
162. Li CS, Vannabouathong C, Sprague S, Bhandari M. The use of carbon-fiber-reinforced (CFR) PEEK material in orthopedic implants: a systematic review. Clin Med Insights Arthritis Musculoskelet Disord. 2015;8:33–45. https://doi.org/10.4137/CMAMD.S20354.
163. Tomé-Bermejo F, Piñera AR, Alvarez L. Osteoporosis and the management of spinal degenerative disease (II). Arch Bone Joint Surg. 2017;5(6):363–74.
164. Fernandes da Silva AL, Borba AM, Simão NR, FLM P, Borges AH, Miloro M. Customized polymethyl methacrylate implants for the reconstruction of craniofacial osseous defects. Case Rep Surg. 2014;2014:358569. https://doi.org/10.1155/2014/358569.
165. Vaishya R, Chauhan M, Vaish A. Bone cement. J Clin Orthop Trauma. 2013;4(4):157–63. https://doi.org/10.1016/j.jcot.2013.11.005.
166. Ruskin J, Caravaggi P, Beebe KS, et al. Steinmann pin augmentation versus locking plate constructs. J Orthop Traumatol Off J Ital Soc Orthop Traumatol. 2016;17(3):249–54. https://doi.org/10.1007/s10195-016-0394-y.
167. Bokov A, Bulkin A, Aleynik A, Kutlaeva M, Mlyavykh S. Pedicle screws loosening in patients with degenerative diseases of the lumbar spine: potential risk factors and relative contribution. Glob Spine J. 2019;9(1):55–61. https://doi.org/10.1177/2192568218772302.
168. Nakashima D, Ishii K, Nishiwaki Y, et al. Quantitative CT-based bone strength parameters for the prediction of novel spinal implant stability using resonance frequency analysis: a cadaveric study involving experimental micro-CT and clinical multislice CT. Eur Radiol Exp. 2019;3:1. https://doi.org/10.1186/s41747-018-0080-3.
169. Galbusera F, Volkheimer D, Reitmaier S, Berger-Roscher N, Kienle A, Wilke H-J. Pedicle screw loosening: a clinically relevant complication? Eur Spine J Off Publ Eur Spine Soc Eur Spinal Deform Soc Eur Sect Cerv Spine Res Soc. 2015;24(5):1005–16. https://doi.org/10.1007/s00586-015-3768-6.

170. Wu X, Shi J, Wu J, et al. Pedicle screw loosening: the value of radiological imagings and the identification of risk factors assessed by extraction torque during screw removal surgery. J Orthop Surg. 2019;14(1):6. https://doi.org/10.1186/s13018-018-1046-0.
171. Zhang B, Li S, Miao D, Zhao C, Wang L. Risk factors of cage subsidence in patients with ossification of posterior longitudinal ligament (OPLL) after anterior cervical discectomy and fusion. Med Sci Monit Int Med J Exp Clin Res. 2018;24:4753–9. https://doi.org/10.12659/MSM.910964.
172. Tsuzuki S, Park SH, Eber MR, Peters CM, Shiozawa Y. Skeletal complications in cancer patients with bone metastases. Int J Urol Off J Jpn Urol Assoc. 2016;23(10):825–32. https://doi.org/10.1111/iju.13170.
173. Rao PJ, Phan K, Giang G, Maharaj MM, Phan S, Mobbs RJ. Subsidence following anterior lumbar interbody fusion (ALIF): a prospective study. J Spine Surg Hong Kong. 2017;3(2):168–75. https://doi.org/10.21037/jss.2017.05.03.
174. Swan J, Hurwitz E, Malek F, et al. Surgical treatment for unstable low-grade isthmic spondylolisthesis in adults: a prospective controlled study of posterior instrumented fusion compared with combined anterior-posterior fusion. Spine J Off J North Am Spine Soc. 2006;6(6):606–14. https://doi.org/10.1016/j.spinee.2006.02.032.
175. Lequin MB, Verbaan D, Bouma GJ. Posterior lumbar interbody fusion with stand-alone trabecular metal cages for repeatedly recurrent lumbar disc herniation and back pain. J Neurosurg Spine. 2014;20(6):617–22. https://doi.org/10.3171/2014.2.SPINE13548.
176. Tokuhashi Y, Ajiro Y, Umezawa N. Subsidence of metal interbody cage after posterior lumbar interbody fusion with pedicle screw fixation. Orthopedics. 2009;32(4).
177. Cho JH, Hwang CJ, Kim H, Joo Y-S, Lee D-H, Lee CS. Effect of osteoporosis on the clinical and radiological outcomes following one-level posterior lumbar interbody fusion. J Orthop Sci Off J Jpn Orthop Assoc. 2018;23(6):870–7. https://doi.org/10.1016/j.jos.2018.06.009.
178. Tedesco G, Gasbarrini A, Bandiera S, Ghermandi R, Boriani S. Composite PEEK/carbon fiber implants can increase the effectiveness of radiotherapy in the management of spine tumors. J Spine Surg Hong Kong. 2017;3(3):323–9. https://doi.org/10.21037/jss.2017.06.20.
179. Laux CJ, Hodel SM, Farshad M, Müller DA. Carbon fibre/polyether ether ketone (CF/PEEK) implants in orthopaedic oncology. World J Surg Oncol. 2018;16(1):241. https://doi.org/10.1186/s12957-018-1545-9.
180. Niu C-C, Liao J-C, Chen W-J, Chen L-H. Outcomes of interbody fusion cages used in 1 and 2-levels anterior cervical discectomy and fusion: titanium cages versus polyetheretherketone (PEEK) cages. J Spinal Disord Tech. 2010;23(5):310–6. https://doi.org/10.1097/BSD.0b013e3181af3a84.
181. Nguyen N-LM, Kong CY, Hart RA. Proximal junctional kyphosis and failure-diagnosis, prevention, and treatment. Curr Rev Musculoskelet Med. 2016;9(3):299–308. https://doi.org/10.1007/s12178-016-9353-8.
182. Hyun S-J, Lee BH, Park J-H, Kim K-J, Jahng T-A, Kim H-J. Proximal junctional kyphosis and proximal junctional failure following adult spinal deformity surgery. Korean J Spine. 2017;14(4):126–32. https://doi.org/10.14245/kjs.2017.14.4.126.
183. O'Leary PT, Bridwell KH, Lenke LG, et al. Risk factors and outcomes for catastrophic failures at the top of long pedicle screw constructs: a matched cohort analysis performed at a single center. Spine. 2009;34(20):2134–9. https://doi.org/10.1097/BRS.0b013e3181b2e17e.
184. Watanabe K, Lenke LG, Bridwell KH, Kim YJ, Koester L, Hensley M. Proximal junctional vertebral fracture in adults after spinal deformity surgery using pedicle screw constructs: analysis of morphological features. Spine. 2010;35(2):138–45. https://doi.org/10.1097/BRS.0b013e3181c8f35d.
185. Hostin R, McCarthy I, O'Brien M, et al. Incidence, mode, and location of acute proximal junctional failures after surgical treatment of adult spinal deformity. Spine. 2013;38(12):1008–15. https://doi.org/10.1097/BRS.0b013e318271319c.
186. Grob D, Daehn S, Mannion AF. Titanium mesh cages (TMC) in spine surgery. Eur Spine J. 2005;14(3):211–21. https://doi.org/10.1007/s00586-004-0748-7.
187. Raisian S, Fallahi HR, Khiabani KS, Heidarizadeh M, Azdoo S. Customized titanium mesh based on the 3D printed model vs. manual intraoperative bending of titanium mesh for reconstructing of orbital bone fracture: a randomized clinical trial. Rev Recent Clin Trials. 2017;12(3):154–8. https://doi.org/10.2174/1574887112666170821165206.
188. Jeyaraj P. Efficacy and versatility of the 3-D titanium mesh implant in the closure of large post-craniectomy osseous defects, and its therapeutic role in reversing the syndrome of the trephined: clinical study of a case series and review of literature. J Maxillofac Oral Surg. 2016;15(1):82–92. https://doi.org/10.1007/s12663-015-0807-0.
189. Lu T, Liang H, Liu C, et al. Effects of titanium mesh cage end structures on the compressive load at the endplate interface: a cadaveric biomechanical study. Med Sci Monit Int Med J Exp Clin Res. 2017;23:2863–70. https://doi.org/10.12659/MSM.905466.
190. Früh HJ, Liebetrau A, Bertagnoli R. Fusion implants of carbon fiber reinforced plastic. Orthopade. 2002;31(5):454–8. https://doi.org/10.1007/s00132-001-0295-4.
191. Sardar Z, Jarzem P. Failure of a carbon fiber–reinforced polymer implant used for transforaminal lumbar interbody fusion. Glob Spine J. 2013;3(4):253–6. https://doi.org/10.1055/s-0033-1343075.

192. Stratton-Powell AA, Pasko KM, Brockett CL, Tipper JL. The biologic response to polyetheretherketone (PEEK) wear particles in total joint replacement: a systematic review. Clin Orthop. 2016;474(11):2394–404. https://doi.org/10.1007/s11999-016-4976-z.
193. Han X, Yang D, Yang C, et al. Carbon fiber reinforced PEEK composites based on 3D-printing technology for orthopedic and dental applications. J Clin Med. 2019;8(2):240. https://doi.org/10.3390/jcm8020240.
194. Heary RF, Kheterpal A, Mammis A, Kumar S. Stackable carbon fiber cages for thoracolumbar interbody fusion after corpectomy: long-term outcome analysis. Neurosurgery. 2011;68(3):810–8; discussion 818-819. https://doi.org/10.1227/NEU.0b013e3182077a9f.
195. Ringel F, Ryang Y-M, Kirschke JS, et al. Radiolucent carbon fiber-reinforced pedicle screws for treatment of spinal tumors: advantages for radiation planning and follow-up imaging. World Neurosurg. 2017;105:294–301. https://doi.org/10.1016/j.wneu.2017.04.091.
196. Nevelsky A, Borzov E, Daniel S, Bar-Deroma R. Perturbation effects of the carbon fiber-PEEK screws on radiotherapy dose distribution. J Appl Clin Med Phys. 2017;18(2):62–8. https://doi.org/10.1002/acm2.12046.
197. Eleraky M, Papanastassiou I, Tran ND, Dakwar E, Vrionis FD. Comparison of polymethylmethacrylate versus expandable cage in anterior vertebral column reconstruction after posterior extracavitary corpectomy in lumbar and thoraco-lumbar metastatic spine tumors. Eur Spine J Off Publ Eur Spine Soc Eur Spinal Deform Soc Eur Sect Cerv Spine Res Soc. 2011;20(8):1363–70. https://doi.org/10.1007/s00586-011-1738-1.
198. Jeyamohan S, Vaccaro A, Harrop J. Use of expandable cages in metastasis to the spine. JHN J. 2009;4(4). https://doi.org/10.29046/JHNJ.004.4.002.
199. Omeis I, Bekelis K, Gregory A, et al. The use of expandable cages in patients undergoing multilevel corpectomies for metastatic tumors in the cervical spine. Orthopedics. 2010;33(2):87–92. https://doi.org/10.3928/01477447-20100104-12.
200. Viswanathan A, Abd-El-Barr MM, Doppenberg E, et al. Initial experience with the use of an expandable titanium cage as a vertebral body replacement in patients with tumors of the spinal column: a report of 95 patients. Eur Spine J Off Publ Eur Spine Soc Eur Spinal Deform Soc Eur Sect Cerv Spine Res Soc. 2012;21(1):84–92. https://doi.org/10.1007/s00586-011-1882-7.
201. Shen FH, Marks I, Shaffrey C, Ouellet J, Arlet V. The use of an expandable cage for corpectomy reconstruction of vertebral body tumors through a posterior extracavitary approach: a multicenter consecutive case series of prospectively followed patients. Spine J. 2008;8(2):329–39. https://doi.org/10.1016/j.spinee.2007.05.002.
202. Crocker M, James G, Ibrahim A, Thomas N, Chitnavis B. Posterior approach vertebrectomy in the thoracolumbar spine with expandable cage reconstruction: indications and techniques based on eight cases. Br J Neurosurg. 2008;22(2):235–40. https://doi.org/10.1080/02688690701837273.
203. Morales Alba NA. Posterior placement of an expandable cage for lumbar vertebral body replacement in oncologic surgery by posterior simple approach: technical note. Spine. 2008;33(23):E901–5. https://doi.org/10.1097/BRS.0b013e31818b8a06.
204. Mica MC, Voronov LI, Carandang G, Havey RM, Wojewnik B, Patwardhan AG. Biomechanics of an expandable lumbar interbody fusion cage deployed through transforaminal approach. Int J Spine Surg. 2017;11(4):24. https://doi.org/10.14444/4024.
205. Liu X, Paulsen A, Giambini H, et al. A new vertebral body replacement strategy using expandable polymeric cages. Tissue Eng Part A. 2017;23(5–6):223–32. https://doi.org/10.1089/ten.TEA.2016.0246.
206. Colman MW, Guss A, Bachus KN, Spiker WR, Lawrence BD, Brodke DS. Fixed-angle, posteriorly connected anterior cage reconstruction improves stiffness and decreases cancellous subsidence in a spondylectomy model. Spine. 2016;41(9):E519–23. https://doi.org/10.1097/BRS.0000000000001312.
207. Kaneda K, Shono Y, Satoh S, Abumi K. New anterior instrumentation for the management of thoracolumbar and lumbar scoliosis. Application of the Kaneda two-rod system. Spine. 1996;21(10):1250–61; discussion 1261-1262. https://doi.org/10.1097/00007632-199605150-00021.
208. Honigmann P, Sharma N, Okolo B, Popp U, Msallem B, Thieringer FM. Patient-specific surgical implants made of 3D printed PEEK: material, technology, and scope of surgical application. Biomed Res Int. 2018;2018:4520636. https://doi.org/10.1155/2018/4520636.
209. Di Prima M, Coburn J, Hwang D, Kelly J, Khairuzzaman A, Ricles L. Additively manufactured medical products – the FDA perspective. 3D Print Med. 2016;2:1. https://doi.org/10.1186/s41205-016-0005-9.
210. Abdullah KA, Reed W. 3D printing in medical imaging and healthcare services. J Med Radiat Sci. 2018;65(3):237–9. https://doi.org/10.1002/jmrs.292.
211. Fernandez de Grado G, Keller L, Idoux-Gillet Y, et al. Bone substitutes: a review of their characteristics, clinical use, and perspectives for large bone defects management. J Tissue Eng. 2018;9:2041731418776819. https://doi.org/10.1177/2041731418776819.
212. Greene AC, Hsu WK. Orthobiologics in minimally invasive lumbar fusion. J Spine Surg. 2019;5(Suppl 1):S11–8. https://doi.org/10.21037/jss.2019.04.15.
213. Wang W, Yeung KWK. Bone grafts and biomaterials substitutes for bone defect repair: a review. Bioact Mater. 2017;2(4):224–47. https://doi.org/10.1016/j.bioactmat.2017.05.007.

214. Albrektsson T, Johansson C. Osteoinduction, osteoconduction and osseointegration. Eur Spine J Off Publ Eur Spine Soc Eur Spinal Deform Soc Eur Sect Cerv Spine Res Soc. 2001;10(Suppl 2):S96–101. https://doi.org/10.1007/s005860100282.
215. Campana V, Milano G, Pagano E, et al. Bone substitutes in orthopaedic surgery: from basic science to clinical practice. J Mater Sci Mater Med. 2014;25(10):2445–61. https://doi.org/10.1007/s10856-014-5240-2.
216. Lopez GD, Hijji FY, Narain AS, Yom KH, Singh K. Iliac crest bone graft: a minimally invasive harvesting technique. Clin Spine Surg. 2017;30(10):439–41. https://doi.org/10.1097/BSD.0000000000000556.
217. Myeroff C, Archdeacon M. Autogenous bone graft: donor sites and techniques. J Bone Joint Surg Am. 2011;93(23):2227–36. https://doi.org/10.2106/JBJS.J.01513.
218. Babbi L, Barbanti-Brodano G, Gasbarrini A, Boriani S. Iliac crest bone graftâ: a 23-years hystory of infection at donor site in vertebral arthrodesis and a review of current bone substitutes. Eur Rev Med Pharmacol Sci. 2016;20(22):4670–6.
219. Carlock KD, Hildebrandt KR, Konda SR, Egol KA. Autogenous iliac crest bone grafting for the treatment of fracture nonunion is equally effective in elderly and nonelderly patients. J Am Acad Orthop Surg. 2019;27(18):696–703. https://doi.org/10.5435/JAAOS-D-18-00322.
220. Boehm KS, Al-Taha M, Morzycki A, Samargandi OA, Al-Youha S, LeBlanc MR. Donor site morbidities of iliac crest bone graft in craniofacial surgery: a systematic review. Ann Plast Surg. 2019;83(3):352–8. https://doi.org/10.1097/SAP.0000000000001682.
221. Morris MT, Tarpada SP, Cho W. Bone graft materials for posterolateral fusion made simple: a systematic review. Eur Spine J Off Publ Eur Spine Soc Eur Spinal Deform Soc Eur Sect Cerv Spine Res Soc. 2018;27(8):1856–67. https://doi.org/10.1007/s00586-018-5511-6.
222. Tuchman A, Brodke DS, Youssef JA, et al. Iliac crest bone graft versus local autograft or allograft for lumbar spinal fusion: a systematic review. Glob Spine J. 2016;6(6):592–606. https://doi.org/10.1055/s-0035-1570749.
223. Elder BD, Ishida W, Goodwin CR, et al. Bone graft options for spinal fusion following resection of spinal column tumors: systematic review and meta-analysis. Neurosurg Focus. 2017;42(1):E16. https://doi.org/10.3171/2016.8.FOCUS16112.
224. Fr N, Pc D, Mp M, Mm M. Vascularized autografts for reconstruction of skeletal defects following lower extremity trauma. A review. Clin Orthop. 1989;243:65–70.
225. Moran CG, Wood MB. Vascularized bone autografts. Orthop Rev. 1993;22(2):187–97.
226. Bohl MA, Almefty KK, Preul MC, et al. Vascularized spinous process graft rotated on a paraspinous muscle pedicle for lumbar fusion: technique description and early clinical experience. World Neurosurg. 2018;115:186–92. https://doi.org/10.1016/j.wneu.2018.04.039.
227. Houdek MT, Rose PS, Bakri K, et al. Outcomes and complications of reconstruction with use of free vascularized fibular graft for spinal and pelvic defects following resection of a malignant tumor. J Bone Joint Surg Am. 2017;99(13):e69. https://doi.org/10.2106/JBJS.16.01458.
228. Bohl MA, Hlubek RJ, Turner JD, Kakarla UK, Preul MC, Reece EM. Far-lateral vascularized rib graft for cervical and lumbar spinal arthrodesis: cadaveric technique description. Plast Reconstr Surg Glob Open. 2019;7(4):e2131. https://doi.org/10.1097/GOX.0000000000002131.
229. Reece EM, Vedantam A, Lee S, et al. Pedicled, vascularized occipital bone graft to supplement atlantoaxial arthrodesis for the treatment of pseudoarthrosis. J Clin Neurosci Off J Neurosurg Soc Australas. 2019; https://doi.org/10.1016/j.jocn.2019.04.014.
230. Saltzman BM, Levy DM, Vakhshori V, DeWald CJ. Free vascularized fibular strut autografts to the lumbar spine in complex revision surgery: a report of two cases. Korean J Spine. 2015;12(3):185–9. https://doi.org/10.14245/kjs.2015.12.3.185.
231. Chacha PB. Vascularised pedicular bone grafts. Int Orthop. 1984;8(2):117–38. https://doi.org/10.1007/bf00265834.
232. Bumbasirevic M, Stevanovic M, Bumbasirevic V, Lesic A, Atkinson HDE. Free vascularised fibular grafts in orthopaedics. Int Orthop. 2014;38(6):1277–82. https://doi.org/10.1007/s00264-014-2281-6.
233. Yanamadala V, Rozman PA, Kumar JI, et al. Vascularized fibular strut autografts in spinal reconstruction after resection of vertebral chordoma or chondrosarcoma: a retrospective series. Neurosurgery. 2017;81(1):156–64. https://doi.org/10.1093/neuros/nyw057.
234. Aldridge JM, Urbaniak JR. Vascularized fibular grafting for osteonecrosis of the femoral head with unusual indications. Clin Orthop. 2008;466(5):1117–24. https://doi.org/10.1007/s11999-008-0201-z.
235. Wilden JA, Moran SL, Dekutoski MB, Bishop AT, Shin AY. Results of vascularized rib grafts in complex spinal reconstruction. J Bone Joint Surg Am. 2006;88(4):832–9. https://doi.org/10.2106/JBJS.E.00409.
236. Tuchman A, Brodke DS, Youssef JA, et al. Autograft versus allograft for cervical spinal fusion. Glob Spine J. 2017;7(1):59–70. https://doi.org/10.1055/s-0036-1580610.
237. Liao Z, Wang C-H, Cui W-L. Comparison of allograft and autograft in lumbar fusion for lumbar degenerative diseases: a systematic review. J Investig Surg Off J Acad Surg Res. 2016;29(6):373–82. https://doi.org/10.3109/08941939.2016.1166534.
238. Godzik J, Ravindra VM, Ray WZ, Schmidt MH, Bisson EF, Dailey AT. Comparison of structural allograft and traditional autograft technique in occipitocervical fusion: radiological and clinical outcomes from a single institution. J

Neurosurg Spine. 2015;23(2):144–52. https://doi.org/10.3171/2014.12.SPINE14535.
239. Chang KY, Hsu WK. Spinal biologics in minimally invasive lumbar surgery. Minim Invasive Surg. 2018;2018:5230350. https://doi.org/10.1155/2018/5230350.
240. Judas F, Saavedra MJ, Mendes AF, Dias R. Cortical strut allografting in reconstructive orthopaedic surgery. Acta Reumatol Port. 2011;36(1):24–8.
241. Park JS, Moon KH. Medium- to long-term results of strut allografts treating periprosthetic bone defects. Hip Pelvis. 2018;30(1):23–8. https://doi.org/10.5371/hp.2018.30.1.23.
242. Emerson RH, Malinin TI, Cuellar AD, Head WC, Peters PC. Cortical strut allografts in the reconstruction of the femur in revision total hip arthroplasty. A basic science and clinical study. Clin Orthop. 1992;285:35–44.
243. Levack AE, Gadinsky N, Gausden EB, Klinger C, Helfet DL, Lorich DG. The use of fibular allograft in complex periarticular fractures around the knee. Oper Tech Orthop. 2018;28(3):141–51. https://doi.org/10.1053/j.oto.2018.07.004.
244. Panegrossi G, Ceretti M, Papalia M, Casella F, Favetti F, Falez F. Bone loss management in total knee revision surgery. Int Orthop. 2014;38(2):419–27. https://doi.org/10.1007/s00264-013-2262-1.
245. Bridwell KH, Lenke LG, McEnery KW, Baldus C, Blanke K. Anterior fresh frozen structural allografts in the thoracic and lumbar spine. Do they work if combined with posterior fusion and instrumentation in adult patients with kyphosis or anterior column defects? Spine. 1995;20(12):1410–8.
246. Kozak JA, Heilman AE, O'Brien JP. Anterior lumbar fusion options. Technique and graft materials. Clin Orthop. 1994;300:45–51.
247. Hildebrand GR, Wright DM, Marston SB, Switzer JA. Use of a fibular strut allograft in an osteoporotic distal humerus fracture: a case report. Geriatr Orthop Surg Rehabil. 2012;3(4):167–71. https://doi.org/10.1177/2151458513477108.
248. Addosooki AI, Alam-Eldin M, Abdel-Wanis ME-S, Yousef MAA, Dionigi P, Kenawey MO. Anterior cervical reconstruction using free vascularized fibular graft after cervical corpectomy. Glob Spine J. 2016;6(3):212–9. https://doi.org/10.1055/s-0035-1558653.
249. Mayr MT, Subach BR, Comey CH, Rodts GE, Haid RW. Cervical spinal stenosis: outcome after anterior corpectomy, allograft reconstruction, and instrumentation. J Neurosurg. 2002;96(1 Suppl):10–6. https://doi.org/10.3171/spi.2002.96.1.0010.
250. Young WF, Rosenwasser RH. An early comparative analysis of the use of fibular allograft versus autologous iliac crest graft for interbody fusion after anterior cervical discectomy. Spine. 1993;18(9):1123–4. https://doi.org/10.1097/00007632-199307000-00002.
251. Fernyhough JC, White JI, LaRocca H. Fusion rates in multilevel cervical spondylosis comparing allograft fibula with autograft fibula in 126 patients. Spine. 1991;16(10 Suppl):S561–4. https://doi.org/10.1097/00007632-199110001-00022.
252. Cheung JPY, Luk KD-K. Complications of anterior and posterior cervical spine surgery. Asian Spine J. 2016;10(2):385–400. https://doi.org/10.4184/asj.2016.10.2.385.
253. Hilibrand AS, Fye MA, Emery SE, Palumbo MA, Bohlman HH. Increased rate of arthrodesis with strut grafting after multilevel anterior cervical decompression. Spine. 2002;27(2):146–51. https://doi.org/10.1097/00007632-200201150-00005.
254. Zhang H, Yang L, Yang X, et al. Demineralized bone matrix carriers and their clinical applications: an overview. Orthop Surg. 2019;11(5):725–37. https://doi.org/10.1111/os.12509.
255. Lee KJH, Roper JG, Wang JC. Demineralized bone matrix and spinal arthrodesis. Spine J. 2005;5(6):S217–23. https://doi.org/10.1016/j.spinee.2005.02.006.
256. Oryan A, Alidadi S, Moshiri A, Maffulli N. Bone regenerative medicine: classic options, novel strategies, and future directions. J Orthop Surg. 2014;9:18. https://doi.org/10.1186/1749-799X-9-18.
257. Tilkeridis K, Touzopoulos P, Ververidis A, Christodoulou S, Kazakos K, Drosos GI. Use of demineralized bone matrix in spinal fusion. World J Orthop. 2014;5(1):30–7. https://doi.org/10.5312/wjo.v5.i1.30.
258. Kadam A, Millhouse PW, Kepler CK, et al. Bone substitutes and expanders in spine surgery: a review of their fusion efficacies. Int J Spine Surg. 2016;10:33. https://doi.org/10.14444/3033.
259. Yang HL, Zhu XS, Chen L, et al. Bone healing response to a synthetic calcium sulfate/β-tricalcium phosphate graft material in a sheep vertebral body defect model. J Biomed Mater Res B Appl Biomater. 2012;100B(7):1911–21. https://doi.org/10.1002/jbm.b.32758.
260. Liu H, Liu B, Gao C, et al. Injectable, biomechanically robust, biodegradable and osseointegrative bone cement for percutaneous kyphoplasty and vertebroplasty. Int Orthop. 2018;42(1):125–32. https://doi.org/10.1007/s00264-017-3674-0.
261. Bai B, Kummer FJ, Spivak J. Augmentation of anterior vertebral body screw fixation by an injectable, biodegradable calcium phosphate bone substitute. Spine. 2001;26(24):2679–83. https://doi.org/10.1097/00007632-200112150-00009.
262. Lykissas M, Gkiatas I. Use of recombinant human bone morphogenetic protein-2 in spine surgery. World J Orthop. 2017;8(7):531–5. https://doi.org/10.5312/wjo.v8.i7.531.
263. Bach D-H, Park HJ, Lee SK. The dual role of bone morphogenetic proteins in cancer. Mol Ther Oncolytics. 2017;8:1–13. https://doi.org/10.1016/j.omto.2017.10.002.
264. Beachler DC, Yanik EL, Martin BI, et al. Bone morphogenetic protein use and cancer risk among patients undergoing lumbar arthrodesis. J Bone

Joint Surg Am. 2016;98(13):1064–72. https://doi.org/10.2106/JBJS.15.01106.
265. Carragee EJ, Chu G, Rohatgi R, et al. Cancer risk after use of recombinant bone morphogenetic protein-2 for spinal arthrodesis. J Bone Joint Surg Am. 2013;95(17):1537–45. https://doi.org/10.2106/JBJS.L.01483.
266. Kelly MP, Savage JW, Bentzen SM, Hsu WK, Ellison SA, Anderson PA. Cancer risk from bone morphogenetic protein exposure in spinal arthrodesis. J Bone Joint Surg Am. 2014;96(17):1417–22. https://doi.org/10.2106/JBJS.M.01190.
267. Schroeder J, Kueper J, Leon K, Liebergall M. Stem cells for spine surgery. World J Stem Cells. 2015;7(1):186–94. https://doi.org/10.4252/wjsc.v7.i1.186.
268. Oliver K, Awan T, Bayes M. Single-versus multiple-site harvesting techniques for bone marrow concentrate: evaluation of aspirate quality and pain. Orthop J Sports Med. 2017;5(8). https://doi.org/10.1177/2325967117724398.
269. Robbins MA, Haudenschild DR, Wegner AM, Klineberg EO. Stem cells in spinal fusion. Glob Spine J. 2017;7(8):801–10. https://doi.org/10.1177/2192568217701102.
270. Kotsias A, Mularski S, Kühn B, Hanna M, Suess O. Does partial coating with titanium improve the radiographic fusion rate of empty PEEK cages in cervical spine surgery? A comparative analysis of clinical data. Patient Saf Surg. 2017;11:13.
271. Walsh WR, Pelletier MH, Bertollo N, Christou C, Tan C. Does PEEK/HA enhance bone formation compared with peek in a sheep cervical fusion model? Clin Orthop Relat Res. 2016;474(11):2364–72.
272. Zajonz D, Franke AC, von der Höh N, et al. Is the radiographic subsidence of stand-alone cages associated with adverse clinical outcomes after cervical spine fusion? An observational cohort study with 2-year follow-up outcome scoring. Patient Saf Surg. 2014;8(1):43.
273. Kim JH, Rhee JM, Enyo Y, Hutton WC, Kim SS. A biomechanical comparison of 360° stabilizations for corpectomy and total spondylectomy: a cadaveric study in the thoracolumbar spine. J Orthop Surg Res. 2015;10:99.
274. Roberto T, Daniele M, Martina C, Tiziano de G, Roberto D. Treatment of thoracolumbar spinal infections through anterolateral approaches using expandable titanium mesh cage for spine reconstruction. ScientificWorldJournal. 2012;2012:545293.

Radiation, Robotics, and Reconstructive Options in Spine Tumor Surgery

21

Matthew L. Goodwin and Daniel M. Sciubba

Introduction

The discovery of X-rays by Wilhelm Roentgen circa 1895 would pave the way for the eventual use of radiographs to aid in diagnoses as well as allow visualization of implanted medical devices [1]. Currently in spine surgery that role has expanded to include multiple modes of intraoperative imaging, including use of intraoperative radiographs, C-arm imaging/fluoroscopy, multiplanar fluoroscopy, intraoperative CT imaging, navigation with pre- or intraop imaging, and robotic-assisted navigation (Fig. 21.1) [2–6]. The choice of what imaging to use during any given procedure is obviously surgeon-dependent, and multiple factors contribute to this decision, including how much radiation the surgeon, operative staff, and patient may be exposed to. In addition to the "traditional use" of imaging modalities both preoperatively and intraoperatively, new advances are rapidly developing in spine tumor surgery for resection of tumors and subsequent reconstruction. These advances include robotic-assisted surgery as well as custom-printed 3D printed implants and cutting guides [7–9].

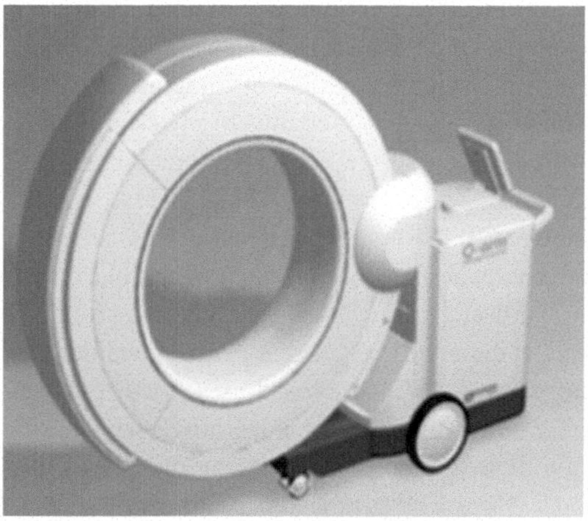

Fig. 21.1 O-arm. Many orthopedic spine surgeons may be more comfortable using C-arm or X-Ray while many neurosurgical surgeons may be more comfortable with modalities like intraoperative CT or "O-arm" imaging. As surgeons continue to "cross-train" in both specialties, these differences are likely to decrease. (Reprinted from Zhang et al. [10], Copyright 2009, with permission from IOS Press. This publication is available at IOS Press through doi: https://doi.org/10.3233/XST-2009-0231. https://content.iospress.com/articles/journal-of-x-ray-science-and-technology/xst00231)

Choice of Intraoperative Modality

Choosing what, if any, intraoperative imaging to use is a surgeon-dependent question. Common considerations include the following: What training has the surgeon had with each modality?

M. L. Goodwin (✉)
Department of Orthopaedics, Washington University, Barnes-Jewish Hospital, Saint Louis, MO, USA

D. M. Sciubba
Department of Neurosurgery, Johns Hopkins Hospital, Baltimore, MD, USA

K. Singh, M. Colman (eds.), *Surgical Spinal Oncology*,
https://doi.org/10.1007/978-3-030-50722-0_21

What is available at the hospital? What is the cost in using/owning each? How much radiation is the surgeon or patient exposed to during use of each modality? Which modality allows the most accurate resection of tumor as well as placement of hardware? Perhaps the first question to address is whether intraoperative imaging is needed at all. Many surgeons have been trained in the "freehand" placement of pedicle screws, relying on local bony anatomy with preoperative imaging to aid in placement of hardware. While many freehand trained surgeons may be wary of a shift to an image-guided operating room, optimizing use of advances in technology is desired by all. For example, a freehand surgeon may place all of her hardware without the use of imaging, and then utilize an imaging modality to check the hardware position before leaving the operating room. Whether with C-arm, traditional X-ray, intraoperative CT, or some other imaging modality, it is advantageous to at a minimum check placement of hardware before leaving the operating room. If this is done, any screw that is questionable may be interrogated and revised as needed. For surgeons in training, it is imperative they master both how to incorporate imaging modalities into their OR as well as how to place freehand screws.

Freehand Placement of Pedicle Screws

While strategies for tumor resection and osteotomies vary depending on the tumor location and available tools, the basic anatomy of the spine and location of safe bony corridors for instrumentation should be well understood by all spine surgeons. It cannot be overemphasized in this chapter that residents and fellows should receive training in how to properly place freehand pedicle screws from C1 to the pelvis. While this chapter cannot serve as an exhaustive review of the numerous studies done on accuracy and complications of freehand versus other techniques, it is worth pointing out that freehand technique should always be used to check any navigation or machine assist, and that in many areas, there are good data suggesting that freehand may actually be better than current navigation assistance. For example, in the placement of C2 pedicle screws, direct visualization of the pars and pedicle has thus far been superior to image guidance [11]. These differences may be due to the addition of added variables when using navigation (additional sources of error), or may result from difficulty in obtaining understandable image planes. However, these factors likely will be minimized as technology improves. Overall, navigation or robotic-assisted surgery are not perfect and are not substitutes for excellent spatial and anatomical awareness from the surgeon.

While we do not intend for this chapter to serve as a tutorial on freehand screw placement, a few key points should be kept in mind at each level. Having preoperative CT images available while operating will maximize successful placement of hardware. Further, for any cervical procedure (even a single level ACDF), the vertebral arteries should be scrutinized on the preoperative MRI to understand dominance and anatomic course abnormalities. The surgeon should recognize locations where the surgical exposure approaches the vertebral arteries and have a plan for control of vertebral bleeding. For example, Fig. 21.2 shows a recent case of ours where a patient suffered a Hangman's fracture and needed fixation. An anomaly in V3 of the left vertebral artery was recognized preoperatively and prevented placement of the usual C1 lateral mass screw. Instead, we exposed above the ring of C1 on the left side and placed our lateral mass screw of C1 *above* the posterior arch. This was critical to have reviewed preoperatively, as this patient was left vertebral arterial dominant, and an injury to the left artery might have had disastrous consequences. Most patients will not require dedicated vascular studies as vertebral arteries are typically easily visualized as flow voids (dark) on standard T2 imaging (Fig. 21.2).

Below is a general guide for freehand placement of hardware in the cervical, thoracic, and lumbar spines:

- C1: At C1, one can choose to remove or not remove the C2 nerve root. We find it helpful to bipolar vessels around the C2 root and then bipolar on either side of the DRG before resecting it. Using this method, we are able to get good visualization of the entire C1/2 joint, which can be drilled before placement of screws, and good hemostasis of a notoriously bloody area. We observe consistent clinical

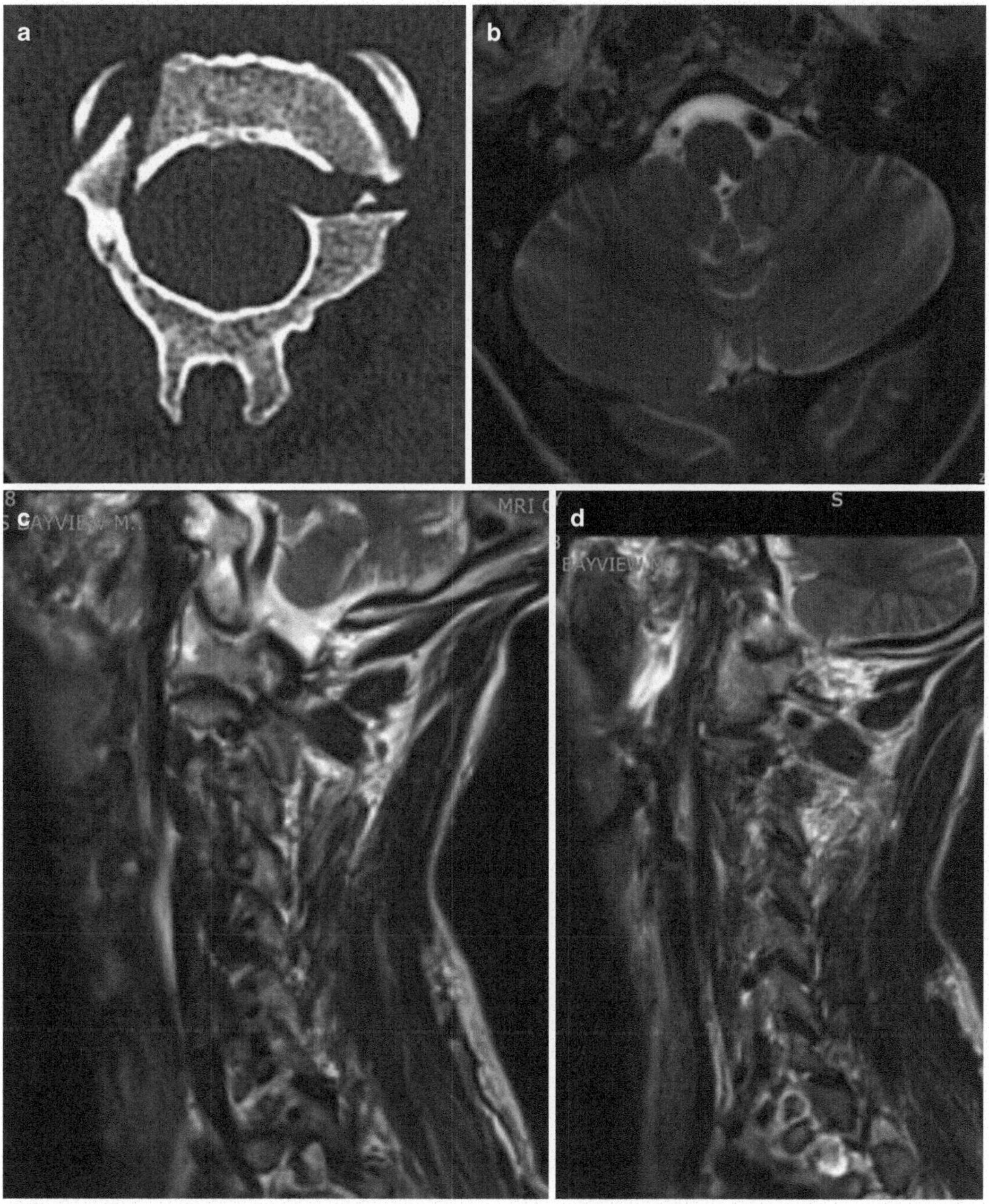

Fig. 21.2 Example of vertebral artery anomaly. Here, a patient suffered from a Hangman's fracture (**a**) and was set to undergo fixation. It was noted that the patient had a left-dominant vertebral artery (**b**). On further review, it was noted that the patient has an anomaly of the V3 segment of the left vertebral artery, where the artery traversed along the inferior surface of the C1 posterior arch rather than the superior surface of it (**c**–**e**). The left C1 screw was placed superior to the posterior arch into the left C1 lateral mass to accommodate (**f**, **g**). Not recognizing this anomaly preoperatively would likely have been catastrophic for this patient

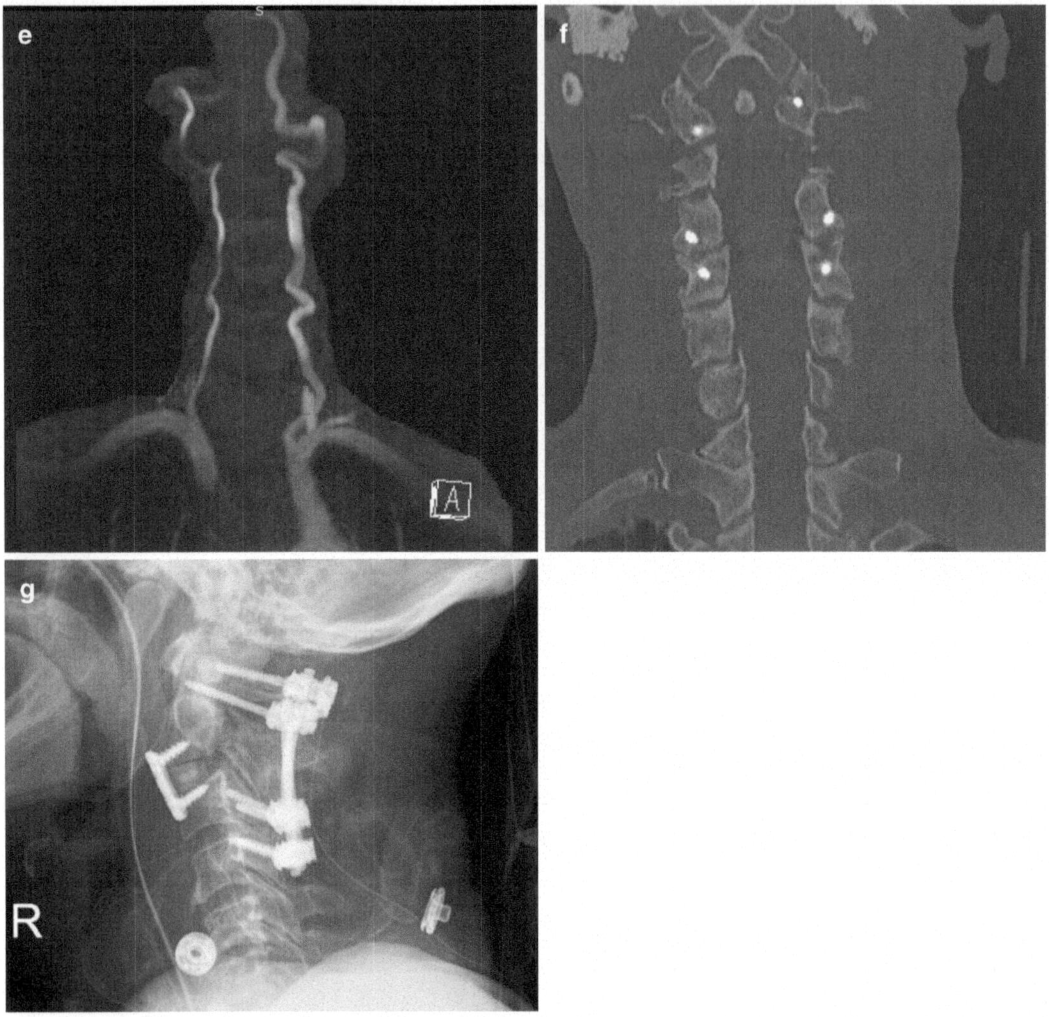

Fig. 21.2 (continued)

results where patients have some numb areas of skin behind the ear but almost never any pain associated with ligation of the C2 roots. Once this area is prepared, one can use the most posterior aspect of the "football"-shaped C1 lateral mass as a guide for optimal placement of the C1 screw start point. This is felt with direct palpation and/or visualization and the axial CT cut at this level helps guide direction along the long axis of the oblong-shaped American "football." We prefer marking the start point with a high-speed burr, then using a drill with guide (often set to no more than 18 mm) based on preoperative measurements to drill the screw pathway (Fig. 21.3).

- C2: At C2, the placement of a screw demands review of a preoperative CT or MRI. Where the vertebral artery traverses the C2 bone, it dictates whether safe placement of a pars/pedicle screw is possible or not. It is our preference to alter the gantry of the axial imaging when viewing this bony corridor to get the best view of both sagittal and axial views. Once it is deemed that there is adequate room, the surgeon should carefully visualize the superior aspect of the pedicle, taking care to stay on the medial aspect of it, away from the vertebral artery. Once the medial wall can be felt with a Penfield number 4, nerve hook, or other instrument, a burr hole is made high on

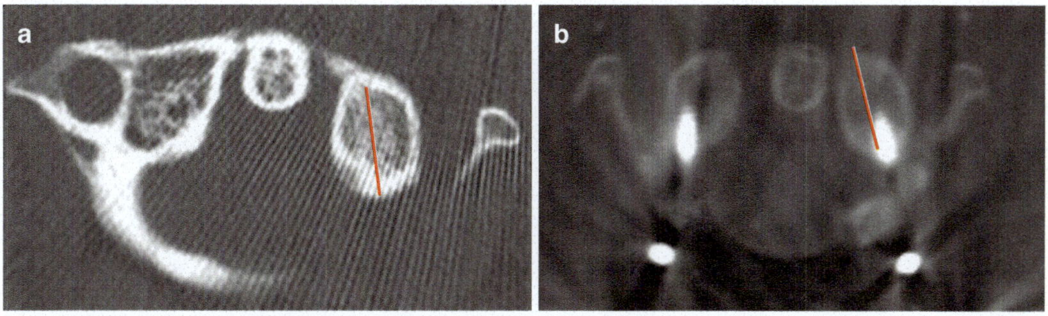

Fig. 21.3 Preoperative (**a**) and postoperative (**b**) CT of a patient undergoing C1 instrumentation. Note the red line indicating the preferred trajectory from the posterior-most aspect of the left lateral mass along the long axis

the posterior aspect and tap and drill guide are used to make the hole. The surgeon should encounter hard medial bone as a guide when placing this. As an alternative, a translaminar screw may need to be used, particularly when the patient has a high-riding vertebral artery, only one vertebral artery (or one very dominant), or if the vertebral artery is injured on placement of the C2 screw on the contralateral side.

- C3-C6: At these levels, lateral mass screws are often used. One should note the location of the vertebral arteries, and also note what length of screw (usually 12 or 14mm) may be placed. Again, adjusting the gantry is helpful in placement planning.
- C7: Although pedicle screws can be placed here, this level is often skipped due to its transitional nature, and the fact that the start point and screw tulip typically impinge upon the C6 lateral mass screw. However, after preoperative MRI and CT review, pedicle screws may be safely placed here. This safe placement is typically facilitated by AP fluoroscopy and/or a limited C6/7 hemilaminotomy to allow direct medial pedicle wall palpation.

Thoracic screws In general, it should be kept in mind that T1 screws start lateral and are medially directed, while T12 screws are typically almost completely vertical. This pattern is helpful to remember when placing these screws. For each individual screw, care should be taken to examine the transition in the bone from lamina to SAP (often demarcated with a bony ridge and often best seen with a small osteotomy removing the overlapping IAP) and the medial and lateral borders of the SAP; start point should never exceed midpoint of the SAP. In the sagittal plane, straightforward screws (vs “anatomic”) are close to parallel with the lamina. Note that reference to the preoperative CT is used to determine start point on the axial. We also look across to the corresponding TP to account for any segmental rotation. With these multiple plane checks, near perfect placement of thoracic screws can be achieved. At T11 and T12, rongeuring off part of the TP allows visualization of the underlying cancellous type pedicle bone.

Lumbosacral Screws Lumbar screw placement is most easily done by looking at the pars above and below along with the midpoint of the TP, recognizing both the changes in transverse trajectory from T12 to L5 as well as the start point with reference to TP from L1 to L5. S1 screws are reproducibly placed by using the alar anatomy, starting just inferolateral to the facet, and aiming medially. We still prefer to refer to our axial CT when placing these.

Pelvic screws Although full discussion of various pelvic screws is beyond this review, it should be noted that well-placed S2 alar-iliac (S2AI) screws line up with S1 and can be consistently

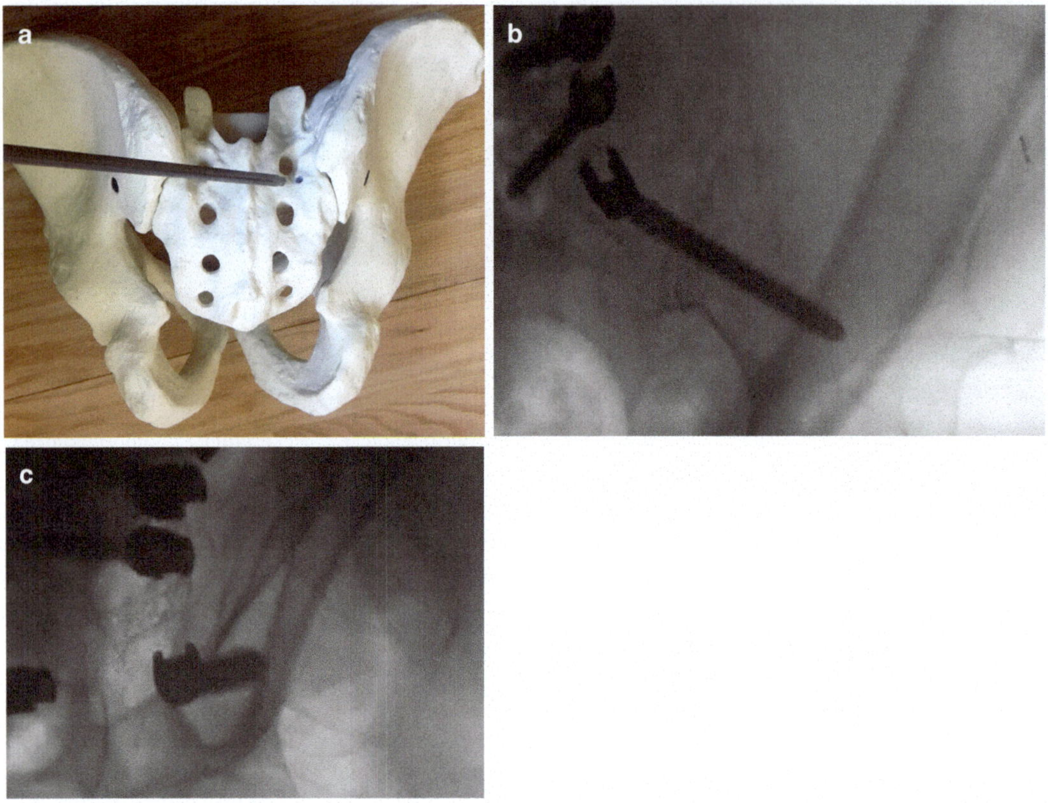

Fig. 21.4 (**a**) The start point for S2AI screws and (**b**) checking placement of S2AI screws on fluoroscopy with iliac oblique and then teardrop view (**c**)

placed freehand. Additionally, the tulip is less prominent, and the screw fixation crosses more cortical bone (through the sacroiliac (SI) joint) than traditional iliac bolts, making them our preferred fixation method at this level. The S1 foramen is easily palpated distal and medial to the S1 screw. Bone of S2 is then palpated and a start point just distal and lateral to the S1 foramen is burred as a start point (Fig. 21.4a). Trajectory can then be estimated by feeling the posterior super iliac spine (PSIS), the greater trochanter, and viewing the CT. The gear shift and then a tap over a guidewire are used. Checking these involves both palpation of a bony corridor, adjusting the tip of the gear shift as needed [12], and visualizing iliac oblique and teardrop views after placing (Fig. 21.4b, c); the sciatic notch should not be violated. Alternatively, our preference is to place all hardware, including the S2AI screws, and then include in our intraoperative 3D imaging spin to check placement.

Use of Fluoroscopy, CT, and Radiographs Intraoperatively

The oldest real-time, image-guided technique for spine surgery is fluoroscopy [13]. This utilizes low-dose radiation for continuous visualization. Actual use and radiation exposure can vary markedly with use of the C-arm. In addition to being sure that the machine is set to the lowest reasonable settings, some surgeons may use C-arm to place each pedicle screw under live fluoroscopy, while others use it only after all hardware is placed freehand, as a quick check with isolated fluoroscopy "spots"; these two different uses are markedly different in their exposure of radiation to patient, staff, and surgeon (see below). Recently, 3D fluoroscopy has also been utilized [4, 14]. Given the heterogeneity with how fluoroscopy is used intraoperatively, comparisons between fluoroscopy and other methods are often complicated by numerous confounding variables.

Many surgeons, rather than placing each screw under fluoroscopy (see radiation exposure section) will instead utilize the C-arm for fluoroscopy spots. This is similar to utilizing a few plain radiographs to check screw placement, albeit with more radiation exposure to the surgeon. In tumor surgery, particularly involving complicated osteotomies, use of both fluoroscopy spots and even live fluoroscopy can be quite useful. However, use of it in this setting often depends on the surgeon's comfort with the imaging as well as the radiology tech's ability to adjust the machine in concert with the surgeon's needs.

While computed tomography (CT) scans introduce a nontrivial amount of radiation, intraoperative CT scans or other 3D imaging systems may deliver considerably less [3, 10]. Images from preoperative CTs are often used by free hand surgeons to optimize placement of screws (e.g., by choosing a starting point with the aid of the preoperative axial view). Combined with knowledge of anatomical landmarks and the localizing intraoperative plain film, placing freehand screws should be both very safe and efficient. Intraoperative 3D imaging is useful as a means of imaging intraoperatively, but many surgeons experience the addition of considerable time to the operation, particularly if one is trying to place hardware while utilizing multiple spins. However, modern use of intraoperative imaging such as multiplanar fluoroscopy is evolving. Workflow efficiency, machine size, and surgeon familiarity with the technology are facilitating more widespread adoption.

Navigation

Navigation involves the application of technology that allows real-time projection of where an instrument is on the patient onto a CT image. This can be most helpful in that it allows trainees a chance to "check" their understanding of freehand placement, it allows accurate screw placement in the event of dysplastic or small pedicles, it allows visualization of the most optimal osteotomy cut, particularly in cases of tumors, and it often allows visualization of other aspects of osteotomies and reconstruction (e.g., what length of screw is appropriate is needed, etc.). Many studies advocate for use of navigation for thoracic pedicle screws given the variation and difficulty placing them freehand. Studies have demonstrated misplaced screws in as high as 55% of thoracic screws [15], improving to 20–30% in several studies with the use of fluoroscopy [16]. Although placement is often checked with AP and lateral plain radiographs in the operating room, ideally placement is checked with an intraoperative 3D scan [17]. Although we support the use of navigation, trainees should use both freehand and navigation to receive adequate training in both methods.

Navigation may be initiated either with intraoperative image acquisition and automatic registration or by linking intraoperative anatomy to preoperative scans using bony landmarks or previously placed fiducials. Either combined with navigation or separately, fiducial markers may be used as a means of orientation. Many surgeons employ preoperatively placed markers as a means to avoid wrong level surgery, particularly in the thoracic spine [18]. In spine tumor surgery, the level is typically easier to localize due to tumor. However, fiducials may be used to improve patient-navigation registration. These efforts are ongoing [18, 19].

Several navigation platforms exist. In most, a reference clamp is placed on an SP (or known landmark) and left in place while an intraoperative scan is performed. The tools can then be registered to a preexisting CT or the intraoperative imaging modality and real-time movements of probes (and in many cases instruments) can be seen on the screen, allowing for near-direct visualization while screws are placed or osteotomy cuts are made [20]. As expected, this has improved accuracy of screw placement in large studies [20]. As technology improves, we might expect this improvement to continue, particularly with the assistance of augmented reality platforms (e.g., Augmedics xvision™ spine (XVS) system [21] and robotic-assisted platforms (see section on "Robotics"). Although beyond the scope of this chapter, machine learning will likely combine with this navigation to make much of the hardware placement and osteotomy cuts near fully automated. However, successful introduction of this technology will require surgeons to be well trained in freehand techniques, as it will ultimately be up to the surgeon to prevent the rare potential catastrophic hardware or software error that may harm the patient. We expect this to be challenging.

On the other hand, the benefits of computer navigation in spine tumor surgery abound. Efficiency and safety of multilevel screw placement, localization of distorted anatomy, and precise assessment of tumor resection margins are all benefits. An infrequently discussed benefit is also that navigation may allow precision placement of screws into novel bony corridors where bone quality is optimal. This is especially germane for spine tumor patients who frequently have tumor-related bone destruction, osteopenia, and frailty.

Finally, the best use of navigation in spine tumor surgery may be in the resection of sacral tumors, where the local anatomy makes bone cuts challenging. We have found navigation to be most useful in these cases, where orientation of the blade throughout a pelvic or sacral cut can be quite difficult. Navigation allows real time feedback on orientation in three planes. Figure 21.5 demonstrates a recent case of ours in which navigation was utilized to spare the S1 bone stock.

Radiation Exposure

Many surgeons opt to use the freehand technique, image-guided, navigation, or more recently, robot-assisted navigation. Even with freehand placement of hardware, decisions must be made as to how this is to be "checked" in the OR. With the rise of minimally invasive surgery (MIS), imaging modalities and radiation exposure to patient and surgeon have come under greater scrutiny, particularly as technology has advanced and allowed the use of powerful imaging modalities like intraoperative CT imaging. Although using navigation requires imaging, it can often be done preoperatively, saving the operating room staff and surgeon exposure to radiation. However, this can be cumbersome or noncompatible with the navigation system, or the surgeon may be unfamiliar altogether with it. Even with navigation, some check of the hardware placement should be performed.

Unfortunately, misinformation abounds when it comes to safe exposure to radiation, both among the public and surgeons. The two major governing bodies, the National Council on Radiation Protection (NCRP) and the International Commission on Radiological Protection (ICRP), have set forth general guidelines for "maximal limits" for those that work with radiation (i.e., surgeons) and those that do not (i.e., patients). These guidelines have been adopted by various professional and societal groups [5, 22–26]:

1. For those that work with radiation, annual dose should not exceed 20 mSv/year averaged over 5 years and should not exceed 50 mSv/year in any 1 year.
2. For those that do not work with radiation, annual dose should not exceed 1 mSv/year in addition to natural background and medical testing.

Determining what level of radiation exposure is "safe" is incredibly challenging and based in large part on exposure to larger amounts of radiation over a smaller time. For example, it is only with ~500 mSv that transient changes to blood cells has been noted; with less than 100 mSv in a year, no change in even cancer risk has been demonstrated [25]. As a point of reference, Table 21.1 shows various amounts of radiation (in mSv) for various exposures. Note that a plain film of the chest is about 0.1 mSv (equivalent to a flight from NYC to LA roundtrip), background radiation on average is around 3 mSv per year on earth, a traditional CT may be ~10 mSv, and intraoperative CT scans can be done for ~2.5 mSv or even less (1 mSv = 100mrem). It must be noted that the limits noted for nonradiation workers (patients) are *in addition to background radiation and medical radiation.* The safe limits of radiation are based

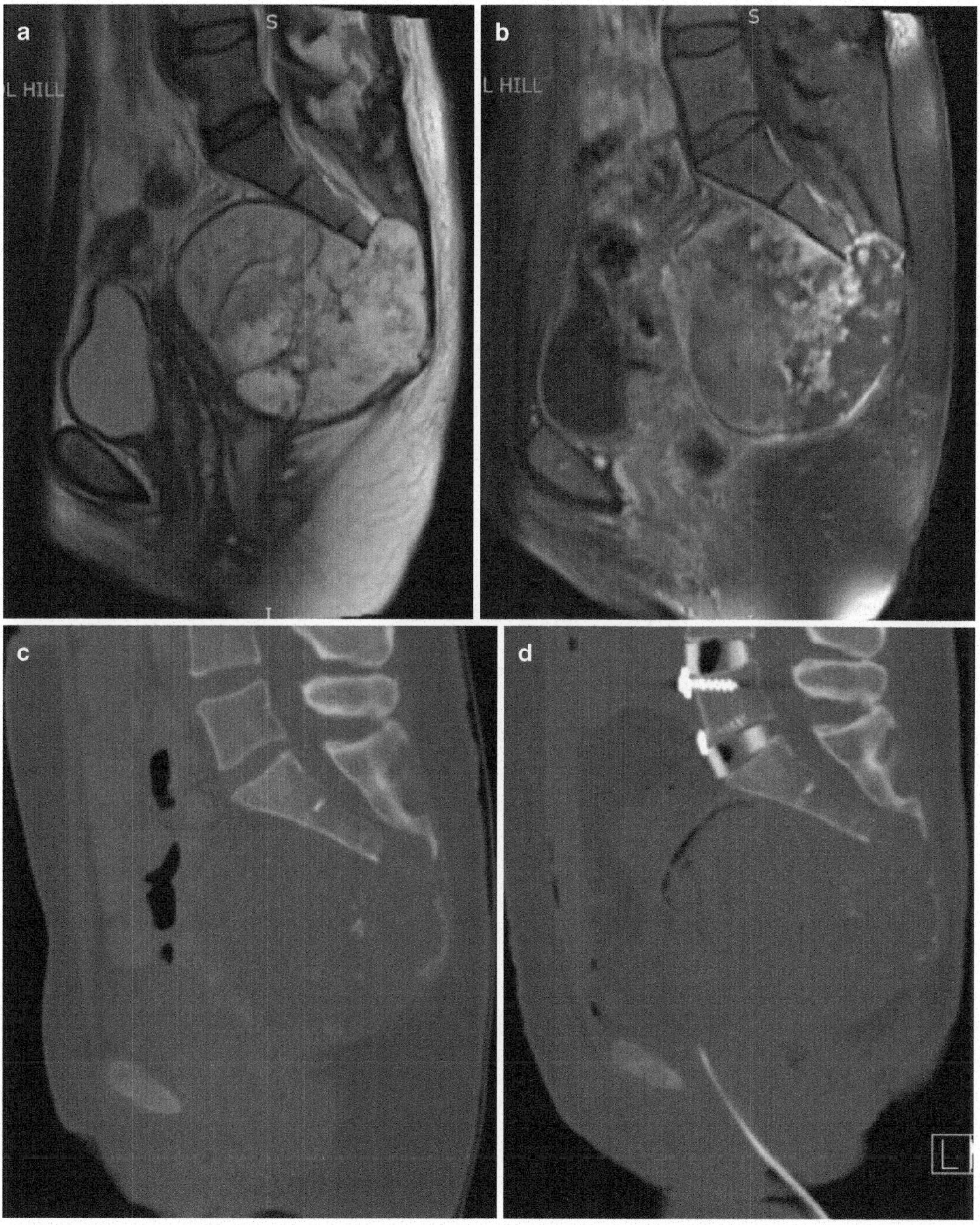

Fig. 21.5 In a 50-year-old patient with a large sacral chondrosarcoma, we elected to use navigation in an effort to maximize preservation of bone at S1. Sagittal (**a**) T2 MRI, (**b**) postcontrast MRI, and (**c**) CT demonstrating a large sacral mass without involvement of S1. Stage 1 involved anterior exposure with ALIFs at L4/5 and L5/1. Poststage 1 CT allows visualization of interbody grafts as well as up-to-date imaging of tumor (**d**). Given efforts to save S1 bone, this was critical, as tumor had grown in the interim, making navigation critical. Note classic popcorn calcifications throughout as well as ureter stents. Postoperative lateral (**e**) and AP (**f**) CT cuts demonstrating the rim of S1 left while removing the tumor en bloc with negative margins. This demonstrates the utility of navigation in spine tumor surgery

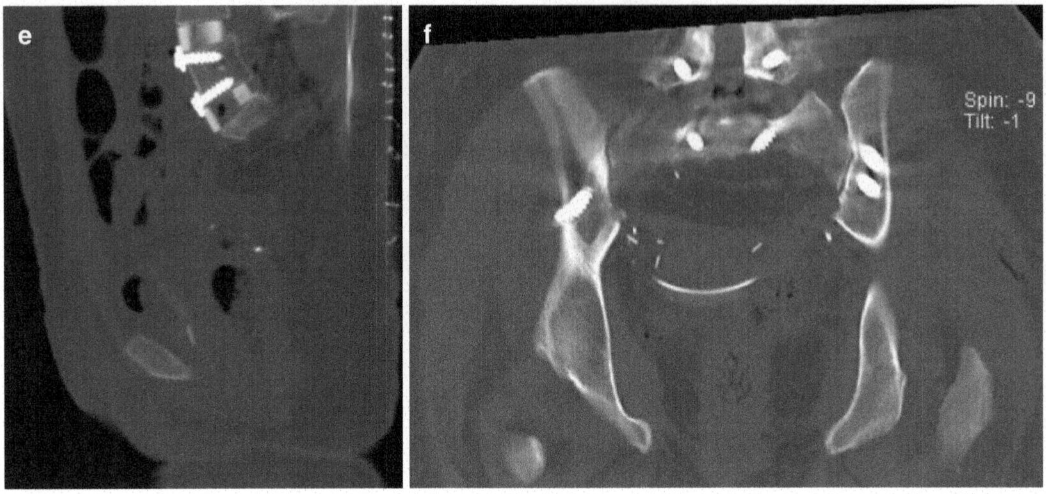

Fig. 21.5 (continued)

Table 21.1 Radiation estimates of various exposures. 1 mSv = 100mrem [4, 5, 10, 25, 28]

Event	Radiation (mSv)
Extremity radiograph	0.001
DEXA	0.001
Chest radiograph	0.1
Flight (NYC to LA), roundtrip	0.1
Lumbar radiographs	0.7
Thoracolumbar radiographs	1.5
O-arm, spine[a]	2.5
Background radiation, Earth	3
CT, spine	10
CTA for PE	10
Coronary angiogram	5–15

[a]Note that the O-arm dose depends on a variety of factors including levels scanned and machine settings. These continue to decrease radiation amount delivered to patient

on theoretical limits that take into account potential short-term (i.e., "deterministic") and long-term (i.e., "stochastic") effects. Given the theoretical nature of these limits, a physician ordering a CT for any medical reason has benefit that already outweighs the small theoretical risk of radiation. As pointed out by the ICRP, "…medical exposure of patients has unique considerations that affect how the fundamental principles are applied. Dose limits are not at all relevant, since ionizing radiation, used at the appropriate level of dose for the particular medical purpose, is an essential tool that will cause more good than harm" [27]. With regard to why medical radiation is not considered as part of the exposure to radiation when discussing safe radiation limits, the American College of Radiology states, "for almost all imaging, benefit outweighs risk for patient" [22, 28]. If we consider that only once we exceed 100 mSv is there any correlation to cancers, receiving 10 mSv for a CT scan to optimally plan a large, high-risk surgery is certainly within reason. Further, intraoperative CT capabilities now allow even less than 2.5 mSv per spin, giving the surgeon the ability to check hardware placement with a CT spin (or two) when needed with little to no risk to the patient or surgical team (as the team steps out of the room for the spin).

Pennington et al. [4] performed an exhaustive review of the amount of intraoperative radiation *per screw* received by patients and surgeons alike for different modalities. Not surprisingly, using intraoperative CT-guided navigation delivered the most radiation to the patient. However, even if the patient were receiving a C2-pelvis procedure, this would only amount to ~10–60 mSv. However, it was 2D fluoroscopy without navigation that delivered the most radiation to the surgeon, which would amount to ~20–30 mSv/year for a busy surgeon. Considering the preceding dose limits, it is the surgeon, not the patient, who is most at risk of exceeding known safe limits of radiation. The exception to this may be in pediatric cases.

One solution is to consider placing hardware freehand and with the use of a preoperative CT (or with navigation), then leaving the room for an intraoperative 3D scan to check once hardware is placed. This minimizes surgeon and staff exposure and is our preferred method.

Robotics

One area of recent rapidly development has been the use of robotics in spine surgery. Currently, most robotic devices in use in spine surgery function to assist the surgeon rather than to function independently. For example, the Excelsius XP (Globus) is a stand-alone machine that integrates navigation with a robotic arm that aligns screw trajectory for the desired surgeon trajectory. Several studies have demonstrated the improved accuracy of screw placement utilizing robotic assistance [29], but data in tumor patients remain limited. For example, Solomiichuk et al. [30] examined robot-assisted hardware placement in patients with metastatic disease and found no difference in accuracy or radiation dose between this cohort and a similar matched cohort. In a similar manner, Hu et al. [31] reported on use of robotic assistance in patients with thoracolumbar tumors, although no comparison group was used. However, limiting the discussion of robotics to robot-assisted hardware placement is likely shortsighted. For example, osteotomy cuts in spine tumor surgery can be challenging. Robotics offers the opportunity to combine navigation with near-perfect, rigid guide placement for complex cuts, like those often needed for sacral tumors. This has already been successfully demonstrated in primary sacral and presacral tumors [32, 33]. Other potential uses for robotics which may evolve in the future include haptic resection feedback or drilling guidance, or controlled manipulative deformity correction maneuvers.

While quickly gaining traction, robotics in spine surgery has lagged behind usage of robotics in urology, gynecology/oncology, and general surgical oncology [9], where the robot has been developed to allow more intricate dissections, greater visibility, and more control around delicate structures. Currently, the mainstream spine surgery robotic devices all function with one arm to guide placement of screws. It is not hard to imagine how this may develop into a system with multiple modular arms, like the Da Vinci, to aid the spine tumor surgeon in the near future. Already, several spine tumor cases have been reported in the literature using the Da Vinci robot, which allows multiple arms and enhanced, precise control by the surgeon when dissecting [34, 35].

Recently, "robotics" has come under some criticism by those not familiar with spine surgery [36]. However, we would contend that navigation and robotics are becoming part of spine surgery and should serve to augment, not interfere or replace, the surgeon's skill. Training the next generation of surgeons to use technology but not rely solely on it will be challenging. One surgeon (personal communication) has started using navigation on every case as a way to allow surgical staff and trainees to become more familiar with the tools, as they are often needed in complex spine tumor cases. The attending positions the monitor so that he can view it, while the resident or fellow sets about placing screws using the freehand technique. In this manner, the attending surgeon is able to better see where the fellow is and how their understanding of free hand placement is progressing. The trainee gains experience in freehand technique while also using navigation, and without sacrificing patient safety. Creative solutions like this will be needed moving forward.

Finally, we must mention augmented reality, an area of growth in spine surgery that involves eyewear that enhances the surgeon's view such that deep structures are visible. A display overlies the deep structures such that the surgeon's view is now enhanced to include deep and superficial anatomic structures. The effect of this technology on spine surgery in the future has yet to be determined.

Reconstructive Options

After a spinal tumor is resected, whether utilizing freehand techniques, fluoroscopy guidance, navigation, or with robotics assistance, the subsequent reconstruction presents its own challenges. Perhaps the most pertinent example is in the case of sacrectomy, where reconstruction varies from minimal bony reconstruction to allograft (and even radiated autograft) to state-of-the-art 3D printed customized implants.

The chosen reconstruction plan depends on numerous factors. Surgeons are forced to think through both how long a patient might live and what function they may need. A patient with a radiated surgical bed and widespread, untreatable metastatic disease may require surgery to decompress and stabilize the spine without increasing OR time and risk with extra efforts to optimize chance of long-term bony fusion. However, an active patient with an isolated primary spinal tumor that undergoes en bloc resection in a radiated surgical bed may require a vascularized graft to optimize chances of fusion. Understanding the patient's needs is paramount, as is understanding the current state of the art for each tumor type; a multidisciplinary tumor board is critical.

For tumors of the mobile spine, reconstructive options also involve a discussion as to whether creating an environment for bony fusion is possible or whether the conditions of the resection or the patient require a reconstruction where fusion is not expected. In these cases, the construct must be placed with the expectation that either it will remain structurally sound for the remainder of the patient's lifespan, or that revision is possible in the future. For example, we recently performed a multilevel corpectomy on a young, healthy 26-year-old male who was almost 7 feet tall. He presented with a destructive spinal coccidiodomycoses (Fig. 21.6). In this case, the patient was

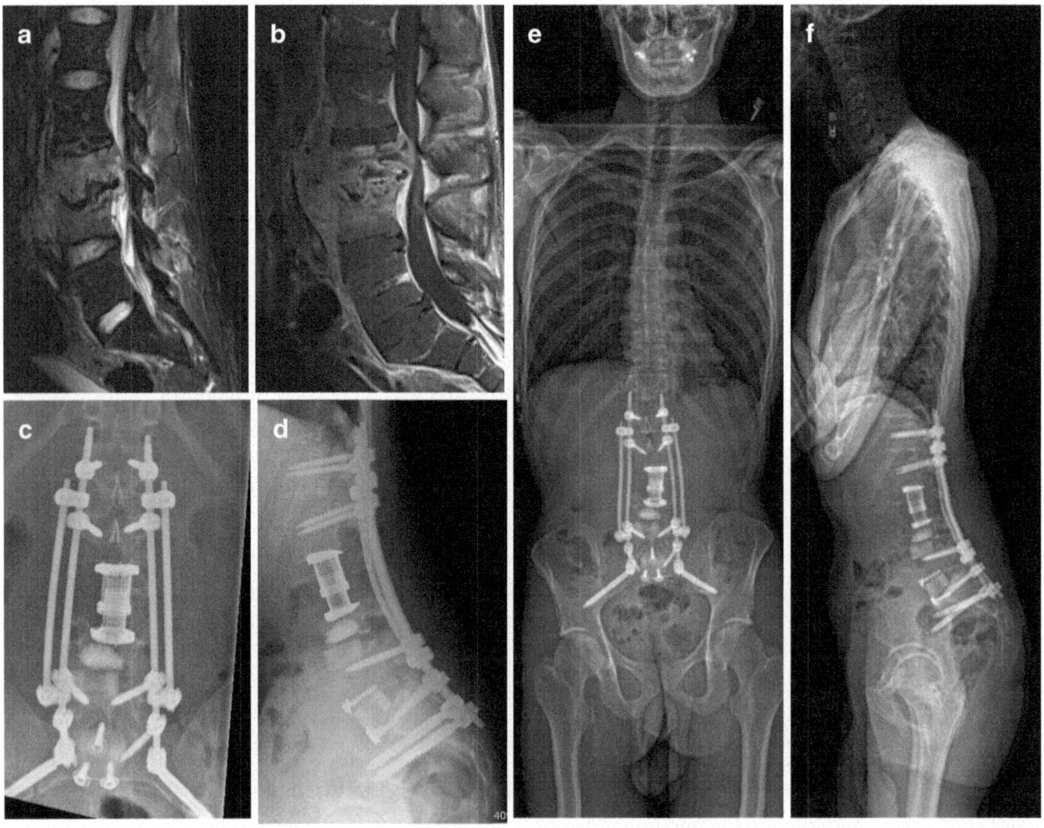

Fig. 21.6 (**a**) T2 and (**b**) postcontrast sagittal MRI demonstrating extensive destruction by a disc-preserving infection, raising suspicion for tuberculosis (TB) vs fungus. The patient had a history of work in a warehouse in Arizona and eventually was discovered to have coccidioidomycosis. Postoperative AP and lateral lumbar films (**c**, **d**) and scoliosis films (**e**, **f**) are shown. Note mild artifact in scoliosis film as they had to be stitched due to patient height. Note quad-rod construct and large, femoral allografts for interbodies at L4/5 and L5/1

young, fit, and active. We were very concerned about the potential for pseudarthrosis and failure after placing a long construct. In this case, the patient had destruction of L3 and part of L4 with soft tissue tracking under the anterior longitudinal ligament that progressed down to the L4/5 disc space with changes visible in the disc on T2 imaging. Beyond the immediate concerns of relieving pressure on nerves and removing infection burden, we were concerned both about having a large or long enough graft/implant, and about his prospects of long-term bony healing. We opted to leave part of L4 that was not affected and place an expandable cage from L2–4. We then performed a discectomy and placed allograft at L4/5. This allowed us to use a shorter implant, preserve some bone stock, and increased our chance of long-term stability. Finally, we had concerns for his long-term prospects at the L5/1 level, since he was young, active, and as noted, almost 7 feet tall. We discussed this at length with the patient and gave him the option of undergoing an L5/1 ALIF, while in the hospital, which he elected to have done (Fig. 21.6).

More traditionally, reconstruction in the spine proceeds with cages, bone graft, and/or cement as needed. For patients with metastatic disease undergoing radiation, reconstruction often does not require long-term bony fusion, and cement may serve as an excellent reconstruction option [37]. However, in patients with improved prognoses, attempts should be made to allow for long-term stability and bony fusion. Our preferred method is with a harms mesh cage with an allograft inside of the cage and augmentation with bone when possible (Fig. 21.7). Others recommend vascularized graft, which may offer the best chance of bony fusion.

In the sacrum, near-full or full sacrectomy remains the standard of care for a primary tumor of the sacrum that involves S1. Once the resection is completed, the surgeon is left to perform a spinopelvic reconstruction. Ideal reconstruction connects the spine to the pelvis, provides long-lasting fixation, and has some bony interface that allows the potential for fusion. Figure 21.8 shows reconstruction with allograft femur and bilateral fibular struts after a complete sacrectomy. This patient underwent radiation and is at risk of nonunion or fracture of graft. Note that pedicle screws were placed into the femoral graft and addition fibular struts were used to improve the bony interface between the spine and pelvis. In patients that undergo radiation pre- or postoperatively, concern for bony healing dominates many of the decisions. In the case of an irradiated field, some have advocated for vascularized autograft fibula. However, harvesting autograft can be morbid and time-consuming, lengthening time in the OR and thus slightly increasing risk of complications in an already lengthy procedure. Whenever possible, native bone in close approximation should be left to increase chance of fusion. For example, Fig. 21.5 shows a patient with a large sacral chondrosarcoma. She underwent sacrectomy, but it was decided to keep part of S1 as a bony bridge between the spine and pelvis, obfuscating the need for more complex reconstruction and decreasing risk of nonunion and hardware failure significantly. In contrast, Fig. 21.9 shows a patient who underwent revision of occipitocervical fusion for broken rods over 1 year out from high cervical chordoma resection with negative margins and no recurrence. The index case was complicated by infection, removal of graft, radiation, and multiple surgeries. In this case, the decision was made after long discussions with the patient to use bone morphogenetic protein (BMP) to aid in our attempts for bony fusion. Given the amount of data that have emerged demonstrating little to no impact of BMP on cancer risk (despite early flawed reports) [38], the patient was well informed and elected to have BMP as part of his procedure (and anything else we could use that could increase the chance of a bony fusion). Figure 21.9 shows our revision construct. He remained cancer free in follow-up.

In some cases, benign lesions erode bone and require intervention ("benign aggressive" lesions). A common example in the sacrum is a vascular malformation that grows and erodes the bone. In these cases, curetting out the lesion should involve preserving bony surfaces that may allow for fusion. For example, Fig. 21.10 shows a patient with erosive and growing benign arteriovenous malformation (AVM) of the sacrum. This lesion was curetted out and she underwent reconstruction. However, care was taken to preserve some S1 endplate and the L5/S1 facet bone, which allowed for fusion across these.

Custom 3D-printed implants can be used for reconstruction, although the dimensions of the implant are premade, making intraoperative adjustments difficult [8, 39]. Further, cost may discourage many from this option. While a 3D implant may not necessarily allow bony fusion *per se* (for example in complete sacrectomy), there is a reliance on the implant to remain fixed and stable over many years, anchored in what is often compromised bone. Custom 3D printing may also be used in the creation of a model of the tumor and/or printing of cutting guides/jigs to achieve desired osteotomies [7]. Even without custom guides or even navigation, a preoperative 3D-printed model of the tumor and surrounding a bony structure may greatly aid the surgeon in planning osteotomies and resection [7, 9].

These reconstructive options are not available everywhere, and out of this grew the radical idea

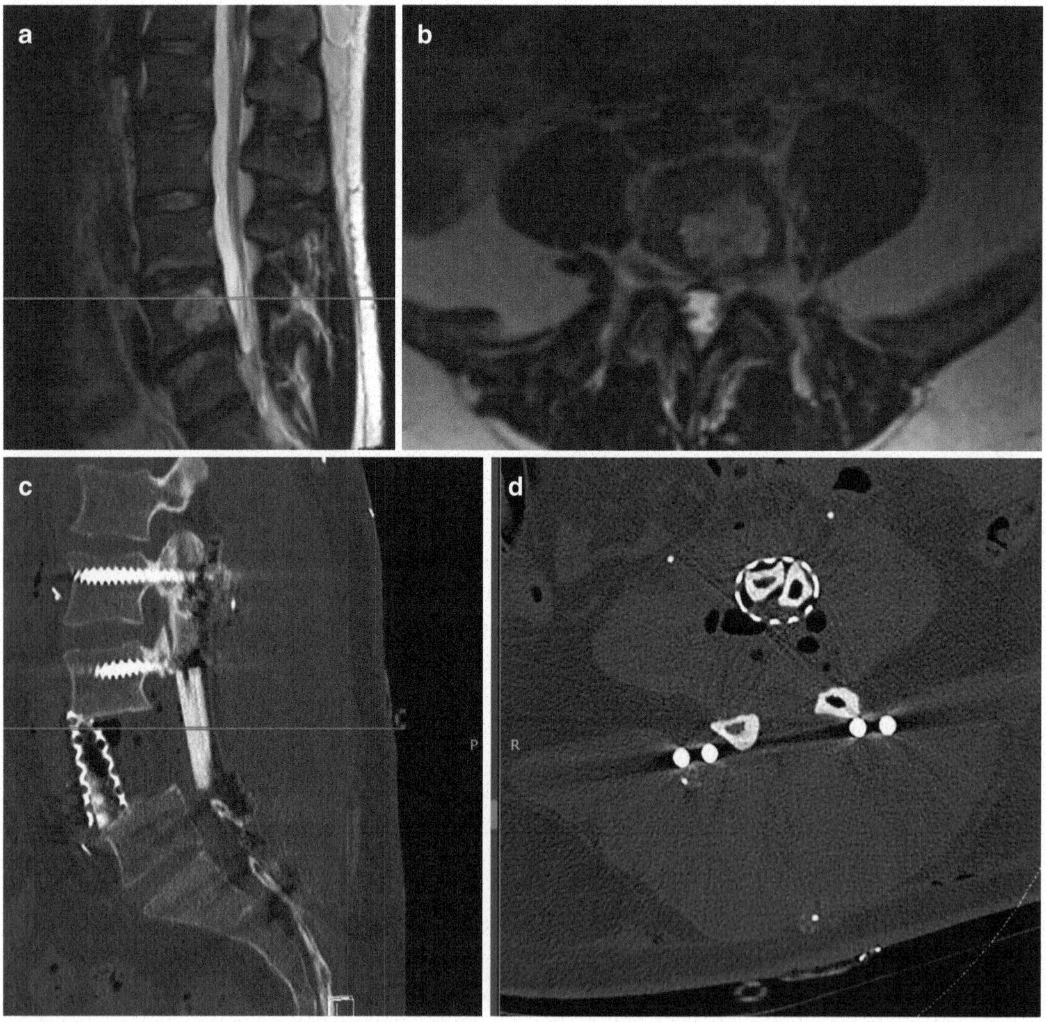

Fig. 21.7 (**a**) T2 sagittal and (**b**) T2 axial MRI demonstrating a chordoma in L4. After instrumenting L2-pelvis from a posterior approach, freeing up above and below L4 during stage 1, we then performed an anterior approach, tumor resection and placement of harms mesh cage with allograft bone inside. Postop CT shown in (**c, d**). Note allograft struts both in the mesh cage and posteriorly. (**e**) Posterior view after stage 1. (**f**) Pathology specimen, with containment within the vertebral body. (**g**) Final construct AP radiograph

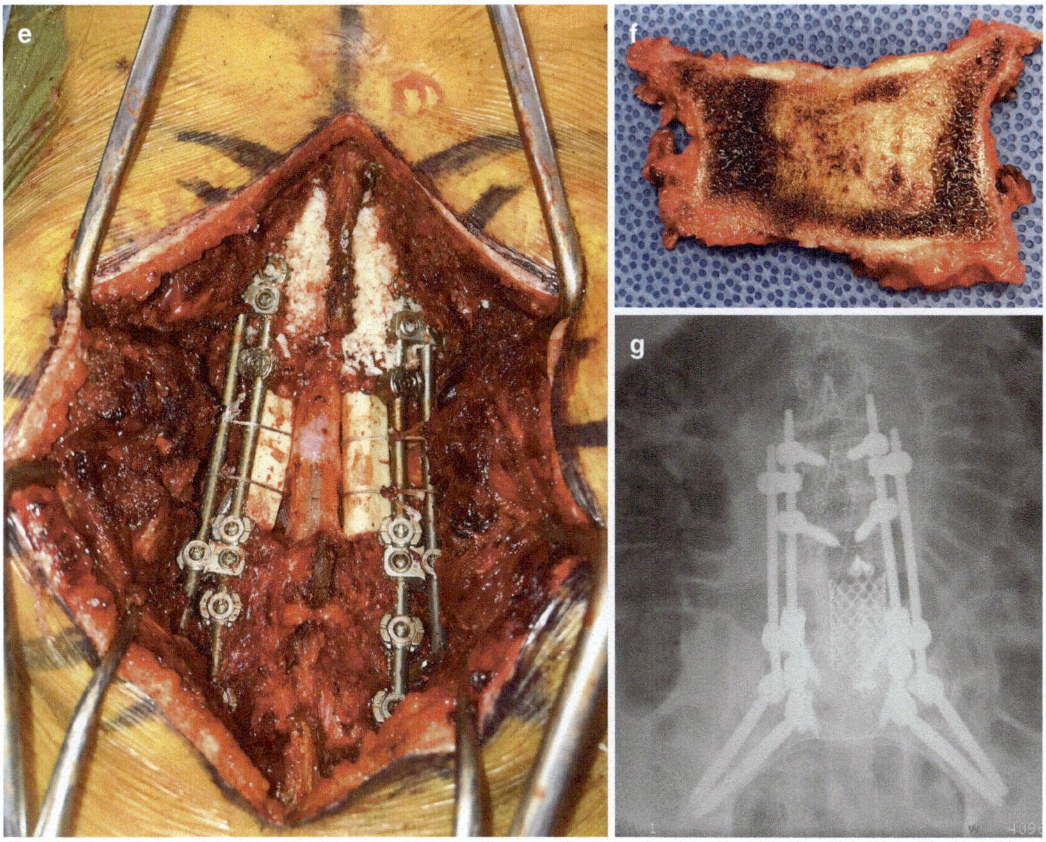

Fig. 21.7 (continued)

that tumor-ridden bone might be removed en bloc, irradiated, and placed back in as a perfectly matched, exact-fitting graft. For example, some cultures in Asia and Africa forbid use of allograft yet cannot afford 3D-printed options. There is also a nonzero rate of disease transmission in using allograft, and maintaining a bone bank for allograft often is not feasible in many countries [40–47]. In 1968, the first "extracorporeal radiation therapy" (ECRT) reconstruction was performed. Remarkably, this method has been only sporadically utilized in the ensuing years [48]. In short, to circumvent the complications with traditional reconstruction when resection of the sacrum is required, the sacrum can be removed en bloc, sent to receive 1 dose of radiation therapy at ~50 Gy, then returned to the OR and implanted into the patient after curetting out the dead tumor cells and cementing the defect (Figs. 21.11 and 21.12). There is good evidence that no live tumor cells remain, and as secondary confirmation of this, recurrence rates with this technique are not higher [49]. The dose of radiation for this procedure should be around 50 Gy, as this is high enough to kill all living cancer cells and yet low enough as to not significantly damage the bone structure [48, 50–56]. There has been recent interest in the reason for high failure rates of allograft bone in these cases [43, 57]; one proposed mechanism is that the allograft bone retains nonmatched MHCs. If this immune-mediated mechanism is correct, using ECRT circumvents this. Further, radiation for ECRT (~50Gy) is high enough to kill all viable cells, yet much lower than traditional allografts (~1000 Gy) and well below the level of irradiation where weakening of the bone is seen (~300 Gy) [55]. While currently not approved in the US, ECRT for reconstruction of tumors of the sacrum remains an appealing, cost-efficient, and effective procedure.

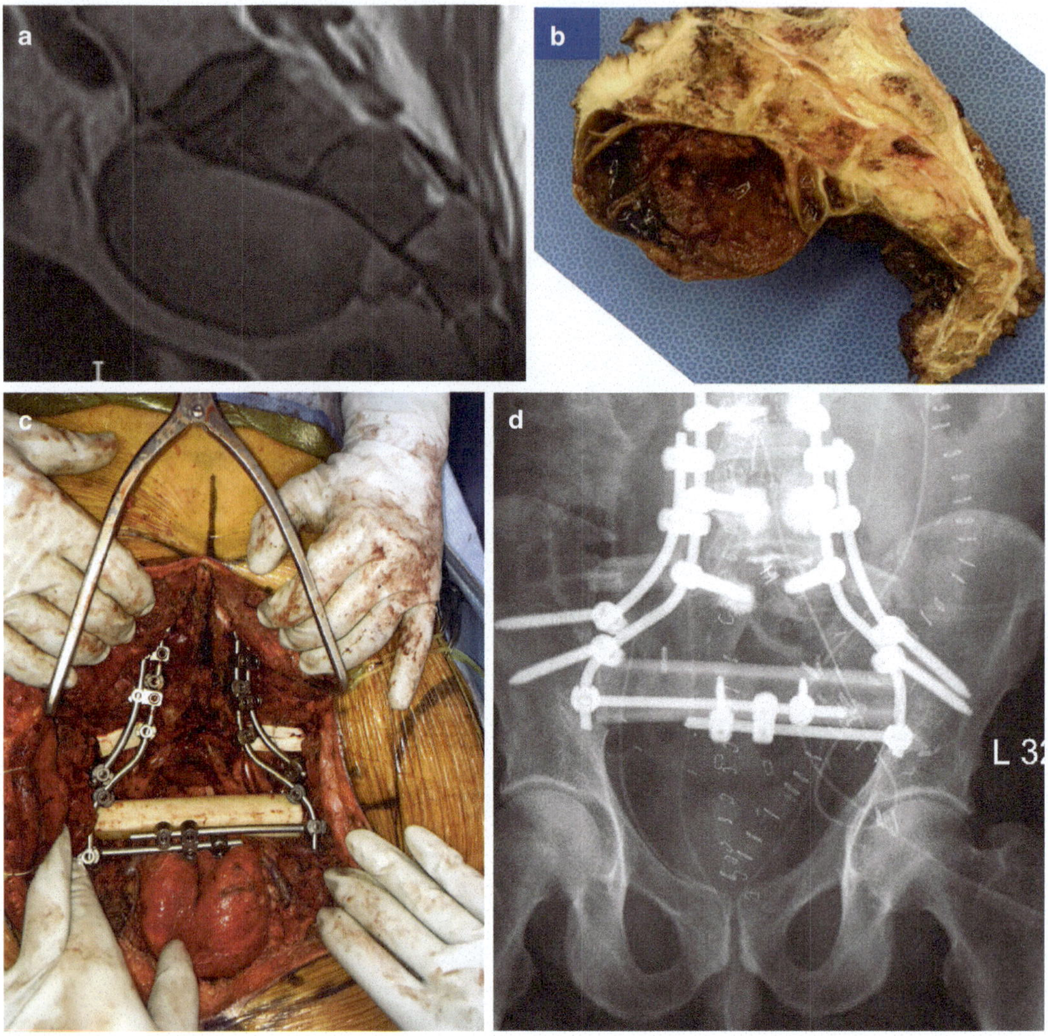

Fig. 21.8 (**a**) MRI and (**b**) final specimen of a large chordoma that required a full sacrectomy. This was done via a staged front-back procedure. Final posterior construct shown in **c** with final radiograph shown in **d**. Note the femoral allograft as well as fibular struts placed between L5 and pelvis

Conclusions and Future Directions

There are many options currently available to aid the spine tumor surgeon in the operating room, from fluoroscopy to robot assistance. In the future there are likely to be even more options. While innovations in technology that augment the surgeon's skills should continually be integrated into practice, care must be taken to ensure that surgeons are integrating these safely. Implementing a new technology that unreasonably lengthens a procedure, has not been demonstrated to be safe and reliable, or does not improve outcomes is an ethical problem which should be avoided. Further, all surgeons should strive to continue teaching anatomy and freehand techniques along with new technology. When new technology errs, it is reliance on these fundamentals that ideally allows recognition of the error in a timely manner, minimizing or avoidng harm to the patient.

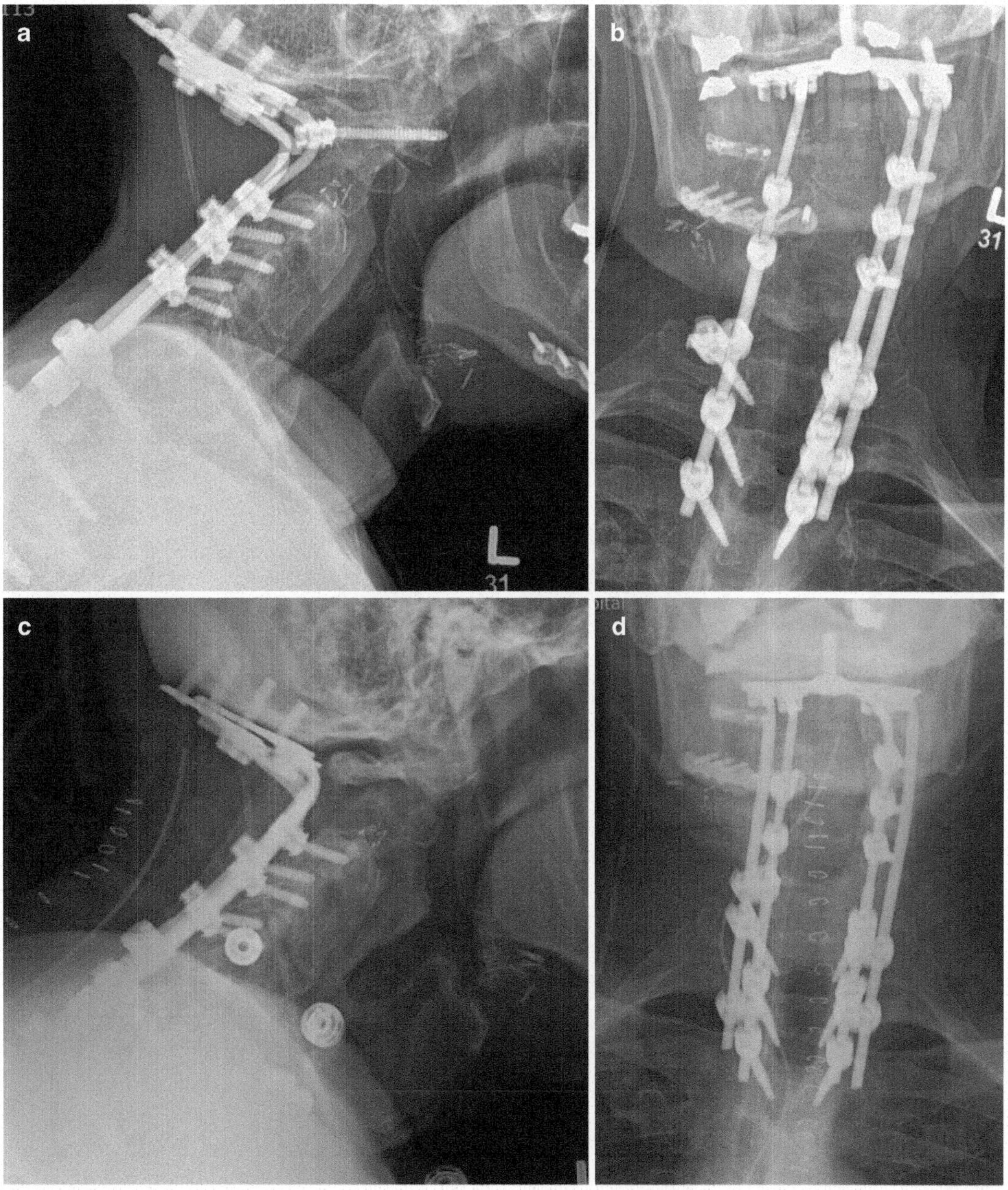

Fig. 21.9 Patient with broken rod at O–C junction (**a**, **b**) over 1 year out from chordoma resection with negative margins and no recurrence. After multiple surgeries, the decision was made to use BMP in addition to our revision construct (**c**, **d**)

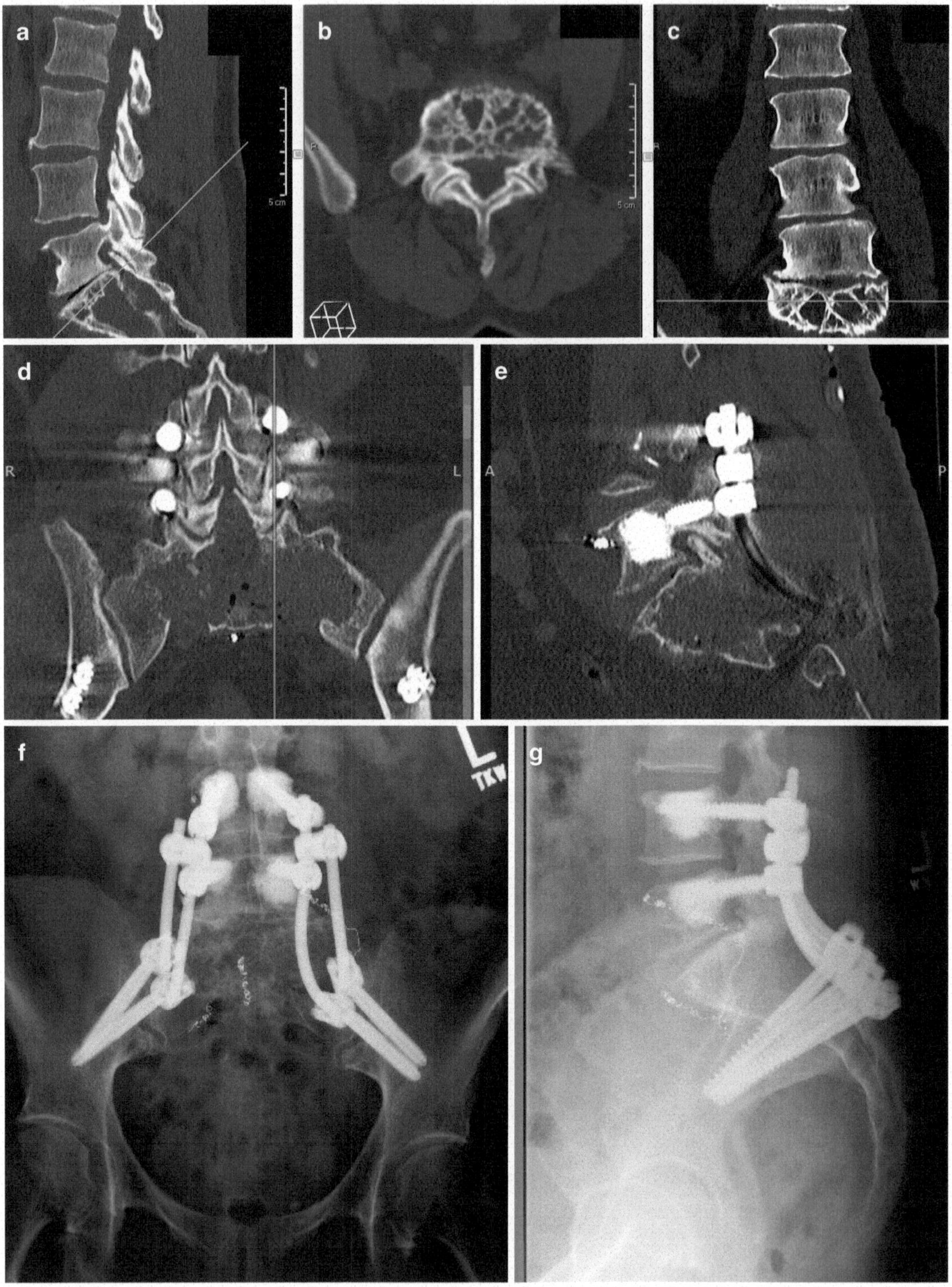

Fig. 21.10 Sagittal (**a**), axial (**b**), and coronal (**d**) images showing expansile destructive lesion of sacrum. Images reveal the classic "honey-comb" type pattern and multiple nondiagnostic biopsies revealed only vascularity and bone, eventually leading to a diagnosis of AVM (**d–g**) Final L4-pelvis construct after curettage and placement of short, quad-rod construct with cemented screws. Note how the L5/S1 joint was left intact and drilled out to aid in bony fusion

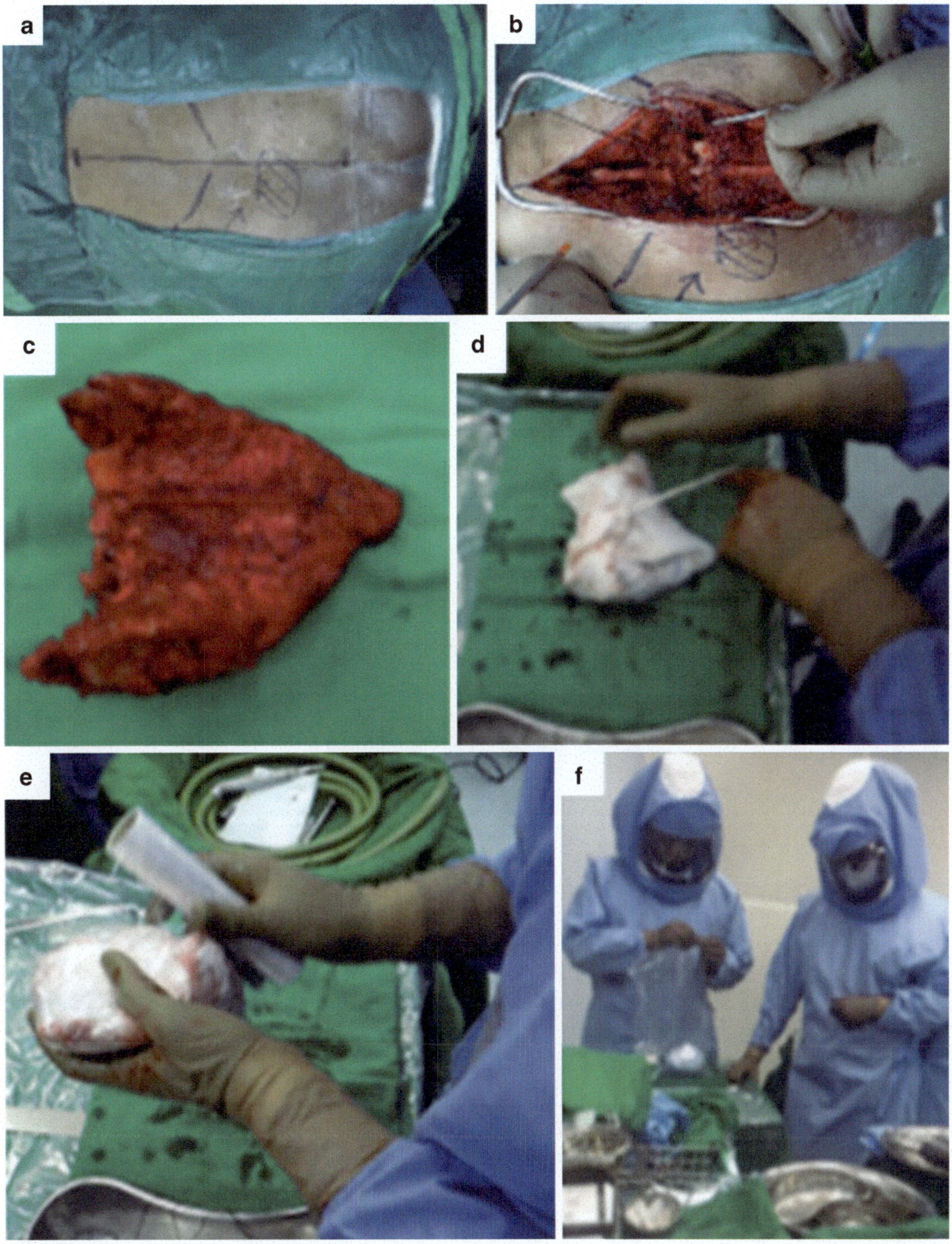

Fig. 21.11 Extracorporeal radiation therapy (ECRT) and reimplantation of sacral tumor. (**a**) shows the process of removing the sacrum (**a**–**c**) and packaging it to be sent to get irradiated (**d**–**g**)

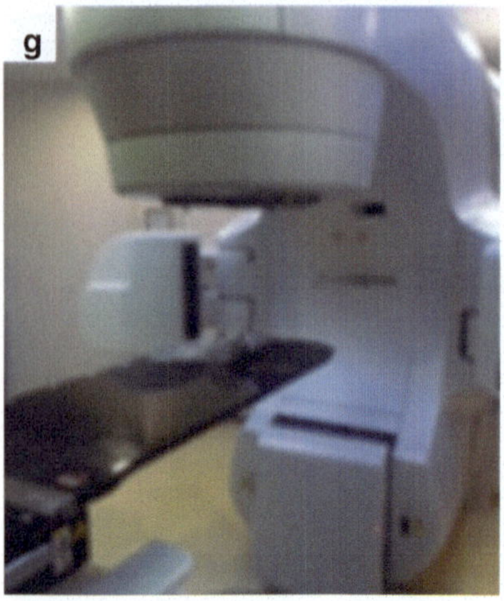

Fig. 21.11 (continued)

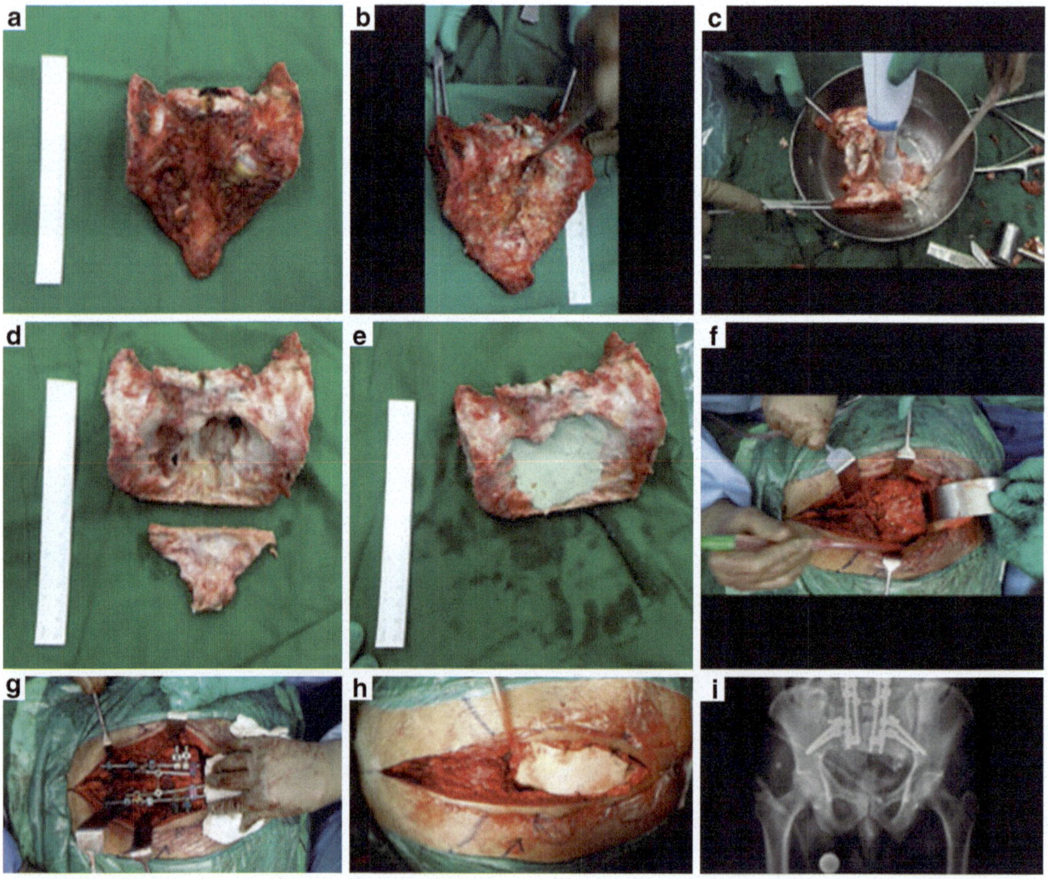

Fig. 21.12 Extracorporeal radiation therapy (ECRT) and reimplantation of sacral tumor. On return from radiation (**a**), dead tumor is curetted out (**b**), the specimen is washed (**c**), nonstructural inferior sacrum and coccyx are removed (**d**), cement is packed into the defect (**e**), and the bone is reimplanted as a perfectly matched, nonreactive graft (**f–i**). (Reproduced here with permission from Goodwin et al. [48])

References

1. Roentgen WC. On a new kind of ray (first report). Munch Med Wochenschr. 1959;101:1237–9.
2. Nasser R, Drazin D, Nakhla J, Al-Khouja L, Brien E, Baron EM, et al. Resection of spinal column tumors utilizing image-guided navigation: a multicenter analysis. Neurosurg Focus. 2016;41(2):E15.
3. Kaissar F, Coudert P, Graillon T, Blondel B, Dufour H, Gille O, et al. Prospective comparative study in spine surgery between O-arm and Airo systems: efficacy and radiation exposure. World Neurosurg. 2018;118:e175–84.
4. Pennington Z, Cottrill E, Westbroek EM, Goodwin ML, Lubelski D, Ahmed AK, et al. Evaluation of surgeon and patient radiation exposure by imaging technology in patients undergoing thoracolumbar fusion: systematic review of the literature. Spine J. 2019;19(8):1397–411.
5. Singer G. Occupational radiation exposure to the surgeon. J Am Acad Orthop Surg. 2005;13(1):69–76.
6. Kelly PD, Zuckerman SL, Yamada Y, Lis E, Bilsky MH, Laufer I, et al. Image guidance in spine tumor surgery. Neurosurg Rev. 2020;43(3):1007–17.
7. Ozturk AM, Ozer MA, Suer O, Derin O, Govsa F. Patient-specific three-dimensional model for a safe surgical pathway in sacral chondrosarcoma. Indian J Surg Oncol. 2019;10(1):107.
8. Wei R, Guo W, Ji T, Zhang Y, Liang H. One-step reconstruction with a 3D-printed, custom-made prosthesis after total en bloc sacrectomy: a technical note. Eur Spine J. 2017;26(7):1902–9.
9. Sayari AJ, Pardo C, Basques BA, Colman MW. Review of robotic-assisted surgery : what the future looks like through a spine oncology lens. Ann Transl Med. 2019;7(10):1–10.
10. Zhang J, Weir V, Fajardo L, Lin J, Hsiung H, Ritenour ER. Dosimetric characterization of a cone-beam O-arm imaging system. J Xray Sci Technol. 2009;17(4):305–17.
11. Hlubek RJ, Bohl MA, Cole TS, Morgan CD, Xu DS, Chang SW, et al. Safety and accuracy of freehand versus navigated C2 pars or pedicle screw placement. Spine J. 2018;18(8):1374–81.
12. Andrade NS, Okafor L, Neuman BJ. Novel technique for sacral alar-iliac (S2AI) fixation. Clin Spine Surg. 2018;31(9):373–6.
13. Mulconrey D. P10. Fluoroscopic radiation exposure in degenerative spinal surgery: in vivo evaluation for operating room personnel. Spine J. 2009;9(10):118S.
14. Villard J, Ryang YM, Demetriades AK, Reinke A, Behr M, Preuss A, et al. Radiation exposure to the surgeon and the patient during posterior lumbar spinal instrumentation: a prospective randomized comparison of navigated versus non-navigated freehand techniques. Spine (Phila Pa 1976). 2014;39(13):1004–9.
15. Xu R, Ebraheim NA, Ou Y, Yeasting RA. Anatomic considerationsof pedicle screw placement in the thoracic spine. Roy-Camille technique versus open-lamina technique. Spine (Phila Pa 1976). 1998;23:1065–8.
16. Liljenqvist UR, Halm HF, Link TM. Pedicle screw instrumentation of the thoracic spine in idiopathic scoliosis. Spine (Phila Pa 1976). 1997;22:2239–45.
17. Weinstein JN, Spratt KF, Spengler D, Brick C, Reid S. Spinal pedicle fixation: reliability and validity of roentgenogram-based assessment and surgical factors on successful screw placement. Spine (Phila Pa 1976). 1988;13:1012–8.
18. Madaelil TP, Long JR, Wallace AN, Baker JC, Ray WZ, Santiago P, et al. Preoperative fiducial marker placement in the thoracic spine: a technical report. Spine. 2017;42(10):E624–8.
19. Kim S, Kazanzides P. Fiducial-based registration with a touchable region model. Int J Comput Assist Radiol Surg. 2017;12:277–89.
20. Overley SC, Cho SK, Mehta AI, Arnold PM. Navigation and robotics in spinal surgery : where are we now? Neurosurgery. 2017;80(3):S86–99.
21. Molina CA, Theodore N, Ahmed AK, Westbroek EM, Mirovsky Y, Harel R, et al. Augmented reality–assisted pedicle screw insertion: a cadaveric proof-of-concept study. J Neurosurg Spine. 2019;29:1–8.
22. Amis ES, Butler PF, Applegate KE, Birnbaum SB, Brateman LF, Hevezi JM, et al. American College of Radiology White Paper on radiation dose in medicine. J Am Coll Radiol. 2007;4(5):272–84.
23. Sinclair WK. Radiation protection: the NCRP guidelines and some considerations for the future. Yale J Biol Med. 1981;54(6):471–84.
24. Rehani MM, Ciraj-Bjelac O, Vañó E, Miller DL, Walsh S, Giordano BD, et al. Radiological protection in fluoroscopically guided procedures performed outside the imaging department. Ann ICRP. 2010;40(6):5–6.
25. Lin EC. Radiation risk from medical imaging. Mayo Clin Proc. 2010;85(12):1142–6.
26. ICRP Publication 105. Radiation protection in medicine. Ann ICRP. 2007;37(6):1–63.
27. Do KH. General principles of radiation protection in fields of diagnostic medical exposure. J Korean Med Sci. 2016;31:S6–9.
28. Amis ES, Butler PF. ACR white paper on radiation dose in medicine: three years later. J Am Coll Radiol. 2010;7(11):865–70.
29. Han X, Tian W, Liu Y, Liu B, He D, Sun Y, et al. Safety and accuracy of robot-assisted versus fluoroscopy-assisted pedicle screw insertion in thoracolumbar spinal surgery: a prospective randomized controlled trial. J Neurosurg Spine. 2019;30(5):615–22.
30. Solomiichuk V, Fleischhammer J, Molliqaj G, Warda J, Alaid A, von Eckardstein K, et al. Robotic versus fluoroscopy-guided pedicle screw insertion for metastatic spinal disease: a matched-cohort comparison. Neurosurg Focus. 2017;42(5):E13.
31. Hu X, Scharschmidt TJ, Ohnmeiss DD, Lieberman IH. Robotic assisted surgeries for the treatment of spine tumors. Int J Spine Surg. 2015;9:1.
32. Oh JK, Yang MS, Yoon DH, Rha KH, Kim KN, Yi S, et al. Robotic resection of huge presacral tumors. J Spinal Disord Tech. 2014;27(4):E151–4.

33. Bederman SS, Lopez G, Ji T, Hoang BH. Robotic guidance for en bloc sacrectomy. Spine (Phila Pa 1976). 2014;39(23):E1398–401.
34. Pacchiarotti G, Wang MY, Kolcun JPG, Chang KH, Al Maaieh M, Reis VS, et al. Robotic paravertebral schwannoma resection at extreme locations of the thoracic cavity. Neurosurg Focus. 2017;42(5):E17.
35. Yang MS, Kim KN, Yoon DH, Pennant W, Ha Y. Robot-assisted resection of paraspinal schwannoma. J Korean Med Sci. 2011;26(1):150–3.
36. Sheetz KH, Dimick JB. Is it time for safeguards in the adoption of robotic surgery? JAMA J Am Med Assoc. 2019;321(20):1971–2.
37. Jordan Y, Buchowski JM, Mokkarala M, Peters C, Bumpass DB. Outcomes and cost-minimization analysis of cement spacers versus expandable cages for posterior-only reconstruction of metastatic spine corpectomies. Ann Transl Med. 2019;7(10):212.
38. Dettori JR, Chapman JR, DeVine JG, McGuire RA, Junge MR, Norvell DC. Longer follow-up continues to reveal no increased risk of cancer with the use of recombinant human bone morphogenetic protein in spine fusion. Spine J. 2019;19(10):1640–7.
39. Wuisman P, Lieshout O, Sugihara S, van Dijk M. Total sacrectomy and reconstruction: oncologic and functional outcome. Clin Orthop Relat Res. 2000;381:192–203.
40. Zhang S, Wang X, Wang J, Xu M. En bloc resection, intraoperative extracorporeal irradiation and re-implantation of involved bone for the treatment of limb malignancies. Mol Clin Oncol. 2017;7(6):1045–52.
41. Araki N, Myoui A, Kuratsu S, Hashimoto N, Inoue T, Kudawara I, et al. Intraoperative extracorporeal autogenous irradiated bone grafts in tumor surgery. Clin Orthop Relat Res. 1999;368:196–206.
42. Hamer A, Strachan J, Black M, Ibbotson C, Stockley I, Elson R. Biomechanical properties of cortical allograft bone using a new method of bone strength measurement. J Bone Joint Surg Br. 1996;78:363–8.
43. Mankin HJ, Hornicek FJ, Raskin KA. Infection in massive bone allografts. Clin Orthop Relat Res. 2005;432:210–6.
44. Matejovsky Z, Matejovsky Z, Kofranek I. Massive allografts in tumour surgery. Int Orthop. 2006;30(6):478–83.
45. Tomford WW. Transmission of disease through transplantation of musculoskeletal allografts. J Bone Joint Surg Ser A. 1995;77(11):1742–54.
46. Yasin NF, Singh VA, Saad M, Omar E. Which is the best method of sterilization for recycled bone autograft in limb salvage surgery: a radiological, biomechanical and histopathological study in rabbit. BMC Cancer. 2015;15(1):1–11.
47. Tomford WW, Mankin HJ. Bone banking: update on methods and materials. Orthop Clin North Am. 1999;30(4):565–70.
48. Goodwin ML, Gundavda MK, Reddy R, Deogaonkar K, Lala M, Baliarsing A, et al. Extracorporeal radiation and reimplantation: a safe and viable option for reconstruction after sacral tumor resection? Ann Transl Med. 2019;7(10):229.
49. Hatano H, Ogose A, Hotta T, Endo N, Umezu H, Morris T. Extracorporeal irradiated autogenous osteochondral graft. J Bone Joint Surg Br. 2005;87:1006–11.
50. Wu P-K, Chen C-F, Chen C-M, Cheng Y-C, Tsai S-W, Chen T-H, et al. Intraoperative extracorporeal irradiation and frozen treatment on tumor-bearing autografts show equivalent outcomes for biologic reconstruction. Clin Orthop Relat Res. 2018;476(4):877–89.
51. Agarwal M, Gundavda M, Gupta R, Reddy R. Does extracorporeal irradiation and reimplantation after acetabular resections result in adequate hip function? A preliminary report. Clin Orthop Relat Res. 2018;476(9):1738–48.
52. Kotb SZ, Mostafa MF. Recycling of extracorporeally irradiated autograft for malignant bone tumors: long-term follow-up. Ann Plast Surg. 2013;71(5):493–9.
53. Sanjay BK, Moreau PG, Younge DA. Reimplantation of autoclaved tumour bone in limb salvage surgery. Int Orthop. 1997;21(5):291–7.
54. Davidson AW. En-bloc resection, extracorporeal irradiation, and re-implantation in limb salvage for bony malignancies. J Bone Joint Surg Br Vol. 2005;87-B(6):851–7.
55. Sabo D, Brocai DRC, Eble M, Wannenmacher M, Ewerbeck V. Influence of extracorporeal irradiation on the reintegration of autologous grafts of bone. J bone Joint Surg. 2000;82–B(1):276–82.
56. Currey J, Foreman J, Laketic I, Mitchell J, Pegg D, Reilly G. Effects of ionizing radiation on the mechanical properties of human bone. Clin Orthop Relat Res. 1997;15:111–7.
57. Lietman SA, Tomford WW, Gebhardt MC, Springfieldand DS, Mankin HJ. Complications of irradiated allografts in orthopaedic tumor surgery. Clin Orthop Relat Res. 2000;375:214–7.

22 Spine Tumors: Technological Advances

Arash J. Sayari, Matthew Colman, and Kern Singh

Introduction

While technological advancements within spinal tumor surgery are vast, they should all serve to support the fundamental goals of the spine oncologist: to obtain tumor control, and to optimize the neurologic and mechanical stability of the spine. With recent advances in technology, it is becoming more feasible to achieve these goals in a wider array of patients. Continuous improvements and new prototypes create paradigm shifts in multiple facets of spine tumor resection. Some of these avenues of improvement include enhanced navigation during surgery, minimally invasive access to targeted sites, more efficient and less ionizing imaging techniques, and the employment of artificial intelligence [1]. Compared to traditional methods in spine surgery, the increased use of fluorescence-guided surgery and the use of machine learning and artificial intelligence have all demonstrated great potential. The following chapter details technological advances that are promising to improve results in the pre-, intra-, and postoperative surgical arenas.

A. J. Sayari · M. Colman · K. Singh (✉)
Department of Orthopaedic Surgery, Rush University Medical Center, Chicago, IL, USA
e-mail: kern.singh@rushortho.com

K. Singh, M. Colman (eds.), *Surgical Spinal Oncology*,
https://doi.org/10.1007/978-3-030-50722-0_22

Three-Dimensional (3D) Technology

Surgical Planning

Using specific design files and increasing the availability of advanced industrial printers have allowed for an expansion of 3D printing (3DP) into the spine and spine tumor arena. CT and MRI alone are often inadequate, but using such imaging software, 3D templating can be implemented as a tool for surgical planning. Specifically, preoperative imaging can be combined to print an exact replica of a patient's anatomy that can be closely analyzed and scrutinized prior to surgery, termed biomodeling [2, 3]. By visualizing pathologic morphology, surgical simulation of complex anatomy allows for accurate planning and execution of spinal surgery. In addition to patient education, models can be sterilized and used intraoperatively for direct surgical reference of bony loss, tumor mass involvement, and adjacent neurovascular structures (Fig. 22.1a–d) [4].

Various applications of patient-specific models have demonstrated successful utility as well. For example, in cases of periacetabular metastases, a 3D-printed biomodel optimized the surgical incision, and reduced operative time owing to more accurate and predictable navigation of the anatomy, inherently minimizing blood loss [5]. Similarly, 3D models have proven their usefulness in complex spinal reconstructive procedures,

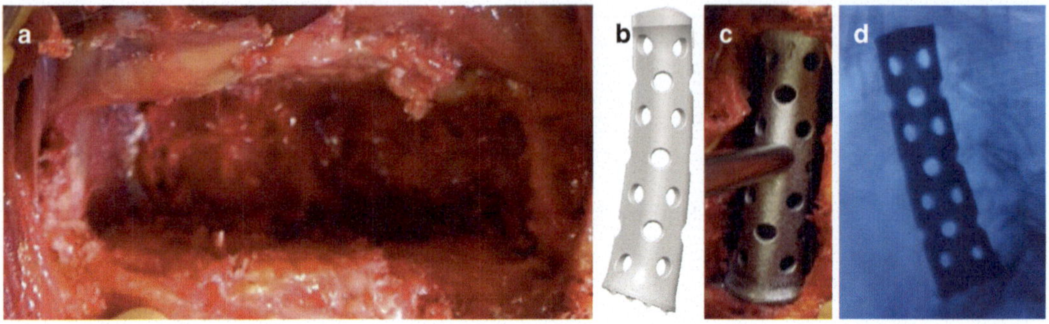

Fig. 22.1 (**a**) Cervical osteotomy site was prepared, (**b**) implant was printed, (**c**) insertion, and (**d**) lateral X-ray to confirm positioning

as explained by Mao et al., who used 3D polystyrene models to assist with instrumentation and successful improvement of coronal and sagittal parameters [6, 7]. Xiao et al. evaluated five patients with malignant tumors of the cervical spine (three with chondrosarcomas, two with chordomas), who underwent en bloc resection with the assistance of 3D models, reporting improved understanding of relationships between normal and pathologic anatomy [8]. Similarly, in 2015, a model was used by Kim et al. to improve surgical planning for en bloc removal of two cases of primary malignant tumors of the thoracic spine [9].

Despite the benefits of 3D modeling in surgical planning, increased costs and delays in production are major deterrents to its use, which can necessitate costs over $1000 and delays of several days [7]. Aside from the improved stereotaxy offered by intraoperative use of 3D-printed models, patients are easily educated with models and they are expected to be more frequently incorporated in the clinical setting as the visual and tactile component lends itself unique and more useful when compared to computer-generated and digital models.

Surgical Guides

Because the spine poses challenging anatomy that is only further clouded by tumors that skew adjacent structures, surgical guides have been implemented to dampen such challenges. 3D guides lend a more unique avenue for tumor excision, reconstruction, and fixation.

Pedicle screw fixation has paved the way in this arena and has been well demonstrated in the literature. In particular, considerations have been made to use 3D-printed templates for pedicle screw placement in an attempt to reduce operative time, complications, and radiation dosing, while improving accuracy [10–13]. Otsuki et al. evaluated custom screw insertion guides in three patients undergoing revision cervical spine surgery with skewed anatomy, with postoperative CT scans demonstrating successful placement of instrumentation [14]. Lin et al. used 3D technology to engineer an osteotomy cutting guide. This enabled them to successfully resect a sacral schwannoma in a 23-year-old female [15]. Using preoperative CT imaging, an osteotomy block was created to mount to the mid-sacrum and safely assist in removing the tumor. Unlike common iterations of robotics and navigation, patient-specific templates and guides are independent of patient positional changes that occur intraoperatively.

3D templates have been created using preoperative imaging to plan screw trajectories, though much of the success of additive technology has been overshadowed by robotics and navigation [16]. Though costs of single-use templates have decreased, such challenges may delay or limit the penetrance of individualized 3D-printed guides as a mainstay of spinal instrumentation.

Surgical Implants

The technology of 3DP has been implemented to create synergism between the increased interest in individualized delivery of medical care and successes of customized implants across various fields such as orthopedics, otolaryngology, and spine surgery [17–19]. 3DP is used to create off-the-shelf (OTS), as well as customized, implants. OTS implants are structurally useful and can be implemented as synthetic cages made from polyethyletherketone (PEEK) or titanium, for example. These implants are obviously less "personalized" though may offer useful components to improve ingrowth and ongrowth surfaces, namely in the cervical spine [20].

OTS implants, however, are not custom made for the patient, and factors around sizing and implantation do not have advantages over traditional mass produced implants (Fig. 22.2a–c). On the other hand, customized implants allow for full customization. Wei et al. used 3DP techniques to create a custom prosthesis to treat a sacral chordoma [21]. In their case, a single-stage en bloc sacrectomy was performed and a custom prosthesis was implanted. Though this was complicated by asymptomatic hardware failure at 1 year, the 3D technology highlighted useful avenues to further applications. Similarly, Kim et al. used 3DP to create a custom titanium hemisacrum for a sacral osteosarcoma, with CT at 1 year demonstrating arthrodesis [22].

The cervical spine has also seen implementation of 3DP technology (Fig. 22.3a–c). In a 12-year-old with a C2 Ewing sarcoma, a 3D-printed vertebral body was used for reconstruction during a staged spondylectomy [23]. In a separate report, a C1–C2 chordoma requiring resection and reconstruction was performed with the aid of 3D-printed implants, whereby the authors reported reduced operative time by avoiding the manual measuring and filling of defects with various graft options [24].

Finally, the thoracolumbar spine, a more frequent location of primary malignancies and metastases, has also been reported in conjunction with 3DP in the literature. In a 14-year-old with a primary T9 tumor and resultant kyphoscoliosis, a patient-specific 3D-printed titanium vertebral body with porous endplates was used not only to fill the defect but also to correct coronal and sagittal balance [25]. Mobbs et al. compared such customized implants to OTS implants in their report on a 64-year-old male with a primary tumor at L5, whereby following en bloc spondylectomy, the defect was filled with a custom-expandable cage, saving the surgeons over 26-fold time during implantation [17]. 3D printing has also demonstrated a role in anterior approaches, osteopenic fractures often encountered in diagnoses of spine tumors, and in the cervical spine [20, 26, 27].

One crucial factor inadequately discussed by most prior authors involves the consideration a surgeon must make to the increased time to production of custom implants. Whereas spine tumor surgery may often be performed on an elective basis, not all clinical situations lend themselves to planning a custom 3D-printed implant, as cord compression, tumor-related pain, or mechanical instability may warrant more urgent care. Increased costs of custom implants are another barrier to more frequent use. However, as the use of 3DP increases and more companies enter the market, costs and time to production are expected to decrease significantly. Furthermore, the implementation of 3D systems that include models, guides, and implants offers a synergistic approach and an exciting future.

Robotic Navigation/Haptics

At present, technological systems such as image guidance (IG), robotics, virtual reality, and augmented reality are becoming more heavily researched. Image guidance and robotic systems have become increasingly widespread as intraoperative enhancers during spinal surgery. Broadly, robotic surgical systems are classified into three major categories: [1] supervisory controlled, [2] telesurgical systems, and [3] shared-control systems [28]. Of these, shared-control systems, which allow for simultaneous control between

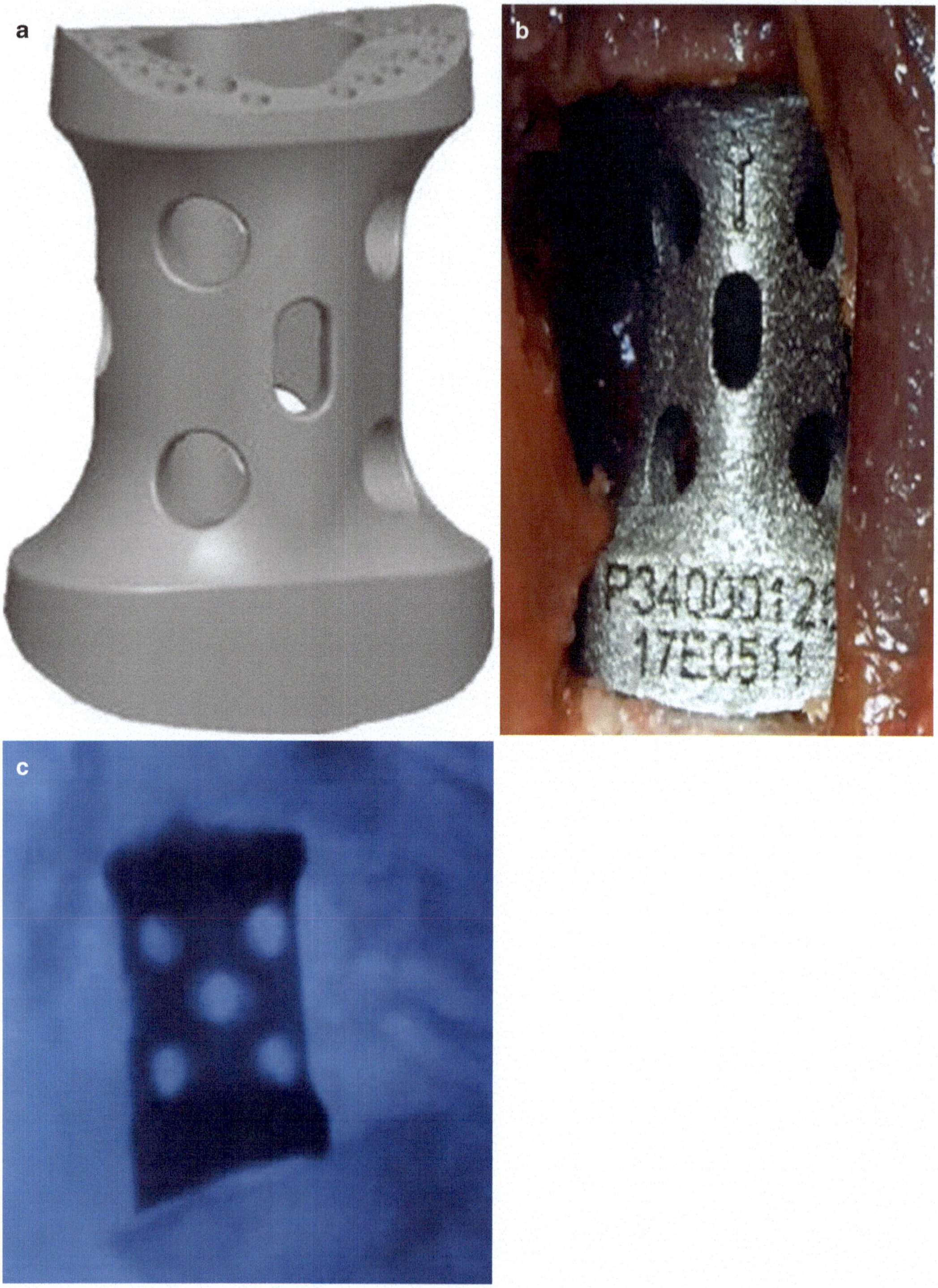

Fig. 22.2 (**a**) Implant, (**b**) insertion of implant, and (**c**) lateral X-ray for confirmation

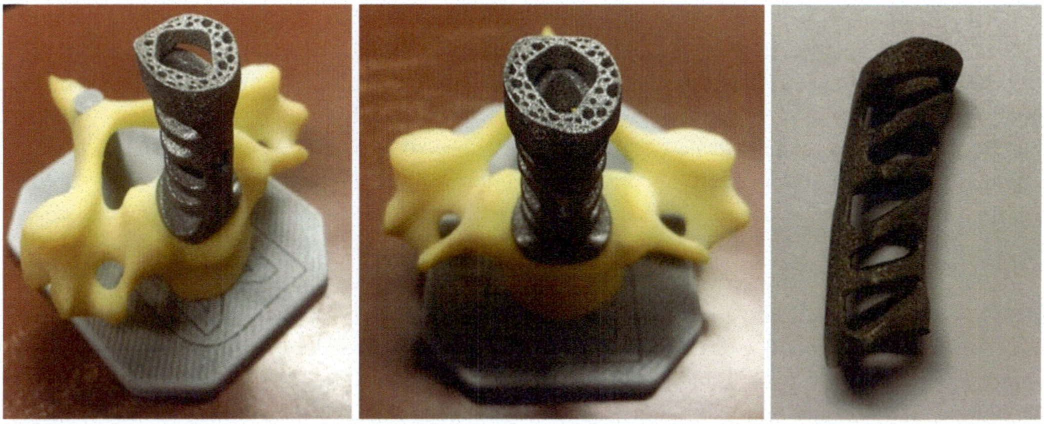

Fig. 22.3 Custom vertebral body replacement cage for two-level cervical vertebrectomy (not FDA approved, proof of concept only)

the surgeon and the robot, are currently the most widely applied and often used during pedicle screw placement [28]. A number of robotic systems have recently been established for use in spine surgery such as the Mazor (Medtronic, Minneapolis, MN, USA), Excelsius GPS (Globus Medical, Audubon, PA, USA), and ROSA Spine (MedTech Surgical, Newark, NJ, USA). Such systems are similar in their ability to assist the surgeon during instrumentation. However, they vary in their registration method, navigation capabilities, registration method, and mounting and setup [16].

The implications of robotic systems on long-term outcomes have yet to be fully determined, especially in the context of neurological injury and reoperation rate for malpositioned screws. A meta-analysis of 23 studies that included a total of 5992 pedicle screws failed to demonstrate statistically significant improvements with the use of IG despite an improved rate of accuracy [29]. Recently, a retrospective single-center clinical outcome analysis demonstrated that the use of multiplanar fluoroscopic-assisted navigation compared to freehand and/or fluoroscopic guidance for thoracolumbar fusion brought about significant decreases in malpositioned pedicle screws, hospital stays, spine-related readmission rates, and risk of hardware failure [30].

In treating spine tumors, robotics and navigation have been increasingly successful. Robotics has been used for precise resection guidance in cases of en bloc sacrectomies and presacral tumor excision, as well as paravertebral tumors [31–33]. Similarly, Hu et al. evaluated nine patients with spinal tumors and neural compression, using image guidance to map planned pedicle screw trajectories with success [34]. Increased precision and more minimally invasive approaches may allow for limited exposures that become relevant in hypervascular bone tumors such as metastatic renal cell and thyroid carcinomas.

Machine Learning/Artificial Intelligence

Current Best Evidence

In the modern operating room, machine learning and artificial intelligence have taken more control over functional systems. The primary purpose of artificial intelligence (AI) is to imitate human learning and thought processes to assist healthcare professionals in making clinical judgments. The formulation of predictive models could anticipate outcomes such as postoperative complications, mortality, and postoperative quality of life [35, 36]. Machine learning (ML) is applied through constant exposure to datasets and algorithms, which allows for the functional evolution of a computer to more efficiently analyze and adapt to new incoming stimuli [37, 38]. Maintenance of algorithm accuracy is typically attained by using a five-fold cross-validation method. This allows for the assessing of overfitting of algorithms for each dataset. The algorithm is developed using a random sample of 80% of the data, and then the model is tested against the remaining 20% of the data. Accuracy is determined by the area under receiver operating curves (AUC) [39].

AI has been applied to several areas of spinal surgery. One study assessed patient clusters and surgeries and used this to develop two-year improvement and complication rates [35]. Algorithms like this may ultimately allow clinicians to choose the best treatment options for patients while minimizing possible surgical risks. Similar systems have been applied to predict survival among patients with metastatic spine disease and risk factors for postoperative spine fusion complications [38, 39]. These models have investigated demographic risk factors as well as postoperative complications such as cardiac problems, wound healing issues, venous thromboembolism, and mortality. When compared to linear regressions, ML implementing logistic regression improves accuracy of identifying risk factors associated with postoperative complications [38].

While linear regressions are simple and easy to use, they assume a normal distribution with a linear correlation, which is not always true of complex data [40]. On the other hand, logistic regressions look at both linear correlations and multi-class classifications, though both systems will provide inaccurate data in case of nonlinear correlations [40]. In contrast, the ML model K-nearest-neighbor (KNN) is a non-parametric model that can identify non-linear associations and improves with higher signal-to-noise ratio; however, it cannot provide confidence intervals and is a slower analytic tool. KNN is similar to decision trees, in that both are non-parametric models. However, decision trees are faster than KNN and can show interactions [40]. The Random Forest is a highly accurate yet slow ML model using multiple decision trees to improve accuracy [41]. These ML models demonstrate that algorithms must be chosen based off the data, and no one model is best in all cases [41].

ML has shown superiority in predictive capability in a broad spectrum of medical settings [36, 42, 43]. Such models have enabled surgeons to utilize risk calculators, such as the American College of Surgeons National Surgical Quality Improvement Program (ACS NSQIP) surgical risk calculator which can improve treatment options for patients while simultaneously reducing morbidity and mortality [44]. Risk calculators can also be used to assess 30-day mortality after major procedures such as lower extremity amputation [45]. Orthopedic surgeons have used such risk calculators to assess the preoperative differences between low- vs. high-risk groups and how this impacts postoperative medical complications in spine surgery candidates [46, 47]. Overall, ML has the potential to make a clinically meaningful impact by providing a better risk assessment for patients, helping to aid in decision-making, and managing patient and clinician expectations of postoperative outcomes.

Neural Mapping

Intraoperative neural mapping is an innovative technique used to accurately resect tumors while maintaining the function of the spinal cord and nerve roots, allowing for improved dissection planes and negative margins [48]. The earliest form of intraoperative neural mapping of the spinal cord involved monitoring somatosensory-evoked potentials (SSEPs) during scoliosis surgery in the hope of predicting the postoperative function of the dorsal column [49, 50]. Later, monitoring of motor-evoked potentials (MEPs) and D waves was developed to assess the corticospinal tract [51, 52]. Both SSEPs and MEPs are actively implemented during spinal tumor surgery, especially when intervention involves the cervicothoracic spine and cephalad lumbar levels in proximity to the spinal cord (Fig. 22.4) [53].

Multimodal monitoring is unique in that it can track both ascending and descending pathways simultaneously during the operative period, and has shown to reduce postoperative neurologic complications [54]. For surgeries involving spinal deformity and those that require

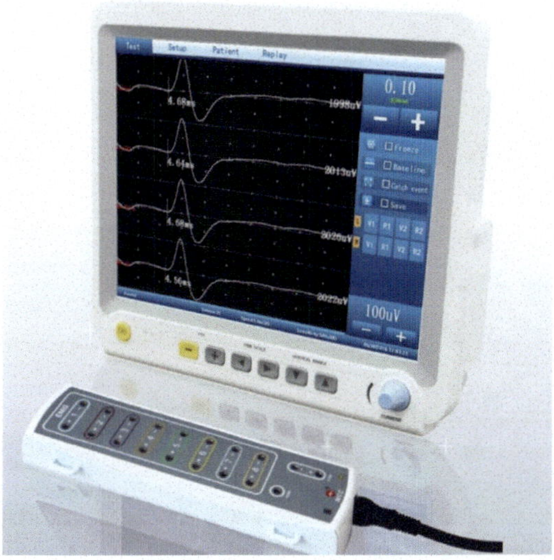

Fig. 22.4 SSEP/MEP neuromonitoring device

removal of spinal cord tumors, MEPs and SSEPs are methods of neural mapping that both have high sensitivity and specificity [55, 56]. Specifically, observing both MEPs and SSEPs demonstrated high sensitivity when measuring poor postoperative outcomes [55]. Not only can neural mapping techniques assist with assessing postoperative outcomes, but it can also help surgeons accurately resect tumors during surgery. These techniques include observing transcranial electric motor-evoked potentials (tcMEPs) and D-waves [57]. Such techniques have demonstrated efficacy in lessening postoperative neurological mishaps during high-risk spinal cord procedures [58].

Magnetoencephalography (MEG) is a newer technique for neural mapping, which functions by measuring lower magnetic fields outside the skull, and therefore providing real-time tracking of brain functionality. Though MEG has previously been utilized among epileptic patients as well as during preoperative neurosurgical evaluations, it has the potential to be applied more broadly and in more clinical settings [59]. Low-intensity focused ultrasound (LIFUS) can track and modify brain activity by downregulating cortical evoked potentials and manipulating cortical oscillatory dynamics. While the utility of LIFUS has not yet been fully established, it may be able to modify neural ion channels and plasma membranes as well, which could broadly be used for neurological clinical applications [60]. Overall, these cutting-edge techniques have not been broadly applied to spine surgery, making it an area of limited research, though the implementation of such technology may allow for improved intraoperative management of spine tumor patients.

Augmented Reality/Virtual Reality

Presently, there are three principal types of simulation systems that have been documented in the literature: (1) virtual reality, in which case the entire simulation is virtual; (2) mixed reality, in which case there is a combination of virtual and physical components; and (3) augmented reality, in which case, a virtual component is superimposed onto a physical reality. As such, surgeons are able to integrate the virtual and physical world in a way where virtual images generated from a computer can then be projected onto the surgeon's physical plane of view. Primarily, AR's utility lies in the fact that surgeons generally prefer not to move their field of vision from the patient during a procedure, and using this technology, they are able to maintain their gaze while assessing the relevant trajectories and anatomy.

Abe et al. assessed the safety and effectiveness of AR in spine models in vivo with a patient population undergoing percutaneous vertebroplasty, noting no pedicle breach [61, 62]. Sparing radiation by using optical cameras and patient motion tracking provides promising technology from AR for applications in spine tumor surgery [63, 64]. Recently, AR has been implemented in anterior and posterior cervical spine procedures, which may lend a useful role in primary and metastatic lesions requiring rapid stabilization and minimal surgical exposure (Fig. 22.5a–c) [65]. Finally, AR models function as useful training tools for junior spine oncologists and trainees [66].

VR has been well established as a learning and training tool that allows surgeons and trainees to learn and master techniques that can be implemented in spine tumor surgery without

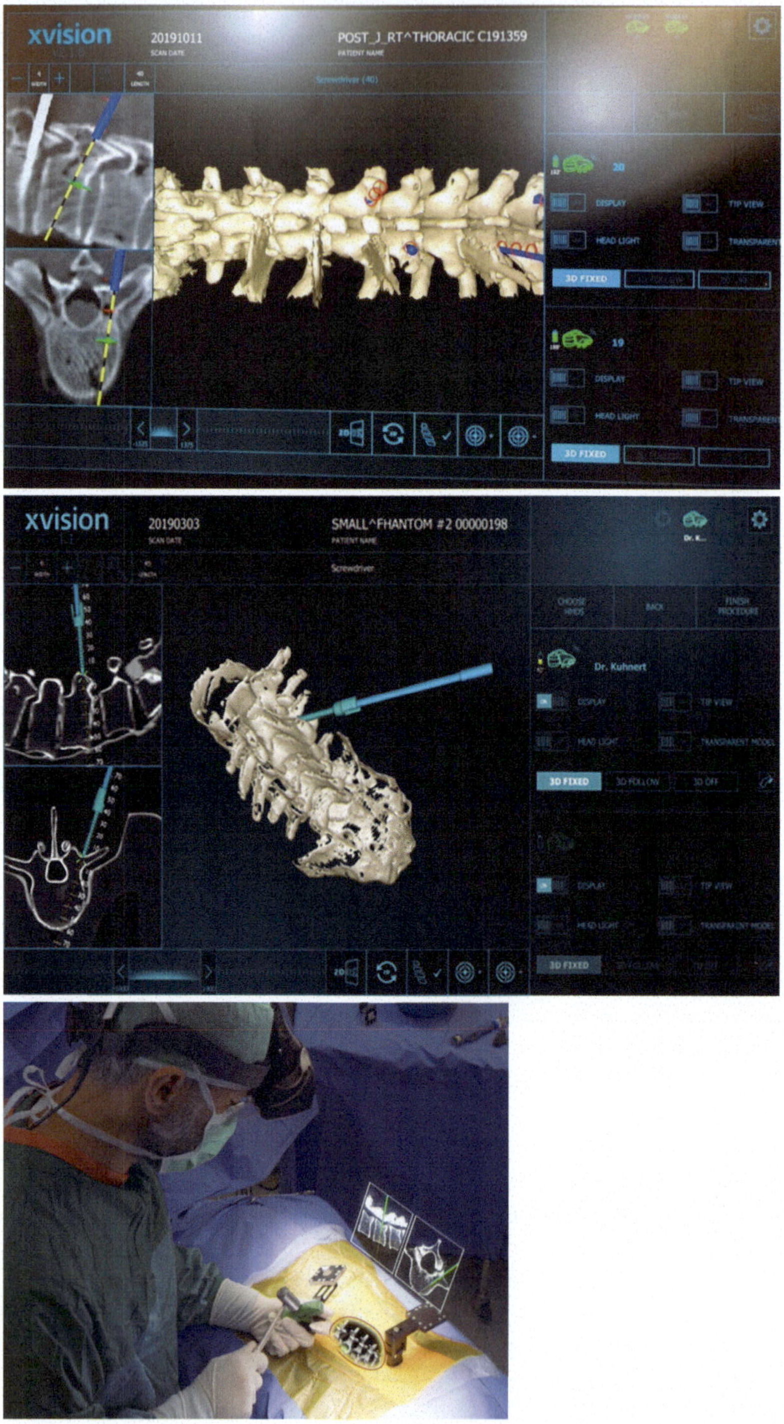

Fig. 22.5 Example applications of augmented reality (AR) in spine surgery

grappling with the potential for making a mistake on a live patient. In a study of medical students practicing lumbar pedicle placements, the researchers sought to explore if there were advantages of VR in contrast to "traditional" methods of learning [67]. One group was to make use of traditional visual and verbal instructions, while the other group made use of an

"ImmersiveTouch" VR simulator. The authors determined that the simulation group outperformed the traditional learning group in all variables including trajectory, depth of screw error, and breach, attributing the results to the sequential learning, enhanced depth perception, and increased 3-dimensional anatomical understanding, though the clinical implications have yet to be determined.

Fluorescence Surgery

Background

Fluorescence occurs when the illumination of material by short-wavelength light is followed by the emission of a longer wavelength. Intraoperatively, fluorescence has been implemented based on properties related to the selective accumulation of dye, metabolic characteristics of tissue, autofluorescence characteristics, or due to fluorescent probes that are engineered to target specific tissues. Various agents can be selected based on their metabolic properties and the ability to emit detectable signals. For example, protoporphyrin IX (PPIX) has a characteristic 635-nm red hue. Fluorescein has a distinctive yellow-green glow at a peak wavelength of 525 nm (the human eye's peak photopic sensitivity of 555 nm), and along with 5-aminolevulinic acid (ALA), has been approved for intraoperative use [68]. Other dyes, such as indocyanine green (ICG) which has a peak emission at 830 nm [69], are not perceivable to the unaided human eye as they fluoresce in the infrared portion of the electromagnetic spectrum.

Fluorescence: Current Best Evidence

Stereotactic neuronavigation was first pioneered by Spiegel and Wycis in 1947 [70], and frameless neuronavigation systems improved this paradigm throughout the 1990s [71, 72]. Interestingly, 5-ALA itself is not fluorescent; rather, it is selectively absorbed by glioma cells of tumors and then metabolized into protoporphyrin IX (PpIX) [73–75]. 5-ALA is a highly sensitive agent, with a positive predictive value of nearly 100% in detecting gliomas, leading to its FDA approval in Europe and the United States [76–85]. Several small retrospective studies have demonstrated 5-ALA-guided resection allows for improved identification of planes between tumor and normal tissue [86–89], more recently focusing on ependymoma resection [90].

Unfortunately, time dependency, cost, and skin sensitization introduces limitations and potential for newer agents, such as sodium fluorescein. This water-soluble dye penetrates damaged blood–brain barriers and concentrates at tumor sites, allowing for visualization with surgical microscopes that utilize specific filters [91]. Fluorescein offers cost savings and a more convenient administration, with fewer side effects, successfully implemented during resection of intramedullary spinal cord tumors (IMSCTs) [91].

Future applications such as epidurally administered fluorophores have been seen with the encapsulated (*E,E*)-1,4-bis(*p*-aminostryl)-2-methoxy benzene (BMB), and may lend itself useful for spine tumor visualization. Similarly, activatable cell-penetrating peptides (ACPP) utilize antibodies bound to fluorophores allowing for shipment of agents into areas with high extracellular cleavage activity, such as the matrix metalloproteinases (MMPs) that are involved in neoplastic growth [92–94]. More recent techniques are able to exploit pH differentials [95]. Antibody-based fluorescence has been utilized against human epidermal growth factor receptor 2 (HER2), vascular endothelial growth factor (VEGF), and embryonic fibroblasts expressing human IGFR-1 and MCF-7 human breast cancer cells [96–99].

References

1. Bourgeois AC, Faulkner AR, Bradley YC, et al. Improved accuracy of minimally invasive transpedicular screw placement in the lumbar spine with 3-dimensional stereotactic image guidance: a comparative meta-analysis. J Spinal Disord Tech. 2015;28:324–9.
2. D'Urso PS, Askin G, Earwaker JS, et al. Spinal biomodeling. Spine. 1999;24:1247–51.

3. Wu A-M, Shao Z-X, Wang J-S, et al. The accuracy of a method for printing three-dimensional spinal models. PLoS One. 2015;10:e0124291.
4. Rankin TM, Giovinco NA, Cucher DJ, et al. Three-dimensional printing surgical instruments: are we there yet? J Surg Res. 2014;189:193–7.
5. Punyaratabandhu T, Liacouras PC, Pairojboriboon S. Using 3D models in orthopedic oncology: presenting personalized advantages in surgical planning and intraoperative outcomes. 3D Print Med. 2018;4:12.
6. Mao K, Wang Y, Xiao S, et al. Clinical application of computer-designed polystyrene models in complex severe spinal deformities: a pilot study. Eur Spine J. 2010;19:797–802.
7. Izatt MT, Thorpe PLPJ, Thompson RG, et al. The use of physical biomodelling in complex spinal surgery. Eur Spine J. 2007;16:1507–18.
8. Xiao J-R, Huang W-D, Yang X-H, et al. En bloc resection of primary malignant bone tumor in the cervical spine based on 3-dimensional printing technology. Orthop Surg. 2016;8:171–8.
9. Kim MP, Ta AH, Ellsworth WA 4th, et al. Three dimensional model for surgical planning in resection of thoracic tumors. Int J Surg Case Rep. 2015;16:127–9.
10. Liu K, Zhang Q, Li X, et al. Preliminary application of a multi-level 3D printing drill guide template for pedicle screw placement in severe and rigid scoliosis. Eur Spine J. 2017;26:1684–9.
11. Sugawara T, Higashiyama N, Kaneyama S, et al. Accurate and simple screw insertion procedure with patient-specific screw guide templates for posterior C1–C2 fixation. Spine. 2017;42:E340–6.
12. Guo F, Dai J, Zhang J, et al. Individualized 3D printing navigation template for pedicle screw fixation in upper cervical spine. PLoS One. 2017;12:e0171509.
13. Chen H, Wu D, Yang H, et al. Clinical use of 3D printing guide plate in posterior lumbar pedicle screw fixation. Med Sci Monit. 2015;21:3948–54.
14. Otsuki B, Takemoto M, Fujibayashi S, et al. Utility of a custom screw insertion guide and a full-scale, color-coded 3D plaster model for guiding safe surgical exposure and screw insertion during spine revision surgery. J Neurosurg Spine. 2016;25:94–102.
15. Lin C-L, Fang J-J, Lin R-M. Resection of giant invasive sacral schwannoma using image-based customized osteotomy tools. Eur Spine J. 2016;25:4103–7.
16. Sayari AJ, Pardo C, Basques BA, et al. Review of robotic-assisted surgery: what the future looks like through a spine oncology lens. Ann Transl Med. 2019;7:224.
17. Mobbs RJ, Choy WJ, Wilson P, et al. L5 En-Bloc vertebrectomy with customized reconstructive implant: comparison of patient-specific versus off-the-shelf implant. World Neurosurg. 2018;112:94–100.
18. Crafts TD, Ellsperman SE, Wannemuehler TJ, et al. Three-dimensional printing and its applications in otorhinolaryngology-head and neck surgery. Otolaryngol Head Neck Surg. 2017;156:999–1010.
19. Wong KC. 3D-printed patient-specific applications in orthopedics. Orthop Res Rev. 2016;8:57–66.
20. Choy WJ, Parr WCH, Phan K, et al. 3-dimensional printing for anterior cervical surgery: a review. J Spine Surg. 2018;4:757–69.
21. Wei R, Guo W, Ji T, et al. One-step reconstruction with a 3D-printed, custom-made prosthesis after total en bloc sacrectomy: a technical note. Eur Spine J. 2017;26:1902–9.
22. Kim D, Lim JY, Shim KW, et al. Sacral reconstruction with a 3D-printed implant after hemisacrectomy in a patient with sacral osteosarcoma: 1-year follow-up result. Yonsei Med J. 2017;58:453–7.
23. Xu N, Wei F, Liu X, et al. Reconstruction of the upper cervical spine using a personalized 3D-printed vertebral body in an adolescent with Ewing sarcoma. Spine. 2016;41:E50–4.
24. Mobbs RJ, Coughlan M, Thompson R, et al. The utility of 3D printing for surgical planning and patient-specific implant design for complex spinal pathologies: case report. J Neurosurg Spine. 2017;26:513–8.
25. Choy WJ, Mobbs RJ, Wilcox B, et al. Reconstruction of thoracic spine using a personalized 3D-printed vertebral body in adolescent with T9 primary bone tumor. World Neurosurg. 2017;105:1032.e13–1032.e17.
26. Mobbs RJ, Parr WCH, Choy WJ, et al. Anterior lumbar interbody fusion using a personalized approach: is custom the future of implants for anterior lumbar interbody fusion surgery? World Neurosurg. 2019. https://doi.org/10.1016/j.wneu.2018.12.144.
27. Siu TL, Rogers JM, Lin K, et al. Custom-made titanium 3-dimensional printed interbody cages for treatment of osteoporotic fracture-related spinal deformity. World Neurosurg. 2018;111:1–5.
28. Nathoo N, Cenk Çavuşoğlu M, Vogelbaum MA, et al. In touch with robotics: neurosurgery for the future. Neurosurgery. 2005;56:421–33.
29. Verma R, Krishan S, Haendlmayer K, et al. Functional outcome of computer-assisted spinal pedicle screw placement: a systematic review and meta-analysis of 23 studies including 5,992 pedicle screws. Eur Spine J. 2010;19:370–5.
30. Xiao R, Miller JA, Sabharwal NC, et al. Clinical outcomes following spinal fusion using an intraoperative computed tomographic 3D imaging system. J Neurosurg Spine. 2017;26:628–37.
31. Bederman SS, Samuel Bederman S, Lopez G, et al. Robotic guidance for en bloc sacrectomy. Spine. 2014;39:E1398–401.
32. Oh JK, Yang MS, Yoon DH, et al. Robotic resection of huge presacral tumors: case series and comparison with an open resection. J Spinal Disord Tech. 2014;27:E151–4.
33. Yang MS, Kim KN, Yoon DH, et al. Robot-assisted resection of paraspinal Schwannoma. J Korean Med Sci. 2011;26:150–3.
34. Hu X, Scharschmidt TJ, Ohnmeiss DD, et al. Robotic assisted surgeries for the treatment of spine

tumors. Int J Spine Surg. 2015;9:1. https://doi.org/10.14444/2001.
35. Ames CP, Smith JS, Pellisé F, et al. Artificial intelligence based hierarchical clustering of patient types and intervention categories in adult spinal deformity surgery: towards a new classification scheme that predicts quality and value. Spine. 2019;44:915–26.
36. Jiang F, Jiang Y, Zhi H, et al. Artificial intelligence in healthcare: past, present and future. Stroke Vasc Neurol. 2017;2:230–43.
37. Shavlik JW, Dietterich T, Dietterich TG. Readings in machine learning. San Mateo (Calif.): Morgan Kaufmann; 1990.
38. Kim JS, Merrill RK, Arvind V, et al. Examining the ability of artificial neural networks machine learning models to accurately predict complications following posterior lumbar spine fusion. Spine. 2018;43:853–60.
39. Paulino Pereira NR, Janssen SJ, van Dijk E, et al. Development of a prognostic survival algorithm for patients with metastatic spine disease. JBJS. 2016;98:1767.
40. Varghese D. Comparative study on classic machine learning algorithms. Medium. 2018 Available at https://towardsdatascience.com/comparative-study-on-classic-machine-learning-algorithms-24f9ff6ab222. Accessed 19 July 2019.
41. Varghese D. Comparative study on classic machine learning algorithms, part-2. Medium. 2018. Available at https://medium.com/@dannymvarghese/comparative-study-on-classic-machine-learning-algorithms-part-2-5ab58b683ec0. Accessed 19 July 2019.
42. Lee S, Mohr N, Street N, et al. Machine learning in relation to emergency medicine clinical and operational scenarios: an overview. West J Emerg Med. 2019;20:219–27.
43. Ahmad T, Lund LH, Rao P, et al. Machine learning methods improve prognostication, identify clinically distinct phenotypes, and detect heterogeneity in response to therapy in a large cohort of heart failure patients. J Am Heart Assoc. 2018;7(8):e008081. https://doi.org/10.1161/jaha.117.008081.
44. Lone Z, Hall S, Terakawa T, et al. Accuracy of American College of Surgeons national surgical quality improvement program universal surgical risk calculator in predicting complications following robot-assisted radical cystectomy at a National Comprehensive Cancer Center. J Endourol. 2019;33:383–8.
45. Jolissaint JS, Shah SK, Martin MC, et al. Risk prediction of 30-day mortality after lower extremity major amputation. J Vasc Surg. 2019;70(6):1868–76. https://doi.org/10.1016/j.jvs.2019.03.036.
46. Kohler J, Glass N, Noiseux NO, et al. Might doctors really "know best"?: utilizing surgeon intuition to strengthen preoperative surgical risk assessment. Iowa Orthop J. 2018;38:203–8.
47. Veeravagu A, Li A, Swinney C, et al. Predicting complication risk in spine surgery: a prospective analysis of a novel risk assessment tool. J Neurosurg Spine. 2017;27:81–91.
48. Scibilia A, Terranova C, Rizzo V, et al. Intraoperative neurophysiological mapping and monitoring in spinal tumor surgery: sirens or indispensable tools? Neurosurg Focus. 2016;41:E18.
49. Owen MP, Brown RH, Spetzler RF, et al. Excision of intramedullary arteriovenous malformation using intraoperative spinal cord monitoring. Surg Neurol. 1979;12:271–6.
50. Macon JB, Poletti CE. Conducted somatosensory evoked potentials during spinal surgery. Part 1: control conduction velocity measurements. J Neurosurg. 1982;57:349–53.
51. Merton PA, Morton HB. Stimulation of the cerebral cortex in the intact human subject. Nature. 1980;285:227.
52. Marsden CD, Merton PA, Morton HB. Direct electrical stimulation of corticospinal pathways through the intact scalp in human subjects. Adv Neurol. 1983;39:387–91.
53. Deletis V, Founder, International Society for Intraoperative Neurophysiology (ISIN). Intraoperative neurophysiology and the motor-evoked potentials methodology. US Neurol. 2008;04:73.
54. Sutter M, Eggspuehler A, Grob D, et al. The diagnostic value of multimodal intraoperative monitoring (MIOM) during spine surgery: a prospective study of 1,017 patients. Eur Spine J. 2007;16(Suppl 2):S162–70.
55. Park T, Park J, Park YG, et al. Intraoperative neurophysiological monitoring for spinal cord tumor surgery: comparison of motor and somatosensory evoked potentials according to tumor types. Ann Rehabil Med. 2017;41:610.
56. Chang SH, Park YG, Kim DH, et al. Monitoring of motor and somatosensory evoked potentials during spine surgery: intraoperative changes and postoperative outcomes. Ann Rehabil Med. 2016;40:470–80.
57. Barzilai O, Lidar Z, Constantini S, et al. Continuous mapping of the corticospinal tracts in intramedullary spinal cord tumor surgery using an electrified ultrasonic aspirator. J Neurosurg Spine. 2017;27:161–8.
58. Sala F, Dvorak J, Faccioli F. Cost effectiveness of multimodal intraoperative monitoring during spine surgery. Eur Spine J. 2007;16(Suppl 2):S229–31.
59. Hari R, Baillet S, Barnes G, et al. IFCN-endorsed practical guidelines for clinical magnetoencephalography (MEG). Clin Neurophysiol. 2018;129:1720–47.
60. Fomenko A, Neudorfer C, Dallapiazza RF, et al. Low-intensity ultrasound neuromodulation: an overview of mechanisms and emerging human applications. Brain Stimul. 2018;11:1209–17.
61. Kirkman MA, Ahmed M, Albert AF, et al. The use of simulation in neurosurgical education and training. J Neurosurg. 2014;121:228–46.

62. Abe Y, Sato S, Kato K, et al. A novel 3D guidance system using augmented reality for percutaneous vertebroplasty. J Neurosurg Spine. 2013;19:492–501.
63. Gottschalk MB, Tim Yoon S, Park DK, et al. Surgical training using three-dimensional simulation in placement of cervical lateral mass screws: a blinded randomized control trial. Spine J. 2015;15:168–75.
64. Halic T, Kockara S, Bayrak C, et al. Mixed reality simulation of rasping procedure in artificial cervical disc replacement (ACDR) surgery. BMC Bioinform. 2010;11(Suppl 6):S11. https://doi.org/10.1186/1471-2105-11-s6-s11.
65. Mascitelli JR, Schlachter L, Chartrain AG, et al. Navigation-linked heads-up display in intracranial surgery: early experience. Oper Neurosurg. 2018;15:184–93.
66. Luciano CJ, Pat Banerjee P, Bellotte B, et al. Learning retention of thoracic pedicle screw placement using a high-resolution augmented reality simulator with haptic feedback. Oper Neurosurg. 2011;69:ons14–9.
67. Gasco J, Patel A, Ortega-Barnett J, et al. Virtual reality spine surgery simulation: an empirical study of its usefulness. Neurol Res. 2014;36:968–73.
68. Kuroiwa T, Kajimoto Y, Ohta T. Development of a fluorescein operative microscope for use during malignant glioma surgery: a technical note and preliminary report. Surg Neurol. 1998;50:41–8; discussion 48–9
69. Raabe A, Beck J, Gerlach R, et al. Near-infrared indocyanine green video angiography: a new method for intraoperative assessment of vascular flow. Neurosurgery. 2003;52:132–9; discussion 139
70. Khoshnevisan A, Allahabadi NS. Neuronavigation: principles, clinical applications and potential pitfalls. Iran J Psychiatry. 2012;7:97–103.
71. Willems PWA, van der Sprenkel JWB, Tulleken CAF, et al. Neuronavigation and surgery of intracerebral tumours. J Neurol. 2006;253:1123–36.
72. Nimsky C, Ganslandt O, Cerny S, et al. Quantification of, visualization of, and compensation for brain shift using intraoperative magnetic resonance imaging. Neurosurgery. 2000;47:1070–9; discussion 1079–80
73. Stummer W, Stocker S, Wagner S, et al. Intraoperative detection of malignant gliomas by 5-aminolevulinic acid-induced porphyrin fluorescence. Neurosurgery. 1998;42:518–25; discussion 525–6
74. Montcel B, Mahieu-Williame L, Armoiry X, et al. Two-peaked 5-ALA-induced PpIX fluorescence emission spectrum distinguishes glioblastomas from low grade gliomas and infiltrative component of glioblastomas. Biomed Opt Express. 2013;4:548–58.
75. Colditz MJ, Jeffree RL. Aminolevulinic acid (ALA)–protoporphyrin IX fluorescence guided tumour resection. Part 1: clinical, radiological and pathological studies. J Clin Neurosci. 2012;19:1471–4.
76. Stummer W, Novotny A, Stepp H, et al. Fluorescence-guided resection of glioblastoma multiforme utilizing 5-ALA-induced porphyrins: a prospective study in 52 consecutive patients. J Neurosurg. 2000;93:1003–13.
77. Zhao S, Wu J, Wang C, et al. Intraoperative fluorescence-guided resection of high-grade malignant gliomas using 5-aminolevulinic acid–induced porphyrins: a systematic review and meta-analysis of prospective studies. PLoS One. 2013;8:e63682.
78. Roberts DW, Valdés PA, Harris BT, et al. Coregistered fluorescence-enhanced tumor resection of malignant glioma: relationships between δ-aminolevulinic acid–induced protoporphyrin IX fluorescence, magnetic resonance imaging enhancement, and neuropathological parameters. J Neurosurg. 2011;114:595–603.
79. Coburger J, Engelke J, Scheuerle A, et al. Tumor detection with 5-aminolevulinic acid fluorescence and Gd-DTPA–enhanced intraoperative MRI at the border of contrast-enhancing lesions: a prospective study based on histopathological assessment. Neurosurg Focus. 2014;36:E3.
80. Valle RD, Solis ST, Gastearena MAI, et al. Surgery guided by 5-aminolevulinic fluorescence in glioblastoma: volumetric analysis of extent of resection in single-center experience. J Neuro-Oncol. 2011;102:105–13.
81. Neurosurgery, 2009. Five-aminolevulinic acid for fluorescence-guided resection of recurrent malignant gliomas: a phase II study. 2009. academic.oup.com. Available at https://academic.oup.com/neurosurgery/article-abstract/65/6/1070/2556044.
82. Yeh S-CA, Sahli S, Andrews DW, et al. 5-aminolevulinic acid induced protoporphyrin IX as a fluorescence marker for quantitative image analysis of high-grade dysplasia in Barrett's esophagus cellular models. J Biomed Opt. 2015;20:036010.
83. Quinones-Hinojosa A, Raza SM. Controversies in neuro-oncology: best evidence medicine for brain tumor surgery. Stuttgart: Thieme; 2013.
84. Lakomkin N, Hadjipanayis CG. Fluorescence-guided surgery for high-grade gliomas. J Surg Oncol. 2018;118:356–61.
85. Valle RD, Hadjipanayis CG, Stummer W. Established and emerging uses of 5-ALA in the brain: an overview. J Neuro-Oncol. 2019;141:487–94.
86. Millesi M, Kiesel B, Woehrer A, et al. Analysis of 5-aminolevulinic acid–induced fluorescence in 55 different spinal tumors. Neurosurg Focus. 2014;36:E11.
87. Eicker SO, Floeth FW, Kamp M, et al. The impact of fluorescence guidance on spinal intradural tumour surgery. Eur Spine J. 2013;22:1394–401.
88. Inoue T, Endo T, Nagamatsu K, et al. 5-Aminolevulinic acid fluorescence-guided resection of intramedullary ependymoma. Oper Neurosurg. 2013;72:ons159–68.
89. Aghakhani N, David P, Parker F, et al. Intramedullary spinal ependymomas: analysis of a consecutive series of 82 adult cases with particular attention to patients with no preoperative neurological deficit. Neurosurgery. 2008;62:1279–85; discussion 1285–6

90. Moreno RG, García LMB, Bastidas HI, et al. Fluorescence guided surgery with 5-aminolevulinic acid for resection of spinal cord ependymomas. Asian Spine J. 2019;13:119–25.
91. Acerbi F, Cavallo C, Schebesch K-M, et al. Fluorescein-guided resection of intramedullary spinal cord tumors: results from a preliminary, multicentric, retrospective study. World Neurosurg. 2017;108:603–9.
92. Talvensaari-Mattila A, Pääkkö P, Turpeenniemi-Hujanen T. Matrix metalloproteinase-2 (MMP-2) is associated with survival in breast carcinoma. Br J Cancer. 2003;89:1270–5.
93. Zhou CX, Gao Y, Johnson NW, et al. Immunoexpression of matrix metalloproteinase-2 and matrix metalloproteinase-9 in the metastasis of squamous cell carcinoma of the human tongue. Aust Dent J. 2010;55:385–9.
94. De la Garza-Ramos R, Bydon M, Macki M, et al. Fluorescent techniques in spine surgery. Neurol Res. 2014;36:928–38.
95. Zhang Y, Li L, Chang L, et al. Design of a new pH-activatable cell-penetrating peptide for drug delivery into tumor cells. Chem Biol Drug Des. 2019;94(5):1884–93. https://doi.org/10.1111/cbdd.13537.
96. van Scheltinga AGTT, van Dam GM, Nagengast WB, et al. Intraoperative near-infrared fluorescence tumor imaging with vascular endothelial growth factor and human epidermal growth factor receptor 2 targeting antibodies. J Nucl Med. 2011;52:1778–85.
97. Rosenthal EL, Kulbersh BD, King T, et al. Use of fluorescent labeled anti-epidermal growth factor receptor antibody to image head and neck squamous cell carcinoma xenografts. Mol Cancer Ther. 2007;6:1230–8.
98. Zhang H, Zeng X, Li Q, et al. Fluorescent tumour imaging of type I IGF receptor in vivo: comparison of antibody-conjugated quantum dots and small-molecule fluorophore. Br J Cancer. 2009;101:71–9.
99. Vandercappellen J, Van Damme J, Struyf S. The role of CXC chemokines and their receptors in cancer. Cancer Lett. 2008;267:226–44.

Index

K. Singh, M. Colman (eds.), *Surgical Spinal Oncology*,
https://doi.org/10.1007/978-3-030-50722-0

D

E

Q

R

S

T

The manufacturer's authorised representative in the EU is Springer Nature Customer Service Centre GmbH, Europaplatz 3, 69115 Heidelberg, Germany. If you have any concerns regarding our products, please contact ProductSafety@springernature.com

Printed and bound by CPI Group (UK) Ltd, Croydon, CR0 4YY
30/09/2026
02225705-0007